Understanding Epilepsy

Understanding Epilepsy

Edited by **Luke Stanton**

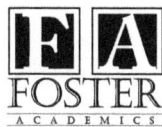

FA
FOSTER
ACADEMICS

New Jersey

Published by Foster Academics,
61 Van Reypen Street,
Jersey City, NJ 07306, USA
www.fosteracademics.com

Understanding Epilepsy
Edited by Luke Stanton

International Standard Book Number: 978-1-63242-459-4 (Hardback)

The publisher's policy is to use permanent paper from mills that operate a sustainable forestry policy. Furthermore, the publisher ensures that the text paper and cover boards used have met acceptable environmental accreditation standards.

Trademark Notice: Registered trademark of products or corporate names are used only for explanation and identification without intent to infringe.

Printed in the United States of America.

Contents

Preface

Epilepsy is characterized by seizures. These seizures can persist for a shorter or longer duration of time. These are generally a set of neurological disorders that result in constant shaking of the body. They may erupt at any point of time and even have the potential to cause physical damage. The causes underneath these attacks are relatively unknown but some of them may occur due to stroke, brain tumors, brain infections or birth defects. Diagnosis and treatment of epilepsy may involve performing blood tests, brain mapping, electroencephalogram and anticonvulsant medications for entire life. In this book, using case studies and examples, constant effort has been made to make the understanding of the difficult concepts of epilepsy as easy and informative as possible, for the readers. This book is a compilation of chapters that discuss the most vital concepts and emerging trends revolving around the symptoms, mechanisms, causes, treatment, and management of this disease. Scientists, neurologists, experts and students actively engaged in this field will find this book full of crucial and unexplored concepts.

This book is a result of research of several months to collate the most relevant data in the field.

When I was approached with the idea of this book and the proposal to edit it, I was overwhelmed. It gave me an opportunity to reach out to all those who share a common interest with me in this field. I had 3 main parameters for editing this text:

1. Accuracy – The data and information provided in this book should be up-to-date and valuable to the readers.

2. Structure – The data must be presented in a structured format for easy understanding and better grasping of the readers.

3. Universal Approach – This book not only targets students but also experts and innovators in the field, thus my aim was to present topics which are of use to all.

Thus, it took me a couple of months to finish the editing of this book.

I would like to make a special mention of my publisher who considered me worthy of this opportunity and also supported me throughout the editing process. I would also like to thank the editing team at the back-end who extended their help whenever required.

Editor

Metabolic Causes of Epileptic Encephalopathy

Joe Yuezhou Yu and Phillip L. Pearl

Department of Neurology, Children's National Medical Center, 111 Michigan Avnue, Washington, DC 20010, USA

Correspondence should be addressed to Phillip L. Pearl; ppearl@childrensnational.org

Academic Editor: Giangennaro Coppola

Epileptic encephalopathy can be induced by inborn metabolic defects that may be rare individually but in aggregate represent a substantial clinical portion of child neurology. These may present with various epilepsy phenotypes including refractory neonatal seizures, early myoclonic encephalopathy, early infantile epileptic encephalopathy, infantile spasms, and generalized epilepsies which in particular include myoclonic seizures. There are varying degrees of treatability, but the outcome if untreated can often be catastrophic. The importance of early recognition cannot be overemphasized. This paper provides an overview of inborn metabolic errors associated with persistent brain disturbances due to highly active clinical or electrographic ictal activity. Selected diseases are organized by the defective molecule or mechanism and categorized as small molecule disorders (involving amino and organic acids, fatty acids, neurotransmitters, urea cycle, vitamers and cofactors, and mitochondria) and large molecule disorders (including lysosomal storage disorders, peroxisomal disorders, glycosylation disorders, and leukodystrophies). Details including key clinical features, salient electrophysiological and neuroradiological findings, biochemical findings, and treatment options are summarized for prominent disorders in each category.

1. Introduction

Inherited metabolic epilepsies are disorders that, while individually rare, are in aggregate a substantial clinical portion of child neurology, as well as a complex field of knowledge for physicians, investigators, and students to tackle. A subset of these disorders can lead to the development of epileptic encephalopathy, that is, a brain disturbance due to highly active clinical or electrographic ictal activity. The epileptologist may view these from the viewpoint of syndromic phenotypes such as early myoclonic encephalopathy, early infantile epileptic encephalopathy, infantile spasms, and myoclonic epilepsies. They have various degrees of treatability at present, with some requiring prompt diagnosis and intervention to avoid otherwise catastrophic outcomes. Careful consideration of metabolic disorders in patients presenting with epileptic encephalopathy is therefore warranted, and to this end, we hope a review may be helpful.

This paper provides an overview of inborn metabolic errors associated with epileptic encephalopathy, summarizing key clinical features and underlying biochemistry, salient electrophysiological and neuroradiological findings,

and primary treatment options where appropriate. Examples of specific disorders are discussed, with full listings of the multiple enzyme defects and diseases in particular categories presented in tables. The range of inherited metabolic disorders has been organized by the category of molecules or the biochemical process involved: for example, small molecule disorders include dysfunction involving amino, organic, or fatty acids, neurotransmitters, the urea cycle, vitamers and cofactors, and disorders of the mitochondria. Large molecule diseases cover defects in glycosylation, lysosomal and peroxisomal function, and leukodystrophies.

2. Small Molecule Disorders

2.1. Amino and Organic Acid Disorders. Amino acidopathies and organic acidemias, resulting from disorders in amino or fatty acid catabolism, present with seizures and cognitive, behavioral, or motor disturbances resulting from the accumulation of toxic intermediaries, or possible structural damage [1]. Some may induce an epileptic encephalopathy. Seizure types and EEG findings vary, though myoclonic epilepsies predominate, and diffuse background slowing is a common EEG finding. More typical EEG findings in metabolic encephalopathies are burst suppression, hypsarrhythmia, and generalized spike-wave discharges. Table 1 lists the protean disorders along with the enzyme defect and metabolites detected on diagnostic studies.

2.1.1. Methylmalonic Acidemia and Cobalamin Deficiencies.
The finding of elevated methylmalonic acid can be caused by a number of distinct disorders including defects in the vitamin B12-related enzymes cobalamin A, B, C, or D and methylmalonyl CoA mutase (MUT). Early myoclonic encephalopathy, as well as other epilepsies and epileptic encephalopathies, has been associated with this finding. The most common methylmalonic acidemia involving cobalamin is cobalamin C deficiency (Figure 1); individuals may present in infancy or early childhood with seizures and progressive encephalopathy. Patients presenting with status epilepticus have also been reported. Treatment with hydroxycobalamin is effective, including prenatal supplementation in affected families but may not reverse existing neurological injury in delayed diagnoses [3].

2.1.2. Propionic Acidemia.
Propionic acidemia (PA) is caused by defects in the enzyme propionyl CoA carboxylase and commonly presents with lethargy, vomiting, metabolic acidemia, and sometimes hyperammonemia [4]. A severe presentation of this disease in infancy with infantile spasms and hypsarrhythmia is reported [5]; myoclonic and generalized seizures are common in early childhood and infancy and typically evolve into mild generalized and absence seizures later in life [6].

2.1.3. Ethylmalonic Acidemia.
Ethylmalonic encephalopathy is usually lethal in infancy or early childhood and has a severe presentation including seizures, brain structural malformations, neurodevelopmental regression, pyramidal and extrapyramidal symptoms, chronic diarrhea, and dermatological findings including petechiae and acrocyanosis. MRI has shown frontotemporal atrophy, enlargement of the subarachnoid spaces, and basal ganglia T2-weighted hyperintensities [7]. EEGs may worsen over time, with multifocal spike and slow waves and background disorganization [8].

2.1.4. 3-Hydroxy-3-Methylglutaric Acidemia.
When untreated, dysfunction of the enzyme 3-hydroxy-3-methylglutaryl CoA lyase (which cleaves 3-hydroxy-3-methylglutaryl CoA into acetyl CoA and acetoacetate) leads to metabolic acidosis with absent ketone production, lactic acidemia, hypoglycemia hepatomegaly, and lethargy, possibly progressing to coma and death. Seizures are linked in most cases to lactic acidemia or hypoglycemia and are associated with multifocal spike-wave discharges on EEG [8]. Some presentations show particular association with white matter lesions, dysmyelination, and cerebral atrophy on neuroimaging [9, 10].

2.1.5. Glutaric Acidemia.
Dysfunction of the enzyme glutaryl CoA dehydrogenase prevents the metabolism of tryptophan, hydroxylysine, and lysine, resulting in increased urine glutaric acid metabolites. This is a cerebral organic acidopathy, with predominantly neurological symptoms featuring macrocephaly, increased subarachnoid spaces, and progressive dystonia and athetosis with striatal injury [11]. Seizures can be a presenting sign and are seen during acute encephalopathic events [12, 13]. EEGs show background slowing with generalized spike-and-wave and mixed multifocal discharges [8, 14]. Therapy using a low-protein diet (especially low lysine and tryptophan), carnitine supplementation, and aggressive emergency management can significantly improve the outcomes. The antiepileptic valproate should be avoided, however, because it is believed to affect acetyl CoA/CoA ratios and may exacerbate metabolic imbalance [13].

2.1.6. 3-Methylglutaconic Acidurias.
Five subtypes of 3-methylglutaconic aciduria (MGA) have been categorized (Table 1); all are cerebral organic acidopathies resulting from defects in the leucine catabolic pathway. Neurological and developmental symptoms are central in all five types although seizures are prominent mainly in Type I. Patients with Type I MGA present with leukoencephalopathy and epileptic encephalopathy with psychosis and depression, in addition to ataxia, optic atrophy, and sensorineural hearing loss. These are often accompanied by systemic issues including cardiomyopathy, liver and exocrine pancreatic dysfunction, and bone marrow failure [15]. EEGs show diffuse slowing and white matter lesions can be seen on MRI, usually in a supratentorial location [8, 15, 16].

2.1.7. Canavan Disease.
Canavan disease is primarily a disease of demyelination. It is thought to be caused by brain acetate deficiency resulting from a defect of N-acetylaspartic acid (NAA) catabolism [17]. Accumulation of NAA, a compound thought to be responsible for maintaining cerebral fluid balance, can lead to cerebral edema and neurological injury. Presentation of Canavan disease includes progressive epileptic encephalopathy with developmental delay, macrocephaly, leukodystrophy, and optic atrophy [18, 19]. Seizures often begin in the second year of life, and treatment is primarily supportive, including antiepileptic medications.

2.1.8. D- and L-2-Hydroxyglutaric Aciduria.
D-2-Hydroxyglutaric aciduria results from the loss of enzyme function in either D-2-hydroglutaric dehydrogenase or hydroxyacid-oxoacid transhydrogenase, which metabolizes GHB (gamma-hydroxybutyrate). Though presentations vary, severe cases manifest in the neonatorum with encephalopathy, intractable epilepsy, and cardiomyopathy. Seizures are present in almost all cases, and MRI findings have included signal alterations in the basal ganglia and diencephalon, as well as agenesis of the corpus callosum.

The enantiomer, L-2-Hydroxyglutaric aciduria, is a disorder of alpha ketoglutarate synthesis. It presents with neurodevelopmental delay, generalized seizures, and progressive ataxia. Multifocal spike-waves and burst suppression can be seen on EEGs [20, 21], and characteristic MRI findings include cerebellar atrophy, subcortical white matter loss, and

TABLE 1: Amino acidemias and organic acidopathies.

Disorder	Defective enzyme	Diagnostic metabolites
Propionic acidemia (PA)	Propionyl CoA carboxylase	Propionylcarnitine (C3; P)* Methylcitrate (U)* 3-Hydroxypropionic acid (U)
Methylmalonic acidemia (MMA)	Methylmalonic mutase Cobalamin A Cobalamin B	Methylmalonic acid (P, U) Propionylcarnitine (C3; P) Methylcitrate (U) 3-Hydroxypropionic acid
Methylmalonic acidemia with homocysteinuria, cobalamin C/D	Cobalamin C Cobalamin D	Methylmalonic acid (P, U) Propionylcarnitine (C3; P) Methylcitrate (U) Total homocysteine (P) 3-Hydroxypropionic acid (U)
Isovaleric acidemia (IVA)	Isovaleryl dehydrogenase	Isovaleric acid (U) Isovalerylcarnitine (C5; P)
3-Methylcrotonylglycinuria (3MCC)	3-Methylcrotonyl CoA carboxylase	3-Hydroxyisovaleric acid (U) 3-Methylcrotonylglycine (U) Hydroxyisovalerylcarnitine (C5OH; P)
3-Hydroxy-3-methylglutaryl CoA lyase deficiency	3-Hydroxy-3-methyl-glutaryl CoA Lyase	Hydroxyisovalerylcarnitine (C5OH; P) 3-Hydroxy-3-methylglutaric acid (U) 3-Methylglutaconic acid (U)
Malonic aciduria	Malonyl CoA decarboxylase	Malonate (U)
2-Methyl-3-hydroxybutyrl CoA dehydrogenase deficiency	2-Methyl-3-hydroxybutyryl CoA dehydrogenase	2-Methyl-3-hydroxybutyrate (U) Tiglylglycine (U)
Ethylmalonic encephalopathy	Branched chain Keto-dehydrogenase	C4 C5 Ethylmalonic acid (U) Methylsuccinic acid C4–C6 acylglycines (P)
Beta-ketothiolase deficiency	3-Methyl acetoacetate thiolase	C5:1 (P) 2-Methyl-3-hydroxybutyrate (U) Tiglylglycine (U) 2-Methyacetoacetate (U)
Biotinidase deficiency and Holocarboxylase synthetase deficiency	Biotinidase Holocarboxylase synthetase	Propionylcarnitine (C3; P) Hydroxyisovalerylcarnitine (C5OH; P) Biotinidase enzyme deficiency (P) Lactate (P, U) 3-Methylcrotonylglycine (U) Methylcitrate (U) 3-Hydroxypropionic acid (U)
2-Methyl butyryl CoA dehydrogenase	2-Methyl butyryl CoA dehydrogenase	2-Methylglycience (U) Isovalerylcarnitine (C5; P)
Glutaric acidemia I	Glutaryl CoA dehydrogenase	Glutaric acid (U) 3-Hydroxyglutaric acid (U) Glutaryl carnitine (C5-DC; P)
3-Methylglutaconic acidurias	3-Methylglutaconyl CoA hydratase (Type I) Barth (Type II) Costeff (Type III) Type IV Type V	3-Methylglutaconic acid (U) Hydroxy-isovalerylcarnitine (P)
Canavan disease	Aspartoacylase	N-Acetylaspartic Acid (U)
L-2-Hydroxyglutaric aciduria	L-2-Hydroxyglutarate dehydrogenase	L-2-Hydroxyglutaric Acid (U) Lysine (CSF)
D-2-Hydroxyglutaric aciduria	D-2-Hydroxyglutarate dehydrogenase Hydroxy-oxoacid transhydrogenase	D-2-Hydroxyglutaric acid (U)
4-Hydroxybutyric Aciduria	Succinate semialdehyde dehydrogenase	Gamma-hydroxybutric acid (U)
Fumaric aciduria	Fumarate hydratase	Fumarate (U)

TABLE 1: Continued.

Disorder	Defective enzyme	Diagnostic metabolites
Maple syrup urine disease (MSUD)	Branched chain Keto-dehydrogenase	Leucine (P) Alloisoleucine (P) Dicarboxylic acids (U)
Dihydrolipoamide dehydrogenase	MSUD III	Leucine (P) Alloisoleucine (P) Dicarboxylic acids (U) Lactic acid (P, U)
Phenylketonuria (PKU)	Phenylalanine hydratase (PAH)	Phenylalanine (P) Low tyrosine (P)

(P): plasma, (U): urine. Adapted from Pearl [2].

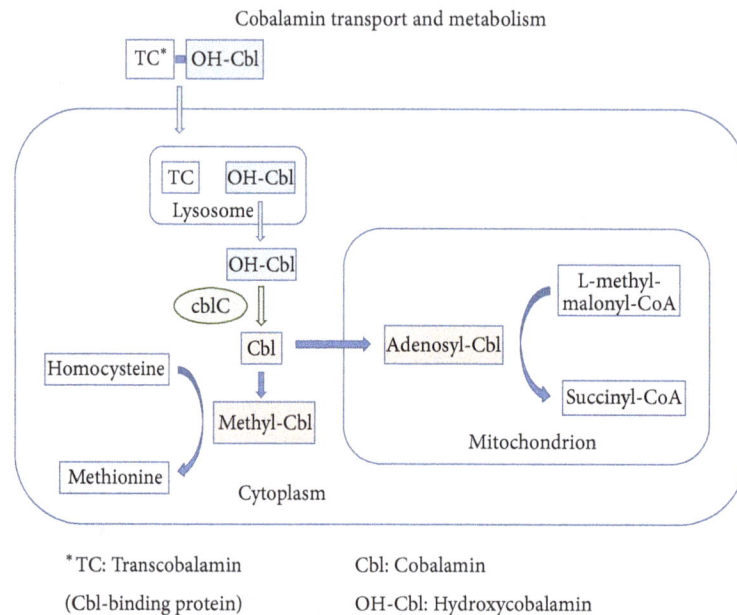

FIGURE 1: Cobalamin transport and metabolism. Hydroxycobalamin (OH-Cbl) enters the cell bound to transcobalamin (TC), a binding protein. The hydroxycobalamin-transcobalamin complex is broken down inside the lysosome, and the enzyme cobalamin C (CblC) removes the hydroxyl group to generate free cobalamin (Cbl), which is synthesized via additional steps into methyl- and adenosyl-cobalamin.

symmetric T2-weighted hyperintensities in the cerebellar dentate nuclei, globus pallidi, and thalami.

2.1.9. Fumaric Aciduria. Seizures are a prominent feature in fumaric aciduria, due to a defect in the conversion of fumarate to malate. The disorder can present prenatally with polyhydramnios and cerebral ventriculomegaly and manifests in infancy and early childhood with epilepsy, serious neurodevelopmental delay, macrocephaly, opisthotonus, and vision loss. Status epilepticus is well reported. Diffuse polymicrogyria, decreased white matter, large ventricles, and open opercula are seen on neuroimaging [22].

2.1.10. Maple Syrup Urine Disease and Dihydrolipoamide Dehydrogenase Deficiency. Dysfunction of the enzyme branched-chain 2-keto dehydrogenase (BCKD) in maple syrup urine disease (MSUD) prevents normal degradation of the branched-chain amino acids leucine, isoleucine, and valine, leading to toxic accumulation of metabolites.

Neurological symptoms present in infancy and include cerebral edema, seizures, lethargy, vomiting, and "bicycling" movements [23]. Seizures are related to the cerebral edema and hyperlycinemia, and these symptoms can progress to coma and death. The EEG may show a characteristic comb-like rhythm (Figure 2). Treatment focuses on removing leucine from blood with dialysis or by reversing catabolism through feeding.

Dihydrolipoamide dehydrogenase deficiency, sometimes referred to as MSUD Type III, is due to a defect in a subunit of BCKD, as well as 3 other essential enzymes. The disorder leads to metabolic acidosis and neurological injury, and patients can present with hypoglycemia, absent ketones, elevated liver transaminases, and seizures [24]. The disorder is often fatal at an early age, representing multienzyme failure.

2.2. Disorders of GABA Metabolism. Seizures are an important problem in disorders of the synthesis or degradation of gamma-aminobutyric acid (GABA), the brain's primary inhibitory neurotransmitter. The most common of

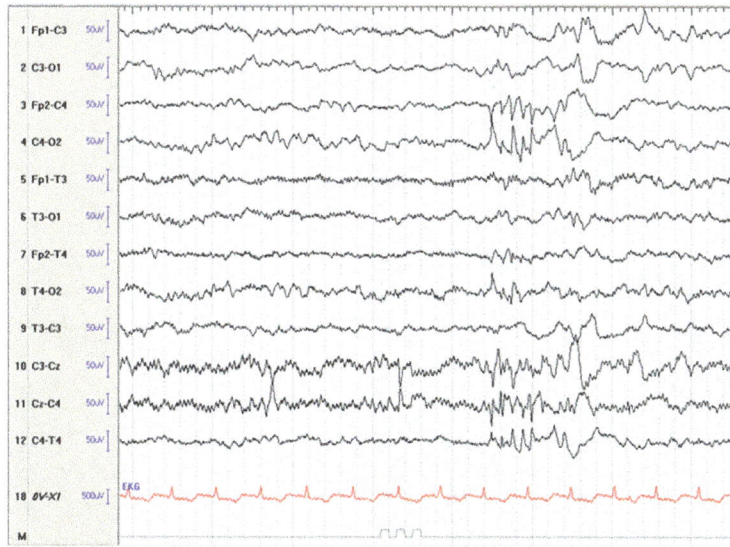

FIGURE 2: EEG of 4-day-old infant with MSUD shows comb-like rhythm over the right central (C4) area. (sensitivity 7 mcv/mm, HFF 70 Hz, time constant 0.5 sec, 8 sec epoch). Pearl [2].

these is succinic semialdehyde dehydrogenase (SSADH) deficiency, though GABA-transaminase deficiency—while extremely rare—features a more severe, progressive epileptic encephalopathy. Both are inherited metabolic disorders affecting GABA degradation.

2.2.1. Succinic Semialdehyde Dehydrogenase Deficiency (4-Hydroxybutyric Aciduria).

Deficiency of the enzyme succinic semialdehyde dehydrogenase (SSADH) results in increased systemic and CSF levels of GABA and its catabolite, 4-hydroxybutyric acid (GHB). Patients present with neurodevelopmental delay, expressive language impairment, hypotonia, hyporeflexia, ataxia, and behavioral disorders that commonly include obsessive compulsive and attention deficit hyperactivity disorders. Over 50% of individuals with SSADH deficiency will develop seizures, most commonly tonic-clonic and atypical absence seizures [25]. Recurring status epilepticus and sudden unexpected death in epilepsy patients (SUDEP) have been reported, the latter associated with escalating seizure frequency and severity [26]. MRIs show increased T2-weighted signals in the globus pallidus, cerebellar dentate nucleus and subthalamic nucleus, and variably cerebral and cerebellar atrophy [27]. EEGs typically show generalized spike-wave activity although some may have partial features and variable hemispheric lateralization (Figure 3). Treatment is currently limited to antiepileptic and behavioral medications. While valproate is generally avoided due to its ability to inhibit any residual enzymatic activity, its use has been associated with improvement in some patients with challenging epilepsy including epileptic encephalopathy.

2.3. Fatty Acid Oxidation Disorders.

Severe seizures can be a presenting sign of defects in fatty acid beta-oxidation, a biochemical process that produces alternatives source of acetyl-CoA and ketone bodies for energy. Fatty acid oxidation

(FAO) disorders (Table 2) are a large category of diseases that particularly endanger the CNS and other organ systems that have high energy demands. Metabolic decompensation can be triggered by physiological stressors such as fasting, fever, or physical exertion, and symptoms can appear at any age. Acute crises resemble Reye syndrome, with cardiomyopathy and arrhythmia, as well as rhabdomyolysis and hypoketotic hypoglycemia [28, 29].

Blood and urine laboratory tests are informative towards a diagnosis, particularly if done while the patient is symptomatic. Treatment is dependent on clinical presentation and include avoidance of fasting with frequent low-fat and carbohydrate-rich intake for nonsymptomatic patients and moderation of physical stress in combination with medium-chain triglyceride (MCT) supplementation for patients symptomatic with myopathy. Patients in metabolic crisis require close management in an inpatient setting, with immediate reversal of the catabolism [30, 31].

2.4. Mitochondrial Diseases.

Epilepsy is a common secondary feature of mitochondrial disease, and disorders in this category (Table 3) have been associated with severe epileptic encephalopathy. Seizures can be a logical consequence of mitochondrial dysfunction: deficient energy generation disrupts the active maintenance of neuronal membrane potential, and seizure-induced cellular hyperactivity adds further oxidative stress to already deficient ATP generation. Up to 60% of patients with mitochondrial disease develop seizures, and many of these can be refractory to treatment [32]. Myoclonic epilepsies are the most commonly reported, but almost all seizure types have been seen, and individual patients can often show multiple types.

2.4.1. POLG1 Disease.

Mutations in the gene POLG1, which facilitates mitochondrial DNA replication, have been linked

(a)

(b)

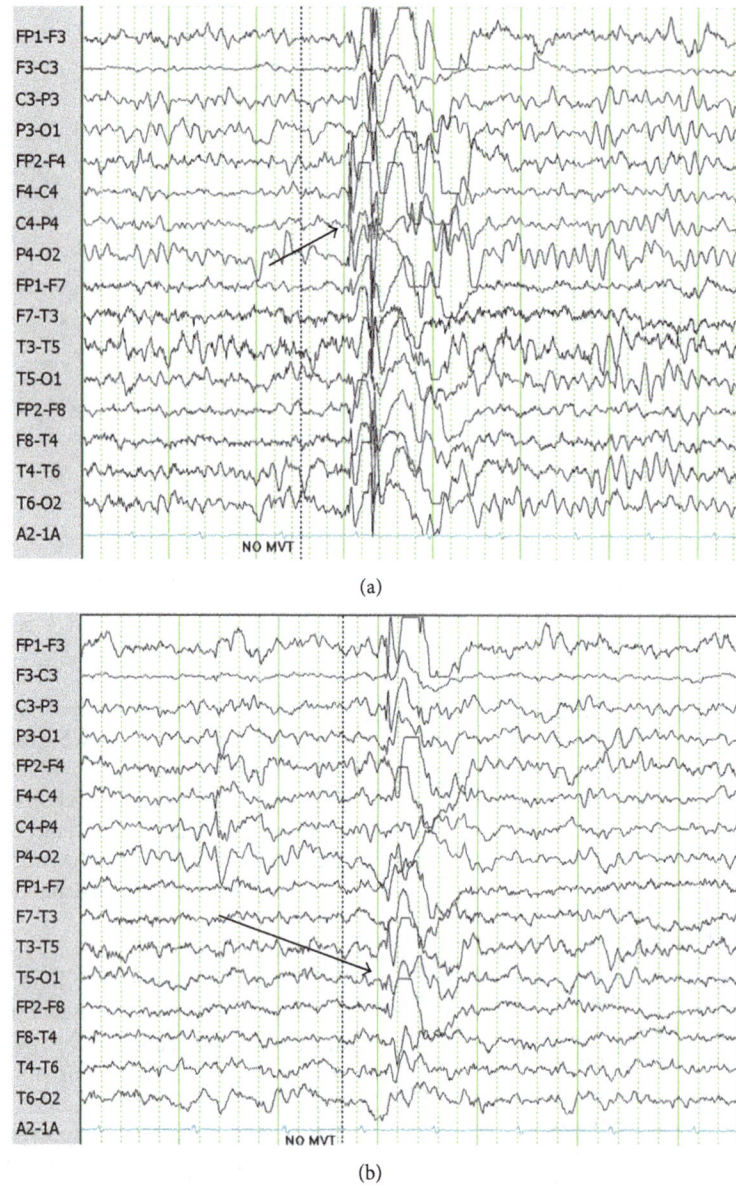

FIGURE 3: (a) EEG of 3-year-old female with SSADH deficiency. Note diffuse spike-wave paroxysm with lead-in over right hemisphere. (b) Same recording as top, showing left-sided spike-wave paroxysm. Pearl [2].

to a range of disease phenotypes, the most prominent being Alpers' disease [33] (Figure 4). Alpers-Huttenlocher disease is a rapidly progressive encephalopathy, causing intractable epilepsy and diffuse neuronal degeneration. Partial complex and myoclonic seizures are most common, although the disorder can evolve to include multiple seizure types [34]. The use of valproate is contraindicated; it has been associated with liver failure in patients with POLG1 mutations, as well as epilepsia partialis continua.

A syndrome of myoclonic epilepsy myopathy sensory ataxia (MEMSA) has also been seen in patients with mutations in POLG1. Seizures, usually focal and often refractory, begin in young adulthood, though other symptoms including sensory neuropathy and cerebellar ataxia may occur in

adolescence. Over time, individuals develop cognitive decline and myopathy [35].

2.4.2. Myoclonic Epilepsy with Ragged Red Fibers (MERRF). Myoclonic epilepsy with ragged red fibers (referring to the appearance of affected muscle cells) is a progressive epilepsy syndrome associated with prominent myoclonus, cognitive decline, optic atrophy, hearing loss, and myopathy [36]. It is associated with mtDNA mutations, and symptoms usually become noticeable in adolescence or young adulthood [37]. EEG findings include focal discharges, atypical spike- or sharp- and slow-wave discharges, and suppression of this activity during sleep [38].

TABLE 2: Fatty acid oxidation disorders and biochemical characteristics.

Disorder	Biochemical characteristics
Carnitine uptake defect (CUD) (Primary/systemic carnitine deficiency, carnitine transporter OCTN2 deficiency)	$\downarrow\downarrow\downarrow$ Carnitine (P)
Carnitine palmitoyltransferase I deficiency (CPT 1A)	$\uparrow$ Ammonia (P) $\uparrow$ Liver enzymes (ALT, AST)
Carnitine palmitoyltransferase II deficiency (CPT II) (i) lethal neonatal (ii) infantile (iii) myopathic	$\uparrow$ C12–C18 acylcarnitines (P)
Carnitine-acylcarnitine translocase deficiency (CACT)	$\uparrow$ Ammonia (P) $\uparrow$ Liver enzymes (ALT, AST) $\uparrow$ Creatine kinase (P) $\uparrow$ Long chain acylcarnitines (P) $\downarrow$ Free carnitine (P)
Mitochondrial trifunction protein deficiency (TFP) (i) Isolated long chain Acyl-CoA Dehydrogenase deficiency (LCHAD)	Hypoketotic hypoglycemia
Very long chain acyl-CoA dehydrogenase deficiency (VLCAD)	Hypoglycemia (ketotic or nonketotic)
Medium chain acyl-CoA dehydrogenase deficiency (MCAD)	Hypoketotic hypoglycemia
Medium chain 3-ketoacyl-CoA thiolase deficiency (MCKAT)	Ketotic lactic aciduria C6–C12 dicarboxylic aciduria
Short chain acyl-CoA dehydrogenase deficiency (SCAD)	$\uparrow$ Ethylmalonic acid (U)
Medium/short chain acyl-CoA dehydrogenase deficiency (M/SCHAD)	Hyperinsulinemic hypoglycemia $\uparrow$ 3-Hydroxybutylcarnitine $\uparrow$ 3-Hydroxy butyric acid (U) $\uparrow$ 3-Hydroxy glutaric acid (U)
Glutaric acidemia Type II	Hypoglycemia Metabolic acidosis
2,4-Dienoyl-CoA reductase deficiency	2-Trans,4-Cis-decadienoylcarnitine (P, U)
Acyl-CoA dehydrogenase 9 deficiency (ACAD9)	Persistent lactic acidosis

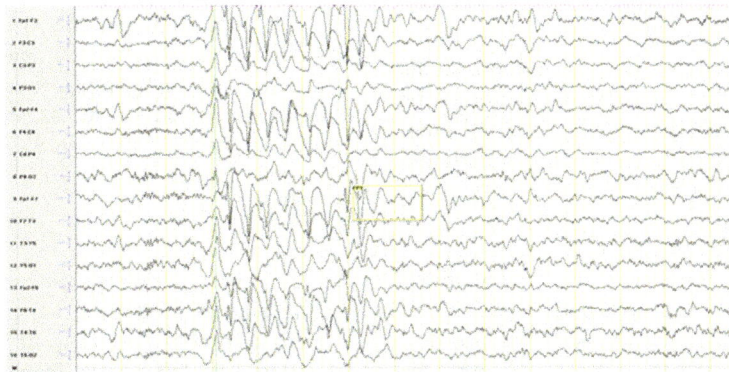

FIGURE 4: 7-year-old boy diagnosed with Alpers' syndrome presented with encephalopathy, tonic-clonic seizures and myoclonic seizures. EEG shows high amplitude anterior poorly formed 2-3 Hertz sharp and slow activity. Pearl [2].

2.4.3. Leigh Syndrome. Leigh syndrome, also known as subacute necrotizing encephalomyopathy, can be seen in disorders involving mitochondrial DNA (as well as nonmitochondrial disorders). Individuals present with neurologic regression with worsening hypotonia, spasticity, and brainstem failure as the disease progresses. Neuroimaging may show bilateral, symmetric lesions in the basal ganglia, thalami, midbrain, and brainstem as well as cortical and cerebellar atrophy [39]. Focal and generalized epilepsy are associated with this phenotype, and epilepsia partialis continua, as well as infantile spasms and hypsarrhythmia, has been described [40].

2.5. Cerebral Folate Deficiency. Cerebral folate deficiency can be a common end result of diverse metabolic and genetic conditions (Table 4). A suspected pathology in primary CFD

TABLE 3: Mitochondrial disorders and epilepsy.

Category of disorder	Syndrome
Mitochondrial complex deficiencies	(i) Complex I deficiency (ii) Complex II deficiency (iii) Complex III deficiency (iv) Complex IV deficiency (v) Complex V deficiency

Mitochondrial DNA disorders	(i) mtDNA depletion syndromes
	  (a) POLG1 disease
	    (1) Alpers-Huttenlocher disease
	    (2) Childhood onset epilepsia partialis continua (EPC)
	    (3) Myoclonic epilepsy myopathy sensory ataxia (MEMSA)
	(ii) mtDNA deletion syndromes
	  (a) Kearns-Sayre syndrome (KSS)
	  (b) Chronic progressive external ophthalmoplegia (CPEO)
	(iii) Myoclonic epilepsy with ragged-red fibers (MERRF)
	(iv) Myoclonic epilepsy, lactic acidosis, and stroke (MELAS)

Other associated syndromes	Leigh syndrome

involves impaired transport of folate across the choroid plexus into the central nervous system. This may be due to one of multiple causes, including loss of function mutations in the folate FR1 receptor, blocking autoantibodies to the folate receptor, or disrupted uptake due to valproic acid. Secondary folate deficiency can also be seen in inborn metabolic diseases, such as Rett syndrome, 3-phosphoglycerate dehydrogenase deficiency (a congenital serine biosynthesis disorder), and mitochondrial disorders such as Kearns-Sayre or Alpers disease [41–44].

Primary cerebral folate deficiency (CFD) is characterized by normal blood but low CSF levels of 5-methylhydrofolate (5-MTHF), the physiologically active form of folate. The common phenotype includes epilepsy, along with neurodevelopmental delay (or regression) and dyskinesias. Individuals with blocking autoantibodies to folate receptors present in early childhood with intractable generalized tonic-clonic seizures. In some cases, treatment with high doses of folinic acid (as opposed to folic acid, which has poor blood-brain barrier entry) has been reported to ameliorate seizures and improve neurological function [45].

2.6. Serine Synthesis Defects.
Lserine, a nonessential amino acid, is synthesized from 3-phosphoglycerate by the sequential activity of three enzymes, each with associated disorders (Table 5). The majority of patients with serine deficiencies are affected by an abnormality in the first step, 3-phosphoglycerate dehydrogenase. The clinical phenotype, which includes congenital microcephaly and psychomotor retardation with refractory seizures and hypsarrhythmia, is nonspecific, likely leading practitioners to suspect in utero processes such as TORCH (Toxoplasmosis, Syphilis, Rubella, Cytomegalovirus, Herpes simplex, HIV) or static perinatal difficulties. MRI findings in infantile onset patients have revealed cortical and subcortical atrophy, as well as delayed myelination [46]. Juvenile onset has also been reported, with presentation at school age with absence seizures and moderate developmental delay [47]. Supplementation with

oral serine and glycine has been reported to significantly improve seizures, spasticity, behavior, and feeding, as well as white matter volume and myelination [48, 49].

2.7. DEND Syndrome (Developmental Delay, Epilepsy, and Neonatal Diabetes).
A syndrome that combines the problems of developmental delay, epilepsy, and neonatal diabetes is an epileptic channelopathy associated with mutations in potassium channel and sulfonylurea receptor genes [50]. These mutations permanently "lock in" the K_{ATP} channel in an open state, leading to insufficient insulin release and severe hyperglycemia within the first six months of life [51–53]. Clinical manifestations include neurodevelopmental delay, dysmorphic features, hypotonia, and seizures starting as early as the neonatorum. Infantile spasms with hypsarrhythmia, as well as severe tonic-clonic and myoclonic epilepsies, are reported. Neonatal hyperglycemia in DEND can be managed with insulin or sulfonylureas, but the latter is capable of bypassing the defective regulation of K_{ATP} channels and may have better efficacy for the neurological phenotype [50, 54, 55].

2.8. Hyperinsulinism-Hyperammonemia (HI-HA).
HI-HA is a syndrome of congenital hyperinsulinism and hyperammonemia that has been related to activating mutations affecting GDH (glutamate dehydrogenase), a participant in the insulin secretion pathway. These defects cause GDH to become insensitive to inhibition, resulting in excess ammonia production and insulin release and neurological sequelae from hypoglycemic insults and hyperammonemia [56]. The clinical constellation of generalized epilepsy, learning disorders, and behavior problems, in the context of hypoglycemia (both postprandial and fasting) and persistent hyperammonemia, is characteristic.

Hypoglycemic seizures may be the first apparent indication. However, some patients have been observed to experience paroxysms, accompanied by generalized electroencephalographic features, without hypoglycemic episodes.

TABLE 4: Cerebral folate deficiencies.

	Disorder or mechanism
Primary cerebral folate deficiency	Folate receptor FR1 defect due to autoantibodies
	Folate receptor FR1 defect due to (FOLR1 gene) mutation
Disorders with secondary cerebral folate deficiency	Aicardi-Goutieres syndrome
	Alpers syndrome
	Isolated Rett syndrome
	Kearns-Sayre syndrome
	Mitochondrial complex I encephalomyopathy
	Valproic acid complications

TABLE 5: Serine synthesis defects.

Disorder	Epilepsy and neuroimaging features	Response to treatment with L-serine and glycine
3-Phosphoglycerate dehydrogenase deficiency	Infantile phenotype:	Infantile phenotype:
	(i) intractable seizures	(i) Seizure control or significantly lowered frequency
	(ii) MRI: hypomyelination and delayed myelination	(ii) Increased white matter volume
	Juvenile phenotype:	Juvenile phenotype:
	(i) absence seizures	(i) Seizure control
	(ii) MRI: no abnormalities	(ii) Prevention of neurological abnormalities
Phosphoserine Aminotransferase deficiency	Symptomatic patient:	Symptomatic patient:
	(i) intractable seizures	(i) No clinical response to treatment
	(ii) MRI: generalized atrophy, including cerebellar vermis and pons, white matter abnormalities	
	Presymptomatic patient:	Presymptomatic patient:
	(i) MRI: no abnormalities	(i) Prevention of all neurological abnormalities
Phosphoserine phosphatase deficiency	Single case, details not reported	Not reported

Adapted from Pearl [2].

This suggests that epilepsy in HI-HA may not be due solely to low CNS glucose availability [57–59]. HI-HA is manageable with a combination of dietary protein restriction, glucagon, antiepileptic medications, and diazoxide, a K_{ATP} channel agonist that inhibits insulin release [60].

2.9. *Glucose Transporter 1 Deficiency.* Glucose transporter type I (Glut-1) facilitates the passage of glucose across the blood-brain barrier, and its dysfunction in the developing brain leads to the development of a metabolic encephalopathy. CSF shows hypoglycorrhachia associated with normal plasma glucose and low-to-normal CSF lactate, measured in a fasting state. A wide array of phenotypes has been associated with this disorder, but 90% of affected children develop epilepsy (of various types, including absence, focal, generalized myoclonic, clonic, tonic, and nonconvulsive status epilepticus) [61]. Microcephaly, ataxia, and psychomotor delay may be present [62], but patients may also suffer from epilepsy without any accompanying motor or cognitive

deficiencies. Haploinsufficiency (of the SLC2A1 gene) is correlated with the severity of symptoms [63]. EEG findings vary and may be normal, but usually include either focal or generalized slowing or attenuation, or spike-and-wave discharges (generalized, focal, or multifocal). Neuroimaging results may demonstrate diffuse atrophy.

Glucose transporter I deficiency has emerged as the leading metabolic indication for the ketogenic diet, a dietary therapy that replaces glucose with ketone bodies as the primary biochemical energy source. Response is rapid, even in the case of formerly refractory seizures, and treatment should be maintained long term. Additionally, there are certain compounds known to inhibit Glut-1, including phenobarbital, diazepam, methylxanthines (theophylline, caffeine), and alcohol, which should be avoided [64].

2.10. *Pyridoxine, Folinic Acid, and Pyridoxal-5'-Phosphate Dependent Epilepsies.* There are various epileptic encephalopathies related to vitamin B6 metabolism (Table 6), and

TABLE 6: Pyridoxine and pyridoxal-5′-phosphate-dependent Epilepsies.

	Pyridoxine- or folinic-acid-dependent epilepsies (PDE)	Pyridoxal-5′-phosphate (PLP-) dependent epilepsy
Deficient enzyme	Antiquitin (ATQ)	Pyridox(am)ine phosphate oxidase (PNPO)
Blood chemistry	Normal, but hypoglycemia and lactic acidosis have been reported	Hypoglycemia and lactic acidosis common
Vanillactic acid (Urine)	Absent	Present
Pipecolic acid (blood, CSF)	↑	Normal
AASA* (blood, urine, CSF)	↑	Normal
Neurotransmitter metabolites (CSF)	(Possible) ↑ 3-Methoxytyrosine	↑ L-DOPA, 3-Methoxytyrosine ↓ Homovanillic acid, 5-Hydroxyindoleacetic acid
Clinical signs	Postnatal refractory seizures, gastrointestinal symptoms, encephalopathy with hyperalertness, sleeplessness	Fetal distress and in utero fetal seizures, postnatal refractory seizures and encephalopathy

*AASA: alpha-aminoadipic semialdehyde. Adapted from Pearl [2].

pyridoxine-dependent epilepsy (PDE) is the prototype, resulting from a loss of the biologically active pyridoxal-5′-phosphate (PLP) due to a dysfunction of the protein antiquitin (*ALDH7A1*) [65]. PDE normally presents within the first hours following birth with serial refractory seizures responsive to pyridoxine administration. Improvement is significant and usually rapidly appreciable on EEG [66]. Variants of the disorder that respond to folinic acid instead of, or in addition to, pyridoxine have also been described, as well as atypical cases with long asymptomatic periods or presenting later in infancy (i.e., weeks or months following birth) [67, 68].

PNPO, or pyridox(am)ine phosphate oxidase, deficiency is a distinct disorder involving refractory seizures responsive not to pyridoxine but to its biologically active form, pyridoxal-5′-phosphate (PLP) [69, 70]. This disorder is due to a defect in the enzyme PNPO, which synthesizes PLP from precursors pyridoxine-P and pyridoxamine-P [71]. Patients may present prenatally with fetal seizures and premature birth and if untreated can progress to status epilepticus and death. Laboratory and genetic testings are available to confirm these diagnoses (Table 6); trials of systemic pyridoxine administration require close cardiorespiratory monitoring.

2.11. Urea Cycle Disorders. The urea cycle (Figure 6), the metabolic mechanism for nitrogen detoxification and removal, is facilitated by six enzymes and a mitochondrial transporter and carrier, each being susceptible to dysfunction (Table 7). In the event of an enzyme or transport defect, the resulting hyperammonemia can lead to overwhelming encephalopathy, often accompanied by seizures and hypotonia that may be exacerbated by metabolic stresses such as fever or infection [72]. EEG monitoring should be initiated early in the course of acute treatment, as seizure activity is thought to be related to hyperammonemic crises or structural damage, and subclinical electrographic seizures are reported. Males with OTC deficiency typically present in the neonatorum and with high mortality, whereas female heterozygotes can vary in the severity and timing of presentation depending on hepatic lyonization [72].

The goals of therapy during metabolic crisis are removal of ammonia through hemodialysis, nitrogen scavenging with agents including sodium benzoate and sodium phenylacetate [73], and reversal of catabolism. Immediate antiepileptic therapy is indicated for optimizing treatment; valproate, however, may interfere with the urea cycle and precipitate metabolic crises [74]. Maintenance therapy of urea cycle defects hinges on the restriction of protein intake while providing sufficient essential amino acids. Orthotopic liver transplant may be curative, but cannot reverse existing neurologic injury.

2.12. Creatine Biosynthesis and Transport Deficiencies. Half of the body's daily requirement of creatine is synthesized from arginine and glycine by the enzymes AGAT (arginine:glycine amidinotransferase) and GAMT (guanidino acetate methyl transferase). A specific creatine transporter, CT1, encoded by an X-linked gene, facilitates the uptake into tissues. Patients with deficiencies in creatine synthesis or transport present with early developmental delay, seizures, neurologic regression, intellectual disability, autistic behavior, hypotonia, and movement disorders. Females with heterozygous mutations of the creatine transporter gene may be symptomatic with more moderate intellectual disability, learning and behavior problems, and epilepsy [75].

Approximately half of individuals with GAMT deficiency, and most males with creatine transporter deficiency, develop epilepsy [76]. Patients with GAMT deficiency have abnormal MRI signals of the globus pallidus and background slowing and generalized spike-and-wave discharges on EEG. Individuals with creatine transporter deficiency present with generalized and partial epilepsy, with EEG usually reported

TABLE 7: Urea cycle defects and biochemical characteristics.

Defective enzyme or component	Citrulline	Arginine	Ammonia	Additional biochemical characteristics
Ornithine transcarbamylase	↓	↓	↑	↑ Glutamine Normal orotic acid
Carbamoylphosphate synthetase I (CPS1)	↓	↓	↑	↑ Glutamine ↑ Orotic acid
N-acetyl glutamate synthase (NAGS)				Reduced CPS1 activity (NAGS is a vital cofactor)
Argininosuccinate synthase (ASS)	↑++ (10–100x normal)	↓	↑	
Argininosuccinate lyase (ASL)	↑	↓	↑	↑ Argininosuccinic acid (unique to ASL deficiency)
Arginase (ARG1)			Normal in absence of metabolic stress	
Ornithine transporter mitochondrial I (ornithine translocase deficiency)			↑	↑ Homocitrulline ↑ Ornithine
Citrin (solute carrier family 5) deficiency	↑			

Adapted from Pearl [2].

as showing generalized polyspike or multifocal epileptiform discharges [77, 78].

Laboratory identification using urine creatine metabolites (Table 8) is necessary to distinguish the three disorders [79]. In the case of creatine synthesis disorders, treatment with oral creatine supplementation can improve seizures and neurological function, and arginine restriction and ornithine supplementation are utilized in GAMT deficiency. Creatine transport disorders, however, are not significantly amenable to therapy other than with traditional antiepileptic medications.

2.13. Glycine Encephalopathy. Glycine encephalopathy is an inherited disorder of glycine degradation resulting from defects in the mitochondrial glycine cleavage system (GCS). The excitatory effects of glycine on the cortex and forebrain, mediated by N-methyl-D-aspartate(NMDA) receptors, lead to excess intracellular calcium accumulation and subsequent neuronal injury with intractable seizures [80]. Based on age at presentation and clinical outcomes, different categories of glycine encephalopathy (GE) can be distinguished. The majority of patients present with a severe neonatal-onset form, with primarily myoclonic and intractable seizures, hypotonia, apnea, and coma [81]. Outcomes are generally poor, particularly in the presence of brain malformations such as corpus callosum hypoplasia. There are attenuated forms, lacking congenital malformations, with a better outcome.

Laboratory analyses reveal elevated plasma and CSF glycine, as well as an increased CSF to plasma glycine ratio. EEG findings include multifocal epileptiform activity, hypsarrhythmia, and burst-suppression patterns (Figure 5) [82]. Treatment with benzoate and a low-protein diet may reduce glycine levels in plasma, and combined antiepileptic treatment is necessary for most individuals.

2.14. Sulfide Oxidase Deficiency/Molybdenum Cofactor Deficiency. Sulfite oxidase deficiency due to molybdenum cofactor deficiency (MOCOD) and isolated sulfite oxidase deficiency (ISOD) are inherited disorders of the metabolism of sulfated amino acids [83]. They typically present in the first days of life with poor feeding following an uneventful pregnancy and delivery. Seizures, primarily myoclonic or tonic-clonic, begin in the first few weeks of life; they can be refractory to therapy and may develop into status epilepticus [84]. Signs of encephalopathy with opisthotonus, apnea, prolonged crying, and provoked erratic eye movements or myoclonias can be seen, and up to 75% of patients will have slight dysmorphia including widely spaced eyes, small nose, puffy cheeks, and elongated face [85].

EEG findings include burst suppression patterns and multifocal spike-wave discharges [86], and neuroimaging results are usually profoundly abnormal, including diffuse cerebral edema evolving into cystic lesions and brain atrophy within weeks [87]. Low total plasma homocysteinemia is associated with both ISOD and MOCOD, and hypouricemia due to secondary xanthine dehydrogenase deficiency can be indicative of MOCOD. Therapy has historically been symptomatic, with combination or monoantiepileptics.

2.15. Homocysteinemias. Disorders involving homocysteine metabolism, specifically methionine and cystathionine synthesis, are characterized by elevated urine and serum homocysteine in the context of neurological symptoms. The spectrum of neurological dysfunction in homocysteine metabolism disorders is wide, including epilepsy, encephalopathy, peripheral neuropathy, ataxia, microcephaly, and psychiatric disorders. Cystathionine beta-synthetase (CBS) deficiency is the most common of the homocysteinemias, with severe defects involving multiple systems due to the essentiality of homocysteine and methionine to normal

TABLE 8: Creatine synthesis defects.

Defective enzyme or component	Urine Creatine	Urine GAA (guanidinoacetate)	Creatine/creatinine ratio	treatment
AGAT (arginine : glycine amidinotransferase)	↓	↓	Normal	(i) Amenable to creatine therapy
GAMT (guanidine acetate methyl transferase)	↓	↑	Normal	(i) Amenable to creatine therapy; (ii) Dietary restriction of arginine, with ornithine supplementation (iii) Antiepileptics may be necessary for seizure control
Creatine transporter	↑	Normal (may be slightly increased in males)	↑	(i) Antiepileptics for seizure control (ii) Creatine supplementation is ineffective

TABLE 9: Biochemical characteristics and treatment of homocysteine metabolism disorders.

Defective enzyme	Homocysteine (U, P)	Additional biochemical characteristics	Treatment
Cystathionine beta-synthase (CBS)	↑	↑ Methionine ↓ Cysteine	Pyridoxine, B12, folate Methionine-restricted diet Cysteine supplementation betaine
Methionine synthase (MTR)	↑	Normal or ↑ Folate Normal or ↑ Cobalamin	High-dose hydroxycobalamin
Methylene tetrahydrofolate reductase (MTHFR)	↑	↓ Methionine	High-dose betaine Methionine supplementation

* (U): urine, (P): plasma.

biochemical function. Focal seizures, stroke, neurodevelopmental delay, and cognitive deficiency, as well as psychosis are common neurological findings. Marfan-like skeletal symptoms, connective tissue abnormalities in the optic lens, and vasculopathies causing thrombosis and multiorgan infarcts may also be present. Treatment and biochemical findings in CBS, as well as other homocysteine disorders are summarized in Table 9.

Autosomal recessively inherited deficiency of methylene tetrahydrofolate reductase (MTHFR) may present in early infancy with severe epileptic encephalopathy [88]. The presentation with hypotonia, lethargy, feeding difficulties, and recurrent apnea may progress from seizures to coma and death. Infantile spasms may also be the presenting feature, with evolution to multiple seizure types including the Lennox-Gastaut syndrome. Status epilepticus, both clinical and subclinical, has been reported. Progressive microcephaly and global encephalopathy may ensue as seizures continue, but there is evidence for reversibility with treatment comprised principally of the methyl donor betaine [89].

2.16. Purine and Pyrimidine Defects. Disorders of purine and pyrimidine metabolism may present with epileptic encephalopathies (Table 10), including adenylosuccinase (adenylosuccinate lyase) deficiency which has a broad phenotypic spectrum including neonatal seizures [90]. Lesch-Nyhan disease, or X-linked hypoxanthine-guanine phosphoribosyltransferase deficiency, may result in epileptic seizures, but these can be difficult to distinguish from the extrapyramidal manifestations, specifically dystonic spasms, tremor, and myoclonus. Generalized tonic-clonic seizures are the most commonly reported epilepsy type in the literature [91, 92]. Treatment with allopurinol is essential for hyperuricemia and may provide some antiepileptic effect. Antiepileptic drug choices must weigh the possibility of exacerbating underlying behavioral irritability with levetiracetam and others. Topiramate and zonisamide are avoided due to the risk of nephrolithiasis.

3. Large Molecule Disorders

3.1. Disorders of Glycosylation. Disorders of protein glycosylation, due to defects in the synthesis of N- and O-linked glycoproteins, are characterized by multiple organ system dysfunction, developmental delay, hypotonia, and epilepsy. Certain of these disorders are associated with severe encephalopathy, particularly those involving alpha-dystroglycan, a protein component of the extracellular matrix, essential to muscle integrity. These are known as dystroglycanopathies.

3.1.1. Walker-Warburg Syndrome. Walker-Warburg syndrome (WWS) is a severe dystroglycanopathy which can present at birth or prenatally with hydrocephalus and encephaloceles on imaging. Seizures and significant structural abnormalities (e.g. cerebellar atrophy, hypoplasia of the corpus callosum), migrational defects (type II lissencephaly), hypomyelination, and ophthalmologic defects are seen. Life expectancy is less than three years [93, 94].

TABLE 10: Purine and pyrimidine metabolism disorders involving epilepsy.

Disorder	Defective enzyme	Biochemical characteristics	Seizure characteristics
Lesch-Nyhan Disease (LSD)	hypoxanthine-guanine phosphoribosyl transferase	↑ Uric acid	Predominantly generalized tonic-clonic, developing in early childhood
Adenylosuccinase deficiency	Adenylosuccinate lyase	↑ succinylaminoimidazole carboxamide riboside ↑ succinyladenosine	Neonatal seizures Severe infantile epileptic encephalopathy

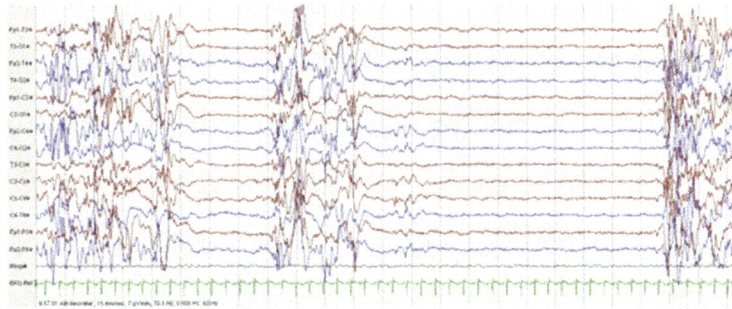

FIGURE 5: EEG of term infant with glycine encephalopathy shows burst-suppression pattern. Pearl [2].

3.1.2. Fukuyama Congenital Muscular Dystrophy. Fukuyama congenital muscular dystrophy (FCMD) classically presents in the neonatorum or even prenatally (poor fetal movement) with frequent seizures and severe brain abnormalities (migration defects, cobblestone lissencephaly, delayed myelination, hypoplasia of the pons, cerebellar cysts). By the age of 3, most patients develop epilepsy. Muscular degeneration and cardiac involvement are progressive [95, 96].

3.2. Lysosomal Storage Disorders. Lysosomal storage disorders (LSD) are a major category of diseases that involve defects in lysosomal enzyme function, lysosomal biogenesis, activation, trafficking, or membrane transporters. Over two-thirds of LSDs are neurodegenerative and some are associated with epileptic encephalopathy. Table 11 lists lysosomal storage disorders by subgroup, and prominent examples are covered below.

3.2.1. Neuronal Ceroid Lipofuscinoses (NCLs). Neuronal ceroid lipofuscinoses are genetically heterogeneous neurodegenerative disorders associated with defects in transmembrane proteins and are characterized by the accumulation of autofluorescent lipopigments in lysosomes. The symptoms include cognitive decline, seizures, vision loss, and motor impairment, though age of onset and clinical course vary [97]. The development of epilepsy can indicate a more severe clinical course, though myoclonic seizures should be distinguished from myoclonus, which is also a frequent and sometimes progressive feature of this disorder [98]. Generalized cerebral and cerebellar atrophy can be seen on neuroimaging [99].

3.2.2. Sphingolipidosis and Gaucher Disease. Defects in the degradation of sphingolipids, an essential component of myelin sheaths and neuronal tissue, lead to progressive neurodegeneration, epilepsy, peripheral neuropathy, extrapyramidal symptoms, and characteristic "cherry-red spots." Subtypes (II and III) of Gaucher Disease, which result from a deficiency in glucocerebrosidase, can cause devastating and rapid neurological deterioration. Neuroimaging is usually normal in patients with Gaucher Disease, but EEG can show several abnormalities including polyspikes with occipital predominance sensitive to photostimulation, diffuse slowing with high-voltage sharp waves during sleep, and multifocal spike-and-wave paroxysms [100, 101].

3.2.3. Gangliosidosis and Tay-Sachs Disease. Tay-Sachs disease is an example of defects involving the degradation of gangliosides, which are vital signaling, transport, and regulatory proteins in the lysosomal membrane. Seizures typically begin within the first year of life and worsen in frequency and severity. They are difficult to control with antiepileptics and can acutely and rapidly progress; in these cases, EEG and clinical deterioration can follow until death [102].

3.3. Peroxisomal Diseases. As a participant in cellular detoxification, lipid metabolism, as well as myelin, neuronal function, migration, and brain development [103], peroxisomes are essential for neuronal health. Nearly all peroxisomal disorders (Table 12) are known to impair neurological function, though peroxisomes are present in almost all eukaryotic cells, and consequently its associated diseases will also manifest in multiple organ systems. Seizures occur particularly in the neonatal period and may be a result of cortical migration defects. Symptomatic treatment using anticonvulsants is the predominant therapy [104, 105].

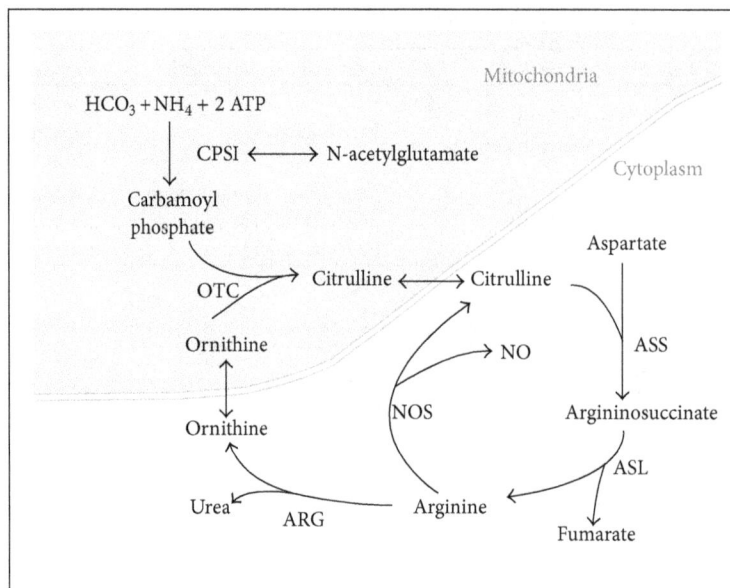

FIGURE 6: The urea cycle. The urea cycle is a pathway of cytosolic and mitochondrial proteins involved in the conversion of ammonia (NH_4) to urea for excretion via the kidneys. The enzymes in the pathway are as follows: carbamoylphosphate synthetase (CPS1), ornithine transcarbamylase (OTC); argininosuccinic acid synthase (ASS); argininosuccinic acid lyase (ASL); arginase I (ARG); nitric oxide synthase (NOS). Pearl [2].

3.3.1. Rhizomelic Chondrodysplasia Punctata. Rhizomelic chondrodysplasia punctata is a peroxisomal biogenesis disorder characterized by white matter abnormalities including inflammatory demyelination and noninflammatory dysmyelination, as well as cerebellar degeneration and loss of Purkinje cells, leading to profound intellectual deficiency. Almost all patients develop seizures, with nonspecific EEG findings. Neurological defects and degeneration are severe, and most individuals do not survive the first two years of life [106].

3.4. Leukodystrophies. Genetic leukoencephalopathies, or inherited white matter disorders, are diseases that primarily affect myelinated structures in the brain and peripheral nervous system. The majority of leukodystrophies primarily feature motor dysfunction rather than encephalopathy, particularly early on in the development of the disease. Epilepsy, however, can be a prominent symptom in certain classic leukodystrophies (Table 13) such as Alexander's disease. This is associated with defects in the GFAPgene encoding astrocyte intermediate filaments. Early onset forms of Alexander's disease (Type I) frequently feature seizures, particularly associated with fever, that are difficult to control. The clinical course of type I Alexander's disease is normally progressive neurodegeneration involving megalencephaly, psychomotor retardation, and spastic paraplegia [107].

4. Conclusion

Epileptic encephalopathies represent a challenging area of pediatric neurology and epilepsy and have a broad differential diagnosis [108]. There are protean inborn errors of metabolism which may lead to epileptic encephalopathies. They have various degrees of treatability at present, with some requiring prompt diagnosis and intervention to avoid otherwise catastrophic outcomes. The epileptologist may view these from the viewpoint of syndromic phenotypes. In general, early myoclonic encephalopathy and myoclonic seizures represent a classic epilepsy syndrome and seizure type, respectively, associated with inborn errors of metabolism. Yet, the phenotypic spectrum of epilepsy caused by hereditary metabolic disorders is wide and includes refractory neonatal seizures, early infantile epileptic encephalopathy (syndrome of Ohtahara), infantile spasms, and progressive myoclonic epilepsies, as well as syndrome variations such as early onset absence epilepsy in glucose transporter deficiency. A careful approach to metabolic disorders is helpful to consider the various diseases that may present and develop into an epileptic encephalopathy.

The small molecule disorders include amino and organic acidopathies such as maple syrup urine disease, homocysteinemia, multiple organic acid disorders, and cobalamin deficiencies. Dietary intervention is key in preventing encephalopathy in maple syrup urine disease and glutaric aciduria, and hydroxycobalamin has a therapeutic role starting in prenatal intervention in cobalamin C deficiency. Neurotransmitter and fatty acid oxidation disorders may result in epileptic encephalopathies, and mitochondrial disorders present with a range of epilepsy phenotypes, including intractable epilepsy and epilepsia partialis continua in polymerase gamma mutations. Cerebral folate deficiency appears to result from a variety of causes but primary deficiency, associated with mutations of the folate receptor or blocking antibodies, has a phenotype of intractable generalized tonic-clonic seizures in infancy which may respond to folinic acid.

TABLE 11: Lysosomal storage disorders.

Storage materials	Diseases	Primary defect
Lipids	Niemann Pick C	Intracellular cholesterol transport
Monosaccharides	Free sialic acid storage disease	Lysosomal transport protein sialin
	(i) infantile free sialic acid storage disease (ISSD)	
	(ii) intermediate salla disease	
	(iii) mild form (salla disease)	
Mucolipidoses	Mucolipidosese	
	(i) type II (I cell disease)	N-acetylglucosamine-1-phosphotransferase
	(ii) type III (pseudo Hurler polydystrophy)	N-acetylglucosamine-1-phosphotransferase
	(iii) type IV	Receptor-stimulated cat ion channel (mucolipidin)
Mucopolysaccharidoses (MPS)	MPS	
Dermatan, heparan sulfate	(i) type IH (Hurler)	L-iduronidase
Dermatan, heparan sulfate	(ii) type II (Hunter)	Iduronate-sulfatase
Heparan sulfate	(i) type III A (Sanfilippo type A)	Heparan-N-sulfatase
	(ii) type III B (Sanfilippo type B)	N-acetyl-α-glucosaminidase
	(iii) type III C (Sanfilippo type C)	α-glucosaminide-acetyl-CoA transferase
	(iv) type III D (Sanfilippo type D)	N-acetylglucosamine-6-sulfatase
Dermatan, heparan, chondroitin sulphate	(i) type VII (Sly)	β-Glucuronidase
Multiple enzyme defects	Multiple sulfatase deficiency	Sulfatase-modifying factor-1 (SUMF1)
	Galactosialidosis	β-Galactosidase and neuraminidase secondary to defect of protective protein, cathepsin A
Neuronal ceroid lipofuscinosis (NCL)	NCL	
	(i) congenital	Cathepsin D (CTSD)
	(ii) infantile (INCL)	Palmitoyl-protein thioesterase-1 (PPT1)
	(iii) late infantile (LNCL)	Tripeptidyl peptidase 1 (TPP1)
	(iv) juvenile (JNCL)	A transmembrane protein
	(v) adult (ANCL)	Ceroid lipofuscinosis neuronal protein 3 (CNT3)
	(vi) Northern epilepsy (NE)	Ceroid lipofuscinosis neuronal protein 8 (CLN8)
Oligosaccharidoses (glycoproteinoses)		
	Alpha-mannosidosis	α-Mannosidase
	Beta-mannosidosis	β-Mannosidase
	Fucosidosis	α-Fucosidase
	Schindler disease	α-N-acetylgalactosaminidase
	Aspartylglucosaminuria (AGU)	Aspartylglucosaminidase
	Sialidosis	
	(i) severe infantile	α-Neuraminidase
	(ii) mild infantile (mucolipidosis I)	α-Neuraminidase
	(iii) adult	α-Neuraminidase
Sphingolipidoses		
Ceramide	Farber disease	Ceramidase
Galactocerebroside	Globoid Cell Leukodystrophy (GLD or Krabbe disease)	β-Galactocerebrosidase
	(i) infantile	
	(ii) late infantile	
	(iii) adult	

TABLE 11: Continued.

Storage materials	Diseases	Primary defect
	(iv) Saposin A deficiency	Sphingolipid activator protein A (SAPA)
Gangliosidoses	GM1 gangliosidoses	β-Galactosidase
	(i) infantile	
	(ii) late infantile	
	(iii) adult	
	GM2 gangliosidoses	β-Hexosaminidase
	(i) Sandhoff disease	β-Hexosaminidase A and B (α-subunit)
	(ii) Tay Sachs	β-Hexosaminidase A (β-subunit)
	(iii) GM2 activator deficiency	β-Hexosaminidase activator
Glucocerebroside	Gaucher disease	β-Glucocerebrosidase
	(i) type II	
	(ii) type III	
	(iii) Saposin C deficiency	Sphingolipid activator protein C
Sphingomyelin	Niemann-Pick	Sphingomyelinase
	(i) type A	
	(ii) type B	
Sulfatide	Metachromatic leukodystrophy (MLD)	Arylsulfatase A
	(i) late infantile	
	(ii) juvenile	
	(iii) adult	
	(iv) Saposin B deficiency	Sphingolipid activator protein B
Multiple sphingolipids	Prosaposin deficiency (pSap)	Precursor of Sphingolipid activator protein

Adapted from Pearl [2].

TABLE 12: Peroxisomal disorders.

Biogenesis disorders	Single enzyme disorders	Contiguous gene syndrome
	X-linked adrenoleukodystrophy (X-ALD)	
	Acyl-coA oxidase deficiency	
Zellweger spectrum disorders (ZSD)	Bifunctional protein deficiency (D-BP)	
(i) Zellweger syndrome (ZS)	Alkyl-DHAP synthase deficiency	
(ii) Neonatal adrenoleukodystrophy (NALD)	DHAP-alkyl transferase deficiency	Contiguous ABCD1 DXS1357E deletion syndrome (CADDS)
(iii) Infantile refsum disease (IRD)	Adult Refsum disease (classic)	
Rhizomelic chondrodysplasia punctata (RCDP)	Glutaric aciduria type III	
	Acatalasemia	
	Hyperoxaluria type I	

Adapted from Pearl [2].

TABLE 13: Leukodystrophies including epilepsy as a manifestation.

Disorder
Alexander's disease
Globoid cell leukodystrophy (Krabbe disease)
X-linked adrenoleukodystrophy
Hereditary diffuse leukoencephalopathy with spheroids
Metachromatic leukodystrophy

Disorders of serine synthesis may respond to pre- and postnatal supplementation with serine and glycine. There are several potassium channelopathies involving the pancreas and brain, presenting either with neonatal diabetes or hypoglycemia, specifically (developmental delay, epilepsy, and neonatal diabetes) DEND and (hyperinsulinism-hyperammonemia) HI-HA with specific therapeutic implications. Glucose transporter deficiency appears to be the prototype of transport defects causing epilepsy and having specific therapy, in this case being the ketogenic diet to supply an alternative brain fuel to glucose, and the disorders related to the pyridoxine vitamers, specifically pyridoxine and pyridoxal-5-phosphate, require prompt identification and therapy to avert a catastrophic outcome. Autosomal recessively inherited deficiency of MTHFR may be reversible with use of betaine, whereas other small molecule defects causing epileptic encephalopathy, for example, glycine encephalopathy and sulfite oxidase deficiency, have no specific therapy at this time.

Large molecule disorders involve a complex constellation of disorders of glycosylation, lysosomal storage diseases, and peroxisomal disorders. Those including severe epilepsy include Walker-Warburg syndrome, Fukuyama congenital muscular dystrophy, gangliosidoses such as Tay-Sachs and Sandhoff diseases, and the neuronal ceroid lipofuscinoses. While epilepsy represents significant gray matter involvement in neurological disease, seizures can be a prominent aspect of leukodystrophies such as Alexander's disease. The epileptologist should consider these hereditary disorders in the investigation of patients with epileptic encephalopathies, leading to specific diagnostic steps and, in some cases, potential therapeutic maneuvers to address the metabolic defect.

References

[1] S. Köker, S. W. Sauer, G. F. Hoffmann, I. Müller, M. A. Morath, and J. G. Okun, "Pathogenesis of CNS involvement in disorders of amino and organic acid metabolism," *Journal of Inherited Metabolic Disease*, vol. 31, no. 2, pp. 194–204, 2008.

[2] P. L. Pearl, *Inherited Metabolic Epilepsies*, Demos Medical, New York, NY, USA, 2013.

[3] R. Biancheri, R. Cerone, M. C. Schiaffino et al., "Cobalamin (Cbl) C/D deficiency: clinical, neurophysiological and neuroradiologic findings in 14 cases," *Neuropediatrics*, vol. 32, no. 1, pp. 14–22, 2001.

[4] W. Fenton, R. Gravel, and D. Rosenblatt, "Disorders of propionate and methylmalonate metabolism," in *The Metabolic & Molecular Basis of Inherited Disease*, C. Scriver, A. Beaudert, W. Sly et al., Eds., pp. 2165–2193, McGraw-Hill, New York, NY, USA, 2001.

[5] L. A. Azuar, J. M. P. Viñas, P. S. Crespo, J. A. P. Perera, and M. T. L. Echeverría, "Infantile spasms as the first manifestation of propionic acidemia," *Anales de Pediatria*, vol. 63, no. 6, pp. 548–550, 2005.

[6] E. Haberlandt, C. Canestrini, M. Brunner-Krainz et al., "Epilepsy in patients with propionic acidemia," *Neuropediatrics*, vol. 40, no. 3, pp. 120–125, 2009.

[7] D. I. Zafeiriou, P. Augoustides-Savvopoulou, D. Haas et al., "Ethylmalonic encephalopathy: Clinical and biochemical observations," *Neuropediatrics*, vol. 38, no. 2, pp. 78–82, 2007.

[8] B. Stigsby, S. M. Yarworth, Z. Rahbeeni et al., "Neurophysiologic correlates of organic acidemias: a survey of 107 patients," *Brain and Development*, vol. 16, pp. 125–144, 1994.

[9] J. Brismar and P. T. Ozand, "CT and MR of the brain in the diagnosis of organic acidemias. Experiences from 107 patients," *Neuropediatrics*, vol. 40, no. 3, pp. 120–125, 2009.

[10] P. T. Ozand, A. Al Aqeel, G. Gascon, J. Brismar, E. Thomas, and H. Gleispach, "3-Hydroxy-3-methylglutaryl-coenzyme A (HMG-CoA) lyase deficiency in Saudi Arabia," *Journal of Inherited Metabolic Disease*, vol. 14, no. 2, pp. 174–188, 1991.

[11] E. Neumaier-Probst, I. Harting, A. Seitz, C. Ding, and S. Kölker, "Neuroradiological findings in glutaria aciduria type I (glutaryl-CoA dehydrogenase deficiency)," *Journal of Inherited Metabolic Disease*, vol. 27, no. 6, pp. 869–876, 2004.

[12] K. A. Strauss, E. G. Puffenberger, D. L. Robinson, and D. H. Morton, "Type I glutaric aciduria, part 1: natural history of 77 patients," *American Journal of Medical Genetics C*, vol. 121, no. 1, pp. 38–52, 2003.

[13] S. Kolker, E. Christensen, J. Leonard et al., "Diagnosis and managament of glutaric aciduria type I-revised recommendations," *Journal of Inherited Metabolic Disease*, vol. 34, no. 3, pp. 677–694, 2011.

[14] V. M. McClelland, D. B. Bakalinova, C. Hendriksz, and R. P. Singh, "Glutaric aciduria type 1 presenting with epilepsy," *Developmental Medicine and Child Neurology*, vol. 51, no. 3, pp. 235–239, 2009.

[15] U. F. H. Engelke, B. Kremer, L. A. J. Kluijtmans et al., "NMR spectroscopic studies on the late onset form of 3-methylglutaconic aciduria type I and other defects in leucine metabolism," *NMR in Biomedicine*, vol. 19, no. 2, pp. 271–278, 2006.

[16] S. Illsinger, T. Lücke, J. Zschocke, K. M. Gibson, and A. M. Das, "3-Methylglutaconic aciduria type I in a boy with fever-associated seizures," *Pediatric Neurology*, vol. 30, no. 3, pp. 213–215, 2004.

[17] P. Arun, C. N. Madhavarao, J. R. Moffett et al., "Metabolic acetate therapy improves phenotype in the tremor rat model of Canavan disease," *Journal of Inherited Metabolic Disease*, vol. 33, no. 3, pp. 195–210, 2010.

[18] M. M. Canavan, "Schilder's encephalitis periaxialis diffusa," *Archives of Neurology and Psychiatry*, vol. 25, no. 2, pp. 299–308, 1931.

[19] R. Segel, Y. Anikster, S. Zevin et al., "A safety trial of high dose glyceryl triacetate for Canavan disease," *Molecular Genetics and Metabolism*, vol. 103, no. 3, pp. 203–206, 2011.

[20] E. Chen, W. L. Nyhan, C. Jakobs et al., "L-2-hydroxyglutaric aciduria: neuropathological correlations and first report of severe neurodegenerative disease and neonatal death," *Journal of Inherited Metabolic Disease*, vol. 19, no. 3, pp. 335–343, 1996.

[21] P. G. Barth, R. J. A. Wanders, H. R. Scholte et al., "L-2-hydroxyglutaric aciduria and lactic acidosis," *Journal of Inherited Metabolic Disease*, vol. 21, no. 3, pp. 251–254, 1998.

[22] J. Kerrigan, K. Aleck, T. J. T et al., "Fumaric aciduria: clinical and imaging features," *Annals of Neurology*, vol. 47, no. 5, pp. 583–588, 2000.

[23] D. T. Chuang and V. Shih, "Maple syrup urine disease (branched chain ketoaciduria)," in *The Metabolic and Molecular Basis of Inherited Disease*, C. Scriver, A. Beaudet, W. Sly et al., Eds., pp. 1971–2005, McGraw-Hill, New York, NY, USA, 2001.

[24] C. Sansaricq, S. Pardo, M. Balwani, M. Grace, and K. Raymond, "Biochemical and molecular diagnosis of lipoamide dehydrogenase deficiency in a North American Ashkenazi Jewish family," *Journal of Inherited Metabolic Disease*, vol. 29, no. 1, pp. 203–204, 2006.

[25] P. L. Pearl, C. Jakobs, and K. M. Gibson, "Disorders of beta- and gamma-amino acids in free and peptide-linked forms," in *Online Molecular and Metabolic Bases of Inherited Disease*, D. Valle, A. Beaudet, B. Vogelstein et al., Eds., 2007, http://www.ommbid.com/.

[26] I. Knerr, K. M. Gibson, G. Murdoch et al., "Neuropathology in succinic semialdehyde dehydrogenase deficiency," *Pediatric Neurology*, vol. 42, no. 4, pp. 255–258, 2010.

[27] P. L. Pearl, K. M. Gibson, M. A. Cortez et al., "Succinic semialdehyde dehydrogenase deficiency: lessons from mice and men," *Journal of Inherited Metabolic Disease*, vol. 32, no. 3, pp. 343–352, 2009.

[28] P. Rinaldo, D. Matern, and M. J. Bennett, "Fatty acid oxidation disorders," *Annual Review of Physiology*, vol. 64, pp. 477–502, 2002.

[29] I. Tein, "Role of carnitine and fatty acid oxidation and its defects in infantile epilepsy," *Journal of Child Neurology*, vol. 17, supplement 3, pp. S57–S82, 2002.

[30] U. Spiekerkoetter, J. Bastin, M. Gillingham, A. Morris, F. Wijburg, and B. Wilcken, "Current issues regarding treatment of mitochondrial fatty acid oxidation disorders," *Journal of Inherited Metabolic Disease*, vol. 33, no. 5, pp. 555–561, 2010.

[31] A. Morris and U. Spiekerkoetter, "Disorders of mitochondrial fatty acid oxidation and related metabolic pathways," in *Inborn Metabolic Diseases: Diagnosis and Treatment*, J. Saudubray, G. vanden Berghe, and J. Walter, Eds., pp. 201–214, Springer, Berlin, Germany, 2012.

[32] D. S. Khurana, L. Salganicoff, J. J. Melvin et al., "Epilepsy and respiratory chain defects in children with mitochondrial encephalopathies," *Neuropediatrics*, vol. 39, no. 1, pp. 8–13, 2008.

[33] B. H. Cohen, P. F. Chinnery, and W. C. Copeland, "POLG-related disorders," in *Genereviews*, R. A. Pagon, T. D. Bird, C. R. Dolan et al., Eds., pp. 1993–2010, University of Washington, Seattle, Wash, USA, 1993.

[34] N. I. Wolf, S. Rahman, B. Schmitt et al., "Status epilepticus in children with Alpers' disease caused by POLG1 mutations: EEG and MRI features," *Epilepsia*, vol. 50, no. 6, pp. 1596–1607, 2009.

[35] J. Finsterer, "Inherited mitochondrial neuropathies," *Journal of the Neurological Sciences*, vol. 304, no. 1-2, pp. 9–16, 2011.

[36] S. DiMauro and E. A. Schon, "Mitochondrial disorders in the nervous system," *Annual Review of Neuroscience*, vol. 31, pp. 91–123, 2008.

[37] D. R. Johns, J. Flier, D. Moller et al., "Mitochondrial DNA and disease," *The New England Journal of Medicine*, vol. 333, no. 10, pp. 638–644, 1995.

[38] L. Canafoglia, S. Franceschetti, C. Antozzi et al., "Epileptic phenotypes associated with mitochondrial disorders," *Neurology*, vol. 56, no. 10, pp. 1340–1346, 2001.

[39] S. DiMauro and D. C. De Vivo, "Genetic heterogeneity in Leigh syndrome," *Annals of Neurology*, vol. 40, no. 1, pp. 5–7, 1996.

[40] S. E. Sabbagh, A. S. Lebre, N. Bahi-Buisson et al., "Epileptic phenotypes in children with respiratory chain disorders," *Epilepsia*, vol. 51, no. 7, pp. 1225–1235, 2010.

[41] D. S. Rosenblatt and W. A. Fenton, "Inherited disorders of folate and cobalamin transport and metabolism," in *The Metabolic and Molecular Bases of Inherited Disease*, C. R. Scriver, A. L. Beaudet, W. S. Sly et al., Eds., p. 3897, McGraw-Hill, New York, NY, USA, 8th edition, 2001.

[42] M. Dougados, J. Zittoun, D. Laplane, and P. Castaigne, "Folate metabolism disorder in Kearns-Sayre syndrome," *Annals of Neurology*, vol. 13, no. 6, p. 687, 1983.

[43] M. Pineda, A. Ormazabal, E. López-Gallardo et al., "Cerebral folate deficiency and leukoencephalopathy caused by a mitochondrial DNA deletion," *Annals of Neurology*, vol. 59, no. 2, pp. 394–398, 2006.

[44] O. Hasselmann, N. Blau, V. T. Ramaekers, E. V. Quadros, J. M. Sequeira, and M. Weissert, "Cerebral folate deficiency and CNS inflammatory markers in Alpers disease," *Molecular Genetics and Metabolism*, vol. 99, no. 1, pp. 58–61, 2010.

[45] P. Moretti, T. Sahoo, K. Hyland et al., "Cerebral folate deficiency with developmental delay, autism, and response to folinic acid," *Neurology*, vol. 64, no. 6, pp. 1088–1090, 2005.

[46] J. Jaeken, "Disorders of serine and proline metabolism," in *Inborn Metabolic Diseases: Diagnosis and Treatment*, J. Saudubray, G. vanden Berghe, and J. Walter, Eds., pp. 360–361, Springer, Berlin, Germany, 2012.

[47] L. Tabatabaie, L. W. Klomp, R. Berger, and T. J. de Koning, "l-Serine synthesis in the central nervous system: a review on serine deficiency disorders," *Molecular Genetics and Metabolism*, vol. 99, no. 3, pp. 256–262, 2010.

[48] T. J. D. Koning, L. W. J. Klomp, A. C. C. V. Oppen et al., "Prenatal and early postnatal treatment in 3-phosphoglycerate-dehydrogenase deficiency," *The Lancet*, vol. 364, no. 9452, pp. 2221–2222, 2004.

[49] T. J. De Koning, J. Jaeken, M. Pineda, L. Van Maldergem, B. T. Poll-The, and M. S. Van der Knaap, "Hypomyelination and reversible white matter attenuation in 3-phosphoglycerate dehydrogenase deficiency," *Neuropediatrics*, vol. 31, no. 6, pp. 287–292, 2000.

[50] K. Shimomura, F. Hörster, H. de Wet et al., "A novel mutation causing DEND syndrome: a treatable channelopathy of pancreas and brain," *Neurology*, vol. 69, no. 13, pp. 1342–1349, 2007.

[51] A. L. Gloyn, E. R. Pearson, J. F. Antcliff et al., "Activating mutations in the gene encoding the ATP-sensitive potassium-channel subunit Kir6.2 and permanent neonatal diabetes," *The New England Journal of Medicine*, vol. 350, no. 18, pp. 1838–1849, 2004.

[52] P. Proks, A. L. Arnold, J. Bruining et al., "A heterozygous activating mutation in the sulphonylurea receptor SUR1 (ABCC8) causes neonatal diabetes," *Human Molecular Genetics*, vol. 15, no. 11, pp. 1793–1800, 2006.

[53] F. M. Ashcroft, "ATP-sensitive K$^+$ channels and disease: from molecule to malady," *American Journal of Physiology*, vol. 293, no. 4, pp. E880–E889, 2007.

[54] L. C. Gurgel, F. Crispim, M. H. S. Noffs, E. Belzunces, M. A. Rahal, and R. S. Moisés, "Sulfonylrea treatment in permanent neonatal diabetes due to G53D mutation in the KCNJ11 gene," *Diabetes Care*, vol. 30, no. 11, p. e108, 2007.

[55] W. Mlynarski, A. I. Tarasov, A. Gach et al., "Sulfonylurea improves CNS function in a case of intermediate DEND syndrome caused by a mutation in KCNJ11," *Nature Clinical Practice Neurology*, vol. 3, no. 11, pp. 640–645, 2007.

[56] M. A. Sperling and R. K. Menon, "Hyperinsulinemic hypoglycemia of infancy: recent insights into ATP-sensitive potassium channels, sulfonylurea receptors, molecular mechanisms, and treatment," *Endocrinology and Metabolism Clinics of North America*, vol. 28, no. 4, pp. 695–708, 1999.

[57] N. Bahi-Buisson, E. Roze, C. Dionisi et al., "Neurological aspects of hyperinsulinism-hyperammonaemia syndrome," *Developmental Medicine and Child Neurology*, vol. 50, no. 12, pp. 945–949, 2008.

[58] F. P. Errazquin, J. S. Fernández, G. G. Martín, M. I. C. Muñoz, and M. R. Acebal, "Hyperinsulinism and hyperammonaemia syndrome and severe myoclonic epilepsy of infancy," *Neurologia*, vol. 26, no. 4, pp. 248–252, 2011.

[59] N. Bahi-Buisson, S. El Sabbagh, C. Soufflet et al., "Myoclonic absence epilepsy with photosensitivity and a gain of function mutation in glutamate dehydrogenase," *Seizure*, vol. 17, no. 7, pp. 658–664, 2008.

[60] A. A. Palladino and C. A. Stanley, "The hyperinsulinism/hyperammonemia syndrome," *Reviews in Endocrine and Metabolic Disorders*, vol. 11, no. 3, pp. 171–178, 2010.

[61] K. Brockmann, "The expanding phenotype of GLUT1-deficiency syndrome," *Brain and Development*, vol. 31, no. 7, pp. 545–552, 2009.

[62] D. C. De Vivo, R. R. Trifiletti, R. I. Jacobson, G. M. Ronen, R. A. Behmand, and S. I. Harik, "Defective glucose transport across the blood-brain barrier as a cause of persistent hypoglycorrhachia, seizures, and developmental delay," *The New England Journal of Medicine*, vol. 325, no. 10, pp. 703–709, 1991.

[63] M. Rotstein, K. Engelstad, H. Yang et al., "Glut1 deficiency: inheritance pattern determined by haploinsufficiency," *Annals of Neurology*, vol. 68, no. 6, pp. 955–958, 2010.

[64] D. Wang, J. M. Pascual, and D. De Vivo, "Glucose transporter type 1 deficiency syndrome," in *GeneReviews*, R. A. Pagon, T. D. Bird, C. R. Dolar et al., Eds., pp. 1993–2002, University of Washington, Seattle, Wash, USA, 2009, Bookshelf ID: NBK1217.

[65] P. B. Mills, E. Struys, C. Jakobs et al., "Mutations in antiquitin in individuals with pyridoxine-dependent seizures," *Nature Medicine*, vol. 12, no. 3, pp. 307–309, 2006.

[66] G. J. Basura, S. P. Hagland, A. M. Wiltse, and S. M. Gospe, "Clinical features and the management of pyridoxine-dependent and pyridoxine-responsive seizures: review of 63 North American cases submitted to a patient registry," *European Journal of Pediatrics*, vol. 168, no. 6, pp. 697–704, 2009.

[67] R. C. Gallagher, J. L. K. Van Hove, G. Scharer et al., "Folinic acid-responsive seizures are identical to pyridoxine-dependent epilepsy," *Annals of Neurology*, vol. 65, no. 5, pp. 550–556, 2009.

[68] P. B. Mills, E. J. Footitt, K. A. Mills et al., "Genotypic and phenotypic spectrum of pyridoxine-dependent epilepsy (ALDH7A1 deficiency)," *Brain*, vol. 133, no. 7, pp. 2148–2159, 2010.

[69] P. L. Pearl and S. M. Gospe, "Pyridoxal phosphate dependency, a newly recognized treatable catastrophic epileptic encephalopathy," *Journal of Inherited Metabolic Disease*, vol. 30, no. 1, pp. 2–4, 2007.

[70] P. Baxter, "Recent insights into pre- and postnatal pyridoxal phosphate deficiency, a treatable metabolic encephalopathy," *Developmental Medicine and Child Neurology*, vol. 52, no. 7, pp. 597–598, 2010.

[71] P. B. Mills, R. A. H. Surtees, M. P. Champion et al., "Neonatal epileptic encephalopathy caused by mutations in the PNPO gene encoding pyridox(am)ine 5'-phosphate oxidase," *Human Molecular Genetics*, vol. 14, no. 8, pp. 1077–1086, 2005.

[72] M. L. Summar, D. Dobbelaere, S. Brusilow, and B. Lee, "Diagnosis, symptoms, frequency and mortality of 260 patients with urea cycle disorders from a 21-year, multicentre study of acute hyperammonaemic episodes," *Acta Paediatrica*, vol. 97, no. 10, pp. 1420–1425, 2008.

[73] M. L. Summar, "Urea cycle disorders overview," in *GeneReviews*, R. A. Pagon, T. D. Bird, C. R. Dolan et al., Eds., pp. 1993–2002, University of Washington, Seattle, Wash, USA, 2005, Bookshelf ID: NBK1217.

[74] M. J. C. C. Dealberto and F. F. A. Sarazin, "Valproate-induced hyperammonemic encephalopathy without cognitive sequelae: a case report in the psychiatric setting," *Journal of Neuropsychiatry and Clinical Neurosciences*, vol. 20, no. 3, pp. 369–371, 2008.

[75] J. M. van de Kamp, G. M. S. Mancini, P. J. W. Pouwels et al., "Clinical features and X-inactivation in females heterozygous for creatine transporter defect," *Clinical Genetics*, vol. 79, no. 3, pp. 264–272, 2011.

[76] F. Nasrallah, M. Feki, and N. Kaabachi, "Creatine and creatine deficiency syndromes: biochemical and clinical aspects," *Pediatric Neurology*, vol. 42, no. 3, pp. 163–171, 2010.

[77] C. Fons, A. Sempere, F. X. Sanmartí et al., "Epilepsy spectrum in cerebral creatine transporter deficiency: letters/commentary," *Epilepsia*, vol. 50, no. 9, pp. 2168–2170, 2009.

[78] V. Leuzzi, "Inborn errors of creatine metabolism and epilepsy: clinical features, diagnosis, and treatment," *Journal of Child Neurology*, vol. 17, supplement 3, pp. S89–S97, 2002.

[79] N. M. Verhoeven, G. S. Salomons, and C. Jakobs, "Laboratory diagnosis of defects of creatine biosynthesis and transport," *Clinica Chimica Acta*, vol. 361, no. 1-2, pp. 1–9, 2005.

[80] A. Hamosh and M. V. Johnston, "Nonketotic hyperglycinemia," in *The Metabolic and Molecular Bases of Inherited Disease*, C. R. Sciver, A. L. Beaudet, W. S. Sly et al., Eds., pp. 2065–2078, McGraw-Hill, New York, NY, USA, 8th edition, 2001.

[81] J. E. Hoover-Fong, S. Shah, J. L. K. van Hove, D. Applegarth, J. Toone, and A. Hamosh, "Natural history of nonketotic hyperglycinemia in 65 patients," *Neurology*, vol. 64, no. 10, pp. 1847–1853, 2004.

[82] S. Rossi, I. Daniele, P. Bastrenta, M. Mastrangelo, and G. Lista, "Early myoclonic encephalopathy and nonketotic hyperglycinemia," *Pediatric Neurology*, vol. 41, no. 5, pp. 371–374, 2009.

[83] E. Bonioli, "Combined deficiency of xanthine oxidase and sulphite oxidase due to a deficiency of molybdenum cofactor," *Journal of Inherited Metabolic Disease*, vol. 19, no. 5, pp. 700–701, 1996.

[84] J. L. Johnson and M. Duran, "Molybdenum cofactor deficiency and isolated sulfite oxidase deficiency," in *The Metabolic and Molecular Bases of Inherited Disease*, C. R. Sciver, A. L. Beaudet, W. S. Sly et al., Eds., pp. 2163–3177, McGraw-Hill, New York, NY, USA, 2001.

[85] A. H. Van Gennip, N. G. G. M. Abeling, A. E. M. Stroomer, H. Overmars, and H. D. Bakker, "The detection of molybdenum cofactor deficiency: clinical symptomatology and urinary metabolite profile," *Journal of Inherited Metabolic Disease*, vol. 17, no. 1, pp. 142–145, 1994.

[86] S. D. Sie, R. C. de Jonge, H. J. Blom et al., "Chronological changes of the amplitude-integrated EEG in a neonate with molybdenum cofactor deficiency," *Journal of Inherited Metabolic Disease*, 2010.

[87] K. Vijayakumar, R. Gunny, S. Grunewald et al., "Clinical neuroimaging features and outcome in molybdenum cofactor deficiency," *Pediatric Neurology*, vol. 45, pp. 246–252, 2011.

[88] A. N. Prasad, C. A. Rupar, and C. Prasad, "Methylenetetrahydrofolate reductase (MTHFR) deficiency and infantile epilepsy," *Brain and Development*, vol. 33, pp. 758–769, 2011.

[89] P. M. Ueland, P. I. Holm, and S. Hustad, "Betaine: a key modulator of one-carbon metabolism and homocysteine status," *Clinical Chemistry and Laboratory Medicine*, vol. 43, no. 10, pp. 1069–1075, 2005.

[90] F. Ciardo, C. Salerno, and P. Curatolo, "Neurologic aspects of adenylosuccinate lyase deficiency," *Journal of Child Neurology*, vol. 16, no. 5, pp. 301–308, 2001.

[91] T. Mizuno, "Long-term follow-up of ten patients with Lesch-Nyhan syndrome," *Neuropediatrics*, vol. 17, no. 3, pp. 158–161, 1986.

[92] J. K. Sass, H. H. Itabashi, and R. A. Dexter, "Juvenile gout with brain involvement," *Archives of Neurology*, vol. 13, no. 6, pp. 639–655, 1965.

[93] J. Vajsar and H. Schachter, "Walker-Warburg syndrome," *Orphanet Journal of Rare Diseases*, vol. 1, no. 1, article 29, 2006.

[94] M. Warburg, "Hydrocephaly, congenital retinal nonattachment, and congenital falciform fold," *American Journal of Ophthalmology*, vol. 85, no. 1, pp. 88–94, 1978.

[95] Y. Fukuyama, M. Osawa, and H. Suzuki, "Congenital progressive muscular dystrophy of the Fukuyama type—clinical, genetic and pathological considerations," *Brain and Development*, vol. 3, no. 1, pp. 1–29, 1981.

[96] E. Mercuri, H. Topaloglu, M. Brockington et al., "Spectrum of brain changes in patients with congenital muscular dystrophy and FKRP gene mutations," *Archives of Neurology*, vol. 63, no. 2, pp. 251–257, 2006.

[97] A. Jalanko and T. Braulke, "Neuronal ceroid lipofuscinoses," *Biochimica et Biophysica Acta*, vol. 1793, no. 4, pp. 697–709, 2009.

[98] S. E. Mole and R. E. Williams, "Neuronal ceroid-lipofuscinoses," in *GeneReviews*, R. A. Pagon, T. C. Bird, C. R. Dolan et al., Eds., pp. 1993–2001, University of Washington, Seattle, Wash, USA, 2005.

[99] P. Santavuori, S. L. Vanhanen, and T. Autti, "Clinical and neuroradiological diagnostic aspects of neuronal ceroid lipofuscinoses disorders," *European Journal of Paediatric Neurology A*, vol. 5, pp. 157–161, 2001.

[100] E. Sidransky, "Gaucher disease: complexity in a "simple" disorder," *Molecular Genetics and Metabolism*, vol. 83, no. 1-2, pp. 6–15, 2004.

[101] A. Tylki-Szymańska, A. Vellodi, A. El-Beshlawy, J. A. Cole, and E. Kolodny, "Neuronopathic Gaucher disease: demographic and clinical features of 131 patients enrolled in the International Collaborative Gaucher Group Neurological Outcomes Subregistry," *Journal of Inherited Metabolic Disease*, vol. 33, no. 4, pp. 339–346, 2010.

[102] G. H. B. Maegawa, T. Stockley, M. Tropak et al., "The natural history of juvenile or subacute GM2 gangliosidosis: 21 new cases and literature review of 134 previously reported," *Pediatrics*, vol. 118, no. 5, pp. e1550–e1562, 2006.

[103] P. Gressens, "Pathogenesis of migration disorders," *Current Opinion in Neurology*, vol. 19, no. 2, pp. 135–140, 2006.

[104] G. V. Raymond, "Peroxisomal disorders," *Current Opinion in Neurology*, vol. 14, no. 6, pp. 783–787, 2001.

[105] N. Shimozawa, "Molecular and clinical aspects of peroxisomal diseases," *Journal of Inherited Metabolic Disease*, vol. 30, no. 2, pp. 193–197, 2007.

[106] A. L. White, P. Modaff, F. Holland-Morris, and R. M. Pauli, "Natural history of rhizomelic chondrodysplasia punctata," *American Journal of Medical Genetics A*, vol. 118, no. 4, pp. 332–342, 2003.

[107] M. Prust, J. Wang, H. Morizono et al., "GFAP mutations, age at onset, and clinical subtypes in Alexander disease," *Neurology*, vol. 77, no. 13, pp. 1287–1294, 2011.

[108] L. Papetti, P. Parisi, V. Leuzzi et al., "Metabolic epilepsy: an update," *Brain and Development*, 2012.

The Peptide Network between Tetanus Toxin and Human Proteins Associated with Epilepsy

Guglielmo Lucchese,[1] **Jean Pierre Spinosa,**[2] **and Darja Kanduc**[3]

[1] *Brain and Language Laboratory, Cluster of Excellence "Languages of Emotions", Free University of Berlin, 14195 Berlin, Germany*
[2] *Faculty of Biology & Medicine, University of Lausanne, CH-1011 Lausanne, Switzerland*
[3] *Department of Biosciences, Biotechnologies and Biopharmaceutics, University of Bari, 70125 Bari, Italy*

Correspondence should be addressed to Darja Kanduc; darja.kanduc@uniba.it

Academic Editor: A. Vezzani

Sequence matching analyses show that *Clostridium tetani* neurotoxin shares numerous pentapeptides (68, including multiple occurrences) with 42 human proteins that, when altered, have been associated with epilepsy. Such a peptide sharing is higher than expected, nonstochastic, and involves tetanus toxin-derived epitopes that have been validated as immunopositive in the human host. Of note, an unexpected high level of peptide matching is found in mitogen-activated protein kinase 10 (MK10), a protein selectively expressed in hippocampal areas. On the whole, the data indicate a potential for cross-reactivity between the neurotoxin and specific epilepsy-associated proteins and may help evaluate the potential risk for epilepsy following immune responses induced by tetanus infection. Moreover, this study may contribute to clarifying the etiopathogenesis of the different types of epilepsy.

1. Introduction

The term epilepsy defines a group of disturbances whose only recognized commonality is the paroxysmal synchronous discharging of groups of neurons. Localization and physiological function of the neuronal populations involved determine the clinical picture, so that (1) clinical manifestations can be extremely subtle and the diagnosis can be challenging also in terms of differential definition; (2) epilepsy(ies) can produce extremely multiform clinical pictures with a large degree of overlap [1–3]. Indeed, epileptic syndromes can also be embedded in larger syndromic clinical pictures, that is, West and Lennox-Gastaut syndromes in tuberous sclerosis complex [4, 5]. This clinical diversity has noteworthy nosological implications. Syndromic or disease status of various forms of epilepsy and the terminology used to define them are indeed still matter of debate [7–9]. Likewise, the molecular etiopathogenesis of epilepsies has to be better defined at the molecular level. Although genetic alterations [10–12], inflammation [13], and viral infections [14–16] have been considered and thoroughly studied, nonetheless,

the molecular basis and the causal mechanisms of epilepsies are still unclear.

Recently, research on epilepsy has also outlined a neurodevelopmental context [17–21]. Spontaneous recurrent seizures have been observed after induction of *status epilepticus* during the second and third postnatal weeks in rodents, by use of chemoconvulsants such as pilocarpine, kainate, and tetanus toxin (TT) [22]. TT seizures as well as experimental febrile seizures and developmental lithium pilocarpine appear to share a common mechanism for enhancing hippocampal network excitability and promoting epilepsy, possibly through alterations in neurotransmitter receptors or voltage-gated ion channels ([23] and further references therein).

Moreover, numerous reports suggest that immune mechanisms might play a role in processes leading to epileptogenesis [15, 24–32]. In fact, antibodies against neural antigens involved in neurotransmission have been detected in epileptic subjects [33–39], and, remarkably, epilepsy was shown to respond to immunotherapeutic approaches [38, 40, 41]. Finally, population-based cohort studies have documented that microbial infections during pregnancy may be a risk factor for epilepsy in offspring [42–45].

In such a multifaceted scientific-clinical context, here we analyze the peptide commonality between TT, a powerful neurotoxin used in animal models of experimental epilepsy [46–50], and human antigens that have been related to epilepsy, searching for possible immunological link(s) that might contribute to epileptogenesis. Indeed, a massive peptide overlap characterizes microbial and human proteomes [51–54] and gives grounds for questioning whether immune response(s) to microbial infections might potentially result in cross-reactions against neuronal antigens [55–58]. Pathogen versus human immune cross-reactivity might contribute to explaining the association between microbial infections and neurological syndromes [59] and assumes a special significance during pregnancy in light of the consequent possible neurodevelopmental alterations in the fetus and offspring [26, 58].

We report that the tetanus neurotoxin and human epilepsy antigens share an ample pentapeptide platform. The bacterial versus human peptide overlap is not random and, importantly, a search through the Immune Epitope Database (IEDB; http://www.immuneepitope.org/) reveals that the shared pentapeptides are part of TT-derived epitopes. The latter datum is relevant also in light of the role of pentapeptides as minimal functional units in cell biology and immunology [60, 61]. On the whole, the results support the possibility that immune cross-reactions may occur between TT and epilepsy-related proteins.

2. Methods

TT protein sequence, UniProtKB/Swiss-Prot accession number: P04958, 1315aa long, from *Clostridium tetani* (NCBI Taxonomic identifier: 212717; further details at http://www.ncbi.nlm.nih.gov/Taxonomy/Browser/wwwtax.cgi) was analyzed for pentapeptide sharing with epilepsy-associated proteins as follows. First, a pentapeptide library was constructed by dissecting the TT primary sequence into pentapeptides offset by one residue, that is, MPITI, PITIN, ITINN, TINNF, INNFR, and so forth. Then, each of the final 1311 pentamers was analyzed for instances of the same match within a library consisting of primary sequences of human proteins that, when altered, have been associated with epilepsy. The number of matches and the human proteins sharing matches were recorded.

Epilepsy-associated proteins were randomly retrieved from UniProtKB Database (http://www.uniprot.org/). An unbiased set of proteins that on whatever basis (i.e., differential regulation, protein modification, or mutation) had been involved in or related to epilepsy was obtained utilizing "epilepsy" and "Homo sapiens" as keywords. Only canonical protein sequences were considered. At the time of this study, the keyword-guided search produced a library of 133 human UniProt entries, for a total of 106,022aa. Epilepsy-associated proteins are reported as UniProtKB/Swiss-Prot entry names throughout the paper, unless when discussed in detail. Any pentapeptide occurrence in the set of epilepsy-associated proteins was termed a match.

A set of proteins associated with Down syndrome, a genetic disease in which infectious agents have no role, was retrieved from UniProtKB Database and used as a comparison sample. This set was formed by the following proteins listed according to the aa length, with UniProtKB/Swiss-Prot entries in parentheses: (1) Down syndrome critical region protein 10 (P59022, DSC10), 87aa; (2) Down syndrome critical region protein 8 (Q96T75, DSCR8), 97aa; (3) Down syndrome critical region protein 4 (P56555, DSCR4), 118aa; (4) Down syndrome critical region protein 9 (P59020, DSCR9), 149aa; (5) Down syndrome critical region protein 5 or phosphatidylinositol N-acetylglucosaminyltransferase subunit P (P57054, PIGP), 158aa; (6) Down syndrome critical region protein 6 or protein ripply3 (P57055, DSCR6), 190aa; (7) Down syndrome candidate region 1-like 1 or regulator of calcineurin 2 (Q14206, RCAN2), 197aa; (8) Down syndrome candidate region 1-like protein 2 or regulator of calcineurin 3 (Q9UKA8, RCAN3), 241aa; (9) Down syndrome critical region protein 1 or regulator of calcineurin 1 (P53805, RCAN1), 252aa; (10) Down syndrome critical region protein 2 or proteasome assembly chaperone 1 (O95456, PSMG1), 288aa; and (11) Down syndrome critical region protein 3 (O14972, DSCR3), 297aa.

The Immune Epitope Database (IEDB; http://www.immuneepitope.org/) was used to search for TT-derived B- and/or T-cell epitopes that had been experimentally validated as positive in the human host.

Expected occurrences for pentapeptide sharing between *C. tetani* neurotoxin and human proteins associated with epilepsy were calculated as follows. First, we considered the number of all possible pentapeptides, N. Since each residue can be any of 20aa, the number of all possible pentapeptides N is given by $N = 20^5 = 3.2 \times 10^5$. Next, we considered the TT and epilepsy-associated proteins as two sets of pentapeptide size m and n. That is, m is the number of pentapeptides present in the TT protein and n is the number of pentapeptides present in the epilepsy-associated protein set. If X is the number of times a pentapeptide is selected in the TT protein of size m and Y is the number of times the same pentapeptide is selected in the epilepsy-associated protein set, then $X = m/N$ and $Y = n/N$. Assuming that X and Y are independent, $XY = mn/N^2$. In other words, the expected number of times that one pentapeptide will be selected simultaneously in both TT and epilepsy-related protein set is given by mn/N^2. Neglecting the relative abundance of aa and assuming $m \ll N$ and $n \ll N$, we obtain a formula derived by approximation where the total number of occurrences in a second sample n (the epilepsy-related protein set) of pentapeptides occurring in the first sample m (TT) is given by $mn/N + m/2$.

3. Results and Discussion

3.1. Description of the Pentapeptide Sharing between TT and Epilepsy-Associated Proteins. Peptide sharing between TT and human epilepsy-associated proteins was analyzed using (1) the pentapeptide module as a matching probe and (2) a library consisting of 133 epilepsy-related protein sequences retrieved from UniProt (see under Methods).

We used pentapeptides as scanning probes in sequence similarity analyses since a grouping of five aa residues may represent a minimal unit of immune recognition in cellular and humoral responses. Indeed, scientific literature indicates that an optimal peptide length for T-cell epitopes ranges between 9 and 15 residues, with the central 5–7 aa representing the specific immune recognition contacts and the flanking residues determining the binding potential to the MHC molecules [62–66]. *De facto*, the HFMPT pentapeptide was reported to be a minimal antigenic determinant for MHC class I-restricted T lymphocytes [65], while the KYVKQ pentapeptide was demonstrated to be a minimal antigenic determinant for CD4(+) T-cell clones [66]; in addition, the IEDB describes numerous pentapeptide epitopes capable of binding MHC molecules (e.g., epitope IEDB IDs: 5740, 7948, 11514, 25472, and 33701) and inducing T-cell proliferation (e.g., epitope IEDB IDs: 815, 40168, 47974, 59947, 107725, 107725, and 110376) (reviewed in [61]). Likewise, humoral immune recognition/reactivity unfolds around short aa motifs ([67–70]; reviewed in [71]). A representative example is a report by Zeng and colleagues [70], according to which the C-terminal pentapeptide (aa sequence: GLRPG) of luteinizing hormone-releasing hormone is a dominant B-cell epitope able to elicit a strong anti-LHRH antibody response and to discriminate between anti-LHRH antibodies present in fertile and nonfertile mice. That is, the pentapeptide GLRPG has immunogenic and antigenic properties and also discriminates antibody specificities associated with reproductive competence.

The analyzed set of 133 human proteins related to epilepsy is listed in Box 1 according to the aa size (i.e., from IR3IP or immediate early response 3-interacting protein 1, 82aa, to GPR98 or monogenic audiogenic seizure susceptibility protein 1 homolog, 6306aa).

Following matching analyses, we found that 42 out of the 133 epilepsy-associated proteins retrieved at random from UniProt database share 58 pentapeptides (68 including multiple occurrences) with the bacterial toxin. Box 2 lists the epilepsy-related proteins that share pentapeptides with TT and the shared pentapeptides. No TT pentapeptide match was found in the comparison set of proteins associated with Down syndrome.

3.2. Nonstochasticity of the Pentapeptide Sharing between TT and Epilepsy-Associated Proteins. The comparative analysis of Boxes 1 and 2 highlights three main points. Firstly, the 68 TT pentapeptide overlap described in Box 2 exceeds the expected value. As detailed under Methods, the expected number of TT pentapeptides that may occur in the epilepsy-related protein set is given by $mn/N + m/2$, where m is the number of pentapeptides contained in TT (1,311), n is the number of pentapeptides contained in the epilepsy-related protein set (105,490), and N is the number of all possible pentapeptides (20^5). Developing the equation gives 43 as expected number of pentapeptide matches, whereas the observed value is 68 (see Box 2). That is, the pentapeptide overlap between TT and epilepsy-related proteins is 1.58 times higher when compared to the expected one.

A second point of note is that the distribution of the pentapeptide overlap through the epilepsy-related proteins is unexpected. According to equation described above, pentapeptide sharing between two samples is as a quantity directly proportional to the number of pentapeptides in the analyzed samples; that is, it is proportional to the protein aa size. Actually, 91 epilepsy-related proteins are excluded from the pentapeptide matching with TT, independently of their length. For example, SPTN1, 2472aa (see Box 1), has no bacterial matches, while LRRC1, 524aa, shares 3 pentapeptides with TT (Box 2).

In summary, a comparative analysis of Boxes 1 and 2 highlights that 68 TT pentapeptide matches are allocated in 42 out 133 human proteins that have been related, when altered, to epilepsy, and no relationship appears to exist between pentapeptide sharing and the human protein size. Applying the equation described above to the set of 42 epilepsy-related proteins sharing 68 pentapeptides with TT and amounting to 50,254aa, the expected pentapeptide overlap is equal to 20, so that the observed occurrence value is 3, 4 times higher.

Finally, a third *punctum saliens* is that nonrandomness characterizes also the distribution of the TT pentapeptides among the 42 epilepsy-associated proteins. Box 2 shows that a few TT pentapeptides are repeated in the 42 epilepsy-associated protein set. Indeed, TT pentapeptides EIIPS, SLSIG, and FCKAL recur twice, and TT pentapeptides FGGQD, KEIEK, and TFLRD occur three times (Box 2; see pentapeptides underlined). Box 2 also shows that MK10 (mitogen-activated protein kinase 10; 464aa); CDKL5 (cyclin-dependent kinase-like 5; 1030aa); and KCMA1 (calcium-activated potassium channel subunit alpha-1; 1236aa) share two sequentially overlapping pentapeptides with TT, that is, share the hexapeptides SVDDAL, KNSFSE, and PKEIEK, respectively. The nonrandom TT pentapeptide sharing clearly emerges from Figure 1, where expected and observed occurrence values are graphically compared.

It can be seen that, in conflict with the theoretical trend of the TT pentapeptide matching as a function of epilepsy-related protein length (Figure 1, columns in gray), the observed to expected ratio of pentapeptide matching shows no relationship with the human protein length (Figure 1, columns in black). For example, contrary to mathematical expectations, MK10 (464aa long) has three pentapeptide matches, whereas VP13A (3174aa long) has one match (see Box 2 and Figure 1).

3.3. Immunologic Potential of the Pentapeptide Sharing between TT and Epilepsy-Associated Proteins. Having defined the TT versus epilepsy-associated proteins pentapeptide overlap, it was next tested whether such a sharing has an immunologic potential. To this aim we used IEDB, a database that describes B- and T-cell epitopes for humans, nonhuman primates, rodents, and other animal species, and searched for TT derived epitopes that had been validated as immunopositive in humans. At the time of the search, we obtained a list of 517 TT-derived epitopes. The pentapeptides common to epilepsy-associated proteins and TT (see Box 2, sequences in italic) were used as probes to scan the 517 TT-derived epitope set in order to define potential cross-reactive peptide sequences. Results are reported in Table 1.

IR3IP (82); CYTB (98); MPC1 (109); OPAL1 (141); ARF6 (175); DYR (187); CP013 (204); GOSR2 (212); RB39B (213); SCN1B (218); THEM4 (240); FOLR1 (257); PNPO (261); CLN8 (286); ROGDI (287); KCTD7 (289); SEN34 (310); CLN6 (311); PPR3C (317); PRS41 (318); GHC1 (323); EPM2A (331); PRRT2 (340); EP2A2 (344); RENR (350); MPRB (354); CLN5 (358); PHF6 (365); LIAS (372); IRK10 (379); CYB (380); AMACR (382); IRK11 (390); NHLC1 (395); ASAH1 (395); SNIP1 (396); ARC (396); NAGAB (411); BCKD (412); SIAT9 (418); STRAA (431); CBPA6 (437); DCX (441); PH4H (452); IDHP (452); GBRD (452); GBRA1 (456); NDUV1 (464); MK10 (464); SRPX2 (465); SEN2 (465); GBRG2 (467); MEF2C (473); GBRB3 (473); SCRB2 (478); AKT1 (480); PUR8 (484); GTR1 (492); KCNA1 (495); KCNV1 (500); ACHB2 (502); ARHG9 (516); JERKY (520); CACB4 (520); D2HDH (521); LRRC1 (524); SEN54 (526); ACHA2 (529); LGI4 (537); AL7A1 (539); LGI2 (545); LGI3 (548); LGI1 (557); TBC24 (559); ARX (562); TPP1 (563); GGT3 (568); PUR9 (592); STXB1 (594); DCE1 (594); EPMIP (607); LBR (615); ACHA4 (627); EFHC1 (640); SL9A9 (645); ITF2 (667); TSEAR (669); SL9A6 (669); SYN1 (705); EFHC2 (749); TRM44 (757); AFG32 (797); BRAT1 (821); PRIC1 (831); PRIC2 (844); KCNQ3 (872); KCNQ2 (872); SOBP (873); MANBA (879); CLCN2 (898); PWP2 (919); GABR1 (961); MIB1 (1006); CDKL5 (1030); AT2A2 (1042); DLGP2 (1054); CASR (1078); AP4E1 (1137); PCD19 (1148); TSC1 (1164); ATN1 (1190); ZEB2 (1214); PLCB1 (1216); KCMA1 (1236); DPOG1 (1239); TPC10 (1259); CNTP2 (1331); ARHGA (1369); NMDE1 (1464); WDR62 (1518); ABCC8 (1581); GCP6 (1819); SCN8A (1980); SCN9A (1988); SCN2A (2005); SCN1A (2009); CAC1E (2313); CAC1H (2353); SPTN1 (2472); VP13A (3174); RELN (3460); CSMD3 (3707); GPR98 (6306)

Box 1: List of the 133 epilepsy-associated proteins analyzed for TT pentapeptide sharing. Proteins were randomly retrieved from UniProtKB (http://www.uniprot.org/) as described under Methods. Proteins are indicated by UniProtKB/Swiss-Prot entry names, and listed according to increasing aa length reported in parentheses.

ROGDI (*LKDKI*); CLN6 (*PALLL*); CLN5 (*VIVHK*); NHLC1 (*TITND*); ASAH1 (*PVLNK*); CBPA6 (*GIPYA*); GBRA1 (*VSFWL*); MK10 (*SVDDAL**, *GAQGI*); GTR1 (*SYLSI*); ARHG9 (*KLEEK*); D2HDH (*GSGLV*); LRRC1 (*NKNEV, SLTDL, FCKAL*); ACHA2 (*NITSL, EIIPS*); LGI2 (*KAKWL*); LGI1 (*GFTEI*); EPMIP (*SGLVS*); ACHA4 (*EIIPS*); EFHC1 (*RVPKV*); SL9A9 (*IMYGF*); TSEAR (*QGYEG*); SL9A6 (*SIMYG, SPTTL*); EFHC2 (*GDFIK*); AFG32 (*DPALL*); CLCN2 (*TFRDL*); PWP2 (*GQYIV, HSLSI*); GABR1 (*EDIDV*); CDKL5 (*KNSFSE**, *SLSIG*); TSC1 (*LKKLE*); KCMA1 (*FCKAL, PKEIEK**); CNTP2 (*DFIKL*); ARHGA (*KLVKA*); NMDE1 (*PALNI*); WDR62 (*LIHVL, KRSYQ, TNGKL*); GCP6 (*SLSIG, KEIEK*); SCN8A (*FGGQD, DTQSK, LRVPK, TFLRD*); SCN9A (*NDMFN*); SCN2A (*FGGQD, TFLRD*); SCN1A (*FGGQD, TFLRD*); VP13A (*ITMTN*); RELN (*SIGSG*); CSMD3 (*EGFNI, KEIEK*); GPR98 (*LISID, ESKDL, VDGSG, TLPND, SGFNS, LSSAN, VQLKN*)

Box 2: Peptide sharing between TT and epilepsy-associated proteins. Proteins reported by UniProtKB/Swiss-Prot entry names and listed according to the aa length. Pentapeptides shared with TT are italic in parentheses. Pentapeptides present more than once in the epilepsy antigen set are underlined. Sharing of two consecutively overlapped pentapeptides (i.e., a hexapeptide) is indicated by an asterisk.

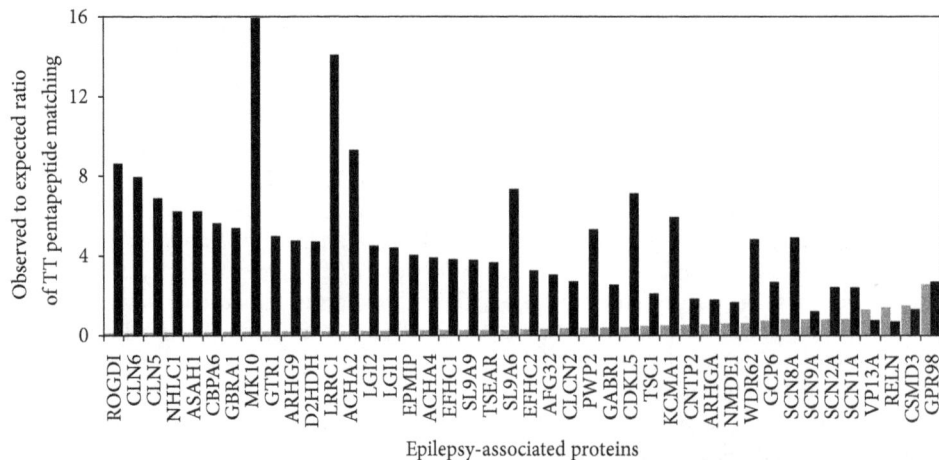

FIGURE 1: Observed versus expected pentapeptide matching between TT and epilepsy-related proteins. The 42 proteins sharing pentapeptides with TT are allocated along the x-axis according to increasing aa length. Gray columns: expected matches calculated according to the formula $mn/N + m/2$, where m is the number of pentapeptides present in the neurotoxin (1,311) and n is the number of pentapeptides present in the epilepsy-associated protein (see Methods). For example, in the case of IR3IP protein, 82aa, the possible pentapeptide overlap is equal to $1{,}311 \times 78/3{,}200{,}000 + 1{,}311/2$. Black columns: observed to expected ratio of the pentapeptide matching. Observed matching values from Box 2.

In essence, Table 1 shows that all of the 58 pentapeptides common to the 42 epilepsy-associated proteins and TT (Box 2, peptide sequences in parentheses and in italic) are present in 116 TT-derived epitopes that had been established to be immunopositive in humans. This datum indicates a potential vulnerability of the 42 epilepsy-associated proteins to cross-reactions following anti-TT immune responses. Moreover, many TT-derived epitopes share fragments with distinct epilepsy-related proteins and are of particular significance to a multiple cross-reactivity risk, since, for example, an immune response targeting the TT epitope fnnftVS-FWLRVPKVsahle (see Table 1, IEDB ID 17207, with shared fragments in capital letter) has the potential to cross-react with the following three crucial proteins related to different forms of epilepsy:

(i) GBRA1 or gamma-aminobutyric acid receptor subunit alpha-1, the major inhibitory neurotransmitter in the vertebrate brain that mediates neuronal inhibition by binding to the GABA/benzodiazepine receptor and opening an integral chloride channel [72],

(ii) SCN8A or voltage-gated sodium channel subunit alpha Nav1.6, a protein that mediates the voltage-dependent sodium ion permeability of excitable membranes [73],

(iii) EFHC1 or myoclonin-1, a protein that may enhance calcium influx through CACNA1E and stimulate programmed cell death [74].

Such a multiple cross-reactivity potential is shown also by other TT-derived epitopes, eg, epitopes IEDB IDs 30436, 48049, 113407, and so forth.

Also, it seems important to highlight that MK10 (mitogen-activated protein kinase 10, also known as stress-activated protein kinase JNK3 or p493F12 kinase), a protein that shows the highest unexpected level of pentapeptide overlap to TT (Figure 1) and also has a high immunologic potential as illustrated in Table 1 (i.e., MK10 pentapeptide(s) are present in 7 TT-derived epitopes), is selectively expressed in a subpopulation of pyramidal neurons in the CA1, CA4, and subiculum regions of the hippocampus, and layers 3 and 5 of the neocortex [75]. That is, there is a potential cross-reactivity risk specifically allocated in brain areas directly linked to epileptogenesis [76, 77].

4. Conclusions

This study describes a vast pentapeptide commonality between TT-derived epitopes and epilepsy-associated proteins. This peptide sharing acquires a relevant pathologic potential in light of the fact that pentapeptide modules have the capacity of inducing immune response(s) and are main players in immune recognition [61–71]. Immunologically, two sequences that share a pentapeptide are potentially subject to a cross-reaction [60].

In the disease model examined here, that is, tetanus infection and epilepsy, the ample cross-reactivity platform between TT-derived epitopes and human epilepsy-associated antigens supports the hypothesis of an immune involvement

in epilepsy. As a matter of fact, all the 42 epilepsy-related proteins listed in Box 2 are potential targets of cross-reactions (see Table 1). Qualitatively, the peptide overlap occurs in human proteins canonically associated with epilepsy such as gamma-aminobutyric acid receptor subunit alpha-1 (GBRA1), gamma-aminobutyric acid type B receptor subunit 1 (GABR1), sodium channel protein subunits (SCN1A, SCN2A. SCN8A, and SCN9A), and calcium-activated potassium channel subunit alpha-1 (KCMA1) (Table 1). Obviously, an immune attack against such epilepsy-associated proteins may cause alterations to neural structures and functions, especially when the neurodevelopmental intrauterine phase is considered. Being of nonsecondary importance, the non-stochastic character of the peptide overlap between TT and epilepsy-associated proteins (Figure 1) indicates that the potential cross-reactivity extent (and the associated risk of developing epilepsy and neurodevelopmental disorders) will increase with the number of anti-TT immune stimulations.

An additional relevant point is the "antigenic patchwork" shown in Table 1. Indeed, the potential peptide crossreactome involved in different extent and in different combinations of 42 epilepsy-associated proteins might help understand the complex neurobiological network that, once hit and perturbed, may underlie different epileptic forms [1–9]. Also, it has to be noted that Table 1 includes proteins such as CNTP2 or contactin-associated protein-like 2, RELN or reelin, and TSC1 or tuberous sclerosis 1 protein, which are also landmark antigens for autism and the associated impairment in communication/language skills and behaviors [78–81]. Hence, Table 1 may provide a mechanistic framework to allocate the occurrence of epilepsy, intellectual disability, and autism spectrum disorder in patients with tuberous sclerosis complex. Likewise, data from Table 1 might contribute to answering a critical question in neuropsychopathology, that is, the coexistence of patients with combined schizophrenia and epilepsy [82–85]. Indeed, Table 1 substantiates the hypothesis according to which the thread joining epilepsy and schizophrenia may reside in neurodevelopmental molecules such as leucine-rich glioma inactivated (LGI) proteins and GPR98, a G protein-coupled receptor, originally known as VLGR1 or very large G protein-coupled receptor [86]. De facto, Table 1 shows that fragments from LGI1, LGI2, and GPR98 are present in 1, 7, and 18 TT-derived epitopes, respectively. In other words, the potential cross-reactivity targeting LGI1, LGI2, and GPR98 following an anti-TT response is high.

Given the caveat that peptide immunoreactivity is influenced by numerous factors, for example, binding affinity [87], cripticity (i.e., determinants embedded in membrane structures do not induce immune responses under physiological conditions) [88], and posttranslational modifications (i.e., citrullination) [89], the present data might contribute to further our understanding of epilepsies. In particular, data from Table 1 might represent a peptide platform to be tested in antibody binding assays using sera from epileptic subjects. Accompanied by parallel immunoassays based on the utilization of epilepsy-related proteins as antigens, such an approach might not only validate the TT-epilepsy link proposed in this study, but also lead to a definition at

TABLE 1: Pentapeptide sharing between TT-derived epitopes and human epilepsy-associated proteins.

IEDB ID[1]	TT-derived epitope[2,3]	Immune context	Epilepsy-associated proteins[4]
1270	afcpeyvptfdnvieNITSL	HLA-Class II, allele undetermined	ACHA2
1389	afrnVDGSGLVSklig	HLA-Class II, allele undetermined	GPR98 D2HDH EPMIP
1501	agevrqiTFRDLpdkfnayl	HLA-Class II, allele undetermined	CLCN2
1929	aihlvnnesseVIVHKamdi	HLA-DRB1*04:01	CLN5
2219	akkqllefDTQSKnilmqyi	HLA-Class II, allele undetermined	SCN8A
3156	amltnliifgpgPVLNKNEV	HLA-Class II, allele undetermined	ASAH1 LRRC1
3418	anskfigiteLKKLEskink	HLA-DRB1*11:01	TSC1
3832	apsyTNGKLniyyrrlyngl	HLA-DRB5*01:01, HLA-DRB1*13:01	WDR62
7603	danLISIDikndlyektl	HLA-DRB1*03:01	GPR98
8734	dinndiisdiSGFNSsvity	HLA-DRB1*01:01	GPR98
8778	diSGFNSsvitypdaqlvpg	HLA-DRB1*15:01	GPR98
/8903	dkisdvstivpyigPALNIv	HLA-DPB1*04:01, HLA-DRB1*15:01	NMDE1
9297	dltfiaeKNSFSEepfqdei	HLA-DRB1*01:01, HLA-DRB1*04:01	CDKL5
9595	DPALLLmheLIHVLhglyg	B-cell HLA-DR2; HLA-Class II, allele undetermined	AFG32 CLN6 WDR62
9595	drLSSANlyingvlmgsaei	B-cell HLA-DR2; HLA-Class II, allele undetermined	GPR98
10472	DTQSKnilqyikanskfigiteLKKLEski	HLA-Class II, allele undetermined	SCN8A TSC1
11980	efDTQSKnilmqyikanskfigitel	B-cell	SCN8A
13095	eLIHVLhglygmqvss	B-cell HLA-DR2; HLA-Class I, allele undetermined	WDR62
13125	eLKKLEskinkvfstpipfs	HLA-Class II, allele undetermined	TSC1
13813	eqdpsgattksamltnliifgpgPVLNKNEV	HLA-Class II, allele undetermined	ASAH1 LRRC1
15087	eysiessmkkHSLSIGSGwsvsl	B-cell	PWP2 GCP6 CDKL5 RELN
15411	fdkdsnGQYIVnedkfqily	HLA-Class II, allele undetermined	PWP2
16155	fiaeKNSFSEepfqdeivsyntk	B-cell	CDKL5
17134	fnaylankwvfiTITNDrls	HLA-Class II, allele undetermined	NHLC1
17205	fnnftVSFWLRVPK	HLA-Class II, allele undetermined	GBRA1 SCN8A
17206	fnnftVSFWLRVPKVsahle	HLA-DR3	GBRA1 SCN8A EFHC1
17207	fnnftVSFWLRVPKVsashle	HLA-DRB1*11:01, HLA-DR, HLA-DR1, HLA-DR5, HLA-DR7, HLA-DR11, HLA-DPw4, HLA-Class II, allele undetermined	GBRA1 SCN8A EFHC1
17208	fnnftVSFWLRVPKVsashleqy	HLA-DRB1*01:01, HLA-DRB1*04:01, HLA-HLA-DRB1*07:01, HLA-DRB1*11:01	GBRA1 SCN8A EFHC1
17487	fqilynSIMYGFTEIelgkk	HLA-Class II, allele undetermined	SL9A6 SL9A9 LGI1
18217	fvksGDFIKLyvsynnnehivgy	B-cell	EFHC2 CNTP2
18356	fwLRVPKVsashleqygtne	HLA-DRB1*11:01	SCN8A EFHC1
19469	gevrqiTFRDLpdkfnaylankw	B-cell	CLCN2
21599	gpdkeqiadeinnlknKLEEKan	B-cell	ARHG9
22769	gtneysiissmkkHSLSIGS	DQB1*06:02, DRB5*01:01	PWP2 GCP6 CDKL5
24238	hLKDKIlgcdwyfvptdegwtnd	HLA-Class II, allele undetermined	ROGDI
25597	idkisdvstivpyigPALNI	HLA-Class II, allele undetermined	NMDE1
25666	idsfvksGDFIKLyvsynnn	HLA-DRB1*15:01	EFHC2 CNTP2
26808	ikiknedltfiaeKNSFSEe	HLA-Class II, allele undetermined	CDKL5
27639	ingkaihlvnnesseVIVHK	HLA-Class II, allele undetermined	CLN5

TABLE 1: Continued.

IEDB ID[1]	TT-derived epitope[2,3]	Immune context	Epilepsy-associated proteins[4]
29241	ivdynlqskiTLPNDrttpv	HLA-Class II, allele undetermined	GPR98
29331	ivkQGYEGnfig	HLA-Class II, allele undetermined	TSEAR
29407	ivpyigPALNIv	HLA-Class II, allele undetermined	NMDE1
29408	ivpyigPALNIvkQGYEGnf	HLA-DRB1*15:01	NMDE1 TSEAR
29843	KAKWLgtvntqfqKRSYQ	HLA-Class II, allele undetermined	LGI2 WDR62
29891	kamdieyNDMFNnftVSFWLrvp	B-cell	SCN9A GBRA1
30269	kdVQLKNitdymyltnapsy	HLA-DRB1*01:01, HLA-DRB1*04:01	GPR98
30436	KEIEKlytSYLSITFLRDpwgnp	B-cell	CSMD3 KCMA1 GCP6 GTR1 SCN1A SCN2A SCN8A CLCN2
30572	keqiadeinnlknKLEEKan	HLA-Class II, allele undetermined	ARHG9
32521	knitdymyltnapsyTNGKL	HLA-Class II, allele undetermined	WDR62
32546	knldcwvdneEDIDVilkkstil	B-cell	GABR1
33527	kstilnldinndiisdiSGFNSs	B-cell	GPR98
34301	kwievyKLVKAKWLgtvntq	HLA-DRB1*01:01	ARHGA LGI2
34887	lankwvfiTITNDrLSSANlyin	B-cell	NHLC1 GPR98
35058	lcikiknedltfiaeKNSFS	HLA-DRB1*04:01	CDKL5
35566	lekryekwievyKLVKAKWL	HLA-Class II, allele undetermined	ARHGA LGI2
35993	lftFGGQDanLISIDikndl	HLA-Class II, allele undetermined	SCN1A SCN2A SCN8A GPR98
36667	lipvassskdVQLKNitdym	HLA-DRB1*11:01	GPR98
38977	lqrITMTNSVDDALinstki	HLA-Class II, allele undetermined	VP13A MK10
40770	lygmqvsshEIIPSkqeiym	HLA-Class II, allele undetermined	ACHA2 ACHA4
41527	mfnnftVSFWLRVPKVsash	HLA-DRB1*11:01	GBRA1 SCN8A EFHC1
42847	mtnSVDDALinstkiysyfp	HLA-DRB1*11:01	MK10
43280	napsyTNGKLniyyrrlynglkf	B-cell	WDR62
43519	ndrLSSANlyingvlmgsae	HLA-Class II, allele undetermined	GPR98
43591	neEDIDVilkkstilnldin	HLA-Class II, allele undetermined	GABR1
43939	nftVSFWLRVPK	HLA-Class II, allele undetermined	GBRA1 SCN8A
43940	nftVSFWLRVPKVsashle	HLA-DRB1*11:01	GBRA1 SCN8A EFHC1
44007	ngkaihlvnnesseVIVHKamdi	B-cell	CLN5
44396	nivkQGYEGnfi	HLA-Class II, allele undetermined	TSEAR
44200	niddntiyqylyaqkSPTTL	HLA-DRB1*01:01	SL9A6
44383	NITSLtigkskyfqDPALLL	HLA-ClassII, allele undetermined	ACHA2 AFG32 CLN6
44557	NKNEVrgivlrvdnknyfpc	HLA-Class II, allele undetermined	LRRC1
44667	nldinndiisdiSGFNSsvi	HLA-Class II, allele undetermined	GPR98
45102	nnftVSFWLRVPKVsashle	HLA-Class II, allele undetermined	GBRA1 SCN8A EFHC1
46136	ntiyqylyaqkSPTTLqrit	HLA-Class II, allele undetermined	SL9A6
46853	PALLLmheLIHVLhglygmq	HLA-Class II, allele undetermined	CLN6 WDR62
46855	PALNIvkQGYEGnfigalet	HLA-Class II, allele undetermined	NMDE1 TSEAR
48049	PKEIEKlytSYLSITFLRDf	HLA-Class II, allele undetermined	GCP6 CSMD3 KCMA1 GTR1 SCN1A SCN2A SCN8A CLCN2
48697	pnrdiliasnwyfnhLKDKIlgc	B-cell	ROGDI
49984	pvtkGIPYApeyksnaastteih	B-cell	CBPA6
51254	qkSPTTLqrITMTNSVDDALIns	B-cell	SL9A6 VP13A MK10
56528	ryekwievyKLVKAKWLgtvntq	B-cell	ARHGA LGI2
57935	sfvksGDFIKLyvsynnneh	HLA-ClassII, allele undetermined	EFHC2 CNTP2
57947	sfwLRVPKVsashle	HLA-DR5, HLA-DRB1*11:01	SCN8A EFHC1
58527	SIGSGwsvslkgnnliwtlk	HLA-DRB1*03:01	RELN
59500	SLTDLggelcikikn	HLA-Class II, allele undetermined	LRRC1

TABLE 1: Continued.

IEDB ID[1]	TT-derived epitope[2,3]	Immune context	Epilepsy-associated proteins[4]
61214	ssmkkHSLSIGSGwsvslkg	HLA-Class II, allele undetermined	PWP2 GCP6 CDKL5 RELN
61354	ssskdVQLKNitdymyltnapsy	B-cell	GPR98
62073	SVDDALinstkiysyfpsviskvnqGAQGIl	HLA-Class II, allele undetermined	MK10
63277	tdymyltnapsyTNGKLniy	HLA-DRB1*01:01, HLA-DRB1*04:01	WDR62
63450	teLKKLEskinkvfstpipf	HLA-DRB1*07:01	TSC1
64514	tiyndtEGFNIESKDLksey	HLA-Class II, allele undetermined	CSMD3 GPR98
65324	TNGKLniyyrrlynglkfii	HLA-Class II, allele undetermined	WDR62
67104	tvntqfqKRSYQmyrsletqvda	B-cell	WDR62
67147	tVSFWLRVPKVsa	HLA-DRB1*11:01, HLA-DRB1*11:04	GBRA1 SCN8A EFHC1
67148	tVSFWLRVPKVsashle	HLA-DRB1*11:01	GBRA1 SCN8A EFHC1
68104	vdynlqskiTLPNDrttpvt	HLA-DQB1*06:02	GPR98
69149	VIVHKamdieyNDMFNnftv	HLA-Class II, allele undetermined	CLN5 SCN9A
69180	vKAKWLgtvntqfqKRSYQm	HLA-DQB1*06:02	LGI2 WDR62
70202	vntqfqKRSYQmyrsleyqv	HLA-DRB1*07:01	WDR62
70165	vnqGAQGIlflqwvrdiidd	HLA-Class II, allele undetermined	MK10
70166	vnqGAQGIlflqwvrdiiddftn	B-cell	MK10
70514	vpyigPALNIvk	HLA-Class II, allele undetermined	NMDE1
70982	vsidkfriFCKALnpk	HLA-DRB1*11:01	LRRC1 SCN8A KCMA1
71155	vstivpyigPALNI	HLA-DR, HLA-DR1, HLA-A*02:01	NMDE1
71156	vstivpyigPALNIvkQGYEGnf	B-cell	NMDE1 TSEAR
72784	wLRVPKVsashleqygtneysie	B-cell	SCN8A EFHC1
76411	yvsidkfriFCKALnPKEIE	HLA-Class II, allele undetermined	LRRC1 KCMA1[5]
76537	yylipvassskdVQLKNitd	HLA-Class II, allele undetermined	GPR98
79808	eLIHVLhglygmq	HLA-DRA*01:01, HLA-DRB1*01:01	WDR62 KCMA1
79816	evyKLVKAKWLgt	HLA-DRA*01:01, HLA-DRB1*01:01	ARHGA LGI2
113407	fnnftVSFWLRVPKVsas	HLA-DR11	GBRA1 SCN8A EFHC1
167585	glygmqvsshEIIPSkqeiy	HLA-DRB1*12:01	ACHA2 ACHA4
167613	kvnqGAQGIlflqwvrdiid	HLA-DRB1*12:01	MK10
167626	nLISIDikndlyektlndyk	HLA-DRB1*12:01	GPR98
167666	shEIIPSkqeiymqhtypis	HLA-DRB1*12:01	ACHA2 ACHA4

[1] One hundred and sixteen linear TT-derived epitopes that had been found to be immunopositive in the human host were analyzed. Epitope number refers to IEDB ID. Further details and references are reported in the Immune Epitope Database (IEDB; http://www.immuneepitope.org/).
[2] Aa sequences given in one-letter code.
[3] Peptide fragments shared with epilepsy-associated proteins in capital.
[4] Epilepsy-associated proteins reported as UniProt/Swiss-prot entries. For details and references, see http://www.uniprot.org/.
[5] TT-derived epitope ID 76411 shares both pentapeptides FCKAL and PKEIE with human KCMA1 (or calcium-activated potassium channel subunit alpha-1).

the molecular level of the repeatedly advanced association between antibodies and epilepsy [33–41]. Moreover, of not less importance, immunoassay validation could also represent a prelude to specific therapies based on peptide modules able to block epileptogenic anti-TT autoantibodies [38–41, 90]. Immunological research in this direction has been programmed in our lab.

Conflict of Interests

The authors declare that there is no conflict of interests regarding the publication of this paper.

Acknowledgment

Guglielmo Lucchese is supported by Deutscher Akademischer Austauschdienst (DAAD).

References

[1] C. D. Ferrie, "Idiopathic generalized epilepsies imitating focal epilepsies," *Epilepsia*, vol. 46, no. 9, pp. 91–95, 2005.

[2] E. C. Wirrell, B. R. Grossardt, E. L. So, and K. C. Nickels, "A population-based study of long-term outcomes of cryptogenic focal epilepsy in childhood: cryptogenic epilepsy is NOT probably symptomatic epilepsy," *Epilepsia*, vol. 52, no. 4, pp. 738–745, 2011.

[3] A. T. Berg, "Epilepsy, cognition, and behavior: the clinical picture," *Epilepsia*, vol. 52, supplement 1, pp. 7–12, 2011.

[4] U. Stephani, "The natural history of myoclonic astatic epilepsy (Doose syndrome) and Lennox-Gastaut syndrome," *Epilepsia*, vol. 47, supplement 2, pp. 53–55, 2006.

[5] C. J. Chu-Shore, P. Major, S. Camposano, D. Muzykewicz, and E. A. Thiele, "The natural history of epilepsy in tuberous sclerosis complex," *Epilepsia*, vol. 51, no. 7, pp. 1236–1241, 2010.

[6] N. Gaspard and L. J. Hirsch, "Pitfalls in ictal EEG interpretation: critical care and intracranial recordings," *Neurology*, vol. 80, supplement 1, pp. S26–S42, 2013.

[7] A. T. Berg, S. F. Berkovic, M. J. Brodie et al., "Revised terminology and concepts for organization of seizures and epilepsies: report of the ILAE Commission on Classification and Terminology, 2005–2009," *Epilepsia*, vol. 51, no. 4, pp. 676–685, 2010.

[8] C. P. Panayiotopoulos, "The new ILAE report on terminology and concepts for the organization of epilepsies: critical review and contribution," *Epilepsia*, vol. 53, no. 3, pp. 399–404, 2012.

[9] G. Avanzini, "A sound conceptual framework for an epilepsy classification is still lacking," *Epilepsia*, vol. 51, no. 4, pp. 720–722, 2010.

[10] R. Ottman, J. F. Annegers, N. Risch, W. A. Hauser, and M. Susser, "Relations of genetic and environmental factors in the etiology of epilepsy," *Annals of Neurology*, vol. 39, no. 4, pp. 442–449, 1996.

[11] X. Wang and Y. Lu, "Genetic etiology of new forms of familial epilepsy," *Frontiers in Bioscience*, vol. 13, no. 8, pp. 3159–3167, 2008.

[12] M. J. Martínez, M. A. López-Aríztegui, N. Puente, I. Rubio, and M. I. Tejada, "CDKL5 gene status in female patients with epilepsy and Rett-like features: two new mutations in the catalytic domain," *BMC Medical Genetics*, vol. 13, article 68, 2012.

[13] A. Vezzani, J. French, T. Bartfai, and T. Z. Baram, "The role of inflammation in epilepsy," *Nature Reviews Neurology*, vol. 7, no. 1, pp. 31–40, 2011.

[14] Y. Takahashi, K. Matsuda, Y. Kubota et al., "Vaccination and infection as causative factors in Japanese patients with Rasmussen syndrome: molecular mimicry and HLA class I," *Clinical and Developmental Immunology*, vol. 13, no. 2–4, pp. 381–387, 2006.

[15] W. H. Theodore, L. Epstein, W. D. Gaillard, S. Shinnar, M. S. Wainwright, and S. Jacobson, "Human herpes virus 6B: a possible role in epilepsy?" *Epilepsia*, vol. 49, no. 11, pp. 1828–1837, 2008.

[16] J. E. Libbey and R. S. Fujinami, "Neurotropic viral infections leading to epilepsy: focus on Theiler's murine encephalomyelitis virus," *Future Virology*, vol. 6, no. 11, pp. 1339–1350, 2011.

[17] Y. Bozzi, S. Casarosa, and M. Caleo, "Epilepsy as a neurodevelopmental disorder," *Frontiers in Psychiatry*, vol. 3, article 19, 2012.

[18] P. Sgadò, M. Dunleavy, S. Genovesi, G. Provenzano, and Y. Bozzi, "The role of GABAergic system in neurodevelopmental disorders: a focus on autism and epilepsy," *International Journal of Physiology, Pathophysiology and Pharmacology*, vol. 3, no. 3, pp. 223–235, 2011.

[19] R. Tuchman and M. Cuccaro, "Epilepsy and autism: neurodevelopmental perspective," *Current Neurology and Neuroscience Reports*, vol. 11, no. 4, pp. 428–434, 2011.

[20] R. J. Hagerman, "Epilepsy drives autism in neurodevelopmental disorders," *Developmental Medicine and Child Neurology*, vol. 55, no. 2, pp. 101–102, 2013.

[21] A. M. van Eeghen, M. B. Pulsifer, V. L. Merker et al., "Understanding relationships between autism, intelligence, and epilepsy: a cross-disorder approach," *Developmental Medicine and Child Neurology*, vol. 55, no. 2, pp. 146–153, 2013.

[22] S. N. Rakhade and F. E. Jensen, "Epileptogenesis in the immature brain: emerging mechanisms," *Nature Reviews Neurology*, vol. 5, no. 7, pp. 380–391, 2009.

[23] C. M. Dubé, A. L. Brewster, C. Richichi, Q. Zha, and T. Z. Baram, "Fever, febrile seizures and epilepsy," *Trends in Neurosciences*, vol. 30, no. 10, pp. 490–496, 2007.

[24] J. Palace and B. Lang, "Epilepsy: an autoimmune disease?" *Journal of Neurology Neurosurgery and Psychiatry*, vol. 69, no. 6, pp. 711–714, 2000.

[25] S. Najjar, M. Bernbaum, G. Lai, and O. Devinsky, "Immunology and epilepsy," *Reviews in Neurological Diseases*, vol. 5, no. 3, pp. 109–116, 2008.

[26] E. Pineda, D. Shin, S. J. You, S. Auvin, R. Sankar, and A. Mazarati, "Maternal immune activation promotes hippocampal kindling epileptogenesis in mice," *Annals of Neurology*, vol. 74, no. 1, pp. 11–19, 2013.

[27] R. Nabbout, "Autoimmune and inflammatory epilepsies," *Epilepsia*, vol. 53, no. 4, pp. 58–62, 2012.

[28] A. Vincent and P. B. Crino, "Systemic and neurologic autoimmune disorders associated with seizures or epilepsy," *Epilepsia*, vol. 52, supplement 3, pp. 12–17, 2011.

[29] T. Granata, H. Cross, W. Theodore, and G. Avanzini, "Immune-mediated epilepsies," *Epilepsia*, vol. 52, supplement 3, pp. 5–11, 2011.

[30] A. Vezzani and S. Rüegg, "The pivotal role of immunity and inflammatory processes in epilepsy is increasingly recognized: introduction," *Epilepsia*, vol. 52, supplement 3, pp. 1–4, 2011.

[31] N. Specchio, L. Fusco, D. Claps, and F. Vigevano, "Epileptic encephalopathy in children possibly related to immune-mediated pathogenesis," *Brain & Development*, vol. 32, no. 1, pp. 51–56, 2010.

[32] K. M. Rodgers, M. R. Hutchinson, A. Northcutt, S. F. Maier, L. R. Watkins, and D. S. Barth, "The cortical innate immune response increases local neuronal excitability leading to seizures," *Brain*, vol. 132, no. 9, pp. 2478–2486, 2009.

[33] H. J. M. Majoie, M. de Baets, W. Renier, B. Lang, and A. Vincent, "Antibodies to voltage-gated potassium and calcium channels in epilepsy," *Epilepsy Research*, vol. 71, no. 2-3, pp. 135–141, 2006.

[34] K. McKnight, Y. Jiang, Y. Hart et al., "Serum antibodies in epilepsy and seizure-associated disorders," *Neurology*, vol. 65, no. 11, pp. 1730–1736, 2005.

[35] C. G. Bien and A. Vincent, "Immune-mediated pediatric epilepsies," *Handbook of Clinical Neurology*, vol. 111, pp. 521–531, 2013.

[36] M. Falip, M. Carreño, J. Miró et al., "Prevalence and immunological spectrum of temporal lobe epilepsy with glutamic acid decarboxylase antibodies," *European Journal of Neurology*, vol. 19, no. 6, pp. 827–833, 2012.

[37] A. Boronat, L. Sabater, A. Saiz, J. Dalmau, and F. Graus, "GABA$_B$ receptor antibodies in limbic encephalitis and anti-GAD-associated neurologic disorders," *Neurology*, vol. 76, no. 9, pp. 795–800, 2011.

[38] V. Nociti, G. Frisullo, T. Tartaglione et al., "Refractory generalized seizures and cerebellar ataxia associated with anti-GAD antibodies responsive to immunosuppressive treatment," *European Journal of Neurology*, vol. 17, no. 1, p. e5, 2010.

[39] C. I. Akman, M. C. Patterson, A. Rubinstein, and R. Herzog, "Limbic encephalitis associated with anti-GAD antibody and common variable immune deficiency," *Developmental Medicine and Child Neurology*, vol. 51, no. 7, pp. 563–567, 2009.

[40] E. Krastinova, M. Vigneron, P. Le Bras, J. Gasnault, and C. Goujard, "Treatment of limbic encephalitis with anti-glioma-inactivated 1 (LGI1) antibodies," *Journal of Clinical Neuroscience*, vol. 19, no. 11, pp. 1580–1582, 2012.

[41] A. M. L. Quek, J. W. Britton, A. McKeon et al., "Autoimmune epilepsy: clinical characteristics and response to immunotherapy," *Archives of Neurology*, vol. 69, no. 5, pp. 582–593, 2012.

[42] M. Nørgaard, V. Ehrenstein, R. B. Nielsen, L. S. Bakketeig, and H. T. Sørensen, "Maternal use of antibiotics, hospitalisation for infection during pregnancy, and risk of childhood epilepsy: a population-based cohort study," *PLoS ONE*, vol. 7, no. 1, Article ID e30850, 2012.

[43] J. F. Bale Jr., "Fetal infections and brain development," *Clinics in Perinatology*, vol. 36, no. 3, pp. 639–653, 2009.

[44] C. S. Wu, L. H. Pedersen, J. E. Miller et al., "Risk of cerebral palsy and childhood epilepsy related to infections before or during pregnancy," *PLoS ONE*, vol. 8, no. 2, Article ID e57552, 2013.

[45] Y. Sun, M. Vestergaard, J. Christensen, A. J. Nahmias, and J. Olsen, "Prenatal exposure to maternal infections and epilepsy in childhood: a population-based cohort study," *Pediatrics*, vol. 121, no. 5, pp. e1100–e1107, 2008.

[46] K. E. Nilsen, M. C. Walker, and H. R. Cock, "Characterization of the tetanus toxin model of refractory focal neocortical epilepsy in the rat," *Epilepsia*, vol. 46, no. 2, pp. 179–187, 2005.

[47] M. Mainardi, M. Pietrasanta, E. Vannini, O. Rossetto, and M. Caleo, "Tetanus neurotoxin-induced epilepsy in mouse visual cortex," *Epilepsia*, vol. 53, no. 7, pp. e132–e136, 2012.

[48] R. C. Wykes, J. H. Heeroma, L. Mantoan et al., "Optogenetic and potassium channel gene therapy in a rodent model of focal neocortical epilepsy," *Science Translational Medicine*, vol. 4, no. 161, Article ID 161ra152, 2012.

[49] W. M. Otte, P. Bielefeld, R. M. Dijkhuizen, and K. P. J. Braun, "Focal neocortical epilepsy affects hippocampal volume, shape, and structural integrity: a longitudinal MRI and immunohistochemistry study in a rat model," *Epilepsia*, vol. 53, no. 7, pp. 1264–1273, 2012.

[50] M. Sedigh-Sarvestani, G. I. Thuku, S. Sunderam et al., "Rapid eye movement sleep and hippocampal theta oscillations precede seizure onset in the tetanus toxin model of temporal lobe epilepsy," *The Journal of Neuroscience*, vol. 34, no. 4, pp. 1105–1114, 2014.

[51] D. Kanduc, A. Stufano, G. Lucchese, and A. Kusalik, "Massive peptide sharing between viral and human proteomes," *Peptides*, vol. 29, no. 10, pp. 1755–1766, 2008.

[52] G. Lucchese, A. Stufano, M. Calabro, and D. Kanduc, "Charting the peptide crossreactome between HIV-1 and the human proteome," *Frontiers in Bioscience*, vol. 3, no. 4, pp. 1385–1400, 2011.

[53] B. Trost, G. Lucchese, A. Stufano, M. Bickis, A. Kusalik, and D. Kanduc, "No human protein is exempt from bacterial motifs, not even one," *Self/Nonself*, vol. 1, no. 4, pp. 328–334, 2010.

[54] G. Lucchese, A. Stufano, and D. Kanduc, "Proposing low-similarity peptide vaccines against mycobacterium tuberculosis," *Journal of Biomedicine and Biotechnology*, vol. 2010, Article ID 832341, 8 pages, 2010.

[55] S. L. Bavaro, M. Calabrò, and D. Kanduc, "Pentapeptide sharing between *Corynebacterium diphtheria* toxin and the human neural protein network," *Immunopharmacology and Immunotoxicology*, vol. 33, no. 2, pp. 360–372, 2011.

[56] D. Kanduc, "Describing the hexapeptide identity platform between the influenza A H5N1 and *Homo sapiens* proteomes," *Biologics*, vol. 4, pp. 245–261, 2010.

[57] R. Ricco and D. Kanduc, "Hepatitis B virus and homo sapiens proteomewide analysis: a profusion of viral peptide overlaps in neuron-specific human proteins," *Biologics: Targets and Therapy*, vol. 4, pp. 75–81, 2010.

[58] G. Lucchese, G. Capone, and D. Kanduc, "Peptide sharing between Influenza A H1N1 hemagglutinin and human axon guidance proteins," *Schizophrenia Bulletin*, vol. 40, no. 2, pp. 362–375, 2014.

[59] A. Hoshino, M. Saitoh, A. Oka et al., "Epidemiology of acute encephalopathy in Japan, with emphasis on the association of viruses and syndromes," *Brain & Development*, vol. 34, no. 5, pp. 337–343, 2012.

[60] D. Kanduc, "Homology, similarity, and identity in peptide epitope immunodefinition," *Journal of Peptide Science*, vol. 18, no. 8, pp. 487–494, 2012.

[61] D. Kanduc, "Pentapeptides as minimal functional units in cell biology and immunology," *Current Protein & Peptide Science*, vol. 14, no. 2, pp. 111–120, 2013.

[62] D. B. Sant'Angelo, E. Robinson, C. A. Janeway Jr., and L. K. Denzin, "Recognition of core and flanking amino acids of MHC classII-bound peptides by the T cell receptor," *European Journal of Immunology*, vol. 32, no. 9, pp. 2510–2520, 2002.

[63] J. B. Rothbard and M. L. Gefter, "Interactions between immunogenic peptides and MHC proteins," *Annual Review of Immunology*, vol. 9, pp. 527–565, 1991.

[64] J. B. Rothbard, R. M. Pemberton, H. C. Bodmer, B. A. Askonas, and W. R. Taylor, "Identification of residues necessary for clonally specific recognition of a cytotoxic T cell determinant," *The EMBO Journal*, vol. 8, no. 8, pp. 2321–2328, 1989.

[65] M. J. Reddehase, J. B. Rothbard, and U. H. Koszinowski, "A pentapeptide as minimal antigenic determinant for MHC class I-restricted T lymphocytes," *Nature*, vol. 337, no. 6208, pp. 651–653, 1989.

[66] B. Hemmer, T. Kondo, B. Gran et al., "Minimal peptide length requirements for CD4$^+$ T cell clones—implications for molecular mimicry and T cell survival," *International Immunology*, vol. 12, no. 3, pp. 375–383, 2000.

[67] K. Landsteiner and J. van der Scheer, "On the serological specificity of peptides. III," *The Journal of Experimental Medicine*, vol. 69, no. 5, pp. 705–719, 1939.

[68] R. Tiwari, K. Geliebter, A. Lucchese, A. Mittelman, and D. Kanduc, "Computational peptide dissection of Melan-a/MART-1 oncoprotein antigenicity," *Peptides*, vol. 25, no. 11, pp. 1865–1871, 2004.

[69] S. Tanabe, "Epitope peptides and immunotherapy," *Current Protein & Peptide Science*, vol. 8, no. 1, pp. 109–118, 2007.

[70] W. Zeng, J. Pagnon, and D. C. Jackson, "The C-terminal pentapeptide of LHRH is a dominant B cell epitope with antigenic and biological function," *Molecular Immunology*, vol. 44, no. 15, pp. 3724–3731, 2007.

[71] G. Lucchese, A. Stufano, B. Trost, A. Kusalik, and D. Kanduc, "Peptidology: short amino acid modules in cell biology and immunology," *Amino Acids*, vol. 33, no. 4, pp. 703–707, 2007.

[72] P. Cossette, L. Liu, K. Brisebois et al., "Mutation of GABRA1 in an autosomal dominant form of juvenile myoclonic epilepsy," *Nature Genetics*, vol. 31, no. 2, pp. 184–189, 2002.

[73] K. R. Veeramah, J. E. O'Brien, M. H. Meisler et al., "*De novo* pathogenic SCN8A mutation identified by whole-genome sequencing of a family quartet affected by infantile epileptic encephalopathy and SUDEP," *American Journal of Human Genetics*, vol. 90, no. 3, pp. 502–510, 2012.

[74] T. Suzuki, A. V. Delgado-Escueta, K. Aguan et al., "Mutations in *EFHC1* cause juvenile myoclonic epilepsy," *Nature Genetics*, vol. 36, no. 8, pp. 842–849, 2004.

[75] A. A. Mohit, J. H. Martin, and C. A. Miller, "p493F12 kinase: a novel MAP kinase expressed in a subset of neurons in the human nervous system," *Neuron*, vol. 14, no. 1, pp. 67–78, 1995.

[76] C. E. Stafstrom, "The role of the subiculum in epilepsy and epileptogenesis," *Epilepsy Currents*, vol. 5, no. 4, pp. 121–129, 2005.

[77] K. Sendrowski and W. Sobaniec, "Hippocampus, hippocampal sclerosis and epilepsy," *Pharmacological Reports*, vol. 65, no. 3, pp. 555–565, 2013.

[78] C. Toma, A. Hervás, B. Torrico et al., "Analysis of two language-related genes in Autism: a case-control association study of FOXP2 and CNTNAP2," *Psychiatric Genetics*, vol. 23, no. 2, pp. 82–85, 2013.

[79] T. D. Folsom and S. H. Fatemi, "The involvement of Reelin in neurodevelopmental disorders," *Neuropharmacology*, vol. 68, pp. 122–135, 2013.

[80] E. Romano, C. Michetti, A. Caruso, G. Laviola, and M. L. Scattoni, "Characterization of neonatal vocal and motor repertoire of reelin mutant mice," *PLoS ONE*, vol. 8, no. 5, Article ID e64407, 2013.

[81] S. Jeste, M. Sahin, P. Bolton, G. Ploubidis, and A. Humphrey, "Characterization of autism in young children with tuberous sclerosis complex," *Journal of Child Neurology*, vol. 23, no. 5, pp. 520–525, 2008.

[82] D. C. Taylor, "Schizophrenias and epilepsies: why? When? How?" *Epilepsy and Behavior*, vol. 4, no. 5, pp. 474–482, 2003.

[83] P. Qin, H. Xu, T. M. Laursen, M. Vestergaard, and P. B. Mortensen, "Risk for schizophrenia and schizophrenia-like psychosis among patients with epilepsy: population based cohort study," *British Medical Journal*, vol. 331, no. 7507, pp. 23–25, 2005.

[84] Y.-T. Chang, P.-C. Chen, I.-J. Tsai et al., "Bidirectional relation between schizophrenia and epilepsy: a population-based retrospective cohort study," *Epilepsia*, vol. 52, no. 11, pp. 2036–2042, 2011.

[85] M. C. Clarke, A. Tanskanen, M. O. Huttunen, M. Clancy, D. R. Cotter, and M. Cannon, "Evidence for shared susceptibility to epilepsy and psychosis: a population-based family study," *Biological Psychiatry*, vol. 71, no. 9, pp. 836–839, 2012.

[86] N. G. Cascella, D. J. Schretlen, and A. Sawa, "Schizophrenia and epilepsy: is there a shared susceptibility?" *Neuroscience Research*, vol. 63, no. 4, pp. 227–235, 2009.

[87] A. Sette, A. Vitiello, B. Reherman et al., "The relationship between class I binding affinity and immunogenicity of potential cytotoxic T cell epitopes," *Journal of Immunology*, vol. 153, no. 12, pp. 5586–5592, 1994.

[88] K. D. Moudgil and E. E. Sercarz, "Understanding crypticity is the key to revealing the pathogenesis of autoimmunity," *Trends in Immunology*, vol. 26, no. 7, pp. 355–359, 2005.

[89] P. Eggleton, R. Haigh, and P. G. Winyard, "Consequence of neo-antigenicity of the 'altered self'," *Rheumatology*, vol. 47, no. 5, pp. 567–571, 2008.

[90] D. Kanduc, "Peptide cross-reactivity: the original sin of vaccines," *Frontiers in Bioscience*, vol. 4, pp. 1393–1401, 2012.

3

Continuous Spikes and Waves during Sleep: Electroclinical Presentation and Suggestions for Management

Iván Sánchez Fernández,[1,2] **Kevin E. Chapman,**[3] **Jurriaan M. Peters,**[1]
Chellamani Harini,[1] **Alexander Rotenberg,**[1] **and Tobias Loddenkemper**[1]

[1] Division of Epilepsy and Clinical Neurophysiology, Department of Neurology, Harvard Medical School,
  Boston Children's Hospital, Boston, MA 02115, USA
[2] Department of Child Neurology, Hospital Sant Joan de Déu, Universidad de Barcelona, 08950 Barcelona, Spain
[3] Department of Neurology, Children's Hospital Colorado, University of Colorado, Aurora, CO 80045, USA

Correspondence should be addressed to Tobias Loddenkemper; tobias.loddenkemper@childrens.harvard.edu

Academic Editor: Elaine Wirrell

Continuous spikes and waves during sleep (CSWS) is an epileptic encephalopathy characterized in most patients by (1) difficult to control seizures, (2) interictal epileptiform activity that becomes prominent during sleep leading to an electroencephalogram (EEG) pattern of electrical status epilepticus in sleep (ESES), and (3) neurocognitive regression. In this paper, we will summarize current epidemiological, clinical, and EEG knowledge on CSWS and will provide suggestions for treatment. CSWS typically presents with seizures around 2–4 years of age. Neurocognitive regression occurs around 5-6 years of age, and it is accompanied by subacute worsening of EEG abnormalities and seizures. At approximately 6–9 years of age, there is a gradual resolution of seizures and EEG abnormalities, but the neurocognitive deficits persist in most patients. The cause of CSWS is unknown, but early developmental lesions play a major role in approximately half of the patients, and genetic associations have recently been described. High-dose benzodiazepines and corticosteroids have been successfully used to treat clinical and electroencephalographic features. Corticosteroids are often reserved for refractory disease because of adverse events. Valproate, ethosuximide, levetiracetam, sulthiame, and lamotrigine have been also used with some success. Epilepsy surgery may be considered in a few selected patients.

1. Introduction

Continuous spikes and waves during sleep (CSWS) is an epileptic encephalopathy, that is, a condition in which the epileptic processes themselves are thought to contribute to the disturbance in cerebral function. CSWS is characterized by (1) seizures, (2) neurocognitive regression, and (3) an electroencephalography (EEG) pattern of electrical status epilepticus during sleep (ESES) [1–6]. ESES is characterized by marked sleep potentiation of epileptiform activity in the transition from wakefulness to sleep that leads to near-continuous bilateral (or occasionally lateralized) slow spikes and waves that occupy a significant proportion of nonrapid eye movement (non-REM) sleep [2, 4].

In this review, we summarize epidemiological, etiological, clinical, and EEG features in CSWS based on available data. We also suggest an approach to manage this syndrome and present it in the framework of a more general childhood seizure susceptibility syndrome.

2. Definitions

The terms "ESES," "CSWS," and "Landau-Kleffner syndrome" have been used interchangeably in the literature to refer to the EEG pattern of frequent spike-waves or to the associated epileptic encephalopathy with regression [6–8]. The EEG pattern and the associated epileptic encephalopathy are different concepts that might require differentiated names. A recent survey in North-America showed that the use of concepts in ESES and CSWS is very heterogeneous, and a common terminology is not available [9]. For the purposes of this review, we will use "ESES" when referring to the EEG pattern, "CSWS" when referring to the epileptic encephalopathy with global regression, and "Landau-Kleffner syndrome" (LKS) when referring to the epileptic encephalopathy with mainly language regression. We use this terminology in order to give unequivocal names to the different concepts, but we acknowledge that terminology is in progress, and it may change in the future.

The main focus of this review is on CSWS, a severe epileptic encephalopathy with (1) ESES on EEG, (2) seizures, and (3) developmental regression in, at least, two domains of development. Therefore, patients with developmental regression in mainly the language domain will be reviewed under the associated condition of "Landau-Kleffner syndrome" [4]. The borders between these entities are often difficult to delineate, and conditions may be considered as different presentations of the same electroclinical spectrum [10].

3. Epidemiology

CSWS is a rare condition that occurs only in children and adolescents. In an outpatient pediatric series, 1 out of 440 (0.2%) epileptic children had CSWS [11]. In tertiary pediatric epilepsy centers, around 0.5%–0.6% of patients were diagnosed with CSWS [12, 13]. Among children and adolescents undergoing epilepsy surgery for intractable seizures, about 1-2% of patients presented with CSWS [14, 15]. The exact frequency of CSWS is difficult to assess because of inconsistent inclusion criteria and study methodologies. Gender distribution in large series and reviews shows a male-to-female ratio of 4 : 3 to 3 : 2 [2, 16–21].

4. Clinical Features

CSWS is an age-related epileptic encephalopathy in which the clinical features evolve over time. The evolving nature of this syndrome allows the recognition of several clinical events: age at seizure onset, age at neurocognitive regression, and age at seizure freedom. These clinical events provide information to identify electroclinical stages in CSWS, namely, dormant stage (from birth to epilepsy onset), prodromal stage (from epilepsy onset to regression), acute stage (from regression to seizure freedom), and residual stage (after seizure freedom) [22–24].

4.1. Seizures. A typical child with CSWS initially has normal or moderately abnormal baseline development and then presents with seizures around 2–4 years of age. Patients with structural lesions of the brain tend to have seizures earlier (around 2 years of age) than patients without lesions (around 4 years of age) [4]. Seizures during the prodromal stage occur typically out of sleep and are frequently clonic or tonic-clonic unilateral seizures that rarely progress to unilateral status epilepticus [6, 16, 25]. During the prodromal stage, two or more seizure types are seen in only 20% of patients [16]. During the acute stage, there is a marked increase in the frequency and types of seizures, which become more difficult to control [2, 6, 16, 25, 26]. Unilateral seizures become rare, while atonic seizures appear and the motor components of the seizures lead to sudden falls. Atypical absence seizures

increase in frequency and severity and may even evolve into absence status epilepticus [6, 16, 25]. The lack of tonic seizures has been classically considered a major feature of this syndrome and allows for differentiation from Lennox-Gastaut syndrome (LGS) [1, 6, 25].

4.2. Neurocognitive Regression. During the dormant stage, neurocognitive development is clinically normal in approximately two-thirds of cases [13, 25, 26]. A severe neurocognitive regression occurs around 5-6 years of age in most patients. Neurocognitive deterioration affects a wide spectrum of developmental and neurocognitive milestones in varying but often severe degrees. Regression domains include language, behavior, learning, memory, attention, social interactions, motor skills, and global intelligence [2, 3, 6, 8, 15, 17, 25, 27–30].

5. Electroencephalographic Features

During wakefulness, the EEG shows focal/multifocal spikes that increase in frequency during the acute stage. The hallmark EEG feature of CSWS is ESES. ESES is characterized by (1) marked potentiation of epileptiform discharges during non-REM sleep, leading to (2) a (near)-continuous, bilateral, or occasionally lateralized slow spikes and waves, (3) and these spikes and waves occur "during a significant proportion" of the non-REM sleep with a threshold ranging from 25% to 85% [1, 6, 15, 19–21, 25, 27, 31–35].

5.1. Evolution of ESES over Time. Abnormal EEG findings are found during the prodromal period or even the dormant stage. Findings always include potentiation of spiking during non-REM sleep. During the acute stage, interictal epileptiform activity becomes much more frequent and severe with more widespread spikes of higher amplitude associated with a more abnormal background. During sleep, the EEG pattern presents as ESES [4]. ESES typically appears about 4–8 years of age and typically remits around 8-9 years of age [8, 17, 19, 35]. The age of detection of the ESES pattern on EEG varies widely in different studies and likely reflects the varied criteria of ESES used as well as the variations of time intervals in which EEGs are performed.

5.2. Cut-Off Value. The initial definitions of ESES proposed that no less than 85% of the total duration of slow sleep should be occupied by slow spike-waves [6, 34]. This cut-off value has been followed by several authors [6–8, 15, 17, 21, 35–39], while other authors used lower cut-off percentages [19, 20, 40, 41]. The International League Against Epilepsy does not refer to any particular threshold and only requires that spike-waves be "continuous" and "diffuse" [1] leading to heterogeneous and variable use of cut-off values by the professionals caring for these children [9].

5.3. Quantification of Epileptiform Activity. The classic measure for the quantification of epileptiform activity is the spike-wave index, expressed as the percentage of sleep occupied by spike-waves. While this percentage has been widely used,

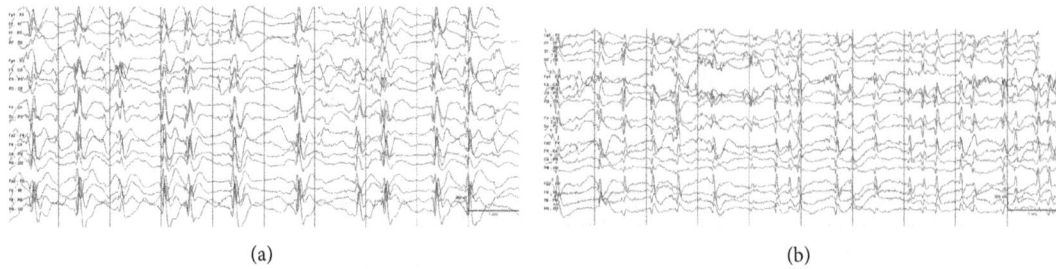

(a)   (b)

FIGURE 1: Different values in the quantification of the epileptiform activity result when using different methods of quantification. Epileptiform activity appears much more frequently in (b) than in (a). Both tracings have a 100% of epileptiform activity if the reader quantifies the epileptiform activity using spike percentage, that is, counting the percentage of 1-second bins occupied by spike-waves. However, if the reader quantifies the epileptiform activity using spike frequency, that is, the total number of individual spike-waves per unit of time (per 10 seconds in this page, per 100 seconds in a longer tracing), epileptiform activity is almost double in (b) than in (a). Note that the tracings have different voltage gains.

the exact method for calculating this value is often not specified [6, 7, 15, 17, 19, 21, 26, 35, 40]. A reproducible way to quantify epileptiform activity is to quantify the percentage of 1-second bins with at least one spike-wave in them, termed spike-wave percentage [24, 36]. Another reproducible method consists in counting the total number of spikes per unit of time, termed spike frequency [24]. A formal comparison between these two methods showed that spike frequency could better detect changes in epileptiform activity in those patients with very active epileptiform discharges (Figure 1) [24]. In addition, spike frequency lends itself better for automated quantification [42]. There is also no formal consensus on which portion of sleep is used for calculating the epileptiform activity with different periods of the night used by different authors [6, 19, 24, 35, 36, 43] and in clinical practice [9]. Regarding lateralized epileptiform activity, there is insufficient evidence to support that unilateral or focal discharges should be quantified differently than symmetric and bilateral discharges [20, 26, 39, 44].

6. Evolution over Time

CSWS evolves over time, and this evolution manifests in all three cardinal manifestations, including clinical seizures, EEG abnormalities, and neurocognitive regression. We therefore describe the evolution of this clinical presentation in these three categories.

6.1. Seizures. Seizures almost always disappear with age, even in patients with a static or progressive encephalopathy [2, 3, 6, 25, 27, 29, 41, 45, 46]. The age of seizure freedom peaks around 6–9 years of age although data on this clinical event are scarce, and the range is wide [27, 29].

6.2. Electroencephalogram Features. ESES progressively resolves with interictal epileptiform discharges during sleep substituted by a progressive return of the physiologic graphoelements and patterns of sleep. Typically, the resolution of the ESES pattern occurs around 8-9 years of age, in parallel with the timing of seizure freedom. However,

ESES can persist and be very active for a period after seizure freedom [3, 24, 25, 29].

6.3. Neurocognitive Features. The initial regression ultimately leads to a plateau in development. Some patients present with moderate improvements after seizure freedom. However, most patients remain severely impaired [2, 3, 6, 47]. The impact of interictal spikes on neurocognitive features is a matter of debate, and it is not clear whether an increased amount of epileptiform activity is associated with a worse cognitive outcome [4, 48, 49].

7. Etiology and Pathophysiology

The exact cause of CSWS is unknown, but there are two factors that have been implicated. First, an association of CSWS with early developmental lesions of the brain has been shown. Second, an increasing number of genetic associations of unclear significance have also been described.

7.1. Early Developmental Lesions. Several case reports and small series described the association between patients with the ESES EEG pattern and early developmental lesions, such as malformations of cortical development [45], or vascular insults [50–52]. Larger series also support this association. In a study of 32 patients with prenatal or perinatal thalamic lesions, sleep potentiation of epileptiform activity occurred in 29 cases (90.6%) [27]. In two large series of patients with ESES, 33 out of 67 patients (49.3%) and 18 out of 44 (40.9%) patients had an early developmental lesion [20, 53]. While these lesions may not be specific for ESES, but for epilepsy in general, a recent series compared 100 patients with ESES and 47 patients with epilepsy without ESES. Patients with ESES had a higher frequency of early developmental lesions (48% versus 19.2%; $P = 0.002$) and a higher frequency of thalamic lesions (14% versus 2.1%; $P = 0.037$). These findings are consistent with other series suggesting that approximately 40–50% of patients with ESES had an early developmental insult [20, 53, 54], with a majority having perinatal lesions of vascular etiology [20, 53, 54]. Interestingly, some authors report that certain cortical malformations may also be related

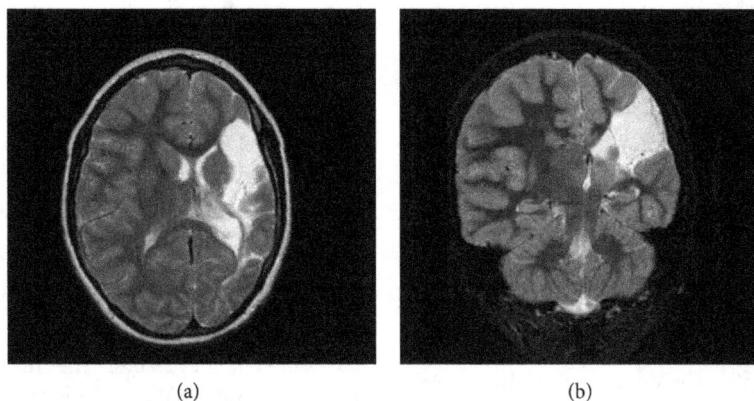

(a)   (b)

FIGURE 2: Early vascular lesions in patients with CSWS. Axial view T2 weighted in (a), coronal view T2 weighted in (b). Extensive cystic encephalomalacia affecting the left hemisphere in the distribution of the left middle cerebral artery consistent with a left middle cerebral artery infarct.

TABLE 1: Genetic factors that have been described in association with CSWS.

Study	Type of study	Association
Beaumanoir et al., 1995 [104]	Case report	CSWS in two monozygotic twins
Praline et al., 2006 [105]	Case report	Two siblings with ESES and different clinical presentations
Verhoeven et al., 2012 [106]	Case report	One patient with CSWS and dysmorphic features carried a de novo 8q12.3q13.2 microdeletion
Godfraind et al., 2008 [107]	Case report	One patient with CSWS carried a G392R mutation in neuroserpin of probable pathogenic significance (the mutation led to a progressive neurodegenerative disease and CSWS)
Nakayama et al., 2012 [108]	Case series (2 patients with CSWS)	Two patients with CSWS and dysmorphic features carried an unbalanced translocation between 8p and 9p
Broli et al., 2011 and Giorda et al., 2009 [109, 110]	Case series (2400 subjects with isolated or syndromic intellectual disability)	Five patients with CSWS carried a Xp11.22-p11.23 duplication
Kevelam et al., 2012 [40]	Case series (13 children with ESES and different clinical presentations)	Two patients with CSWS carried copy number variations in CHRNA7 and PCYT1B genes of probable pathogenic significance
Mefford et al., 2011 [111]	Case series (315 patients with different epileptic encephalopathies, 29 had CSWS or Landau-Kleffner syndrome)	One patient with CSWS carried a copy number variant in the DOK5 gene of uncertain pathogenic significance
Reutlinger et al., 2010 [112]	Case series (3 patients with ESES and different clinical presentations)	Three patients with ESES and different clinical presentations and dysmorphic features carried a deletion in 16p13.2p13.13
Atkins and Nikanorova, 2011 [66]	Case series (20 patients with ESES and different clinical presentations)	One patient with ESES (no further details on clinical presentation) carried a partial trisomy 13/21

Legend: CSWS: continuous spikes and waves during sleep. ESES: electrical status epilepticus in sleep.

to early vascular insults [55]. In particular, early developmental lesions that involve the thalamus are strongly associated with CSWS (Figure 2) [54].

7.2. Genetic Factors. Familial antecedents of seizures (including febrile seizures) are found in around 10–15% of patients with CSWS [6, 25]. Although genetic predisposition seems to play a minor role in CSWS, a growing number of case reports and small series describe associations with copy number variations and different mutations in several chromosomes

(Table 1). The etiological role of these genetic factors in CSWS is largely undefined to date. It is likely that these genetic variants are associated not with CSWS *per se*, but with different neurological conditions that result in the final common pathway of CSWS. A similar theory is suggested for hypsarrhythmia in West syndrome.

7.3. Pathophysiology. Animal models are providing insights into the basic pathophysiology of sleep-potentiated spiking

[56]. Cortical lesions have been found to weaken the neuro-transmission between corticothalamic neurons and the reticular nucleus of the thalamus without weakening the circuit between corticothalamic and thalamocortical neurons [57–59]. Therefore, reticular neurons do not have the normal loop interaction with the corticothalamic neurons that provides a feed-forward inhibition to thalamocortical neurons [57]. In contrast, a pathological loop with thalamocortical neurons is created which promotes a robust oscillatory network in the cortico-thalamo-cortical loop [57–59]. Breaking this pathological loop by selective inhibition of the thalamocortical neurons is a promising approach that has been found to work in an animal model [59]. The deficiency of the GluA4 AMPA receptor in a $Gria4^{-/-}$ mouse model similarly weakens the normal output of the reticular neurons leading to the development of spike-wave discharges [57]. It can be hypothesized that lesions in the reticular nucleus of the thalamus may also lead to a potentiation of oscillatory discharges in the cortico-thalamo-cortical network. Supporting this hypothesis, marked sleep potentiation of epileptiform activity has been found in patients with early developmental lesions affecting the thalamus [27, 54]. The only study that evaluated the specific thalamic areas that were injured showed that the reticular nucleus was the most frequently affected structure and it was involved in 91% of the cases [27].

8. Management

8.1. To Treat or Not to Treat Epileptiform Activity. The relationship of epileptiform activity in the EEG with neuropsychological function is a matter of debate. Near-continuous epileptiform discharges are considered to be related to neurocognitive regression in CSWS [6, 48, 49, 60]. Many studies demonstrate that epileptiform activity is deleterious for learning and memory under certain experimental conditions [48, 49, 60–65], indirectly supporting the option of treatment. A recent study associated epileptiform activity during ESES with activation in the thalamocortical network and deactivation in the default mode network [38]. Since these networks seem prominent in neuropsychological processes and consolidation of memory traces during sleep, it is possible that epileptic spikes may contribute to regression in CSWS. On the other hand, the impact of interictal epileptiform activity on cognitive function may not be severe enough to serve as the sole explanation for the degree of neurocognitive regression [48, 65]. Many studies suggest that long-term neurocognitive function may significantly improve if epileptiform activity in the EEG can be reduced with antiepileptic drugs [3, 6, 7, 17, 19, 49], but this effect remains to be proven. Therefore, whether to treat epileptiform activity without a direct clinical correlate and, especially, to what extent to treat EEG findings is unclear. As a rule of thumb, we always treat the patient while considering the clinical presentation as a whole, not solely the EEG or other isolated laboratory values.

8.2. Modification of the Natural Course of the Disease by Treatment. Treatment goals of CSWS include not only improved seizure control, but also a reduction in EEG abnormalities

and potentially improvement of neurocognitive function or at least prevention of further regression. There is evidence in the literature supporting a beneficial effect of treatment on seizure frequency and severity [7, 19, 26, 36, 66–70] and epileptiform activity [19, 21, 71, 72]. Several studies suggest that long-term neurocognitive function can significantly improve once epileptiform discharges are reduced, and this effect has been related to treatment with antiepileptic drugs [3, 6, 7, 17, 19, 73–77]. However, to date, there is no scientific evidence for or against treatment of interictal spikes.

8.3. Antiepileptic Drugs. The most common antiepileptic drugs used for CSWS include valproate, ethosuximide, and levetiracetam [78]. In a series of 15 patients with CSWS treated with high-dose valproate alone or with valproate and ethosuximide, 10 cases (67%) responded with long-term control of their epilepsy and partial recovery of cognitive function [19]. In a separate study, the combination of valproate and ethosuximide was effective in 2 additional patients [7]. In contrast, other series did not report similar improvements after treatment with comparable medication regimes. Valproate was reported as not effective in 28 patients [26]; valproate and benzodiazepines did not achieve any improvement in 7 patients and were associated with adverse behavioral reactions in 3 children [30], and several case reports describe no significant improvement with valproate [67, 68, 79]. Ethosuximide was also found to lack efficacy in 7 patients with CSWS [26] and to exert only a modest effect in 3 [67]. The efficacy of levetiracetam is supported by several case reports in the literature [26, 36, 66–68, 70]. The only placebo-controlled double-blind crossover study in patients with ESES showed that treatment with levetiracetam reduced epileptiform activity (from a spike index of 56 to 37) in a series of 18 patients, although 3 other patients discontinued treatment because of negative cognitive side effects [80]. Other drugs that have been reported as effective in small series include sulthiame [26, 81] and lamotrigine [45, 82]. Phenytoin, phenobarbital, and, especially, carbamazepine and oxcarbazepine are generally avoided because they have been associated with exacerbations of epileptiform discharges in patients with ESES [82–85].

8.4. High-Dose Benzodiazepines. Benzodiazepines have demonstrated efficacy in reducing epileptiform activity in the short term. Transitory resolution of the ESES pattern was observed after the administration of clonazepam [19, 21]. Diazepam has a shorter half-life than clonazepam, which can be advantageous in a condition such as CSWS where more severe epileptiform activity occurs during the night. In a series of 4 patients with CSWS refractory to valproate and ethosuximide, a short cycle of high-dose oral or intrarectal diazepam (0.5–1 mg/Kg per day for 6-7 days) was effective in the short term in two patients [19]. In a series of 15 patients with CSWS, all patients responded to the treatment with high-dose rectal diazepam [86]. High-dose oral diazepam (0.75–1 mg/Kg/day for 3 weeks) was also efficacious in 3 out of 8 (37.5%) patients, but the response was temporary [26]. In 29 patients with ESES and different clinical presentations, the mean epileptiform activity decreased from 77% to 41% after a nocturnal administration of 1 mg/Kg of oral diazepam [72]. This reduction in epileptiform activity persisted for some months [87], but whether this reduction in epileptiform activity is accompanied by a sustained improvement in clinical features remains to be proven. Other series show that 9 out of 10 patients did not respond to valproate and benzodiazepines, and 3 patients experienced an adverse behavioral reaction [30]. Adverse effects of high-dose diazepam treatment are generally considered mild and self-limited [72, 86], but severe behavioral disinhibition and even the need for discontinuation have also been described in few children [3, 87].

8.5. Immune Modulation Therapy. Corticosteroids and intravenous immunoglobulins have shown improvement in selected cases and, in some cases, lead to complete resolution of CSWS. Once CSWS is recognized, usually during the acute phase, corticosteroid treatment should be considered. In a series of 44 children with a pattern of ESES and clinical presentations of variable severity, prolonged corticosteroid treatment (hydrocortisone 5 mg/kg/day during the first month, 4 mg/kg/day during the second month, 3 mg/kg/day during the third month, and 2 mg/kg/day during the next 9 months, followed by slow withdrawal for a total treatment duration of 21 months) led to reductions of seizures or neuropsychological improvement in 34/44 (77.3%) cases, with 34 achieving complete control of seizures and normalization of EEG abnormalities in 21 patients. The long-term remission rate was 45% [53]. However, the inclusion of milder clinical presentations could make these results difficult to compare to other series where all or most patients had clear CSWS [53]. In another series, a positive response to different corticosteroids (prednisone, methylprednisolone, or adrenocorticotrophic hormone) was observed in 11 out of 17 patients with CSWS [26]. The intramuscular administration of 0.001–0.04 mg/kg/day of adrenocorticotrophic hormone was reported to be effective in 1 out of 4 patients [19]. The side effects of corticosteroid treatments usually limit its long-term use. Only a handful of patients treated with intravenous immunoglobulins have been reported in the literature. Intravenous immunoglobulin treatment was associated with improvements in 3 out of 9 patients with CSWS [26]. In another series, the neurocognitive function of 1 out of 3 patients with CSWS improved following the administration of intravenous immunoglobulins [88]. However, there is probably a publication bias of positive results, and the high cost and risk of complications associated with immunoglobulins make their role in the treatment of CSWS unclear.

8.6. Surgical Treatment. Although classically epilepsy surgery was performed on patients with focal discharges, it has also been successfully applied to select patients with generalized discharges [89, 90]. Some patients with CSWS may also benefit from surgical treatment. Surgical interventions include multiple subpial transections (MSTs), focal resective surgery of the epileptogenic zone, hemispherectomy and corpus callosotomy. MST consists of multiple small superficial parallel cuts in the cortex that theoretically severs only the local corticocortical connections in an attempt to disrupt local epileptic circuitry without altering the vertical neural columns and their function. It has been reported to lead to recovery of age-appropriate speech in 7 patients out of a series of 14 patients with Landau-Kleffner syndrome [89], whereas a less dramatic language improvement was found in other series [91, 92]. Two patients with CSWS secondary to neonatal stroke markedly improved after hemispherectomy [93]. In another study, two patients with CSWS secondary to early developmental lesions in the thalamus became seizure-free after a hemispherectomy in one and after an extensive corticectomy around a large porencephalic cyst in the other [27]. A study evaluated epilepsy surgery in 13 patients with CSWS secondary to different early developmental lesions who underwent various surgical procedures including anterior callosotomy (6 patients), complete callosotomy (3 patients), hemispherectomy (2 patients), and lobar resection (2 patients). Subjects achieved an overall improvement in seizure control and EEG features in most patients [8].

Improvements may be related to the type of surgery performed. The cognitive deterioration may be halted in most patients; however, while there was some cognitive recovery, patients did not return to baseline. In a series of 8 patients with CSWS secondary to perinatal infarction (7 patients) and a malformation of cortical development (1 patient), 6 patients underwent a hemispherectomy, and 2 underwent focal resection. Results included disappearance of the pattern of ESES (all 8 patients), seizure freedom (6 patients), marked improvement in seizure control (2 patients), and an overall improvement in cognitive function (in 3 out of 5 patients with neuropsychological evaluation) [15]. Patients with CSWS should undergo epilepsy surgery only after a careful evaluation of potential benefits and risks in the individual patient. A tendency toward neurocognitive improvement was found in 3 out of 5 patients with CSWS after epilepsy surgery [15]. However, data on the long-term neurocognitive outcome of surgically managed CSWS patients are not available.

8.7. General Suggestions for Managing Patients with CSWS (Figure 3). Current literature does not permit the development of an evidence-based management approach to CSWS. Most of the drugs used for CSWS are selected based on individual experience, case reports, or small case series that claim efficacy for a specific drug. Responses to treatment in uncontrolled case reports or case series should be interpreted with caution as any treatment for a disorder with a fluctuating natural course tends to be initiated at the peak of severity, so that some improvement can be attributed to the natural fluctuations of the disease. In addition, other series report a lack of efficacy for commonly used treatment options for CSWS. There is no evidence on the efficacy of the ketogenic diet in patients with CSWS. Here, we provide a practical treatment approach based on case series in the literature (Figure 3). In practice, most patients with CSWS were already

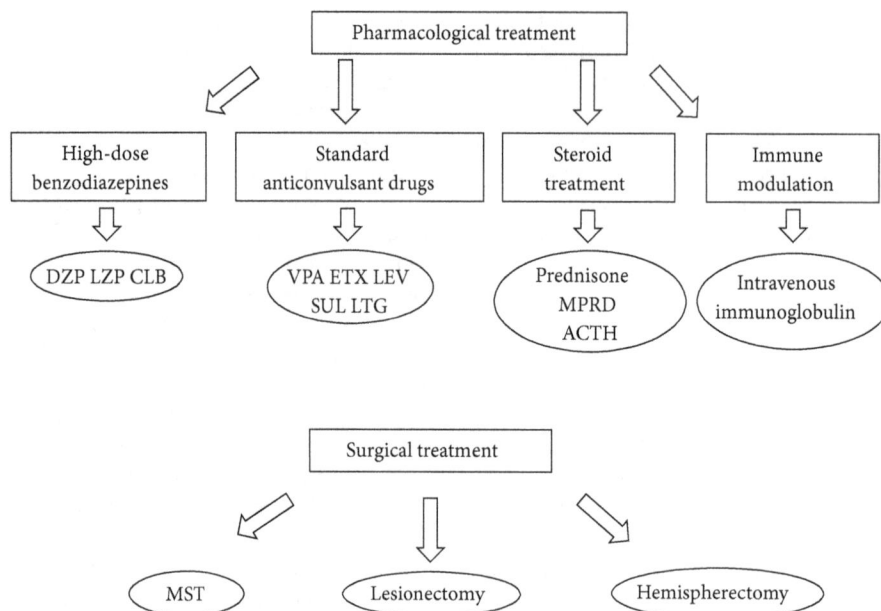

FIGURE 3: Options for the management of patients with CSWS. Options for chronic management are high-dose benzodiazepines, standard antiepileptic drugs in different combinations, and corticosteroids and immune-modulating agents. These options are considered as first choices by different authors, although standard antiepileptic drugs are generally used before the recognition of CSWS. Epilepsy surgery is reserved for few selected refractory cases. Legend: ACTH: adrenocorticotrophic hormone. CLB: clobazam. DZP: diazepam. ETX: ethosuximide. LEV: levetiracetam. LTG: lamotrigine. LZP: lorazepam. MPRD: methylprednisolone. MST: multiple subpial transection. SUL: sulthiame. VPA: valproate.

on some standard antiepileptic drug (valproate, levetirac-etam, or similar) when their seizures first began and before their condition was recognized as CSWS. Once in the acute phase, standard antiepileptic drugs, corticosteroids, and ben-zodiazepines can be considered as first choices depending on the particular patient and the familiarity of the physician with these drugs. Several groups have reported the usefulness of benzodiazepines [19, 26, 72, 86], and a frequent protocol used at our institutions is nocturnal Diazepam 1 mg/Kg during the first night followed by 0.5 mg/Kg every following night for 1–3 months [87]. For the chronic management of CSWS and par-ticularly for seizure control standard antiepileptic drugs such as valproate, ethosuximide, levetiracetam, sulthiame, and lamotrigine are frequently used. Polytherapy is often needed. Medication selection should be guided by presenting seizure types [7, 19, 26, 30, 36, 45, 66–68, 70, 78–82]. Other options include treatment with corticosteroids, adrenocorticotrophic hormone, or intravenous immunoglobulin [19, 26, 53, 88]. Epilepsy surgery should be considered, especially in patients with an early unilateral developmental lesion, even when the epileptiform activity on EEG is generalized [8, 15, 27, 89–93]. For the acute control of very active nighttime epileptiform discharges, high-dose benzodiazepines have been used over a period of a few months [19, 21, 26, 72, 86]. While adequate control of seizures improves the quality of life of the patients and should be pursued, it is unknown how aggressively inter-ictal epileptiform activity in relationship with neurocognitive regression should be treated. Only prospective studies that correlate the response to treatment of interictal epileptiform

activity with the improvement in neurocognitive function will be able to answer that relevant question.

9. Related Conditions

ESES, the EEG pattern that characterizes CSWS, can be found in other electroclinical conditions. CSWS might represent the most severe end of a continuum in which Landau-Kleffner syndrome would be an intermediate condition and "benign" focal epilepsy syndromes of childhood would be at the most benign end of the spectrum.

9.1. Landau-Kleffner Syndrome. It is an age-related epilep-tic encephalopathy where regression occurs mainly in the language spectrum and the EEG abnormalities are more centered around the temporal-parietal regions [94]. Seizures are not a prominent part of this syndrome, and they are either infrequent or do not even occur in 20–30% of cases [3, 74]. Contrary to CSWS, structural brain lesions in LKS are an exception to the rule [94]. Most antiepileptic drugs are effective for seizure control in LKS [7, 18, 21]. Corticosteroids have been reported to markedly improve the evolution of the disease [18, 53, 77], and intravenous immunoglobulins demonstrated promising results in very few cases, although immunoglobulins are expensive and associated with poten-tially serious side effects [88, 95–99]. Resective surgery is not an option because the focus of epileptiform activity frequently involves eloquent cortex, including language areas. The technique of multiple subpial transections has led to variable results [91, 92, 100]. Similar to CSWS, seizures and EEG abnormalities normalize over time, but most patients do not recover their baseline language status [76].

9.2. "Benign" Pediatric Focal Epileptic Syndromes. They include "Benign" epilepsy of childhood with central-temporal spikes, Panayiotopoulos syndrome, and Gastaut-type late-onset childhood occipital epilepsy. These syndromes share features such as a strong genetic predisposition, age-related appearance and disappearance of electroclinical manifestations, and a relatively "benign" clinical course. As in the previous syndromes, interictal epileptiform activity may be disproportionately severe in comparison with the seizure correlation. Neurocognitive dysfunction, if present, is mild. The individual description of each particular syndrome is beyond the scope of this review and can be found elsewhere [101, 102]. Because of their main features, "benign" pediatric focal epileptic syndromes may be considered as part of the electroclinical spectrum of CSWS [101, 102].

9.3. Seizure (or Spikes) Susceptibility Syndrome. CSWS, Landau-Kleffner syndrome and "benign" pediatric focal epilepsy syndromes share a series of common features: (1) an electroclinical syndrome consisting of seizures, interictal epileptiform activity, and neuropsychological deficits of different severities, (2) an age-related evolution with onset in early childhood and spontaneous improvement before puberty, (3) interictal epileptiform activity becomes markedly potentiated during non-REM sleep, (4) interictal epileptiform activity is disproportionately severe in comparison with the seizure correlate, and (5) interictal epileptiform activity frequently persists after seizure freedom. Overlap between these clinical presentations has led to the hypothesis of a common seizure susceptibility syndrome. In this syndrome, the different electroclinical presentations reflect different severities of a common underlying pathophysiology, similar to what happens with the different clinical presentations of hypsarrhythmia. A genetic or acquired disruption of the neural networks early in development would create hyperexcitable neural networks [57, 58] that, depending on its severity and localization, could manifest as different electroclinical presentations in the spectrum [27, 54, 56, 101, 103].

10. Conclusions

CSWS is an age-related epileptic encephalopathy that represents the most severe end of the childhood seizure susceptibility syndrome. Its characterizing features are (1) seizures, (2) interictal epileptiform activity that becomes prominent during sleep leading to the electroencephalogram pattern of ESES, and (3) neurocognitive regression. The etiology of CSWS is unknown, but early developmental lesions play a major role in around half of the cases. The neurocognitive outcome is generally poor, and it is currently unknown whether treatment can modify it. High-dose benzodiazepines have been used successfully to decrease very active epileptiform discharges. Polytherapy with combinations of valproate, ethosuximide, levetiracetam, sulthiame or lamotrigine, and corticosteroids is frequently used. Epilepsy surgery can be considered in a few very selected number of patients. A better understanding of the response to treatment, the electroclinical spectrum, and the underlying pathophysiology may allow for the development of an evidence-based management approach in the future.

Conflict of Interests

The authors do not have any conflict of interests relevant to this paper to disclose.

Acknowledgments

Iván Sánchez Fernández is funded by a grant for the study of Epileptic Encephalopathies from "Fundación Alfonso Martín Escudero." Kevin E. Chapman performs, interprets, and bills for clinical neurophysiology procedures, including EEGs, at Children's Hospital Colorado. Jurriaan M. Peters is supported by National Institutes of Health P20 RFA-NS-12-006 and 1U01NS082320-01 Grants, by the World Federation of Neurology Grant-in-Aid Competition, and by a Faculty Development Fellowship from the "Eleanor and Miles Shore 50th Anniversary Fellowship Program for Scholars in Medicine," Boston Children's Hospital, Department of Neurology, 2012-2013. He performs video-EEG long-term monitoring, EEGs, and other electrophysiological studies at Boston Children's Hospital and bills for these procedures. Chellamani Harini performs, interprets, and bills for clinical neurophysiology procedures, including EEGs, at Boston Children's Hospital. Alexander Rotenberg performs, interprets, and bills for clinical neurophysiology procedures, including EEGs, at Boston Children's Hospital. Dr. Rotenberg's salary and research are supported by grants, unrelated to the present paper, from the Department of Defense, NIH NINDS, the Epilepsy Therapy Project, CIMIT, the AlRashed Family Foundation, the Fisher Family Foundation, and the Translational Research Program at Boston Children's Hospital. He serves as an Associate Editor at the Journal of Pediatric Neurology. Tobias Loddenkemper serves on the Laboratory Accreditation Board for Long-Term (Epilepsy and ICU) Monitoring (ABRET); he serves as a Member of the American Clinical Neurophysiology Council (ACNS) and serves on the American Board of Clinical Neurophysiology and serves as an Associate Editor of Seizure. He performs Video EEG long-term monitoring, EEGs, and other electrophysiological studies at Children's Hospital Boston and bills for these procedures and receives support from NIH/NINDS 1R21NS076859-01 (2011–2013). He is supported by a Career Development Fellowship Award from Harvard Medical School and Children's Hospital Boston, by the Program for Quality and Safety at Children's Hospital Boston, the Translational Research Project, and by the Payer Provider Quality Initiative. He receives funding from the Epilepsy Foundation of America (EF-213583 & EF-213882), from the Center for Integration of Medicine & Innovative Technology (CIMIT), Citizens United for Research in Epilepsy (CURE), the Epilepsy Therapy Project, and an infrastructure grant from the American Epilepsy Society and received investigator initiated research support from Eisai Inc. and Lundbeck.

References

[1] "Commission on Classification and Terminology of the International League Against Epilepsy. Proposal for revised classification of epilepsies and epileptic syndromes," *Epilepsia*, vol. 30, pp. 389–399, 1989.

[2] T. Loddenkemper, I. Sánchez Fernández, and J. M. Peters, "Continuous spike and waves during sleep and electrical status epilepticus in sleep," *Journal of Clinical Neurophysiology*, vol. 28, pp. 154–164, 2011.

[3] K. Nickels and E. Wirrell, "Electrical Status Epilepticus in Sleep," *Seminars in Pediatric Neurology*, vol. 15, no. 2, pp. 50–60, 2008.

[4] I. Sánchez Fernández, T. Loddenkemper, J. M. Peters, and S. V. Kothare, "Electrical status epilepticus in sleep: clinical presentation and pathophysiology," *Pediatric Neurology*, vol. 47, pp. 390–410, 2012.

[5] C. A. Tassinari, G. Cantalupo, B. Dalla Bernardina et al., "Encephalopathy related to status epilepticus during slow sleep (ESES) including Landau-Kleffner syndrome," in *Epileptic Syndromes in Infancy, Childhood and Adolescence*, M. Bureau, P. Genton, C. Dravet et al., Eds., pp. 255–275, John Libbey Eurotext, London, UK, 5th edition, 2012.

[6] C. A. Tassinari, G. Rubboli, L. Volpi et al., "Encephalopathy with electrical status epilepticus during slow sleep or ESES syndrome including the acquired aphasia," *Clinical Neurophysiology*, vol. 111, no. 2, supplement, pp. S94–S102, 2000.

[7] E. Liukkonen, E. Kantola-Sorsa, R. Paetau, E. Gaily, M. Peltola, and M.-L. Granström, "Long-term outcome of 32 children with encephalopathy with status epilepticus during sleep, or ESES syndrome," *Epilepsia*, vol. 51, no. 10, pp. 2023–2032, 2010.

[8] M. E. Peltola, E. Liukkonen, M.-L. Granström et al., "The effect of surgery in encephalopathy with electrical status epilepticus during sleep," *Epilepsia*, vol. 52, no. 3, pp. 602–609, 2011.

[9] I. Sánchez Fernández, K. E. Chapman, J. M. Peters et al., "The tower of Babel: survey on concepts and terminology in electrical status epilepticus in sleep and continuous spikes and waves during sleep in North America," *Epilepsia*, vol. 54, pp. 741–750, 2013.

[10] J. Engel Jr., "Report of the ILAE classification core group," *Epilepsia*, vol. 47, no. 9, pp. 1558–1568, 2006.

[11] U. Kramer, Y. Nevo, M. Y. Neufeld, A. Fatal, Y. Leitner, and S. Harel, "Epidemiology of epilepsy in childhood: a cohort of 440 consecutive patients," *Pediatric Neurology*, vol. 18, no. 1, pp. 46–50, 1998.

[12] Y. Eksioglu, E. Tas, M. Takeoka et al., "Clinical presentation and acute treatment of electrical status epilepticus in sleep and sleep potentiated spikes," *Neurology*, vol. 72, 2009.

[13] T. Morikawa, M. Seino, Y. Watanabe, M. Watanabe, and K. Yagi, "Clinical relevance of continuous spike-waves during slow wave sleep," in *Advances in Epileptology*, S. Manelis, E. Bental, J. Loeber, and F. Dreifuss, Eds., pp. 359–363, Raven Press, New York, NY, USA, 1989.

[14] A. S. Harvey, J. H. Cross, S. Shinnar, and G. W. Mathern, "Defining the spectrum of international practice in pediatric epilepsy surgery patients," *Epilepsia*, vol. 49, no. 1, pp. 146–155, 2008.

[15] T. Loddenkemper, G. Cosmo, P. Kotagal et al., "Epilepsy surgery in children with electrical status epilepticus in sleep," *Neurosurgery*, vol. 64, no. 2, pp. 328–337, 2009.

[16] M. Bureau, "Outstanding cases of CSWS and LKS: analysis of the data sheets provided by the participants," in *Continuous Spikes and Waves during Slow Sleep*, A. Beaumanoir, M. Bureau, L. Deonna, L. Mira, and C. A. Tassinari, Eds., pp. 213–216, John Libbey, London, UK, 1995.

[17] R. H. Caraballo, L. Bongiorni, R. Cersósimo, M. Semprino, A. Espeche, and N. Fejerman, "Epileptic encephalopathy with continuous spikes and waves during sleep in children with shunted hydrocephalus: a study of nine cases," *Epilepsia*, vol. 49, no. 9, pp. 1520–1527, 2008.

[18] A. S. Galanopoulou, A. Bojko, F. Lado, and S. L. Moshé, "The spectrum of neuropsychiatric abnormalities associated with electrical status epilepticus in sleep," *Brain and Development*, vol. 22, no. 5, pp. 279–295, 2000.

[19] M. Inutsuka, K. Kobayashi, M. Oka, J. Hattori, and Y. Ohtsuka, "Treatment of epilepsy with electrical status epilepticus during slow sleep and its related disorders," *Brain and Development*, vol. 28, no. 5, pp. 281–286, 2006.

[20] M. Van Hirtum-Das, E. A. Licht, S. Koh, J. Y. Wu, W. D. Shields, and R. Sankar, "Children with ESES: variability in the syndrome," *Epilepsy Research*, vol. 70, supplement, pp. S248–S258, 2006.

[21] X. Yan Liu and V. Wong, "Spectrum of epileptic syndromes with electrical status epilepticus during sleep in children," *Pediatric Neurology*, vol. 22, no. 5, pp. 371–379, 2000.

[22] X. De Tiège, S. Goldman, S. Laureys et al., "Regional cerebral glucose metabolism in epilepsies with continuous spikes and waves during sleep," *Neurology*, vol. 63, no. 5, pp. 853–857, 2004.

[23] X. De Tiège, N. Ligot, S. Goldman, N. Poznanski, A. de Saint Martin, and P. Van Bogaert, "Metabolic evidence for remote inhibition in epilepsies with continuous spike-waves during sleep," *NeuroImage*, vol. 40, no. 2, pp. 802–810, 2008.

[24] I. Sánchez Fernández, J. M. Peters, S. Hadjiloizou et al., "Clinical staging and electroencephalographic evolution of continuous spikes and waves during sleep," *Epilepsia*, vol. 53, no. 7, pp. 1185–1195, 2012.

[25] M. Bureau, ""Continuous spikes and waves during slow sleep" (CSWS): definition of the syndrome," in *Continuous Spikes and Waves During Slow Sleep*, A. Beaumanoir, M. Bureau, L. Deonna, L. Mira, and C. A. Tassinari, Eds., pp. 17–26, John Libbey, London, UK, 1995.

[26] U. Kramer, L. Sagi, H. Goldberg-Stern, N. Zelnik, A. Nissenkorn, and B. Ben-Zeev, "Clinical spectrum and medical treatment of children with electrical status epilepticus in sleep (ESES)," *Epilepsia*, vol. 50, no. 6, pp. 1517–1524, 2009.

[27] F. Guzzetta, D. Battaglia, C. Veredice et al., "Early thalamic injury associated with epilepsy and continuous spike-wave during slow sleep," *Epilepsia*, vol. 46, no. 6, pp. 889–900, 2005.

[28] L. Mira, B. Oxilia, and A. Van Lierde, "Cognitive assessment of children with CSWS syndrome: a critical review of data from 155 cases submitted to the Venice colloquium," in *Continuous Spikes and Waves During Slow Sleep*, A. Beaumanoir, M. Bureau, L. Deonna, L. Mira, and C. A. Tassinari, Eds., pp. 229–242, John Libbey, London, UK, 1995.

[29] T. Morikawa, M. Seino, and M. Watanabe, "Long-term outcome of CSWS syndrome," in *Continuous Spikes and Waves during Slow Sleep*, A. Beaumanoir, M. Bureau, L. Deonna, L. Mira, and C. A. Tassinari, Eds., pp. 27–36, John Libbey, London, UK, 1995.

[30] F. B. J. Scholtes, M. P. H. Hendriks, and W. O. Renier, "Cognitive deterioration and electrical status epilepticus during slow sleep," *Epilepsy and Behavior*, vol. 6, no. 2, pp. 167–173, 2005.

[31] A. Beaumanoir, "EEG data," in *Continuous Spikes and Waves during Slow Sleep*, A. Beaumanoir, M. Bureau, L. Deonna, L. Mira, and C. A. Tassinari, Eds., pp. 217–223, John Libbey, London, UK, 1995.

[32] B. Dalla Bernardina, C. A. Tassinari, and C. Dravet, "Benign focal epilepsy and "electrical status epilepticus" during sleep," *Revue d'E.E.G. et de Neuro-Physiologie Clinique*, vol. 8, no. 3, pp. 350–353, 1978.

[33] G. Laurette and G. Arfel, "Electrical "status epilepticus" during afternoon sleep," *Revue d'E.E.G. et de Neuro-Physiologie Clinique*, vol. 6, no. 1, pp. 137–139, 1976.

[34] G. Patry, S. Lyagoubi, and C. A. Tassinari, "Subclinical "electrical status epilepticus" induced by sleep in children. A clinical and electroencephalographic study of six cases," *Archives of Neurology*, vol. 24, no. 3, pp. 242–252, 1971.

[35] S. Saltik, D. Uluduz, O. Cokar, V. Demirbilek, and A. Dervent, "A clinical and EEG study on idiopathic partial epilepsies with evolution into ESES spectrum disorders," *Epilepsia*, vol. 46, no. 4, pp. 524–533, 2005.

[36] A. Aeby, N. Poznanski, D. Verheulpen, C. Wetzburger, and P. Van Bogaert, "Levetiracetam efficacy in epileptic syndromes with continuous spikes and waves during slow sleep: experience in 12 cases," *Epilepsia*, vol. 46, no. 12, pp. 1937–1942, 2005.

[37] J. R. Hughes, "A review of the relationships between Landau-Kleffner syndrome, electrical status epilepticus during sleep, and continuous spike-waves during sleep," *Epilepsy and Behavior*, vol. 20, no. 2, pp. 247–253, 2011.

[38] M. Siniatchkin, K. Groening, J. Moehring et al., "Neuronal networks in children with continuous spikes and waves during slow sleep," *Brain*, vol. 133, no. 9, pp. 2798–2813, 2010.

[39] P. Veggiotti, F. Beccaria, R. Guerrini, G. Capovilla, and G. Lanzi, "Continuous spike-and-wave activity during slow-wave sleep: syndrome or EEG pattern?" *Epilepsia*, vol. 40, no. 11, pp. 1593–1601, 1999.

[40] S. H. G. Kevelam, F. E. Jansen, E. V. Binsbergen et al., "Copy number variations in patients with electrical status epilepticus in sleep," *Journal of Child Neurology*, vol. 27, no. 2, pp. 178–182, 2012.

[41] K. Kobayashi, H. Hata, M. Oka et al., "Age-related electrical status epilepticus during sleep and epileptic negative myoclonus in DRPLA," *Neurology*, vol. 66, no. 5, pp. 772–773, 2006.

[42] V. Chavakula, I. Sanchez Fernandez, J. M. Peters et al., "Automated quantification of spikes," *Epilepsy & Behavior*, vol. 26, pp. 143–152, 2013.

[43] R. Massa, A. De Saint-Martin, E. Hirsch et al., "Landau-Kleffner syndrome: sleep EEG characteristics at onset," *Clinical Neurophysiology*, vol. 111, no. 2, supplement, pp. S87–S93, 2000.

[44] I. Sánchez Fernández, J. Peters, M. Takeoka et al., "Patients with electrical status epilepticus in sleep share similar clinical features regardless of their focal or generalized sleep potentiation of epileptiform activity," *Journal of Child Neurology*, vol. 28, pp. 83–89, 2013.

[45] R. Guerrini, P. Genton, M. Bureau et al., "Multilobar polymicrogyria, intractable drop attack seizures, and sleep-related electrical status epilepticus," *Neurology*, vol. 51, no. 2, pp. 504–512, 1998.

[46] Y. Ohtsuka, A. Tanaka, K. Kobayashi et al., "Childhood-onset epilepsy associated with polymicrogyria," *Brain and Development*, vol. 24, no. 8, pp. 758–765, 2002.

[47] C. Seegmüller, T. Deonna, C. Mayor Dubois et al., "Long-term outcome after cognitive and behavioral regression in nonlesional epilepsy with continuous spike-waves during slow-wave sleep," *Epilepsia*, vol. 53, pp. 1067–1076, 2012.

[48] A. P. Aldenkamp and J. Arends, "Effects of epileptiform EEG discharges on cognitive function: is the concept of "transient cognitive impairment" still valid?" *Epilepsy and Behavior*, vol. 5, no. 1, supplement, pp. S25–S34, 2004.

[49] C. A. Tassinari, G. Cantalupo, L. Rios-Pohl, E. D. Giustina, and G. Rubboli, "Encephalopathy with status epilepticus during slow sleep: "the penelope syndrome"," *Epilepsia*, vol. 50, no. 7, supplement, pp. 4–8, 2009.

[50] G. Incorpora, P. Pavone, P. G. Smilari, P. Trifiletti, and E. Parano, "Late primary unilateral thalamic hemorrhage in infancy: report of two cases," *Neuropediatrics*, vol. 30, no. 5, pp. 264–267, 1999.

[51] A. Kelemen, P. Barsi, Z. Gyorsok, J. Sarac, A. Szucs, and P. Halász, "Thalamic lesion and epilepsy with generalized seizures, ESES and spike-wave paroxysms—report of three cases," *Seizure*, vol. 15, no. 6, pp. 454–458, 2006.

[52] J. P. Monteiro, E. Roulet-Perez, V. Davidoff, and T. Deonna, "Primary neonatal thalamic haemorrhage and epilepsy with continuous spike-wave during sleep: a longitudinal follow-up of a possible significant relation," *European Journal of Paediatric Neurology*, vol. 5, no. 1, pp. 41–47, 2001.

[53] M. Buzatu, C. Bulteau, C. Altuzarra, O. Dulac, and P. Van Bogaert, "Corticosteroids as treatment of epileptic syndromes with continuous spike-waves during slow-wave sleep," *Epilepsia*, vol. 50, no. 7, supplement, pp. 68–72, 2009.

[54] I. Sánchez Fernández, M. Takeoka, and E. Tas, "Early thalamic lesions in patients with sleep-potentiated epileptiform activity," *Neurology*, vol. 78, pp. 1721–1727, 2012.

[55] A. J. Barkovich, R. Guerrini, R. I. Kuzniecky, G. D. Jackson, and W. B. Dobyns, "A developmental and genetic classification for malformations of cortical development: update 2012," *Brain*, vol. 135, no. 5, pp. 1348–1369, 2012.

[56] M. P. Beenhakker and J. R. Huguenard, "Neurons that fire together also conspire together: is normal sleep circuitry hijacked to generate epilepsy?" *Neuron*, vol. 62, no. 5, pp. 612–632, 2009.

[57] J. T. Paz, A. S. Bryant, K. Peng et al., "A new mode of corticothalamic transmission revealed in the Gria4 -/- model of absence epilepsy," *Nature Neuroscience*, vol. 14, no. 9, pp. 1167–1175, 2011.

[58] J. T. Paz, C. A. Christian, I. Parada, D. A. Prince, and J. R. Huguenard, "Focal cortical infarcts alter intrinsic excitability and synaptic excitation in the reticular thalamic nucleus," *Journal of Neuroscience*, vol. 30, no. 15, pp. 5465–5479, 2010.

[59] J. T. Paz, T. J. Davidson, and E. S. Frechette, "Closed-loop optogenetic control of thalamus as a tool for interrupting seizures after cortical injury," *Nature Neuroscience*, vol. 16, pp. 64–70, 2013.

[60] G. L. Holmes and P.-P. Lenck-Santini, "Role of interictal epileptiform abnormalities in cognitive impairment," *Epilepsy and Behavior*, vol. 8, no. 3, pp. 504–515, 2006.

[61] B. K. Bölsterli, B. Schmitt, T. Bast et al., "Impaired slow wave sleep downscaling in encephalopathy with status epilepticus during sleep (ESES)," *Clinical Neurophysiology*, vol. 122, no. 9, pp. 1779–1787, 2011.

[62] S. Diekelmann and J. Born, "The memory function of sleep," *Nature Reviews Neuroscience*, vol. 11, no. 2, pp. 114–126, 2010.

[63] E. A. Licht, R. H. Jacobsen, and D. G. Fujikawa, "Chronically impaired frontal lobe function from subclinical epileptiform discharges," *Epilepsy and Behavior*, vol. 3, no. 1, pp. 96–100, 2002.

[64] K. Majak and A. Pitkänen, "Do seizures cause irreversible cognitive damage? Evidence from animal studies," *Epilepsy and Behavior*, vol. 5, no. 1, supplement, pp. S35–S44, 2004.

[65] J. Nicolai, S. Ebus, D. P. L. J. J. G. Biemans et al., "The cognitive effects of interictal epileptiform EEG discharges and short nonconvulsive epileptic seizures," *Epilepsia*, vol. 53, pp. 1051–1059, 2012.

[66] M. Atkins and M. Nikanorova, "A prospective study of levetiracetam efficacy in epileptic syndromes with continuous spikes-waves during slow sleep," *Seizure*, vol. 20, no. 8, pp. 635–639, 2011.

[67] G. Capovilla, F. Beccaria, S. Cagdas, A. Montagnini, R. Segala, and D. Paganelli, "Efficacy of levetiracetam in pharmacoresistant continuous spikes and waves during slow sleep," *Acta Neurologica Scandinavica*, vol. 110, no. 3, pp. 144–147, 2004.

[68] T. Hoppen, T. Sandrieser, and M. Rister, "Successful treatment of pharmacoresistent continuous spike wave activity during slow sleep with levetiracetam," *European Journal of Pediatrics*, vol. 162, no. 1, pp. 59–61, 2003.

[69] P. G. Larsson, K. A. Bakke, H. Bjørnæs et al., "The effect of levetiracetam on focal nocturnal epileptiform activity during sleep - A placebo-controlled double-blind cross-over study," *Epilepsy and Behavior*, vol. 24, pp. 44–48, 2012.

[70] S.-B. Wang, W.-C. Weng, P.-C. Fan, and W.-T. Lee, "Levetiracetam in continuous spike waves during slow-wave sleep syndrome," *Pediatric Neurology*, vol. 39, no. 2, pp. 85–90, 2008.

[71] N. Bahi-Buisson, R. Savini, M. Eisermann et al., "Misleading effects of clonazepam in symptomatic electrical status epilepticus during sleep syndrome," *Pediatric Neurology*, vol. 34, no. 2, pp. 146–150, 2006.

[72] I. Sánchez Fernández, S. Hadjiloizou, Y. Eksioglu et al., "Short-term response of sleep-potentiated spiking to high-dose diazepam in electric status epilepticus during sleep," *Pediatric Neurology*, vol. 46, no. 5, pp. 312–318, 2012.

[73] D. Brazzo, M. C. Pera, M. Fasce, G. Papalia, U. Balottin, and P. Veggiotti, "Epileptic encephalopathies with status epilepticus during sleep: new techniques for understanding pathophysiology and therapeutic options," *Epilepsy Research and Treatment*, vol. 2012, Article ID 642725, 6 pages, 2012.

[74] L. Nieuwenhuis and J. Nicolai, "The pathophysiological mechanisms of cognitive and behavioral disturbances in children with Landau-Kleffner syndrome or epilepsy with continuous spike-and-waves during slow-wave sleep," *Seizure*, vol. 15, no. 4, pp. 249–258, 2006.

[75] R. O. Robinson, G. Baird, G. Robinson, and E. Simonoff, "Landau-Kleffner syndrome: course and correlates with outcome," *Developmental Medicine and Child Neurology*, vol. 43, no. 4, pp. 243–247, 2001.

[76] P. Giovanardi Rossi, A. Parmeggiani, A. Posar, M. C. Scaduto, S. Chiodo, and G. Vatti, "Landau-Kleffner syndrome (LKS): long-term follow-up and links with electrical status epilepticus during sleep (ESES)," *Brain and Development*, vol. 21, no. 2, pp. 90–98, 1999.

[77] D. B. Sinclair and T. J. Snyder, "Corticosteroids for the treatment of Landau-Kleffner syndrome and continuous spike-wave discharge during sleep," *Pediatric Neurology*, vol. 32, no. 5, pp. 300–306, 2005.

[78] P. Veggiotti, M. C. Pera, F. Teutonico, D. Brazzo, U. Balottin, and C. A. Tassinari, "Therapy of encephalopathy with status epilepticus during sleep (ESES/CSWS syndrome): an update," *Epileptic Disorders*, vol. 14, no. 1, pp. 1–11, 2012.

[79] Ç. Okuyaz, K. Aydin, K. Gücüyener, and A. Serdaroğlu, "Treatment of electrical status epilepticus during slow-wave sleep with high-dose corticosteroid," *Pediatric Neurology*, vol. 32, no. 1, pp. 64–67, 2005.

[80] P. G. Larsson, K. A. Bakke, H. Bjørnæs et al., "The effect of levetiracetam on focal nocturnal epileptiform activity during sleep—a placebo-controlled double-blind cross-over study," *Epilepsy and Behavior*, vol. 24, pp. 44–48, 2012.

[81] E. Wirrell, A. W.-C. Ho, and L. Hamiwka, "Sulthiame therapy for continuous spike and wave in slow-wave sleep," *Pediatric Neurology*, vol. 35, no. 3, pp. 204–208, 2006.

[82] A. Van Lierde, "Therapeutic data," in *Continuous Spikes and Waves during Slow Sleep*, A. Beaumanoir, M. Bureau, L. Deonna, L. Mira, and C. A. Tassinari, Eds., pp. 225–227, John Libbey, London, UK, 1995.

[83] P. Lerman, "Seizures induced or aggravated by anticonvulsants," *Epilepsia*, vol. 27, no. 6, pp. 706–710, 1986.

[84] C. Marescaux, E. Hirsch, S. Finck et al., "Landau-Kleffner syndrome: a pharmacologic study of five cases," *Epilepsia*, vol. 31, no. 6, pp. 768–777, 1990.

[85] O. C. Snead III and L. C. Hosey, "Exacerbation of seizures in children by carbamazepine," *New England Journal of Medicine*, vol. 313, no. 15, pp. 916–921, 1985.

[86] M. De Negri, M. G. Baglietto, F. M. Battaglia, R. Gaggero, A. Pessagno, and L. Recanati, "Treatment of electrical status epilepticus by short diazepam (DZP) cycles after DZP rectal bolus test," *Brain and Development*, vol. 17, no. 5, pp. 330–333, 1995.

[87] I. Sánchez Fernández, J. M. Peters, S. An et al., "Long-term response to high-dose diazepam treatment in continuous spikes and waves during sleep," *Pediatric Neurology*, 2013.

[88] W. F. M. Arts, F. K. Aarsen, M. Scheltens-De Boer, and C. E. Catsman-Berrevoets, "Landau-Kleffner syndrome and CSWS syndrome: treatment with intravenous immunoglobulins," *Epilepsia*, vol. 50, no. 7, pp. 55–58, 2009.

[89] A. Moosa, T. Loddenkemper, and E. Wyllie, "Epilepsy surgery for congenital or early lesions," in *Pediatric Epilepsy Surgery: Preoperative Assessment and Surgical Intervention*, O. Cataltepe and G. Jallo, Eds., pp. 14–23, Thieme Medical Publishers, New York, NY, USA, 2010.

[90] E. Wyllie, D. K. Lachhwani, A. Gupta et al., "Successful surgery for epilepsy due to early brain lesions despite generalized EEG findings," *Neurology*, vol. 69, no. 4, pp. 389–397, 2007.

[91] J. H. Cross and B. G. R. Neville, "The surgical treatment of Landau-Kleffner syndrome," *Epilepsia*, vol. 50, no. 7, supplement, pp. 63–67, 2009.

[92] K. Irwin, J. Lees, C. Polkey et al., "Multiple subpial transection in Landau-Kleffner syndrome," *Developmental Medicine and Child Neurology*, vol. 43, no. 4, pp. 248–252, 2001.

[93] D. Battaglia, P. Veggiotti, D. Lettori et al., "Functional hemispherectomy in children with epilepsy and CSWS due to unilateral early brain injury including thalamus: sudden recovery of CSWS," *Epilepsy Research*, vol. 87, no. 2-3, pp. 290–298, 2009.

[94] W. M. Landau and F. R. Kleffner, "Syndrome of acquired aphasia with convulsive disorder in children," *Neurology*, vol. 7, no. 8, pp. 523–530, 1957.

[95] M. N. Fayad, R. Choueiri, and M. Mikati, "Landau-kleffner syndrome: consistent response to repeated intravenous γ-globulin doses: a case report," *Epilepsia*, vol. 38, no. 4, pp. 489–494, 1997.

[96] L. G. Lagae, J. Silberstein, P. L. Gillis, and P. J. Casaer, "Successful use of intravenous immunoglobulins in Landau-Kleffner syndrome," *Pediatric Neurology*, vol. 18, no. 2, pp. 165–168, 1998.

[97] M. A. Mikati and R. Saab, "Successful use of intravenous immunoglobulin as initial monotherapy in Landau-Kleffner syndrome," *Epilepsia*, vol. 41, no. 7, pp. 880–886, 2000.

[98] M. A. Mikati, R. Saab, M. N. Fayad, and R. N. Choueiri, "Efficacy of intravenous immunoglobulin in Landau-Kleffner syndrome," *Pediatric Neurology*, vol. 26, no. 4, pp. 298–300, 2002.

[99] M. A. Mikati and A. N. Shamseddine, "Management of Landau-Kleffner syndrome," *Pediatric Drugs*, vol. 7, no. 6, pp. 377–389, 2005.

[100] F. Morrell, W. W. Whisler, M. C. Smith et al., "Landau-Kleffner syndrome. Treatment with subpial intracortical transection," *Brain*, vol. 118, no. 6, pp. 1529–1546, 1995.

[101] C. P. Panayiotopoulos, M. Michael, S. Sanders, T. Valeta, and M. Koutroumanidis, "Benign childhood focal epilepsies: assessment of established and newly recognized syndromes," *Brain*, vol. 131, no. 9, pp. 2264–2286, 2008.

[102] I. Sánchez Fernández and T. Loddenkemper, "Pediatric focal epilepsy syndromes," *Journal of Clinical Neurophysiology*, vol. 29, pp. 425–440, 2012.

[103] M. Koutroumanidis, "Panayiotopoulos syndrome: an important electroclinical example of benign childhood system epilepsy," *Epilepsia*, vol. 48, no. 6, pp. 1044–1053, 2007.

[104] "Case reports," in *Continuous Spikes and Waves during Slow Wave Sleep*, A. Beaumanoir, M. Bureau, L. Deonna, L. Mira, and C. A. Tassinari, Eds., pp. 169–210, John Libbey, London, UK, 1995.

[105] J. Praline, M.-A. Barthez, P. Castelnau et al., "Atypical language impairment in two siblings: relationship with electrical status epilepticus during slow wave sleep," *Journal of the Neurological Sciences*, vol. 249, no. 2, pp. 166–171, 2006.

[106] W. M. A. Verhoeven, J. I. M. Egger, I. Feenstra, and N. de Leeuw, "A de novo 3.57 Mb microdeletion in 8q12.3q13.2 in a patient with mild intellectual disability and epilepsy," *European Journal of Medical Genetics*, vol. 55, pp. 358–361, 2012.

[107] C. Godfraind, M. Coutelier, S. Andries et al., "Neuroserpin mutation causes electrical status epilepticus of slow-wave sleep," *Neurology*, vol. 71, no. 1, pp. 64–66, 2008.

[108] T. Nakayama, S. Nabatame, Y. Saito et al., "8p deletion and 9p duplication in two children with electrical status epilepticus in sleep syndrome," *Seizure*, vol. 21, no. 4, pp. 295–299, 2012.

[109] M. Broli, F. Bisulli, M. Mastrangelo et al., "Definition of the neurological phenotype associated with dup (X)(p11.22-p11.23)," *Epileptic Disorders*, vol. 13, no. 3, pp. 240–251, 2011.

[110] R. Giorda, M. C. Bonaglia, S. Beri et al., "Complex segmental duplications mediate a recurrent dup(X)(p11.22-p11.23) associated with mental retardation, speech delay, and EEG anomalies in males and females," *American Journal of Human Genetics*, vol. 85, no. 3, pp. 394–400, 2009.

[111] H. C. Mefford, S. C. Yendle, C. Hsu et al., "Rare copy number variants are an important cause of epileptic encephalopathies," *Annals of Neurology*, vol. 70, no. 6, pp. 974–985, 2011.

[112] C. Reutlinger, I. Helbig, B. Gawelczyk et al., "Deletions in 16p13 including GRIN2A in patients with intellectual disability, various dysmorphic features, and seizure disorders of the rolandic region," *Epilepsia*, vol. 51, no. 9, pp. 1870–1873, 2010.

4

Choice of Antiepileptic Drugs in Idiopathic Generalized Epilepsy: UAE Experience

Taoufik Alsaadi, Haytham Taha, and Fatema Al Hammadi

Department of Neurology, Sheikh Khalifa Medical City, Abu Dhabi 51900, UAE

Correspondence should be addressed to Taoufik Alsaadi; talsaadi@live.ca

Academic Editor: József Janszky

We retrospectively reviewed the electroencephalogram (EEG) reports of patients at our EEG lab from the years 2005–2010 to identify patients referred from the epilepsy clinic, with a confirmed diagnosis of idiopathic generalized epilepsy (IGE) by EEG criteria. We sought to report our experience in UAE of how often patients with IGE are placed on nonspecific antiepileptic drugs (AEDs) before being evaluated at an epilepsy referral clinic. 109 patients with a confirmed diagnosis of IGE based on EEG criteria were identified. When initially seen, 32.11% were taking a broad-spectrum (specific) AED only, 25.69% were taking a narrow-spectrum (nonspecific) AED, and 15.59% were placed on various combinations. Of the total patients who were receiving nonspecific AEDs, 35.71% were seizure-free and 64.28% were poorly controlled accounting for "pseudointractability status." When converted to broad-spectrum (specific) AEDs, 50% became well controlled. Furthermore, 26.6% of patients, who were previously on no AED prior to the clinic visit, became well controlled once placed on specific AED.

1. Introduction

Idiopathic generalized epilepsy (IGE) comprises a wide variety of epileptic syndromes that are believed to have a strong genetic basis [1] and, as a group, have the highest rate of complete seizure control with the use of broad-spectrum (specific) antiepileptic drugs (AEDs) [2]. Patients with IGE often have a family history of epilepsy that tend to present during childhood or adolescence, although they may not be diagnosed or begin until adulthood (adult onset IGE) [1, 3–5]. They often have normal intelligence, normal neurological examination, and normal magnetic resonance imaging (MRI) scan. The electroencephalogram (EEG) is the only definitive test to confirm the diagnosis of IGE and, when abnormal, it can be very characteristic of the syndrome, showing generalized spikes and polyspike complexes of 3-4 Hz, or faster frequency, superimposed on a normal EEG background [6–8]. In general, IGEs respond well to treatment, with 70–80% being fully controlled. However, not all AEDs are equally effective in treating IGE. The use of narrow-spectrum (nonspecific) AEDs, such as carbamazepine (CBZ) and phenytoin (PHT), either in monotherapy or in combination, is a common wrong practice, which could account for the seemingly difficult to control seizures "pseudointractability" in some reported series [1, 9–11].

2. Methods

We retrospectively reviewed the EEG reports of all patients seen at our EEG lab in the period from the years 2005–2010. Patients with EEG criteria consistent with a diagnosis of IGE and referred from the epilepsy clinic at SKMC were identified. For those identified patients, we reviewed their charts, demographic data, workup for epilepsy, age of onset, seizure types, seizure frequency, and their history of AED use, prior to their evaluation at a specialized epilepsy clinic. This clinic was established in mid June 2006, with the objective of providing a comprehensive evaluation for patients with refractory epilepsy. The clinic is managed by an epileptologist along with other neurologists and supportive staff. We recorded the seizure response rate based on the patients' last 6 months clinic visits and compared it to a 6-month period following their evaluation at the epilepsy

TABLE 1: Patient demographics.

Total number	109
Mean age	26
Male	50
Female	59
Duration of seizures (mean)	10 years
Age of onset (mean)	16
Age >20	24 (22.01%)
EEG (IGE alone)	96 (88.07%)
EEG (IGE + Focality)	13 (11.92%)
Family History of seizures, excluding febrile Sz	17 (15.59%) 1st degree relatives, 5 (4.58%) 2nd degree relatives

TABLE 2: Epilepsy/seizure types.

Epilepsy type	Seizure types	Total patients
Idiopathic generalized epilepsy with generalized tonic clonic seizures	(89) 100% GTCs	89 (81.65%)
Juvenile myoclonic epilepsy	15 (88%) GTCs 17 (100%) myoclonic	17 (15.59%)
Juvenile absence epilepsy	3 (100%) GTCS 3 (100%) absences	3 (2.75%)

TABLE 3: Prior AED use.

Patients on no prior AED	29 (26.60%)
Patients on specific AED	35 (32.11%)
Patients on nonspecific AED	28 (25.69%)
Patients on combination of specific and nonspecific AED	17 (15.59%)

TABLE 4: Prior adequate AED use.

Patients on specific AED	35 patients
(1) Valproate	22 (62.85%)
(2) Topiramate	3 (8.57%)
(3) Lamotrigine	3 (8.57%)
(4) Levetiracetam	3 (8.57%)
(5) Combination	4 (11.43%)

TABLE 5: Prior nonspecific AED use.

Patients on nonspecific AED	28 patients
(1) Carbamazepine	15 (53.57%)
(2) Phenytoin	3 (10.71%)
(3) Gabapentin	1 (3.57%)
(4) Phenobarbital	1 (3.57%)
(5) Oxcarbazepine	1 (3.57%)
(6) Combination	7 (25.0%)

TABLE 6: Treatment response in nonspecific AED group.

28 patients	Prior nonspecific AED	Change adequate AED
Adequately controlled seizures	10 (35.71%)	14 (50.0%)
Poorly controlled seizures	18 (64.28%)	8 (28.57%)
Missed to follow up		6 (21.42%)

clinic and initiation of the "broad-spectrum" AED, if indicated. We have divided the types of AED use into broad-spectrum (specific) and narrow-spectrum (nonspecific). It is well established that certain AEDs are more specific than the others for the treatment of IGE, namely, valproate (VPA), lamotrigine (LTG), topiramate (TPM), and levetiracetam (LEV) [10–16]. On the other hand, the group of "nonspecific" AEDs include phenytoin (PHT), carbamazepine (CBZ), oxcarbazepine (OXC), and gabapentin (GBP). We have used the International League Against Epilepsy 1989 classification to classify the different epilepsy types [17, 18].

The primary objective of our study was to report our experience in UAE of how often patients with IGE are misdiagnosed and/or mistreated with nonspecific AEDs prior to being evaluated by the epilepsy clinic. The secondary objective was to determine the percentage of patients who become adequately controlled after evaluation at the epilepsy clinic and switched to the "right" choice of AEDs.

3. Results

109 patients were identified, 50 males and 59 females, aged 12–56 with mean age of 26 and mean seizure duration of 10 years (Table 1). According to the International League Against Epilepsy classification, 89 patients (81.65%) had idiopathic generalized epilepsy, 17 patients (15.59%) had juvenile myoclonic epilepsy (JME), and 3 patients (2.75%) had juvenile absence epilepsy (JAE) (Table 2).

When initially seen, 29 patients (26.6%) were not on any AED, and 35 patients (32.11%) were using specific AED (Table 3); of those, 62.85% were on VPA, 8.57% were on TPM, 8.57% were on LTG, 8.57% were on LEV, and 11.43% were on various combinations of specific AEDs (Table 4). On the other hand, 28 patients (25.69%) were taking narrow-spectrum (nonspecific) AEDs (Table 3); of those, 53.57% were on CBZ, 10.71% were on PHT, 3.57% were on GBP, 3.57% were on PB, 3.57% were on OXZ, and 25% were on various combinations of these nonspecific AEDs (Table 5). The remaining 17 patients (15.59%) were on a combination of both specific and nonspecific AEDs (Table 3).

Of the total 28 patients who were receiving nonspecific AEDs, seizures were adequately controlled in 10 patients

(35.71%), while 18 patients (64.28%) had poorly controlled seizures (Table 6). When these patients' AED regimens were changed from nonspecific to a specific AED, 14 patients (50.0%) became fully controlled, 8 patients (28.57%) appeared to be truly intractable to all medication regimens, and 6 patients (21.42%) have missed followup (Table 6).

4. Discussion

To our knowledge, this is the first study in the Middle-East region that demonstrates the percentage of IGE patients who seemingly have difficult to control seizures (pseudointractable), but, in reality, they were using "nonspecific" AEDs. Our findings underscore the importance of establishing accurate diagnosis based on syndromic classification. As a matter of fact, the International League Against Epilepsy explicitly recommends that the classification of syndromes be "used daily in communication between colleagues" and be the "subject of clinical trials and other investigations."

Our findings in our region are similar to other series, where 30% of patients with IGE were on nonspecific medications and 65% of them had poorly controlled seizures. When switched to more specific AEDs, 50% became seizure-free. This shows the importance of thorough and comprehensive evaluation of patients with difficult to control seizures before they are deemed refractory to AEDs. Interestingly, however, 34% of IGE patients treated with "nonspecific" drugs, such as CBZ or PHT, were seizure-free. Of note, all these patients had GTCs as the predominant seizure type, and none of them had associated absence or myoclonic seizures. It is well established that these latter seizure types may worsen with the use of certain AEDs, whereas GTCs may respond well to a narrow-spectrum (nonspecific) AEDs [2, 11, 16].

Our study has clinical implications as most patients with generalized tonic clonic (GTC) seizures are assumed to have focal seizures with secondary generalization, especially if their seizures start in adult life [19]. Indeed, 22% of our IGE patients had their seizures beginning after the age of 20. This emphasizes the need to keep an open mind approach, when evaluating these patients, and to consider using broad-spectrum AEDs if in doubt about the underlying syndromic diagnosis.

We realize that our study has its limitations. It is relatively small, single center, and retrospective. Some patients were missed to follow-up. Moreover, it has a selection bias, as specialty epilepsy clinics tend to evaluate patients that are doing poorly. Indeed, and as illustrated in our cohorts, a significant proportion of our patients were doing poorly at the time of referral, and 28.57% of them have remained intractable despite a trial of several AEDs.

5. Conclusion

Our findings confirm the previous views that a poor choice of AED is still the main cause of IGEs that are seemingly difficult to control and show the importance of establishing specialized epilepsy clinics to evaluate these patients and make the appropriate changes. In our region, the inappropriateness of some AEDs for IGE is still not well recognized in a significant proportion of our patients.

Conflict of Interests

The authors declare that there is no conflict of interests.

References

[1] C. Marini, M. A. King, J. S. Archer, M. R. Newton, and S. F. Berkovic, "Idiopathic generalised epilepsy of adult onset: clinical syndromes and genetics," *Journal of Neurology Neurosurgery and Psychiatry*, vol. 74, no. 2, pp. 192–196, 2003.

[2] S. R. Benbadis, W. O. Tatum, and M. Gieron, "Idiopathic generalized epilepsy and choice of antiepileptic drugs," *Neurology*, vol. 61, no. 12, pp. 1793–1795, 2003.

[3] H. O. Luders, "Classification of epileptic seizures and epilepsies," in *Textbook of Epilepsy Surgery*, H. O. Luders, Ed., p. 245, Informa UH, London, UK, 2008.

[4] A. Nicolson, D. W. Chadwick, and D. F. Smith, "A comparison of adult onset and 'classical' idiopathic generalized epilepsy," *Journal of Neurology, Neurosurgery and Psychiatry*, vol. 75, no. 1, pp. 72–74, 2004.

[5] F. Andermann and S. F. Berkovic, "Idiopathic generalized epilepsy with generalized and other seizures in adolescence," *Epilepsia*, vol. 42, no. 3, pp. 317–320, 2001.

[6] S. Yenjun, A. S. Harvey, C. Marini et al., "EEG in adult-onset idiopathic generalized epilepsy," *Epilepsia*, vol. 44, pp. 252–256, 2003.

[7] J. M. Rho, R. Sankar, and J. E. Cavazos, *Epilepsy: Scientific Foundations of Clinical Practice*, Marcel Dekker, New York, NY, USA, 2004.

[8] R. Mohanraj and M. J. Brodie, "Outcomes of newly diagnosed idiopathic generalized epilepsy syndromes in a non-pediatric setting," *Acta Neurologica Scandinavica*, vol. 115, no. 3, pp. 204–208, 2007.

[9] R. H. Mattson, "Drug treatment of uncontrolled seizures," *Epilepsy Research*, no. 5, pp. 29–35, 1992.

[10] A. Nicolson, R. E. Appleton, D. W. Chadwick, and D. F. Smith, "The relationship between treatment with valproate, lamotrigine, and topiramate and the prognosis of the idiopathic generalised epilepsies," *Journal of Neurology, Neurosurgery and Psychiatry*, vol. 75, no. 1, pp. 75–79, 2004.

[11] E. Perucca, "The management of refractory idiopathic epilepsies," *Epilepsia*, vol. 42, supplement 3, pp. 31–35, 2001.

[12] V. Biton, G. D. Montouris, F. Ritter et al., "A randomized, placebo-controlled study of topiramate in primary generalized tonic-clonic seizures," *Neurology*, vol. 52, no. 7, pp. 1330–1337, 1999.

[13] M. Mazurkiewicz-Bełdzińska, M. Szmuda, and A. Matheisel, "Long-term efficacy of valproate versus lamotrigine in treatment of idiopathic generalized epilepsies in children and adolescents," *Seizure*, vol. 19, no. 3, pp. 195–197, 2010.

[14] D. Atakli, D. Sözüer, T. Atay, S. Baybas, and B. Arpaci, "Misdiagnosis and treatment in juvenile myoclonic epilepsy," *Seizure*, vol. 7, no. 1, pp. 63–66, 1998.

[15] J. P. Leach and M. J. Brodie, "Lamotrigine clinical use," in *Antiepileptic Drugs*, pp. 889–895, Raven Press, New York, NY, USA, 1995.

[16] S. R. Benbadis, "Practical management issues for idiopathic generalized epilepsies," *Epilepsia*, vol. 46, no. 9, pp. 125–132, 2005.

[17] R. S. Fisher, W. van Emde Boas, W. Blume et al., "Epileptic seizures and epilepsy: definitions proposed by the International League Against Epilepsy (ILAE) and the International Bureau for Epilepsy (IBE)," *Epilepsia*, vol. 46, no. 4, pp. 470–472, 2005.

[18] "Proposal for revised classification of epilepsies and epileptic syndromes. Commission on Classification and Terminology of the International League Against Epilepsy," *Epilepsia*, vol. 30, no. 4, pp. 389–399, 1989.

[19] S. R. Benbadis, "Observations on the misdiagnosis of generalized epilepsy as partial epilepsy: causes and consequences," *Seizure*, vol. 8, no. 3, pp. 140–145, 1999.

5

Temporal Lobe Resective Surgery for Medically Intractable Epilepsy: A Review of Complications and Side Effects

Iordanis Georgiadis,[1] **Effie Z. Kapsalaki,**[2] **and Kostas N. Fountas**[1,3]

[1] Departments of Neurosurgery, University Hospital of Larisa, Faculty of Medicine, University of Thessaly, Biopolis, Larissa 41110, Greece
[2] Departments of Neurosurgery & Diagnostic Radiology, University Hospital of Larisa, Faculty of Medicine,
  University of Thessaly, Larissa, Greece
[3] CERETETH, Center for Research and Technology of Thessaly, Larissa 38500, Greece

Correspondence should be addressed to Kostas N. Fountas; fountas@med.uth.gr

Academic Editor: Louis Lemieux

Object. It is widely accepted that temporal resective surgery represents an efficacious treatment option for patients with epilepsy of temporal origin. The meticulous knowledge of the potential complications, associated with temporal resective procedures, is of paramount importance. In our current study, we attempt to review the pertinent literature for summating the complications of temporal resective procedures for epilepsy. *Method.* A PubMed search was performed with the following terms: "behavioral," "cognitive," "complication," "deficit," "disorder," "epilepsy," "hemianopia," "hemianopsia," "hemorrhage," "lobectomy," "medial," "memory," "mesial," "neurobehavioral," "neurocognitive," "neuropsychological," "psychological," "psychiatric," "quadranopia," "quadranopsia," "resective," "side effect," "surgery," "temporal," "temporal lobe," and "visual field." *Results.* There were six pediatric, three mixed-population, and eleven adult surgical series examining the incidence rates of procedure-related complications. The reported mortality rates varied between 0% and 3.5%, although the vast majority of the published series reported no mortality. The cumulative morbidity rates ranged between 3.2% and 88%. *Conclusions.* Temporal resective surgery for epilepsy is a safe treatment modality. The reported morbidity rates demonstrate a wide variation. Accurate detection and frank reporting of any surgical, neurological, cognitive, and/or psychological complications are of paramount importance for maximizing the safety and improving the patients' overall outcome.

1. Introduction

It is well known that epilepsy constitutes one of the most common neurological clinico-pathological entities, affecting approximately 1% of the general population [1]. It has been estimated, that its prevalence in North America varies between 5 and 10 per 1000 people, and it affects people from all races, ethnicities, and socioeconomic backgrounds [1]. Therefore, epilepsy represents a common clinical condition with significant medical sequences but also serious social and economic ramifications. It has been demonstrated that temporal lobe epilepsy represents by far the most common form of focal epilepsy in adults, while it is one of the most common forms of epilepsy in children [2–7]. Temporal lobe epilepsy usually presents with simple and/or complex partial seizures, although the underlying pathology may be any of a wide spectrum of pathological entities, such as hippocampal sclerosis, low grade glial tumors (dysembryoplastic neuroepithelial tumor, ganglioglioma, and oligodendroglioma), neuronal migrational disorders (cortical dysplasia), and vascular lesions (cavernous malformation and arteriovenous malformation), while in a significant number of cases no structural abnormalities can be found despite the exhausting imaging workup.

A large number of clinical and epidemiological studies have shown that approximately a third of adult patients suffering from epilepsy will eventually develop medically refractory epilepsy, despite proper administration of the indicated anticonvulsants [1, 7, 8]. Similarly, approximately 10–20% of children with epilepsy will develop, at some point, medically refractory epilepsy [9–11]. It has been adequately demonstrated, that surgical treatment of patients with medically intractable epilepsy is the method of choice for managing them, particularly in cases of temporal lobe epilepsy [1, 12, 13]. Wiebe et al. in prospective, randomized, and controlled studies have clearly shown that surgical treatment of patients with epilepsy of temporal origin is superior to any kind of medical treatment [1]. Besides, it offers to those patients a good chance to become seizure-free, while it significantly improves their quality of life. Despite the rapidly growing body of evidence regarding the efficacy of epilepsy surgery in cases of temporal epilepsy, the number of the performed epilepsy cases in North America and Europe remains disproportionally low, compared to the temporal lobe epilepsy cases [14, 15]. This underutilization of epilepsy surgery may be related to the fact that many patients, and their referring physicians, face with a lot of skepticism of a possible surgical intervention, due to the associated complications.

Indeed, temporal epilepsy surgery may be associated with complications as any other neurosurgical procedure. The occurrence of a temporal epilepsy surgery-associated neurological complication becomes even more dramatic, since the vast majority of the surgical candidates are neurologically intact. The resection or the disconnection of theoretically normal brain tissue, which is part of epilepsy surgery strategy, may lead to a behavioral and/or cognitive deficit [16]. Therefore, accurate knowledge of all potential complications of temporal lobe epilepsy surgery is of paramount importance for preventing them, if possible, or appropriately managing them when they occur. Furthermore, a well and accurately informed surgical candidate may rationally face the risks of any surgical interventions and properly weight them against the risks of no surgical intervention. Moreover, understanding of the underlying mechanisms of many of these complications may eventually lead to the development of imaging, neurophysiological, or surgical techniques, which may prevent their occurrence.

Although the published number of temporal epilepsy surgery series is geometrically increasing, the number of publications regarding surgical or other procedure-related complications remains quite limited. This may be related to the fact that for several years many of the temporal epilepsy surgery-associated complications were considered as expected, inevitable, or acceptable complications [17]. Additionally, the existence of various classification schemes regarding complications and the utilization of different terms (complication or side effect) make the interpretation of the reported complication rates extremely difficult. Furthermore, the existing confusion along with the heterogeneity of the reported series makes almost impossible their comparison regarding the complication rates.

In our current study, we attempted to systematically review the existent literature regarding the temporal lobe epilepsy surgery associated complications and to identify, whenever possible, their underlying pathophysiologic mechanisms. We also attempted to summate all techniques and strategies reported in different surgical series, for providing a guide for preventing or minimizing the incidence of any temporal lobe resective surgery-related complications.

2. Material and Methods

An extensive literature search was performed in the PubMed medical database. The following terms were used for our search: "behavioral," "cognitive," "complication," "deficit," "disorder," "epilepsy," "hemianopia," "hemianopsia," "hemorrhage," "lobectomy," "medial," "memory," "mesial," "neurobehavioral," "neurocognitive," "neuropsychological," "psychological," "psychiatric," "quadranopia," "quadranopsia," "resective," "side effect," "surgery," "temporal," "temporal lobe," and "visual field," in any possible combination. Our search was limited within the last 23 years (1990–present). Furthermore, only papers published in English language and published in peer-reviewed journals were considered. All the retrieved titles and abstracts were meticulously reviewed. In addition, the reference lists from the retrieved papers were carefully reviewed to identify any additional pertinent papers for inclusion. Case reports were excluded from our current study. Moreover, complications associated with invasive preoperative monitoring were excluded from our current study, since the target of our analysis was solely resective-surgery associated complications.

Every possible effort was made to identify any repetition of cases among the published surgical series and any overlaps of series reported in different journals. In such occasions, only the original or the largest, regarding the number of participants, surgical series were included in our study. It has to be mentioned, however, that despite our efforts in identifying such repetitions, this task was not easy and the reader must be aware of potential redundancies in the reported data.

We attempted in our review to separate pediatric from adult surgical series. Frequently, the pediatric series included adolescents (12–18 yr), while other series had purely pediatric (≤12 yr) populations. In a few rare occasions, the reported surgical series included mixed, pediatric, and adult populations, without providing data regarding the percentage of each component. In these series that mixed populations are included, this is clearly indicated in our current study. Furthermore, the reported complications were grouped as surgical, neurological, and neuropsychological for presentation purposes, and a percentage was calculated whenever the total number of patients included in the surgical series was available. Additionally, a cumulative complication rate was calculated by adding the number of all complicated cases in each surgical series.

Unfortunately, temporal lobe resective surgery for epilepsy is an extremely wide term, describing a spectrum of surgical procedures and varying from simple neocortical lesionectomy to extensive anterior temporal lobectomy (ATL) and ipsilateral amygdalohippocampectomy (AH). In a large number of the reviewed surgical series there was a single surgical procedure performed and its associated complications were reported. However, in a few occasions there were various surgical techniques utilized, targeting the neocortex of the temporal lobe or the mesial temporal structures, or both of them. We took into consideration this variability and we provided this information whenever available. In a large number of the published surgical series, there were mixed data regarding temporal and extratemporal resective procedures, or temporal resective procedures, hemispherectomies, and corpus callosotomies. In these series that data for distinct groups were provided, the temporal lobe resective procedures and their complication rates were calculated, while those series, in which data from temporal and extratemporal surgical procedures were mixed, we excluded them from our study. Every effort was made to summate and present every procedure-associated complication, without characterizing them as major or minor, since such classification is not unanimously accepted. We also attempted to include in our report the permanent or transient character of each of the reported complications, whenever this information was provided in the published paper.

3. Results

Different combinations of the utilized search terms provided a total of 1681 papers, of which the combination of "temporal lobe epilepsy surgery complications" provided the largest number of papers (1325 abstracts), while the search "temporal lobe epilepsy surgery hemianopia" provided the smallest number of retrieved papers (26 abstracts). We meticulously reviewed all the retrieved abstracts and we carefully selected 55 papers reporting on temporal lobe surgical series complications. Subsequently, the reference lists of all the retrieved papers were meticulously reviewed and were crossed checked for any additional pertinent papers. Finally, a total of 58 full papers met our inclusion criteria and were analyzed in our current study.

3.1. Pediatric Surgical Series. All the retrieved pediatric surgical series reported no procedure-related deaths [6, 9, 13, 18–21]. The observed cumulative morbidity rates varied between 0–9.3% in the reviewed series [6, 9, 13, 18–21] (Table 1).

3.1.1. Neurological Complications. Analysis of the reported complications confirms that the most common neurological complication is the development of postoperative visual field deficit (VFD) [6, 9, 18, 20]. Kim et al. [9] found that the incidence of postoperative superior quadranopsia in their cohort was 22.0%. However, Lopez-Gonzalez et al. [6] reported a significantly lower (1.5%) incidence of postoperative VFDs. Likewise, Erba et al. [18] reported postoperative hemianopsia in 4.3% of their patients and Terra-Bustamante et al. [20] in 2.9% of their series. Interestingly, Sinclair et al. [19] and Vadera et al. [13] reported no postoperative VFDs.

Postoperative hemiparesis occurred in 4.3% of the patients reported by Erba et al. [18], while the respective rate was 8.5% in the series reported by Kim et al. [9]. Transient speech difficulties occurred in 0.7% of the patients reported by Lopez-Gonzalez et al. [6], while Sinclair et al. [19] reported the development of postoperative stroke in 3.1% of their series. Erba et al. documented transient ipsilateral oculomotor nerve palsy in 2.1% of their patients [18].

3.1.2. Surgical Complications. Postoperative hydrocephalus requiring surgical management occurred in 3.1% of the patients reported by Sinclair et al. [19]. Postoperative

meningitis and/or surgical wound infections seemed to not be major problems in the reported series. Sinclair et al. [19] found postoperative bone flap infections in 3.1% of their patients, Erba et al. [18] reported superficial wound infections in 2.1% of their cohort, while Lopez-Gonzalez et al. [6] reported wound infection in 1.5% of their patients. Kim et al. reported slightly higher (8.5%) wound infection rate and meningitis rate of 3.4% [9]. However, in all the reported series infections were successfully managed with antibiotic administration, with no further sequelae.

3.1.3. Neuropsychological Complications. The development of cognitive, behavioral, and/or psychiatric postoperative symptoms represents another procedure-related complication, even among children [6, 9, 18]. Erba et al. found that 4.3% of their patients developed postoperatively a syndrome of hypergraphia, hyperreligiosity, and sticky personality, while another 4.3% developed postoperative depression with suicidal ideation [18]. Similarly, Kim et al. [9] documented the development of postoperative psychosis in 5.1% of their patients, while Lopez-Gonzalez et al. [6] found that 10% of their patients developed postoperative *de novo* depression.

3.2. Mixed Population (Pediatric and Adult) Surgical Series. There are a few surgical series reporting on the complication rate of temporal resections in adult and pediatric patients [16, 22, 23] (Table 2). There were no deaths in the reported series, with the exception of Lee et al. who reported 3.5% mortality rate in their series [22]. They reported one death after developing severe hypoxic brain damage postoperatively caused most probably, according to the authors, by the induced hypoventilation for treating severe postoperative headache [22]. The cumulative complication rates including neurological, surgical, neuropsychological, and psychiatric complications varied between 3.8% and 26.1% [16, 22, 23].

3.2.1. Neurological Complications. Salanova et al. reported that the most common complication in their series was the development of transient postoperative language difficulties, occurring in 3.7% of their patients [23]. The respective incidence of transient dysphasia (lasting less than 12 months), in the series reported by Tanriverdi et al. was 0.6% [16]. Salanova et al. [23] found that transient cranial nerve deficits occurred in 3.2% of their patients, while the respective rate reported by Tanriverdi et al. [16] was 0.3%. The incidence of postoperative hemiparesis ranged between 0.1% and 0.9% [16, 23]. Postoperative VFDs, hemianopsia, or superior quadranopsia were reported by Salanova et al. [23] in 0.4% of their patients and in 0.2% by Tanriverdi et al. [16].

3.2.2. Surgical Complications. Surgical wound infection reported by Salanova et al. [23] in 1.3% of their patients, while Tanriverdi et al. [16] reported 0.5%, including cases of meningitis and cerebral abscess (0.3%). Tanriverdi et al. also reported the development of postoperative hematomas in 0.6% of their patients, postoperative transient brain edema in 0.2%, postoperative hydrocephalus in 0.1%, while 0.4% of their patients had subgaleal fluid collections and another

Table 1: Synopsis of data of pediatric temporal lobe epilepsy surgical series and their reported complications.

Series/year of publication	Study characteristics	Number of pts	Surgical procedure	Mortality	Mean followup	Seizure-free outcome	Complications	Cumulative complication rate*	Behavioral/cognitive/psychiatric complications
Erba et al., 1992 [18]	Prospective, pediatric & adolescent	46	Standard ATL + AH	0%	5 years	85%	Infection: 2.1% Hemiparesis/hemianopsia: 4.3% C.N. Palsy: 2.1%	17.1%	Depression: 4.3% Behavioral syndrome: 4.3%
Sinclair et al., 2003 [19]	Retrospective, pediatric	32	Standard ATL	0%	6.9 years	76%	Infection: 3.1% Hydrocephalus: 3.1% Stroke: 3.1%	9.3%	N/A
Terra-Bustamante et al., 2005 [20]	Prospective, pediatric & adolescent	35	Standard ATL + AH	0%	3.5 years	77.1%	Hemianopsia: 2.9%	2.9%	N/A
Kim et al., 2008 [9]	Prospective, pediatric	59	Standard ATL + AH	0%	62.3 months	69%	VFDs: 22.0% Hemiparesis: 8.5% Wound infection: 8.5% Meningitis: 3.4%	47.5%	Psychosis: 5.1%
Lopez-Gonzalez et al., 2012 [6]	Retrospective, pediatric	130	Cortico-amygdalo-hippocampectomy (CAH), Lesionectomy + CAH, Lesionectomy, neocortical resection, tailored ATL + AH, selective AH	0%	2 years	72%	VFDs: 1.5% Transient speech Difficulties: 0.7% Infection: 1.5%	17%	Depression: 10%
Vadera et al., 2012 [13]	Retrospective, pediatric	45	Standard ATL + AH	0%	60.2 months	69%	None	0%	N/A

*This rate includes the behavioral/cognitive/psychiatric complications. ATL: anterior temporal lobectomy; AH: amygdalohippocampectomy; VFDs: visual field deficits; C.N.: cranial nerve.

TABLE 2: Synopsis of data of mixed pediatric and adult temporal lobe epilepsy surgical series and their reported surgical complications.

Series/year of publication	Study characteristics	Number of pts	Surgical procedure	Mortality	Mean followup	Seizure-free outcome	Complications	Cumulative complication rate*	Behavioral/ cognitive/ psychiatric complications
Salanova et al., 2002 [23]	Prospective	215	Temporal resective surgery	0%	7 years	69%	Dysphasia: 3.7% Hemiparesis: 0.9% C.N. palsy: 3.2% VFDs: 0.4% Infection: 1.3%	26.1%	Verbal memory deficits: 8.8% Depression: 5.5% Psychosis: 2.3%
Lee et al., 2008 [22]	Retrospective	28	ATL + AH	3.5%	N/A	N/A	N/A	10.6%	N/A
Tanriverdi et al., 2009 [16]	Retrospective	1232	ATL + AH, Selective AH	0%	At least 1 year	N/A	Dysphasia: 0.6% Hemiparesis: 0.1% C.N. palsy: 0.3% VFDs: 0.2% Infection: 0.5% Hematomas: 0.6% Hydrocephalus: 0.1% Subgaleal Collections: 0.4% CSF Leakage: 0.1% Suture Detachment: 0.1%	3.8%	N/A

*This rate includes the behavioral/cognitive/psychiatric complications. ATL: anterior temporal lobectomy; AH: amygdalohippocampectomy; VFDs: visual field deficits; C.N.: cranial nerve.

0.2% had problems with CSF leak through their surgical wound or skin suture detachment [16].

3.2.3. Neuropsychological Complications. Salanova et al. found that the most common neuropsychological complication in their series was the development of postoperative verbal memory difficulties, in 8.8% of their patients [23]. They also noticed that 5.5% of their patients developed postoperatively depression, while another 2.3% developed postoperative psychosis [23]. Unfortunately, Tanriverdi et al. did not include in their detailed series their neuropsychological complications [16].

3.3. Adult Surgical Series. No deaths were reported in the retrieved adult surgical series [1, 4, 5, 15, 17, 24–30] (Table 3).

3.3.1. Neurological Complications. The development of postoperative neurological deficits remains a major concern in epilepsy surgery. The occurrence of hemiparesis postoperatively has been reported to vary between 0 and 5%, with a wide range of severity, duration, and rehabilitation rates [4, 17, 21, 24, 26, 28, 30, 31]. This could be attributed either to the development of postoperative ischemia secondary to edema, ischemia secondary to cerebral vasospasm development, and excessive manipulation of the middle and/or dominant anterior choroidal arteries during resection [5, 17, 24, 28]. It has to be mentioned, that vasospasm has been detected by transcranial Doppler sonography in 32.7% of patients undergoing selective AH [32]. Engel et al. [30] reported that 21.4% of their patients demonstrated cerebral ischemic

changes in their postoperative MRIs, although these were clinically significant in only 7.1% of their cases.

Dysphasic or more rarely aphasic postoperative symptomatology occurs in 1.7%–7.7% of the reported cohorts [4, 24, 26, 29, 31]. In the vast majority of cases, these symptoms are transient, and usually resolve within the first few postoperative weeks with no further consequences. However, in rare instances these deficits may be permanent. Falowski et al. [4] reported 0.9% incidence of permanent postoperative dysphasia, while Grivas et al. [26] found that the incidence of permanent dysphasia in their series (patients older than 50 yr) was 3.8%.

Cranial nerve deficits and mostly trochlear nerve palsy are usually responsible for the development of postoperative diplopia in patients undergoing ATL + AH. The incidence of trochlear nerve palsy has been reported to vary between 2.6% and 19% [17, 24, 26, 31, 33, 34]. In the vast majority of the reported cases, postoperative diplopia spontaneously resolved with no further sequelae [17, 24, 26, 31, 33, 34]. Contrariwise, the observed postoperative VFDs are permanent. Their incidence presents a high variation, with rates ranging from 1.8% to 69% [24, 26, 28, 33, 33, 34]. In the vast majority of the reported series, these VFDs were superior quadranopsia [23, 35–37]. However, Heller et al. [28] reported 1.8% incidence of complete contralateral homonymous hemianopsia, while Grivas et al. [26] found similar findings in 5.8% of their patients. It has to be mentioned that in several surgical series the exact incidence of VFDs is not available, since many epilepsy surgeons consider the occurrence of VFDs postoperatively inevitable [4, 17].

Table 3: Synopsis of data of adult temporal lobe epilepsy surgical series and their reported surgical complications.

Series/year of publication	Study characteristics	Number of pts	Surgical procedure	Mortality	Mean followup	Seizure-free outcome	Complications	Cumulative complication rate*	Behavioral/cognitive/psychiatric complications
Wiebe et al., 2001 [1]	Prospective	40	ATL + AH	0%	12 months	54%	None	5%	5% memory deficits
Cohen-Gadol et al., 2003 [33]	Prospective	47	ATL + AH	0%	6 months	N/A	Diplopia: 19% VFDs: 69%	88%	N/A
Oertel et al., 2004 [31]	Prospective	60	Transcortical selective AH	0%	N/A	N/A	Hemiparesis: 5% Aphasia: 1.7% C.N. palsy: 5% Infections: 1.7%	13.4%	N/A
Grivas et al., 2006 [26]	Retrospective	52	AH, lesionectomy + AH	0%	33 months	71%	Hemiparesis: 3.8% Aphasia: 3.8% C.N. palsy: 5.8% VFDs: 5.8% Hematomas: 3.8% Pneumonia: 1.9% Pulmonary embolism: 1.9%	53.4%	Decline in neuropsychological status: 26.5% (Verbal memory decline in 29.4%, visual memory decline in 32.4%)
Sindou et al., 2006 [17]	Retrospective	100	Tailored ATL + AH	0%	53 months	85%	Hemiparesis: 2% C.N. palsy: 5% Hydrocephalus: 2% Meningitis: 3% Hematomas: 3% Pulmonary embolism: 1%	19%	Permanent neuropsychological impairment: 3%
Roberti et al., 2007 [15]	Retrospective	42	Tailored ATL + AH	0%	60 months	64%	Frontal branch of facial n. palsy: 2.4% Bone flap reabsorption: 2.3%	4.7%	N/A
Acar et al., 2008 [24]	Retrospective	39	Transcortical selective AH	0%	25.9 months	82%	Hemiparesis: 2.6% Dysphasia: 7.7% VFDs: 10.3% C.N. palsy: 2.6% Hemotympanum: 2.6% Frontal branch of facial n. palsy: 2.6%	33.5%	Memory difficulties: 5.1%
Elsharkawy et al., 2009 [25]	Retrospective	483	ATL + AH	0%	2 years	72.3%	Permanent deficits: 2.3% Temporary deficits: 2.3% Hemiparesis: 1.8% Stroke: 5.5%	5%	N/A
Heller et al., 2009 [28]	Retrospective	55	Tailored ATL + AH	0%	N/A	N/A	VFDs: 1.8% Hematomas/hygromas: 3.6% Meningitis: 1.8% Deep venous thrombosis: 1.8%	16.3%	N/A

TABLE 3: Continued.

Series/year of publication	Study characteristics	Number of pts	Surgical procedure	Mortality	Mean followup	Seizure-free outcome	Complications	Cumulative complication rate*	Behavioral/ cognitive/psychiatric complications
Ipekdal et al., 2011 [5]	Retrospective	58	ATL + AH	0%	N/A	N/A	Stroke: 1.7% Frontal branch of Facial n. palsy: 1.7% Infections: 4.7% Subdural effusion: 1.7%	14.9%	Psychosis: 1.7% Depression: 1.7% Anxiety disorders: 1.7%
Falowski et al., 2012 [4]	Retrospective	222	Tailored AH	0%	5.4 years	70%	Dysphasia: 0.9% Infections: 1.4% Deep venous thrombosis: 0.9%	3.2%	N/A

*This rate includes the behavioral/cognitive/psychiatric complications. ATL: anterior temporal lobectomy; AH: amygdalohippocampectomy; VFDs: visual field deficits; C.N.: cranial nerve.

3.3.2. Surgical Complications. The formation of postoperative hematomas, either intraparenchymal or epi-/subdural, was quite rare among the reported series. Sindou et al. reported postoperative hematoma in 3% of their patients [17]. These were hematomas of the resection cavity, which were developed within the first 24 postoperative hours. They had to surgically evacuate them, with no further sequelae for their patients [17]. Likewise, Grivas et al. reported 3.8% incidence of postoperative hematomas in a series of elderly (≥50 yr) patients undergoing AH or cortical lesionectomy and AH [26]. They had to surgically intervene and evacuate all these hematomas, with no further consequences [26]. Heller et al. reported 1.8% incidence of postoperative epidural hematoma, which required surgical evacuation, while another 1.8% of their patients developed postoperative hygromas [28]. Ipekdal et al. reported that 1.7% of their patients developed postoperative subdural effusion, which was spontaneously resolved [5]. An interesting finding was the development of immediate (within the first few hours) postoperative cerebellar hemorrhage in cases of ATL + AH [38, 39]. Toczek et al. [39] reported 4.9% incidence rate of cerebellar hemorrhage, while de Paola et al. [38] found that the occurrence of cerebellar hemorrhage was slightly lower (2.5%) in their cohort. Although the exact pathophysiologic mechanism responsible for this complication remains unclear, it has been postulated that undetected blood coagulation abnormalities, which may be present in epileptic patients with chronic use of anticonvulsant medications could be responsible for this distant hematoma formation [39]. The intraoperative drainage of large amounts of CSF during ATL, in association with the rapid volume change of intracranial compartments, could be another mechanism responsible for the postoperative development of distant hematomas [39–41]. A similar mechanism may well be responsible for the development of lumbar subdural hematomas in cases of ATL + AH [35]. It has been reported that these spinal subdural hematomas were developed after the third postoperative day and required no surgical intervention [35].

Sindou et al. reported that in 2% of their patients, hydrocephalus developed postoperatively, for which shunt insertion was necessary [17]. Engel et al. [30] reported 7.1% incidence of postoperative hydrocephalus in their cohort. Complications related to the skin incision and to the dissection of the soft tissues during craniotomy have been reported in many series [5, 15, 24]. Characteristically, Roberti et al. reported palsy of the frontal branch of the facial nerve in 2.4% of their patients, while another 2.3% experienced problems with bone flap reabsorption [15]. Likewise, Ipekdal et al. reported frontal branch injury and postoperative palsy in 1.7% of their patients [5]. Acar et al. reported similar rates of frontal branch palsy (2.6%), while in another 2.6% hemotympanum occurred secondary to opening of the air mastoid cells during the craniotomy [24].

Infections in the postoperative period represented either superficial wound infections or meningitis. The reported postoperative infection rates ranged between 1% and 4.7% [4, 5, 17, 28, 31]. Sindou et al. [17] reported 3% meningitis rate, while Heller et al. [28] found 1.8% cases of bacterial meningitis, and Ipekdal et al. [5] in 4.7% of their patients.

However, in none of the reported cases antibiotic treatment of meningitis failed.

Other various procedure-related complications were also reported in the reviewed surgical series [4, 26, 28]. Heller et al. [28] reported deep venous thrombosis (DVT) in 1.8% of their patients, while Falowski et al. [4] found that DVT occurred in 0.9% of their cohort. Grivas et al. reported pneumonia in 1.9% and pulmonary embolism in another 1.9% of their patients [26].

3.3.3. Neuropsychological Complications. Postoperative memory decline constitutes one of the most worrisome temporal resective surgery complications, particularly in cases of the dominant temporal lobe. Ojemann and Dodrill emphasized the negative effect of dominant hemisphere temporal lobectomy in the patient's verbal memory [42]. In their original series, they found 22% verbal memory decline at one month after surgery and 11% at the completion of the first postoperative year [36]. Gleissner et al. [43] reported their results from a series of adult patients, who underwent detailed verbal and visual memory evaluations before and then at 3 months postoperatively. They found that there was 51% loss of verbal memory in left-sided cases, while the respective percentage among right-sided resections was 32%. The postoperative visual memory loss was approximately 27% in their series. They noticed that the verbal memory loss was more frequent among males [43]. Comparable memory loss rates were documented by Grivas et al. in their series [26]. They found postoperative verbal memory decline in 29.4%, while the visual memory loss was 32.4% in their patients [26]. Acar et al. [24] reported 5.1% memory deficits in their series, while Helmstaedter et al. [12] found that there was significant postoperative verbal learning recognition deficit in their left-sided lobe resections. Similarly, Bell et al. [2] found significant postoperative loss of verbal ability in their patients undergoing left-sided ATL + AH for nonlesional epilepsy.

During the last two decades, the number of published series examining the development of *de novo* postoperative psychiatric entities or investigating the role of temporal resective surgery in the exacerbation of preoperative psychiatric conditions has been exponentially growing [5, 26, 44–53]. The reported psychiatric clinical entities include psychosis, depression, anxiety disorders, and obsessive-compulsive disorders [5, 26, 44–53]. Older reports stated that the actual incidence of postoperative psychosis was approximately 8%, which was at the lower edge of the previously published series [54]. Indeed, Leinonen et al. [48] reported that *de novo* psychosis occurred in 5.3% of their series of patients undergoing temporal lobectomy. Grivas et al. [26] reported 5.8% incidence of postoperative organic psychological syndrome. Shaw et al. [51], in a recent series, found that the incidence of *de novo* psychosis among patients undergoing ATL + AH was 3.4%. They also found that there was a clustering of psychosis development within the first 12 postoperative months. Christodoulou et al. [45] reported even lower incidence of postoperative psychosis in their series (1.1%), while Malmgren et al. [49] found 0.5% incidence of *de novo* psychosis and Ipekdal et al. [5] reported 1.7%

incidence of *de novo* psychosis. However, it has to be emphasized that temporal resections may exacerbate preexisting psychosis [44, 46, 49]. Blumer et al. [44] found worsening of the pre-existing psychiatric conditions in 24% of their patients.

Naylor et al. [50] found 10.8% of postoperative depression in their series. They reported that the vast majority of these were *de novo* cases (8%), while the remaining (2.8%) represented worsening of a pre-existing condition. Blumer et al. [44] found that in their cohort, 42.1% of their preoperatively intact from psychiatric standpoint patients developed depression after temporal lobectomy. Wrench et al. [53] reported 10% incidence of *de novo* postoperative depression. However, Ipekdal et al. [5] found significantly lower rates (1.7%) of postoperative depression in their series. Malmgren et al. [49] found that the incidence of anxiety disorders increased from 1.4% preoperatively to 17% postoperatively. Likewise, the occurrence of affective disorders in their series increased from 1.4% before surgery to 17% after surgery. Ipekdal et al. [5] found postoperative anxiety disorders in 1.7% of their patients, while Kulaksizoglu et al. [47] reported the postoperative development of *de novo* obsessive-compulsive disorders in patients undergoing temporal resections.

4. Discussion

Reviewing of complications associated with resective temporal surgery for epilepsy is a quite complicated issue. This is related to the fact that the reported series used different surgical techniques, with or without neocortical resection, with different extent of hippocampal resection, and with varying anatomical avenues for resecting the mesial temporal structures. The underlying temporal lobe pathology also varied significantly among the published series, while the patients' groups of the published series are far from being considered homogenous and comparable. Occasionally, even in the same series there is utilization of different surgical techniques and/or participation of more than one epilepsy surgeon. Thus, comparison between the reported complication rates is almost impossible. In addition, many of the commonly observed complications (visual field deficits, cognitive, and psychiatric postoperative changes) of temporal lobectomy are underreported, since for a long period of time were considered from many epilepsy surgeons as either inevitable complications or acceptable side effects and, therefore, were excluded from their complication reports. However, detailed and accurate knowledge of the potential complications is of paramount importance for appropriately informing the surgical candidates during the decisionmaking process for avoiding complications' development if possible and for identifying them in a timely fashion and properly managing them.

Moreover, the published rates of certain complications may be greatly affected by the utilized method for detecting them. The detection of a postoperative superior quadranopsia may be undetected during a confrontational clinical visual field examination. The employment of official visual field examination may increase the incidence of postoperative

VFDs. Even the employment of different VF examination methodologies may provide different rates of VFDs [36, 55]. Manji and Plant [36] reported 47% incidence of VFD when their patients were examined with the Eastman method, while VFDs were documented in 54% of the patients in the same series when the Goldman perimeter was used.

Similarly, the actual incidence of postoperative cognitive deficits may be higher when detailed pre- and postoperative cognitive evaluations will be employed. This may well explain the observed variation between the reported postoperative memory decline rates among the different series. Another confounding factor in determining the accuracy of the reported memory decline rates may be the exact time of postoperative cognitive evaluation. The adaptation of a widely accepted cognitive pre- and postoperative evaluation methodology could provide comparable results among different series and a more realistic estimate about the true incidence of memory decline. Similar inaccuracies are applicable in regard to the incidence of postoperative psychiatric complications. Although, many reports have pointed out the occurrence of psychosis, depression, and anxiety disorders after temporal lobectomy, their actual incidence remains still controversial [44–47, 49–53, 56–62]. The differentiation of *de novo* from relapsing, preexisting, or preoperatively undetected cases remains a major problem, in determining the exact rate of postoperative psychiatric complications. Detailed pre- and postoperative psychiatric evaluation of all surgical candidates may define the true occurrence of postoperative psychopathology and improve the patients' surgical outcome and their quality of life.

Several parameters have been identified by various clinical investigators in the reported temporal lobectomy series as predisposing factors for complications' development. The patient's age has been recognized as an important factor in the temporal lobectomy-associated morbidity [21, 23, 26]. This may be attributed to the employment of preoperative invasive monitoring more frequently in pediatric patients or may be related to the patients' age [21]. Younger adult patients seemed to have lower complication rates than older adults in several of the reported series [23, 26]. Contrariwise, Sindou et al. [17] found no significant correlation between their complication rate and the patient's age, the side, or the extent of temporal resection. Heller et al. [28] identified in their study the surgeon's experience as an important factor in the development of complications. Oertel et al. [31] identified the utilization of a neuronavigational system as a factor decreasing their complication rate. Furthermore, the exact role of structural lesions versus nonlesional temporal cases in the development of postoperative complications remains to be defined.

The development of cognitive, neuropsychological, and/or psychiatric complications has been associated with various factors [2, 43, 46, 49, 51, 53]. Gleissner et al. [43] found that postoperative loss of visual memory decline was associated with the patient's gender and the laterality of resection (patients with left-sided resections had more commonly verbal memory loss). The positive history for anxiety and/or depression disorders, the positive family history for psychiatric disorders, the presence of mood disturbances preoperatively, the postoperative continuation of seizures, the difficulty in postoperative psychosocial adjustment, the diffuse epileptogenicity, and the presence of secondary generalized tonic-clonic seizures preoperativel have all been identified as predisposing factors for developing postoperative psychiatric complications [46, 49, 53]. Shaw et al. [51] have demonstrated that patients with histopathology other than mesial temporal sclerosis, the presence of bilateral EEG abnormalities, and the small size of the contralateral amygdala may all predispose to postoperative psychosis development. However, there are reports implicating the large size of the contralateral to the resection amygdala in the pathogenesis of postoperative psychosis [52]. The exact role of the side of resection, the extent of the mesial and neocortical temporal resection, the underlying histopathology, and the presence of previous temporal surgeries in the development of postoperative cognitive and psychiatric complications remains to be accurately defined in the future.

The development of newer imaging modalities and the wider application of intraoperative electrophysiological methodologies may contribute in preventing or minimizing the possibility of VFDs after temporal resective surgery [37, 63, 64]. The employment of preoperative advanced MR imaging techniques, such as diffusion tensor imaging (DTI) and fiber tracking (FT), may help in outlining the visual tracts [37, 63, 64]. Registration of the DTI data on the preoperative neuronavigational planning may protect the visual pathway, without compromising though the extent of the resection. Additionally, the intraoperative employment of visual evoked potential monitoring and application of direct subcortical electrical stimulation may further increase the accuracy of resection along the visual pathway and thus may minimize the chance of postoperative VFDs. Similarly, the employment of careful dissection along the trochlear nerve and the avoidance of even gentle retraction on the nerve may prevent or minimize the incidence of postoperative diplopia [24, 33].

The occurrence of postoperative hemiparesis after temporal lobectomy has been attributed to the development of vasospasm of the middle cerebral or of the dominant anterior choroidal arteries or the development of cerebral edema secondary to surgical manipulation [26, 28, 65]. The selective employment of intraoperative micro-Doppler in high-risk patients may identify those who are predisposed to vasospasm development. The early pharmacological treatment of these patients with nimodipine could prevent the development of clinically symptomatic vasospasm and thus prevent the development of ischemic strokes and postoperative hemiparesis. Likewise, the issue of administering perioperative antibiotics for preventing any infections and the selection of the proper antibiotic prophylaxis regimen remains controversial. Although the vast majority of epilepsy surgeons administer perioperative antibiotic prophylaxis, there are reports questioning its role [16]. Surgical complications related to the skin incision or the craniotomy may be prevented by employing interfascial dissection for avoiding any injuries to the frontal branch of the facial nerve and thus accomplish a better postoperative cosmetic result [15].

5. Conclusions

Temporal resective surgery for medically refractory epilepsy constitutes an extremely safe procedure, with mortality rates approaching zero. The reported procedure-associated complications may be classified into three large groups: surgical, neurological, and neurocognitive/psychological. The most common surgical complications include infection (surgical wound, meningitis, and cerebral abscess), postoperative hematoma formation (resection cavity hematoma, intraparenchymal adjacent to the resective site, distant cerebral or spinal, or epi/subdural), palsy of the frontal branch of the facial nerve secondary to intraoperative injury, postoperative hydrocephalus, CSF leakage, and wound healing problems. Although these complications are rare, modification of the surgical technique by employing careful interfascial dissection during the craniotomy, meticulous hemostasis at the completion of the resection, and routine evaluation of the patient's coagulation profile preoratively, intraoperatively, and for the first 2-3 days postoperatively may further decrease their incidence.

The neurological complications include postoperative VFDs, hemiparesis, dysphasia/aphasia, cerebral ischemic changes, and cranial nerve paresis or palsy. More sensitive detection and more accurate documentation of VFDs are necessary for understanding their actual postoperative incidence. Application of advanced MR imaging techniques, such as DTI and FT, and intraoperative neurophysiologic monitoring may decrease the incidence of postoperative VFDs. The employment of intraoperative micro-Doppler and postoperative transcranial Doppler for early detection of cerebral vasospasm may prevent or minimize the incidence of postoperative ischemic events and thus the occurrence of postoperative hemiparesis. The importance of minimal and gentle manipulations of the adjacent vascular structures during resection cannot be overemphasized.

Postoperative cognitive and psychological deficits include decline of preoperative verbal and visual memory, as well as exacerbation of preexisting or *de novo* development of psychosis, depression, and anxiety disorders. Early diagnosis of postoperative psychological and cognitive disturbances may help in their more efficient management and may improve the patients' overall outcome. Finally, proper identification of any predisposing to psychopathology factors preoperatively may help in the early diagnosis of such psychiatric complications and may help in their prompt treatment.

References

[1] S. Wiebe, W. T. Blume, J. P. Girvin, and M. Eliasziw, "A randomized, controlled trial of surgery for temporal-lobe epilepsy," *The New England Journal of Medicine*, vol. 345, no. 5, pp. 311–318, 2001.

[2] M. L. Bell, S. Rao, E. L. So et al., "Epilepsy surgery outcomes in temporal lobe epilepsy with a normal MRI," *Epilepsia*, vol. 50, no. 9, pp. 2053–2060, 2009.

[3] W. T. Blume, "Temporal lobe epilepsy surgery in childhood: rationale for greater use," *Canadian Journal of Neurological Sciences*, vol. 24, no. 2, pp. 95–98, 1997.

[4] S. M. Falowski, D. Wallace, A. Kanner, M. Smith, M. Rossi, A. Balabanov et al., "Tailored temporal lobectomy for medically intractable epilepsy: evaluation of pathology and predictors of outcome," *Neurosurgery*, vol. 71, pp. 703–709, 2012.

[5] H. I. Ipekdal, O. Karadas, E. Erdogan, and Z. Gokcil, "Spectrum of surgical complications of temporal lobe epilepsy surgery: a single. Center study," *Turkish Neurosurgery*, vol. 21, no. 2, pp. 147–151, 2011.

[6] M. A. Lopez-Gonzalez, J. A. Gonzalez-Martinez, L. Jehi, P. Kotagal, A. Warbel, and W. Bingaman, "Epilepsy surgery of the temporal lobe in pediatric population: a retrospective analysis," *Neurosurgery*, vol. 70, pp. 684–692, 2012.

[7] S. Spencer and L. Huh, "Outcomes of epilepsy surgery in adults and children," *The Lancet Neurology*, vol. 7, no. 6, pp. 525–537, 2008.

[8] S. U. Schuele and H. O. Lüders, "Intractable epilepsy: management and therapeutic alternatives," *The Lancet Neurology*, vol. 7, no. 6, pp. 514–524, 2008.

[9] S.-K. Kim, K.-C. Wang, Y.-S. Hwang et al., "Epilepsy surgery in children: outcomes and complications," *Journal of Neurosurgery*, vol. 1, no. 4, pp. 277–283, 2008.

[10] S.-K. Kim, K.-C. Wang, Y.-S. Hwang et al., "Pediatric intractable epilepsy: the role of presurgical evaluation and seizure outcome," *Child's Nervous System*, vol. 16, no. 5, pp. 278–286, 2000.

[11] G. Morrison, M. Duchowny, T. Resnick et al., "Epilepsy surgery in childhood. A report of 79 patients," *Pediatric Neurosurgery*, vol. 18, no. 5-6, pp. 291–297, 1992.

[12] C. Helmstaedter, S. Richter, S. Röske, F. Oltmanns, J. Schramm, and T.-N. Lehmann, "Differential effects of temporal pole resection with amygdalohippocampectomy versus selective amygdalohippocampectomy on material-specific memory in patients with mesial temporal lobe epilepsy," *Epilepsia*, vol. 49, no. 1, pp. 88–97, 2008.

[13] S. Vadera, V. R. Kshettry, P. Klaas, and W. Bingaman, "Seizure-free and neuropsychological outcomes after temporal lobectomy with amygdalohippocampectomy in pediatric patients with hippocampal sclerosis," *Journal of Neurosurgery*, vol. 10, pp. 103–107, 2012.

[14] J. Engel Jr. and D. A. Shewmon, "Overview: who should be considered a surgical candidate?" in *Surgical Treatment of the Epilepsies*, J. Engel Jr., Ed., pp. 23–24, Raven Press, New York, NY, USA, 2nd edition, 1993.

[15] F. Roberti, S. J. Potolicchio, and A. J. Caputy, "Tailored anteromedial lobectomy in the treatment of refractory epilepsy of the temporal lobe: long term surgical outcome and predictive factors," *Clinical Neurology and Neurosurgery*, vol. 109, no. 2, pp. 158–165, 2007.

[16] T. Tanriverdi, A. Ajlan, N. Poulin, and A. Olivier, "Morbidity in epilepsy surgery: an experience based on 2449 epilepsy surgery procedures from a single institution: clinical article," *Journal of Neurosurgery*, vol. 110, no. 6, pp. 1111–1123, 2009.

[17] M. Sindou, M. Guenot, J. Isnard, P. Ryvlin, C. Fischer, and F. Mauguière, "Temporo-mesial epilepsy surgery: outcome and complications in 100 consecutive adult patients," *Acta Neurochirurgica*, vol. 148, no. 1, pp. 39–45, 2006.

[18] G. Erba, K. R. Winston, J. R. Adler, K. Welch, R. Ziegler, and G. W. Hornig, "Temporal lobectomy for complex partial seizures that began in childhood," *Surgical Neurology*, vol. 38, no. 6, pp. 424–432, 1992.

[19] D. B. Sinclair, K. E. Aronyk, T. J. Snyder et al., "Pediatric Epilepsy Surgery at the University of Alberta: 1988–2000," *Pediatric Neurology*, vol. 29, no. 4, pp. 302–311, 2003.

[20] V. C. Terra-Bustamante, L. M. Inuzuca, R. M. F. Fernandes et al., "Temporal lobe epilepsy surgery in children and adolescents: clinical characteristics and post-surgical outcome," *Seizure*, vol. 14, no. 4, pp. 274–281, 2005.

[21] W. J. Hader, J. Tellez-Zenteno, A. Metcalfe, L. Hernandez-Ronquillo, S. Wiebe, C. S. Kwon et al., "Complications of epilepsy surgery: a systematic review of focal surgical resections and invasive EEG monitoring," *Epilepsia*, vol. 54, pp. 840–847, 2013.

[22] J. H. Lee, Y. S. Hwang, J. J. Shin, T. H. Kim, H. S. Shin, and S. K. Park, "Surgical complications of epilepsy surgery procedures: experience of 179 procedures in a single institute," *Journal of Korean Neurosurgical Society*, vol. 44, no. 4, pp. 234–239, 2008.

[23] V. Salanova, O. Markand, and R. Worth, "Temporal lobe epilepsy surgery: outcome, complications, and late mortality rate in 215 patients," *Epilepsia*, vol. 43, no. 2, pp. 170–174, 2002.

[24] G. Acar, F. Acar, J. Miller, D. C. Spencer, and K. J. Burchiel, "Seizure outcome following transcortical selective amygdalohippocampectomy in mesial temporal lobe epilepsy," *Stereotactic and Functional Neurosurgery*, vol. 86, no. 5, pp. 314–319, 2008.

[25] A. E. Elsharkawy, A. H. Alabbasi, H. Pannek et al., "Long-term outcome after temporal lobe epilepsy surgery in 434 consecutive adult patients: clinical article," *Journal of Neurosurgery*, vol. 110, no. 6, pp. 1135–1146, 2009.

[26] A. Grivas, J. Schramm, T. Kral et al., "Surgical treatment for refractory temporal lobe epilepsy in the elderly: seizure outcome and neuropsychological sequels compared with a younger cohort," *Epilepsia*, vol. 47, no. 8, pp. 1364–1372, 2006.

[27] W. Harkness, "Temporal lobe resections," *Child's Nervous System*, vol. 22, no. 8, pp. 936–944, 2006.

[28] A. C. Heller, R. V. Padilla, and A. N. Mamelak, "Complications of epilepsy surgery in the first 8 years after neurosurgical training," *Surgical Neurology*, vol. 71, no. 6, pp. 631–637, 2009.

[29] A. P. Smith, S. Sani, A. M. Kanner et al., "Medically intractable temporal lobe epilepsy in patients with normal MRI: surgical outcome in twenty-one consecutive patients," *Seizure*, vol. 20, no. 6, pp. 475–479, 2011.

[30] J. Engel Jr., M. P. McDermott, S. Wiebe et al., "Early surgical therapy for drug-resistant temporal lobe epilepsy: a randomized trial," *Journal of the American Medical Association*, vol. 307, no. 9, pp. 922–930, 2012.

[31] J. Oertel, M. R. Gaab, U. Runge, H. W. S. Schroeder, W. Wagner, and J. Piek, "Neuronavigation and complication rate in epilepsy surgery," *Neurosurgical Review*, vol. 27, no. 3, pp. 214–217, 2004.

[32] P. Lackner, F. Koppelstaetter, P. Ploner, M. Sojer, J. Dobesberger, G. Walser et al., "Cerebral vasospasm following temporal lobe epilepsy surgery," *Neurology*, vol. 78, pp. 1215–1220, 2012.

[33] A. A. Cohen-Gadol, J. A. Leavitt, J. J. Lynch, W. R. Marsh, and G. D. Cascino, "Prospective analysis of diplopia after anterior temporal lobectomy for mesial temporal lobe sclerosis," *Journal of Neurosurgery*, vol. 99, no. 3, pp. 496–499, 2003.

[34] D. M. Jacobson, J. J. Warner, and K. H. Ruggles, "Transient trochlear nerve palsy following anterior temporal lobectomy for epilepsy," *Neurology*, vol. 45, no. 8, pp. 1465–1468, 1995.

[35] K. Mursch, M.-E. Halatsch, B. J. Steinhoff, and J. Behnke-Mursch, "Lumbar subdural haematoma after temporomesial resection in epilepsy patients-report of two cases and review of the literature," *Clinical Neurology and Neurosurgery*, vol. 109, no. 5, pp. 442–445, 2007.

[36] H. Manji and G. T. Plant, "Epilepsy surgery, visual fields, and driving: a study of the visual field criteria for driving in patients after temporal lobe epilepsy surgery with a comparison

of Goldmann and Esterman perimetry," *Journal of Neurology Neurosurgery and Psychiatry*, vol. 68, no. 1, pp. 80–82, 2000.

[37] G. P. Winston, P. Daga, J. Stretton et al., "Optic radiation tractography and vision in anterior temporal lobe resection," *Annals of Neurology*, vol. 71, no. 3, pp. 334–341, 2012.

[38] L. de Paola, A. R. Troiano, F. M. B. Germiniani et al., "Cerebellar hemorrhage as a complication of temporal lobectomy for refractory medial temporal epilepsy: report of three cases," *Arquivos de Neuro-Psiquiatria*, vol. 62, no. 2 B, pp. 519–522, 2004.

[39] M. T. Toczek, M. J. Morrell, G. A. Silverberg, and G. M. Lowe, "Cerebellar hemorrhage complicating temporal lobectomy: report of four cases," *Journal of Neurosurgery*, vol. 85, no. 4, pp. 718–722, 1996.

[40] A. Konig, R. Laas, and H.-D. Herrmann, "Cerebellar haemorrhage as a complication after supratentorial craniotomy," *Acta Neurochirurgica*, vol. 88, no. 3-4, pp. 104–108, 1987.

[41] S. Yoshida, Y. Yonekawa, K. Yamashita, I. Ihara, and Y. Morooka, "Cerebellar hemorrhage after supratentorial craniotomy. Report of three cases," *Neurologia Medico-Chirurgica*, vol. 30, no. 10, pp. 738–743, 1990.

[42] G. A. Ojemann and C. B. Dodrill, "Verbal memory deficits after left temporal lobectomy for epilepsy. Mechanism and intraoperative prediction," *Journal of Neurosurgery*, vol. 62, no. 1, pp. 101–107, 1985.

[43] U. Gleissner, C. Helmstaedter, J. Schramm, and C. E. Elger, "Memory outcome after selective amygdalohippocampectomy: a study in 140 patients with temporal lobe epilepsy," *Epilepsia*, vol. 43, no. 1, pp. 87–95, 2002.

[44] D. Blumer, S. Wakhlu, K. Davies, and B. Hermann, "Psychiatric outcome of temporal lobectomy for epilepsy: incidence and treatment of psychiatric complications," *Epilepsia*, vol. 39, no. 5, pp. 478–486, 1998.

[45] C. Christodoulou, M. Koutroumanidis, M. J. Hennessy, R. D. C. Elwes, C. E. Polkey, and B. K. Toone, "Postictal psychosis after temporal lobectomy," *Neurology*, vol. 59, no. 9, pp. 1432–1435, 2002.

[46] R. A. Cleary, P. J. Thompson, Z. Fox, and J. Foong, "Predictors of psychiatric and seizure outcome following temporal lobe epilepsy surgery," *Epilepsia*, vol. 53, pp. 1705–1712, 2012.

[47] I. B. Kulaksizoglu, N. Bebek, B. Baykan et al., "Obsessive-compulsive disorder after epilepsy surgery," *Epilepsy and Behavior*, vol. 5, no. 1, pp. 113–118, 2004.

[48] E. Leinonen, A. Tuunainen, and U. Lepola, "Postoperative psychoses in epileptic patients after temporal lobectomy," *Acta Neurologica Scandinavica*, vol. 90, no. 6, pp. 394–399, 1994.

[49] K. Malmgren, J.-E. Starmark, G. Ekstedt, H. Rosén, and C. Sjöberg-Larsson, "Nonorganic and organic psychiatric disorders in patients after epilepsy surgery," *Epilepsy and Behavior*, vol. 3, no. 1, pp. 67–75, 2002.

[50] A. S. Naylor, B. Rogvi-Hansen, L. Kessing, and C. Kruse-Larsen, "Psychiatric morbidity after surgery for epilepsy: short term follow up of patients undergoing amygdalohippocampectomy," *Journal of Neurology Neurosurgery and Psychiatry*, vol. 57, no. 11, pp. 1375–1381, 1994.

[51] P. Shaw, J. Mellers, M. Henderson, C. Polkey, A. S. David, and B. K. Toone, "Schizophrenia-like psychosis arising de novo following a temporal lobectomy: timing and risk factors," *Journal of Neurology, Neurosurgery and Psychiatry*, vol. 75, no. 7, pp. 1003–1008, 2004.

[52] L. Tebartz Van Elst, D. Baeumer, L. Lemieux et al., "Amygdala pathology in psychosis of epilepsy: a magnetic resonance imaging study in patients with temporal lobe epilepsy," *Brain*, vol. 125, no. 1, pp. 140–149, 2002.

[53] J. M. Wrench, S. J. Wilson, M. F. O'Shea, and D. C. Reutens, "Characterising de novo depression after epilepsy surgery," *Epilepsy Research*, vol. 83, no. 1, pp. 81–88, 2009.

[54] M. Koch-Weser, D. C. Garron, D. W. Gilley et al., "Prevalence of psychologic disorders after surgical treatment of seizures," *Archives of Neurology*, vol. 45, no. 12, pp. 1308–1311, 1988.

[55] D. Nilsson, K. Malmgren, B. Rydenhag, and L. Frisén, "Visual field defects after temporal lobectomy: comparing methods and analysing resection size," *Acta Neurologica Scandinavica*, vol. 110, no. 5, pp. 301–307, 2004.

[56] L. Altshuler, R. Rausch, S. Delrahim, J. Kay, and P. Crandall, "Temporal lobe epilepsy, temporal lobectomy, and major depression," *Journal of Neuropsychiatry and Clinical Neurosciences*, vol. 11, no. 4, pp. 436–443, 1999.

[57] S. Anhoury, R. J. Brown, E. S. Krishnamoorthy, and M. R. Trimble, "Psychiatric outcome after temporal lobectomy: a predictive study," *Epilepsia*, vol. 41, no. 12, pp. 1608–1615, 2000.

[58] E. S. Cankurtaran, B. Ulug, S. Saygi, A. Tiryaki, and N. Akalan, "Psychiatric morbidity, quality of life, and disability in mesial temporal lobe epilepsy patients before and after anterior temporal lobectomy," *Epilepsy and Behavior*, vol. 7, no. 1, pp. 116–122, 2005.

[59] O. Devinsky, W. B. Barr, B. G. Vickrey et al., "Changes in depression and anxiety after resective surgery for epilepsy," *Neurology*, vol. 65, no. 11, pp. 1744–1749, 2005.

[60] Y. Inoue and T. Mihara, "Psychiatric disorders before and after surgery for epilepsy," *Epilepsia*, vol. 42, no. 8, pp. 13–18, 2001.

[61] M. Quigg, D. K. Broshek, S. Heidal-Schiltz, J. W. Maedgen, and E. H. Bertram III, "Depression in intractable partial epilepsy varies by laterality of focus and surgery," *Epilepsia*, vol. 44, no. 3, pp. 419–424, 2003.

[62] H. A. Ring, J. Moriarty, and M. R. Trimble, "A prospective study of the early postsurgical psychiatric associations of epilepsy surgery," *Journal of Neurology Neurosurgery and Psychiatry*, vol. 64, no. 5, pp. 601–604, 1998.

[63] X. Chen, D. Weigel, O. Ganslandt, M. Buchfelder, and C. Nimsky, "Prediction of visual field deficits by diffusion tensor imaging in temporal lobe epilepsy surgery," *NeuroImage*, vol. 45, no. 2, pp. 286–297, 2009.

[64] H. W. R. Powell, G. J. M. Parker, D. C. Alexander et al., "MR tractography predicts visual field defects following temporal lobe resection," *Neurology*, vol. 65, no. 4, pp. 596–599, 2005.

[65] C. Schaller, A. Jung, H. Clusmann, J. Schramm, and B. Meyer, "Rate of vasospasm following the transsylvian versus transcortical approach for selective amygdalohippocampectomy," *Neurological Research*, vol. 26, no. 6, pp. 666–670, 2004.

6

Electroencephalogram of Age-Dependent Epileptic Encephalopathies in Infancy and Early Childhood

Lily C. Wong-Kisiel and Katherine Nickels

Division of Child and Adolescent Neurology, Department of Neurology, Mayo Clinic College of Medicine, 200 First St. SW, Rochester, MN 55905, USA

Correspondence should be addressed to Lily C. Wong-Kisiel; wongkisiel.lily@mayo.edu

Academic Editor: Elaine Wirrell

Epileptic encephalopathy syndromes are disorders in which the epileptiform abnormalities are thought to contribute to a progressive cerebral dysfunction. Characteristic electroencephalogram findings have an important diagnostic value in classification of epileptic encephalopathy syndromes. In this paper, we focus on electroencephalogram findings of childhood epileptic encephalopathy syndromes and provide sample illustrations.

1. Introduction

Epilepsy electroclinical syndromes have characteristic seizure semiology, frequency, duration, inciting factors, and age of seizure onset and are often associated with specific electroencephalogram (EEG) findings. Epileptic encephalopathies are syndromes in which the epileptiform abnormalities are thought to contribute to a progressive cerebral dysfunction. The ictal and interictal EEG patterns can help define the electroclinical syndromes, identify potential etiologies, and guide treatment. A detailed description of each genetic etiology is beyond the scope of this review. This review focuses on the neurophysiological features, including variant patterns relevant to selected etiologies (Table 1).

2. Neonatal/Infantile Onset Epilepsy Syndromes

2.1. Early Infantile Epileptic Encephalopathy

2.1.1. Clinical Presentation. Ohtahara first recognized early infantile epileptic encephalopathy (EIEE) in neonates who suffered frequent tonic seizures and subsequently developed significant intellectual disability [1]. Later studies of infants with EIEE show average seizure onset within 2-3 months after birth. Brief tonic seizures occur hundreds of times per day,

often in clusters of 10 to 40 seizures. Focal seizures present as tonic eye deviation or unilateral clonic contractions. Myoclonic seizures are not a prominent feature [2].

2.1.2. Long-Term Prognosis. Mortality in EIEE is high during childhood, with 50% dying during the first 2 years of life [2]. Survivors into childhood have pharmacoresistant epilepsy with severe intellectual disability. EIEE evolves to West syndrome during infancy in 75%, Lennox-Gastaut syndrome in older children, or focal epilepsy [3].

2.1.3. Etiologies. Cerebral structural abnormality is the most common etiology of EIEE. However, in 13–38% of patients, STXBP1 mutation results in synaptic vesicle protein with impaired neurotransmitter release [4–6]. Children with STXBP1 mutation develop a paroxysmal movement disorder during infancy, which persists beyond the intractable phase of the epilepsy [6].

2.1.4. Interictal EEG. Suppression burst pattern is a distinct EEG feature during the early phase of EIEE. This EEG pattern is characterized by a suppression phase less than 10 μV lasting from 3 to 5 seconds with paroxysms of high-voltage 150–350 μV delta-theta bursts of spikes, polyspikes, and sharp waves that alternate at regular intervals [1]. The suppression

TABLE 1: Summary of clinical characteristics and EEG features at presentation in early and childhood onset epileptic encephalopathy.

Epilepsy syndrome	Clinical features				EEG features at presentation		
	Age of seizure onset	Seizure types	Underlying etiology	Prognosis	Background	Interictal	Ictal
Early infantile epileptic encephalopathy (ohtahara syndrome)	First 2 weeks of life	Tonic seizures	Cerebral structural abnormality, genetic abnormalities (i.e., STXBP1)	25% die by 2 years or evolves to West syndrome and profound disability	Suppression burst pattern in awake and sleep	High voltage (150–350 uV) paroxysm	Generalized paroxysms or focal discharges
Early myoclonic encephalopathy	First weeks of life	Myoclonic seizures (erratic/fragmentary/generalized); focal seizures	Metabolic genetic etiologies (nonketotic hyperglycinemia, pyridoxine/pyridoxal-5-phosphate dependency, molybdenum cofactor deficiency, organic aciduria, amino-acidopathies)	50% die within first year or profound disability	Suppression burst pattern, enhanced by sleep	High voltage (150–350 uV) paroxysm	Generalized paroxysms or focal discharges
Migrating focal seizures in infancy	3 months	Focal motor seizures with autonomic manifestations	Unknown; SCN1A, PLCB1, KCNT1 mutations; 2q24, 16p11.2 copy number variants	High mortality before 1 year or profound disability (cortical visual impairment; acquired microcephaly)	Hemispheric background slowing	Multifocal discharges, maximal in temporal and rolandic regions	Rhythmic, monomorphic alpha or theta discharges in noncontiguous brain regions
West syndrome	3–8 months	Epileptic spasms	Heterogenous (congenital cortical malformations, tuberous sclerosis, trisomy 21, trisomy 18, CDKL5, ARX, MECP2)	Depends on etiology; other seizure types evolve by about 5 years	Poorly organized, high amplitude (500–1000 mV), generalized slowing	Multifocal epileptiform discharges with generalized electrodecrement	Generalized sharp wave followed by electrodecrement
Dravet syndrome	6 months	Febrile status epilepticus, alternating hemiconvulsions → absence, and myoclonic seizures	80% SCN1A mutation	Mortality in childhood 10%, intellectual disability, or crouched gait without spasticity in adults	Normal, generalized or focal slowing	Generalized, multifocal or focal discharges; photoparoxysmal response	Generalized paroxysms or focal discharges
ESES-related syndromes	5–8 years	Focal seizures	CSWS structural; LKS unknown	Relapsing-remitting course or age limiting by teenage years	Normal or focal/diffuse slowing	Focal/multifocal/generalized discharges; marked sleep activation with increased interictal spatial distribution or bilateral synchrony; sleep spike wave index >85%; CSWS-frontal predominant LKS-temporal predominant	Focal discharges

TABLE 1: Continued.

Epilepsy syndrome	Clinical features				EEG features at presentation		
	Age of seizure onset	Seizure types	Underlying etiology	Prognosis	Background	Interictal	Ictal
Lennox-Gastaut syndrome	1–8 years	Multiple (tonic, atonic, absences, myoclonic, or focal)	Heterogenous	Intellectual disability	Normal or generalized slowing	Frequent slow spike waves 1.5–2.5 Hz or multifocal	Absence-low spike and waves; tonic-generalized attenuation with recruiting rhythm; atonic-generalized polyspike/spike waves, or attenuation; myoclonic-generalized polyspike/spike waves
Myoclonic-atonic epilepsy	7 months–6 years	Multiple (atonic, myoclonic, absences, or rarely tonic)	No consistent etiology	50% normal cognition at last followup	Normal or mild diffuse/focal slowing	Generalized polyspike-and-wave discharges; photoparoxysmal response	Generalized spike or polyspike-and-wave
Progressive myoclonic epilepsies	Varies by etiology	Prominent myoclonic seizures	Inborn errors of metabolism and mitochondrial disorders (Tay-Sachs, Alpers syndrome, Lafora disease, Unverricht-Lundborg disease, or neuronal ceroid lipofuscinosis)	Developmental regression/dementia; mortality depends on etiology	Generalized slowing	Generalized/multifocal discharges; photoparoxysmal response in Unverricht-Lundborg and neuronal ceroid lipofuscinosis	Generalized discharges

ESES: electrical status epilepticus in slow wave sleep; CSWS: continuous spike wave in sleep; LKS: Landau-Kleffner syndrome.

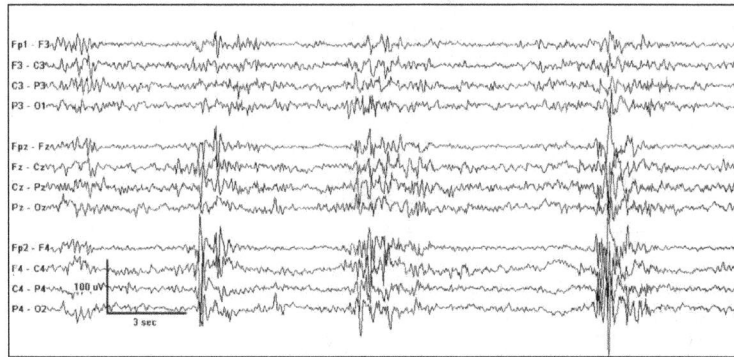

FIGURE 1: Increased burst amplitude over the right hemisphere in an one-month-old girl with right frontal cortical dysplasia.

burst pattern continues during both awake and sleep states. This pattern does not imply specific etiology and can also be seen due to hypoxic ischemic encephalopathy, metabolic derangement, medication effects, and hypothermia.

For those who survive, EEG wake-sleep differentiation occurs from 40 days to 5 months, with more apparent suppression burst in sleep [7]. During wakefulness, suppression burst pattern evolves into hypsarrhythmia pattern, diffuse slowing, multifocal abnormalities, or pseudoperiodic pattern with improved background organization [8]. Asynchronous attenuations present during wakefulness become more synchronized during sleep. Focal slowing, interictal focal spikes, and increased amplitude bursts may lateralize over the side of the structural abnormality (Figure 1). By one year of life, the EEG shows generalized background slowing and generalized or focal paroxysmal fast activity.

2.1.5. Ictal EEG. The burst activities of the suppression burst pattern coincide with tonic seizures [7]. Focal seizures may start as focal rhythmic spike and wave activity followed by tonic seizures. Ictal discharges for focal seizures show no particular localization and any focus can be involved.

2.1.6. EEG Variants. Compared to other etiologies, EEGs of affected patients with STXBP1 mutation have longer periods of suppression and bursts [6].

2.2. Early Myoclonic Encephalopathy

2.2.1. Clinical Presentation. Neonates with early myoclonic encephalopathy (EME) have no apparent perinatal complications or insults and present shortly after birth with progressive decreased alertness and hypotonia. Myoclonic seizures are the initial semiology, followed by focal seizures or epileptic spasms. Myoclonic seizures may begin as fragmentary or focal erratic myoclonus involving regions of the face and limbs, at times nearly continuously, and then become more generalized with time. Focal seizures may manifest as gaze deviation or autonomic disturbances. Between 3 and 4 months of age, seizures evolve into epileptic spasms [9].

2.2.2. Long-Term Prognosis. The long-term prognosis of EME is poor. Approximately 50% of infants die in the first year [1]. Those who survive have profound intellectual disability.

2.2.3. Etiologies. Unlike EIEE, metabolic and genetic etiologies are more common than structural abnormalities. EME has classically been associated with nonketotic hyperglycinemia. However, the etiology is unknown in up to 50% and investigations for pyridoxine or pyridoxal-5-phosphate dependency, molybdenum cofactor deficiency, organic aciduria, and amino acidopathies should also be completed [10, 11].

2.2.4. Interictal EEG. The interictal EEG shows the characteristic suppression burst background initially (Figure 2). In contrast with EIEE, the suppression burst pattern in EME is enhanced by sleep with shorter burst duration. The EEG evolves to atypical hypsarrhythmia or multifocal epileptiform discharges with profound slowing of the background EEG activity at age from 3 to 5 months. Hypsarrhythmia pattern may persist for months before a return to burst suppression pattern [12].

2.2.5. Ictal EEG. The ictal EEG often shows no correlation with the presenting erratic myoclonia [12] (Figure 3). When focal seizures or epileptic spasms occur, the EEG correlate is not different from focal neonatal seizures seen in nonsyndromic cases.

2.3. Migrating Focal Seizures in Infancy

2.3.1. Clinical Presentation. Migrating focal seizures in infancy is also known as malignant migrating partial epilepsy of infancy, first described by Coppola in 1995 [13]. The mean age of seizure onset is 3 months but can occur as early as the neonatal period [14]. Infants have normal development before seizure onset. At presentation, there are sporadic focal motor seizures with rapid evolution to bilateral convulsive seizures. Autonomic manifestations such as apnea, flushing, or cyanosis often occur. The seizures increase in frequency and become nearly continuous multifocal or bihemispheric seizures. Ictal semiology reflects the affected cortical regions. Epilepsy becomes intractable. Profound psychomotor developmental delay ensues. Seizures of multifocal onset may evolve into epileptic spasms, with or without interictal hypsarrhythmic pattern [13, 15–17].

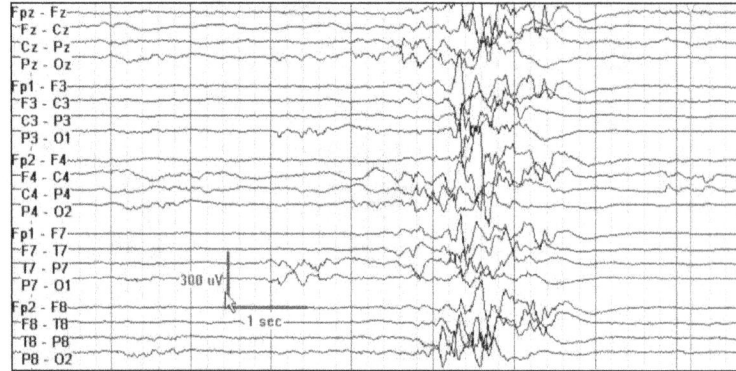

FIGURE 2: Generalized suppression burst pattern in a newborn with early myoclonic encephalopathy.

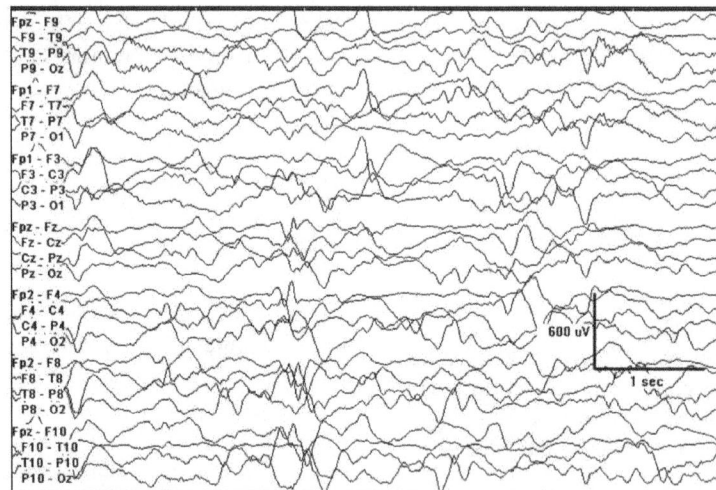

FIGURE 3: High amplitude poorly organized slow background with multifocal epileptiform discharges and intermittent generalized electrodecrement, consistent with hypsarrhythmia at age 4 months in a child with early myoclonic encephalopathy due to nonketotic hyperglycinemia.

2.3.2. Long-Term Prognosis. Although better seizure control may be accomplished between 12 and 14 months, neurologic regression and stagnation continue. Children develop cortical visual impairment. Acquired microcephaly or evidence of brain atrophy is seen during followup. There is high mortality before 1 year of age. Illnesses easily trigger clusters of seizures or occasional status epilepticus.

2.3.3. Etiologies. The etiology is heterogeneous and often is unknown. Genetic etiologies include SCN1A mutations, duplication of 16p11.2, homozygous deletion of the PLCB1 gene, and KCNT1 de novo gain-of-function mutation. Deletion in 2q24 was reported in a single patient [18–22].

2.3.4. Interictal EEG. The EEG at seizure onset shows increased background slowing for several months. The background slow waves shift from one hemisphere to the other. Shortly after initial seizures, multifocal discharges emerge and are present during wakefulness and sleep [23]. Epileptiform discharges are most prominent in the temporal and rolandic areas. As seizure frequency subsides after age one year, the EEG shows a low voltage "burnt out" slowing [24].

2.3.5. Ictal EEG. Ictal onset shifts in consecutive seizures from one lobe to another and from one hemisphere to another (Figure 4). Although the involved ictal regions vary, the ictal pattern is very similar. Ictal EEG shows rhythmic, monomorphic alpha or theta frequency discharges in a localized cortical area, then expand to contiguous regions, or may develop independently in different areas [13]. Tandem seizures in different noncontiguous brain regions may occur, with one seizure beginning before the waning of the other. Ictal and interictal EEGs almost overlap. The original ictal EEG discharges may persist or fade and be replaced by new patterns, thus producing a very complex multifocal status epilepticus.

2.4. West Syndrome

2.4.1. Clinical Presentation. West syndrome refers to the triad of epileptic spasms, intellectual disability, and EEG hypsarrhythmia. Spasm onset is between 3 and 8 months, characterized by brief truncal and neck flexion coinciding with bilateral arm abduction, typically occurring in clusters. Developmental regression occurs.

(a)

(b)

(c)

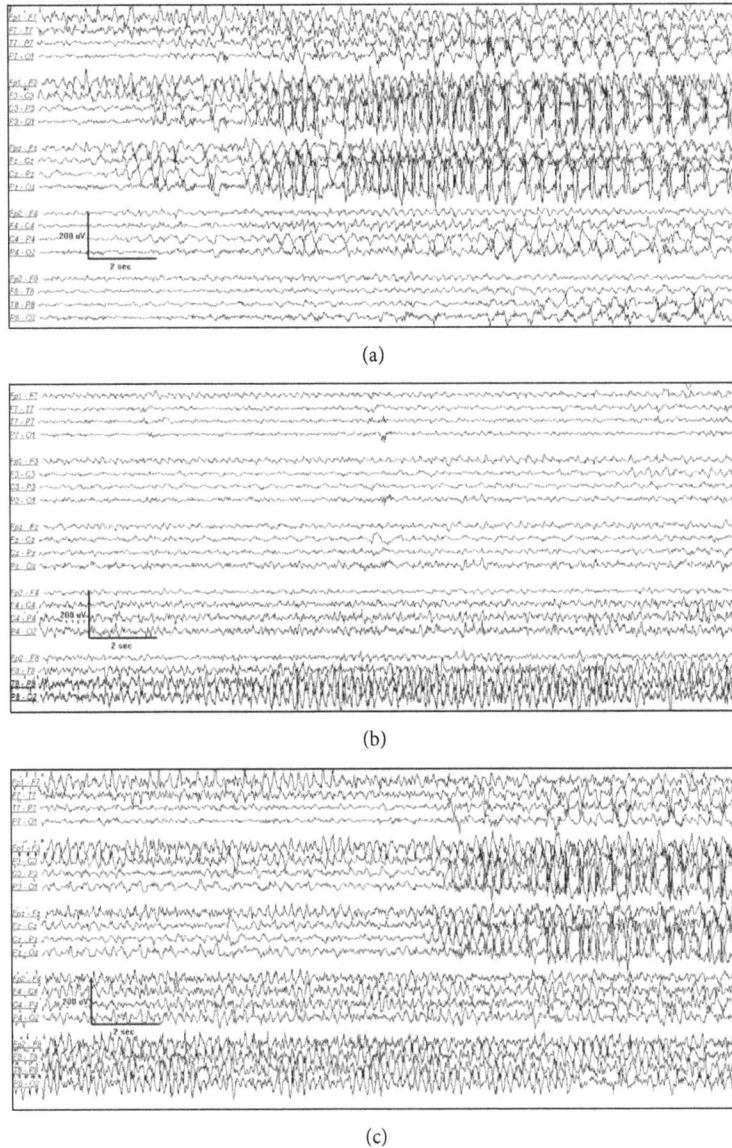

FIGURE 4: 3-month-old female with migrating focal seizures in infancy. (a) Left central onset seizure, (b) right temporal onset seizure 2 minutes later, and (c) independent left central onset seizure with ongoing right temporal lobe seizure 15 minutes later.

2.4.2. Long-Term Prognosis. The long-term prognosis of West syndrome is poor, especially if not treated early. Epileptic spasms typically resolve by age 5 years. Other seizure types often emerge and children may develop Lennox-Gastaut syndrome. Learning disorders, intellectual disability, and autistic features are common. Although an etiology is found in the majority of children with epileptic spasms, those of unknown etiology can have a more favorable prognosis if early effective treatment is provided [25].

2.4.3. Etiologies. Epileptic spasm etiologies are heterogeneous and include structural, metabolic, and genetic causes. Classically, tuberous sclerosis complex (TSC) has been associated with epileptic spasms and must be excluded at initial evaluation. Asymmetric spasms characterized by unilateral head turn, asymmetric upper extremity flexion or extension, or automatisms suggest lateralized structural abnormality. Congenital central nervous system malformation or TSC accounts for more than half of the cases of epileptic spasms, followed by 15% due to chromosomal abnormalities including trisomy 21 and trisomy 18. Monogenic etiologies including X-linked CDKL5, ARX, and MECP2 are increasingly recognized, particularly in children with seizure onset less than 3 months of age and atypical Rett-like features [25]. Hypermotor-tonic-spasm sequence is not diagnostic for a specific etiology but should raise a suspicion for CDKL5 mutation [26].

2.4.4. Interictal EEG. The classic hypsarrhythmia is an interictal EEG pattern of a poorly organized, high amplitude (500–1000 μV), slow background with accompanying multifocal epileptiform discharges, and generalized electrodecrement

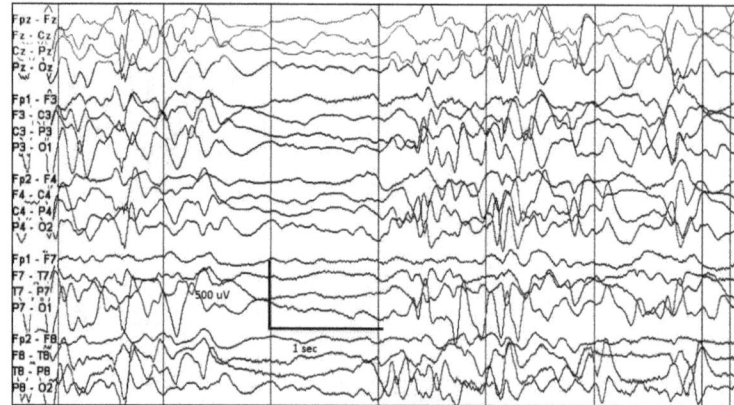

FIGURE 5: Interictal EEG recording of typical hypsarrhythmia in a two-year-old girl with West syndrome due to genetic mutation.

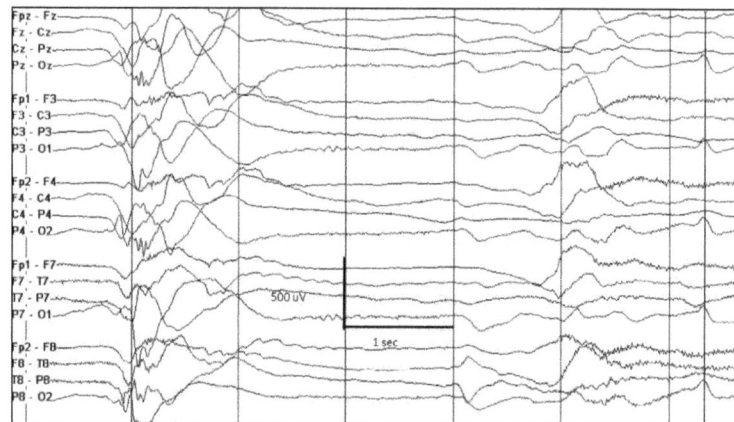

FIGURE 6: Ictal EEG recording of epileptic spasms in a two-year-old girl with West syndrome due to genetic mutation.

(Figure 5). There may be generalized discharges on the interictal recording, but repetitive trains of generalized discharges are uncommon. Lack of hypsarrhythmia in the routine outpatient EEG does not exclude the diagnosis of epileptic spasms. The characteristic EEG features may be present only during non-REM sleep, particularly early in the course of the epilepsy. Prolonged video EEG with recorded spasms and a sleep recording remains an essential diagnostic tool.

2.4.5. Ictal EEG. The EEG during the epileptic spasms typically demonstrates a high amplitude generalized sharp wave followed by generalized electrodecrement (Figure 6). The electrodecrement differentiates short spasms from myoclonic seizures.

2.4.6. EEG Variants. Variant patterns of classic hypsarrhythmia, including more organized or synchronous background, voltage lower than 500 μV, and persistently focal features or asymmetries are often referred to as "modified hypsarrhythmia" but may occur in up to 1/3 of epileptic spasms [27, 28]. In partially treated spasms, especially in older children, the background may be more organized, synchronous, and of lower voltage (Figures 7 and 8). Persistent asymmetry of the ictal or interictal EEG suggests a focal lesion (Figure 9). However, the EEG and semiology may lack lateralizing or localizing features, despite focal structural etiology. Therefore, all children with intractable epileptic spasms due to structural etiology should be evaluated for possible resective surgery, regardless of the presence or absence of localizing EEG features [29, 30].

The EEG in children with CDKL5 initially demonstrates multifocal epileptiform discharges with gradual evolution to hypsarrhythmia or modified hypsarrhythmia, which persists well into early childhood. The prolonged duration of hypsarrhythmia is not typically seen in other causes of West syndrome [6, 31, 32].

The presence of prehypsarrhythmia patterns remains controversial. Retrospective analysis of serial EEGs prior to onset of hypsarrhythmia has demonstrated gradual evolution of multifocal potentially epileptogenic discharges with nearly normal background to frequent bihemispheric discharges with abnormal background [33]. Children who demonstrate worsening EEG background and an increase in bihemispheric epileptiform discharges should be considered at risk for developing epileptic spasms.

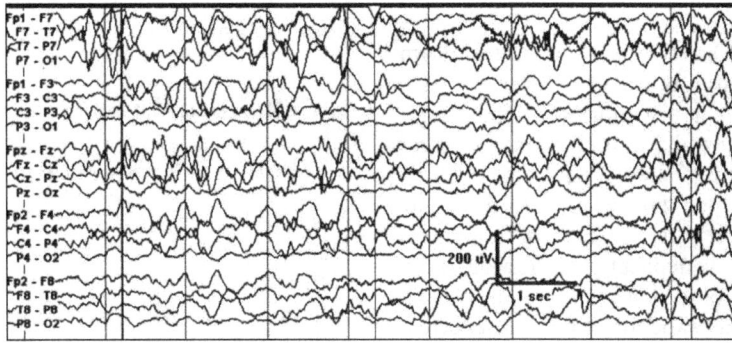

Figure 7: Interictal EEG recording of modified hypsarrhythmia in an 8-month-old child with partially treated epileptic spasms; note the lower amplitude of the background.

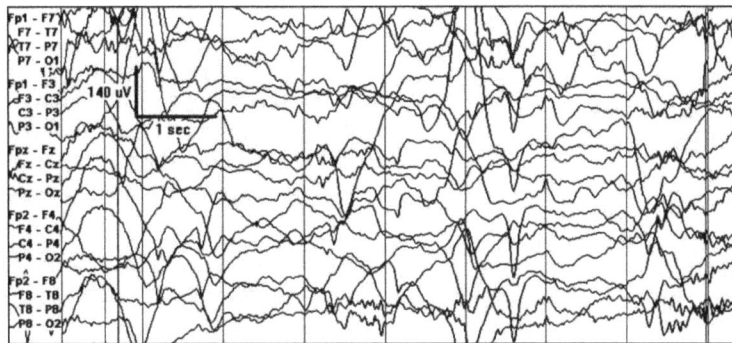

Figure 8: Ictal EEG recording of epileptic spasms with modified hypsarrhythmia.

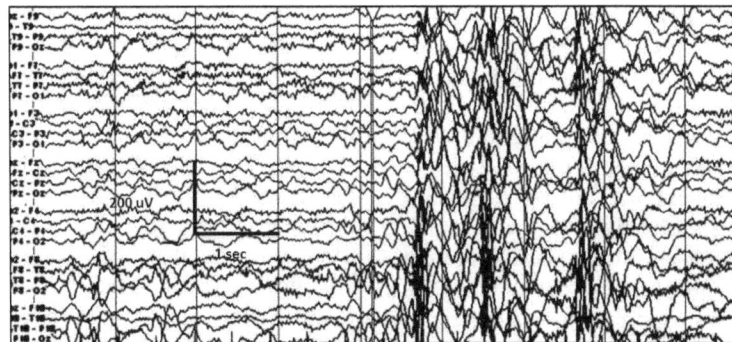

(a) Interictal EEG

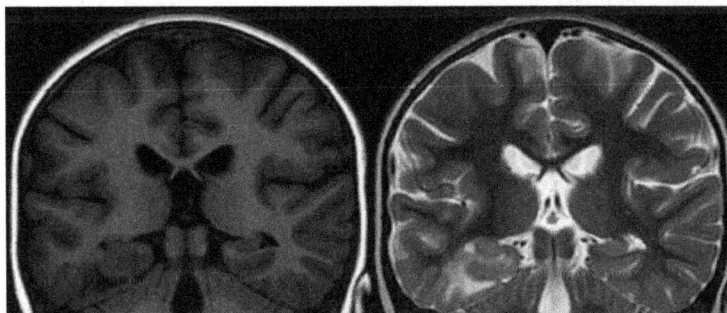

(b) MRI of right temporal lesion

Figure 9: Asymmetric spasm: (a) interictal EEG showing synchronous generalized discharges consistently having maximal amplitude on the right, which corresponds to (b) right temporal focal lesion (WHO 1 ganglioglioma).

2.5. Dravet Syndrome

2.5.1. Clinical Presentation. Dravet syndrome is also known as severe myoclonic epilepsy of infancy. Febrile status epilepticus manifests in previously normal infants prior to age 1 year either as generalized tonic-clonic seizures or a hemiconvulsion involving alternating sides. Afebrile seizures of multiple types then follow and are medically refractory. Head sensitivity, both to fever and ambient temperature, is a hallmark. Antiepileptic medications such as carbamazepine, oxcarbazepine, and phenytoin exacerbate seizures. Development stagnates and may regress. Intellectual disability, impulsivity, and ataxia emerges [34].

2.5.2. Long-Term Prognosis. The prognosis for Dravet syndrome is typically poor although there is phenotypic variability. Frequent intractable seizures and recurrent refractory status epilepticus occur throughout childhood. Seizures often improve in adulthood, but nocturnal convulsive seizures continue [35]. Mortality is reported in up to 10%, and death often occurs due to seizure-related complications [36, 37].

2.5.3. Etiologies. SCN1A mutations are found in 80% of patients with Dravet syndrome although mutations in SCN1B, SCN2A, and GABRG2 have also been reported. A minority of children with clinically diagnosed Dravet syndrome have no mutation found.

2.5.4. Interictal EEG. The EEG findings in Dravet syndrome evolve with age. During the first year of life, the background EEG may be normal or show nonspecific slowing. Generalized or focal slowing may be present if the EEG is done after a prolonged seizure. The interictal epileptiform abnormalities increase between the second and fifth years of life and are typically generalized spike and polyspike and wave discharges. Multifocal or focal abnormalities are also present in the frontocentral or centrotemporal and vertex regions and likely represent fragments of diffuse discharges [38]. Photosensitivity and/or pattern sensitivity may be present in up to 40% of patients [34, 38]. In approximately 19–25% of children, generalized paroxysms and photosensitivity may decrease or disappear with age [39]. Focal and multifocal abnormalities may appear only during sleep [38].

2.5.5. Ictal EEG. The ictal EEG findings depend on the seizure type. Pseudorhythmic spike and wave discharges with periodic attenuations can be present in hemiconvulsion or focal seizures with evolution to bilateral convulsive seizures [38]. Atypical absence seizures are seen within the first year after seizure onset and may be associated with eyelid myoclonus and generalized myoclonus. The EEG shows 2–4 Hz generalized spike wave discharges [40]. Myoclonic seizures can occur in clusters associated with generalized 3 Hz or faster spike wave with frontocentral predominance. Erratic, or segmental, myoclonia involving distal extremities and areas of the face, which are more palpable than visible, are epileptic seizures even though there is no EEG correlation [34]. Tonic seizures are rare in Dravet syndrome. The ictal EEGs in tonic seizures show a generalized fast rhythm lasting from 2 to 3 seconds.

3. Childhood Onset Epilepsy Syndromes

3.1. Electrical Status Epilepticus in Slow Wave Sleep Syndromes

3.1.1. Clinical Presentation. Continuous spike wave in sleep syndrome (CSWS) and Landau Kleffner syndrome (LKS) both present in school-aged children with developmental and behavioral regression. Regression in CSWS is more global with significant executive dysfunction. A history of brain insult or abnormal development can be present before seizure onset and regression. Children with LKS are developmentally normal and then experience a regression in receptive language called acquired auditory agnosia.

3.1.2. Long-Term Prognosis. With treatment, development and seizures improve although clinical and EEG relapses are common. As the child approaches adolescence, the seizures and EEG abnormalities in both CSWS and LKS spontaneously resolve. However, development does not normalize.

3.1.3. Etiologies. Children with LKS have normal neuroimaging and normal development prior to onset of symptoms. There is no known cause of LKS. In contrast, children with CSWS are often found to have genetic, metabolic, or structural etiologies [41].

3.1.4. Interictal EEG. Both syndromes are associated with electrical status epilepticus in slow wave sleep (ESES) defined by nearly continuous epileptiform discharges during slow wave sleep. This EEG pattern must be present to make the diagnosis.

The EEG in CSWS demonstrates focal or diffuse slowing of the background with or without interictal discharges during wakefulness. Epileptiform discharges are focal, multifocal, or generalized. The epileptiform discharges in CSWS are often maximally present over the frontal regions, which may correlate with the observed executive dysfunction of these patients. There is significant activation if spike wave discharges during sleep, typically maximal over the frontal and frontocentral head regions. Furthermore, focal and multifocal discharges often have a broad distribution during sleep (Figure 10).

The EEG in LKS during wakefulness may be normal or may demonstrate focal epileptiform discharges that are maximal over the frontotemporal or temporal regions. Like the children with CSWS, there may be focal or generalized slowing of the background activity. The EEG during sleep demonstrates nearly continuous spike wave discharges that are often maximal over the temporal regions (Figure 11) [41].

3.1.5. Ictal EEG. Children with CSWS and LKS may or may not have seizures, making these unique epilepsy syndromes. The ictal EEG is similar to other focal seizures and is not diagnostic.

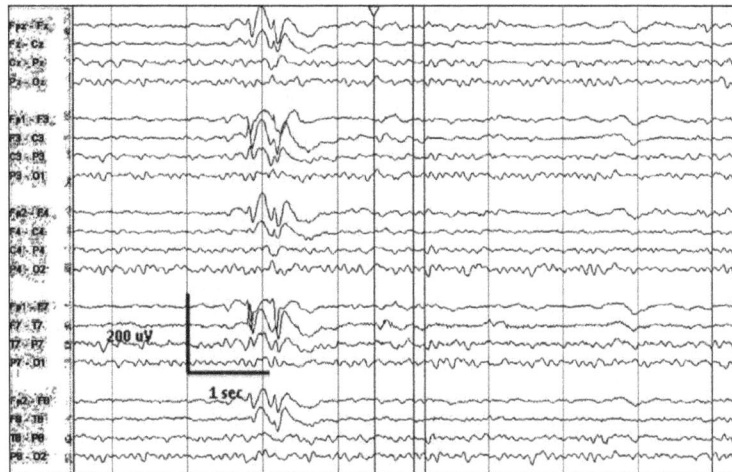

(a) Awake EEG in CSWS

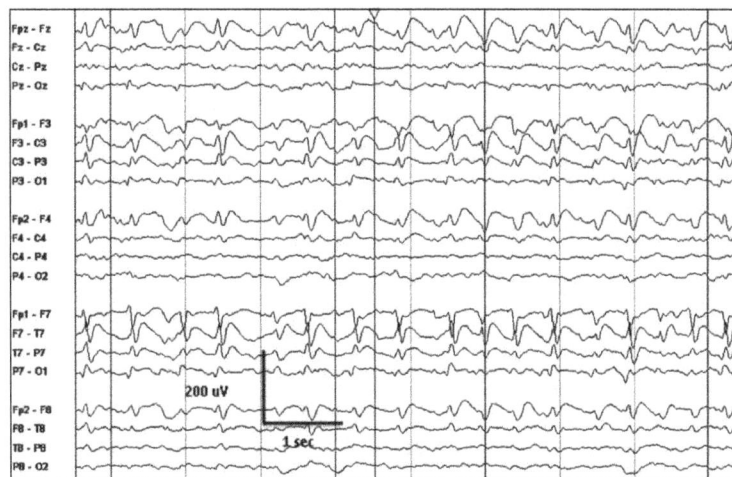

(b) Sleep EEG in CSWS

FIGURE 10: EEG in a patient with CSWS and history of left neonatal intraventricular hemorrhage: (a) awake interictal EEG in CSWS demonstrating generalized epileptiform discharges, maximal left, and (b) asleep interictal EEG demonstrating continuous epileptiform discharges maximally present over the frontocentral head regions, maximal left.

3.2. Lennox-Gastaut Syndrome

3.2.1. Clinical Presentation. Lennox-Gastaut syndrome (LGS) manifests in children from 1 to 8 years of age. The most common seizures are tonic, atonic, and absence seizures. All seizure types may not be present simultaneously or at onset. The presence of other seizure types such as myoclonic seizures, unilateral clonic seizures, or focal seizures with or without evolution to bilateral convulsive seizures does not exclude LGS [42]. LGS can evolve from epileptic spasms. Developmental delay is present in 20–60% of patients at onset and increases to 75–95% after 5 years [43].

3.2.2. Long-Term Prognosis. The long-term prognosis for Lennox-Gastaut syndrome is poor. Refractory seizures may improve with time but do not resolve. Recurrent status epilepticus also continues. Intellectual disability continues throughout life. Those with early onset epilepsy, especially

those with a prior history of West syndrome, have the worst prognosis [44].

3.2.3. Etiologies. Etiologies for LGS are heterogeneous. Up to 1/3 of children have no known cause of their epilepsy. Structural lesions are a common cause of LGS and may be due to congenital malformation so of cortical development, hypoxic-ischemic encephalopathy or other cerebrovascular events, and tuberous sclerosis complex. Genetic and metabolic disorders are also associated with LGS, but less frequently [44].

3.2.4. Interictal EEG. At seizure onset, the interictal EEG may demonstrate a slow and poorly organized background during wakefulness with normal EEG during sleep. The degree of slowing tends to correlate with severity of intellectual impairment. Diffuse slow spike wave discharges then occur in repetitive sequences but can be irregular infrequency,

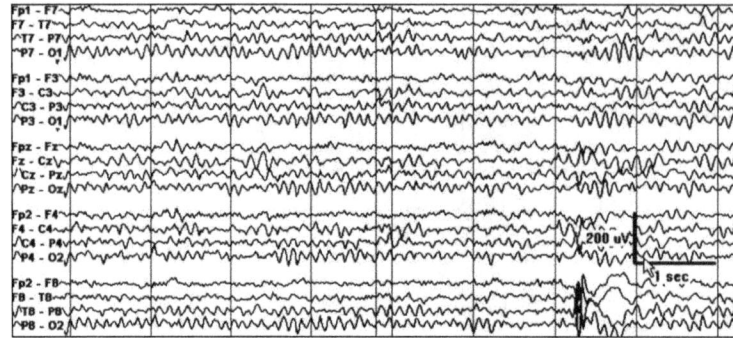

(a) Awake interictal EEG in LKS

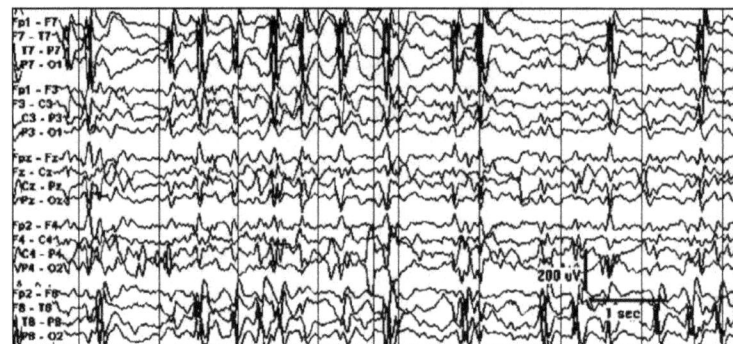

(b) Asleep interictal EEG in LKS

FIGURE 11: EEG in a nine-year old with LKS: (a) awake interictal EEG demonstrating infrequent potentially epileptiform discharges over the right temporal region and (b) asleep interictal EEG demonstrating nearly continuous discharges maximally present over the bilateral temporal regions.

amplitude, morphology, and distribution. Slow spike wave discharges (SSW) consist of a spike (<70 ms) or a sharp wave (70–200 ms), followed by a positive deflection and a sinusoidal negative slow wave of 300–500 ms (Figure 12) [44]. SSWs repeat between 1 and 4 Hz, but typically at 1.5–2.5 Hz [45]. SSWs are abundant and at times prolonged without apparent clinical changes. Hyperventilation and photic stimulation do not generally increase SSW. Focal and multifocal epileptiform discharges are seen in 14–18% of patients [44].

In adulthood, the awake EEG may be normal or show generalized slowing. Generalized fast activity persists in sleep, but the SSW are present only in a minority of adults with LGS [46]. Many EEGs evolve to show independent multifocal spike wave discharges [47].

3.2.5. Ictal EEG.
The ictal EEG pattern depends on the recorded seizure type. Bursts of nearly continuous SSW may be associated with decreased responsiveness, representing atypical absence seizures. The ictal EEG shows high amplitude 1.5–2.5 Hz and is difficult to distinguish from the interictal pattern. Tonic seizures are associated with generalized voltage attenuation (electrodecremental pattern) or bursts of low-amplitude fast (15–25 Hz) activity with increasing amplitude 50–100 μV ("recruiting" rhythm), followed by generalized delta slowing for several seconds before returning to baseline (Figure 13). Atonic seizures can be characterized

by generalized spike-wave activity, generalized polyspike-and-wave activity, generalized voltage attenuation, or runs of low- or high- voltage fast activity (Figure 14). Myoclonic seizures may show generalized spike or polyspike and wave discharge corresponding to the myoclonic jerk. In adulthood, the tonic seizures and accompanying diffuse fast rhythms continue during sleep [48].

Status epilepticus occurs in more than 2/3 of all patients with LGS. Tonic status and atypical absence status are the most common. The EEG during status epilepticus may be difficult to appreciate from the abnormal interictal pattern of abundant SSW. Ictal spike wave discharges are more persistent and the EEG becomes more desynchronous and absence of posterior background activity [42].

3.3. Myoclonic-Atonic Epilepsy

3.3.1. Clinical Presentation.
Myoclonic-atonic epilepsy (MAE) is also known as myoclonic-astatic epilepsy, or Doose syndrome. Seizure onset is between 7 months and 6 years in previously normally developing children. It is more common in males by twofold, except in the first year of life during which the ratio is similar. Myoclonic-atonic seizures are characterized by initial vocalization or grunt, caused by quick contracture of the diaphragm, followed by atonic head or body drop. The presence of the myoclonic-atonic sequence accounts for 10% of children with MAE; 50% have isolated

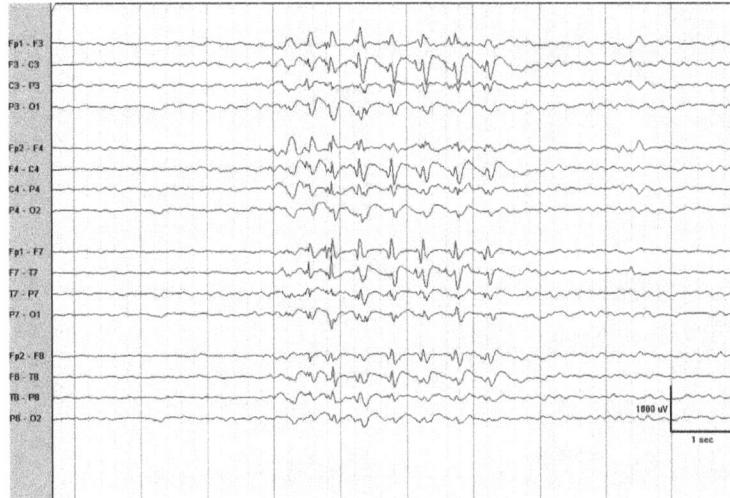

FIGURE 12: Slow spike and wave discharges in a four-year-old child with Lennox-Gastaut syndrome. Note the high amplitude of the generalized, anteriorly predominant, slow spike and wave discharges.

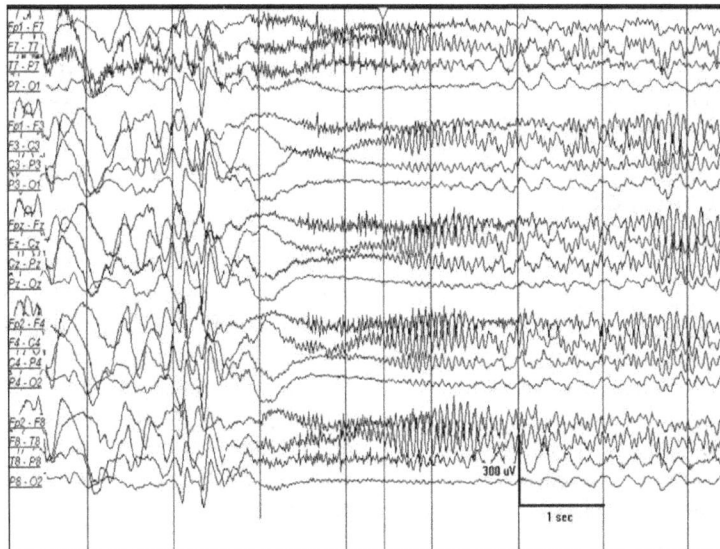

FIGURE 13: A 17-year-old man with history of autism spectrum disorder with a tonic seizure. Generalized voltage attenuation (electrodecremental pattern), bursts of low amplitude fast activity (15–25 Hz) with increasing amplitude from 50 to 100 μV with a "recruiting" rhythm.

myoclonic seizures and 30% have isolated atonic seizures [49]. Other seizure types present include absence seizures, clonic seizures, and generalized tonic-clonic seizures. Tonic seizures are only rarely present. Status epilepticus of absence seizures and myoclonic-atonic seizures is common.

3.3.2. Long-Term Prognosis. The prognosis of MAE is variable. If effective treatment is found early, some children can become seizure-free and have a good cognitive outcome. Although prognosis cannot be predicted at initial presentation, those children with status epilepticus and cognitive decline have a poorer outcome. EEG features that suggest less favorable outcome include persistence of abnormal background slowing and failure of alpha rhythm to develop.

3.3.3. Etiologies. There is no known cause of MAE identified although there may be a possible genetic link to the generalized epilepsy with febrile seizures plus (GEFS+) family [50].

3.3.4. Interictal EEG. The EEG is initially normal. Diffuse or focal theta activities have been described. Brief bursts of generalized polyspike and wave epileptiform activity at 2–5 Hz are noted. Occipital 4 Hz activity may also be seen and can be attenuated by eye opening [50]. Photoparoxysmal responses are associated with 3–7 Hz generalized spike and wave complexes.

3.3.5. Ictal EEG. All ictal EEGs demonstrate generalized spike or polyspike and wave complexes. Persistent focal EEG

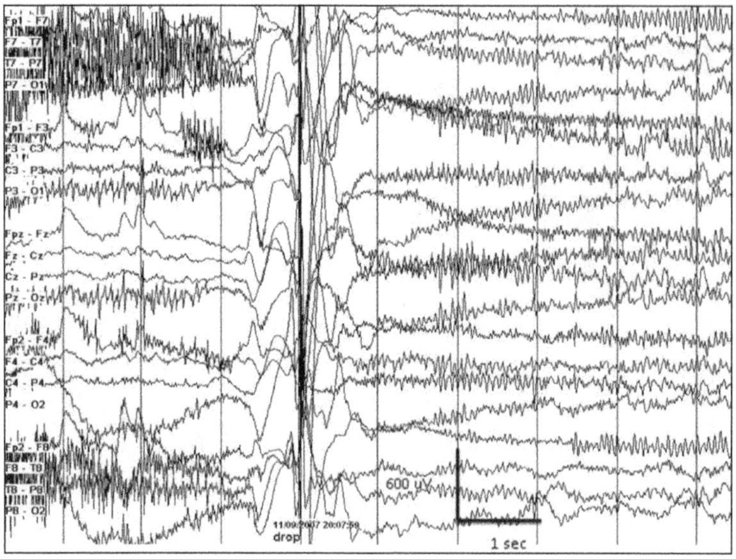

FIGURE 14: A 7-year-old girl with Lennox-Gastaut syndrome. Atonic seizure associated with generalized polyspike-and-wave, generalized voltage attenuation, and runs of low voltage fast activity.

findings are not typically seen in MAE although apparent focal abnormalities or shifting laterality may be present and are likely fragments of generalized discharges [50].

4. Epilepsy Syndromes with Variable Age of Onset

4.1. Progressive Myoclonic Epilepsies. Progressive myoclonic epilepsies are rare disorders caused by metabolic, genetic, and neurodegenerative diseases. Children can present at all ages with multiple seizure types, worsening myoclonus, and developmental regression. Long-term prognosis and mortality depend on the specific etiology. The interictal EEG in the progressive myoclonic epilepsies demonstrates generalized slowing of the background with frequent generalized and multifocal epileptiform discharges. The myoclonus is associated with a generalized spike and wave discharge on EEG. Photosensitivity is common and can increase interictal and ictal discharges. These patterns are neither specific nor sensitive for determining specific etiology [51] although there are some clinical and neurophysiologic findings that can be helpful in determining etiology.

4.1.1. Tay-Sachs. Tay-Sachs is due to hexosaminidase a deficiency and typically presents during infancy with exaggerated startle reflex to sound a developmental regression. The EEG can demonstrate fast spikes over the central head region [52].

4.1.2. Myoclonic Epilepsy with Ragged Red Fibers. Mitochondrial disorders result in metabolic energy failure. The cerebral involvement manifests as seizures. Myoclonic epilepsy with ragged red fibers is an example of a mitochondrial disease that presents with multiple neurologic signs in addition to myoclonic epilepsy, including deafness, myopathy, optic atrophy, and cerebellar ataxia. The EEG is nonspecific,

demonstrating slowing of the background with generalized and focal epileptiform discharges [51].

4.1.3. POLG1 Mutation. Mutation in the nuclear encoded mitochondrial POLG1 gene may manifest as Alpers disease or as ataxia syndromes such as myoclonus, epilepsy, myopathy, sensory ataxia (MEMSA) syndromes in older individuals. Alpers disease causes recurrent prolonged status epilepticus, hepatic failure, and cognitive decline. The EEG in Alpers disease demonstrates a slow or absent posterior dominant rhythm with multifocal and generalized epileptiform activity [53] (Figure 15). Status epilepticus is common and may have an EEG correlation of high amplitude delta activity that is maximal over the posterior head regions with superimposed epileptiform activity [54].

4.1.4. Lafora Disease. During adolescence, Lafora disease causes recurrent seizures and cognitive regression. Early in the course of Lafora disease, the generalized epileptiform discharges occur at a frequency of approximately 3 Hz. As the disease progresses, there is slowing of the background and the frequency of the discharges increases from 3 Hz up to 6–12 Hz [51].

4.1.5. Unverricht-Lundborg Disease. Similar to Lafora disease, Unverricht-Lundborg disease is also associated with adolescent onset epilepsy with cognitive regression. The EEG in Unverricht-Lundborg disease is nonspecific during wakefulness, showing the expected generalized slowing, epileptiform discharges, and photoparoxysmal response. However, the sleep EEG patterns remain essentially normal, which is not a typical finding in other progressive myoclonic epilepsies [51].

4.1.6. Neuronal Ceroid Lipofuscinosis. Neuronal ceroid lipofuscinosis (NCL) also presents in adolescence with refractory

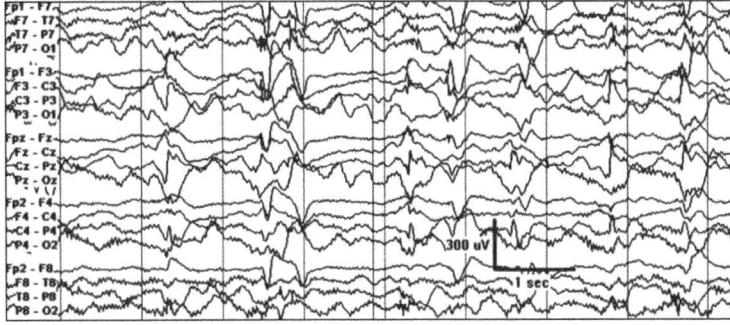

FIGURE 15: Interictal EEG in Alper's disease due to POLG1 mutation demonstrating high-amplitude generalized epileptiform discharges and suppressed background.

seizures and regression, as well as visual loss. As in other storage diseases, there is progressive slowing of the background activity on the EEG, leading to loss or "vanishing" of EEG activity in NCL [52]. Photosensitivity with a photoparoxysmal response below 3 Hz may also be present [55].

4.2. Immune-Mediated Syndromes.
Autoimmune-mediated etiologies for epilepsy are increasingly recognized and should be suspected in patients with multifocal neurologic signs and symptoms, including intractable epilepsy, psychiatric disorder, cognitive dysfunction, movement disorders, sleep disturbance, or autonomic dysfunction with acute or subacute onset and a progressive course. There may be personal or family history of autoimmunity or symptom onset after illness or immunizations.

4.2.1. Rasmussen's Encephalitis.
Rasmussen's encephalitis is an autoimmune-mediated progressive focal epilepsy with associated increasing contralateral hemiatrophy. The EEG may show lateralized background slowing ipsilateral to the hemiatrophy. Epilepsia partialis continua is common and may not have an EEG correlation (Figure 16).

4.2.2. Voltage-Gated Potassium Channel Complex Antibodies.
Voltage-gated potassium channel (VGKC) complex antibodies are associated with intractable epilepsy and encephalopathy in children. LGI1 and CASPR2 are the two most commonly identified VGKC target antigens. The interictal EEG demonstrates nonspecific slowing of the background and multifocal or generalized epileptiform discharges. Faciobrachial dystonic seizures are characterized by brief unilateral facial grimace with concurrent ipsilateral arm dystonia that occurs many times per day and is often seen in children and adults with VGKC-related encephalopathy [56]. The ictal EEG demonstrates contralateral rhythmic frontotemporal spike wave discharges.

4.2.3. NMDA Receptor Antibodies.
NMDA receptor (NMDAR) antibodies are also associated with intractable epilepsy and encephalopathy in children. The EEG in patients with NMDAR antibodies demonstrates diffuse nonspecific slowing but often does not reveal potentially epileptogenic discharges. In a minority of patients, nearly

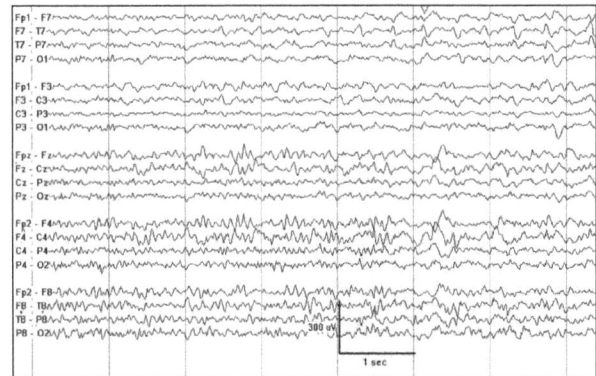

(a) Focal left temporal interictal discharges with decreased amplitude over the left hemisphere

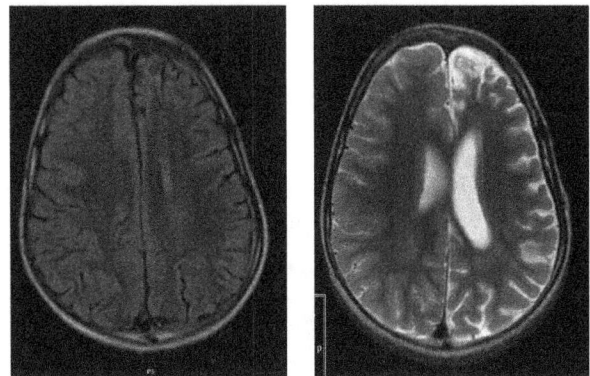

(i)   (ii)

(b) Progressive cerebral atrophy at (i) 8 months and (ii) 15 months after seizure onset

FIGURE 16: EEG in a previously well child presenting with epilepsia partialis continua, progressive hemiparesis, and contralateral cerebral atrophy, consistent with Rasmussen's syndrome.

continuous 1–3 Hz delta activity with superimposed bursts of beta frequency fast activity is present, termed "extreme delta brush" because it is reminiscent of the spindle delta brush pattern seen in premature infants [57].

4.3. Specific EEG Findings in Other Childhood Developmental Disabilities.
Rarely, neurodevelopmental syndromes are

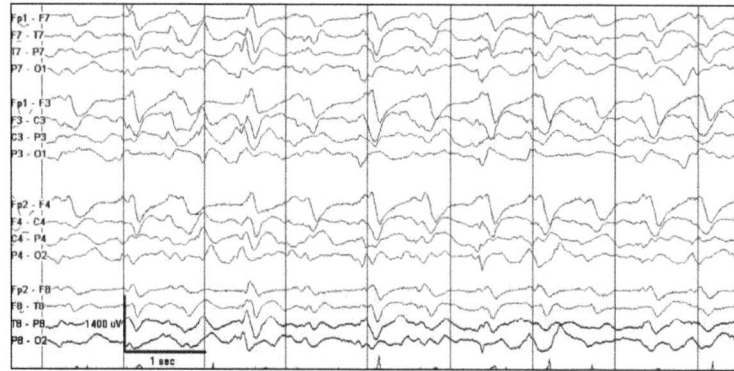

FIGURE 17: A 5 year-old girl with Angelman syndrome. The notched-delta pattern, a variant of ill-defined slow spike-and-wave complexes, in which spikes are superimposed on the ascending or the descending phase of the slow wave giving it a notched appearance.

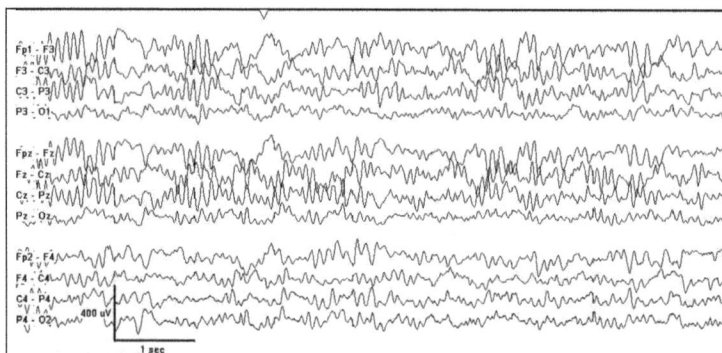

(a) Diffuse alpha and beta activity greater than $100\,\mu V$

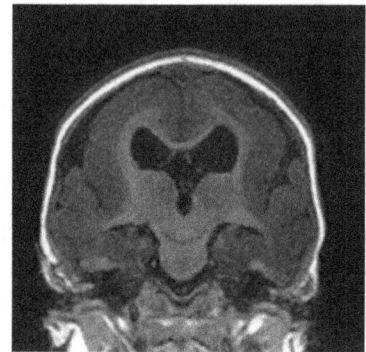

(b) MRI showing lissencephaly

FIGURE 18: Lissencephaly due to *DCX* mutation in a 6 month-old male.

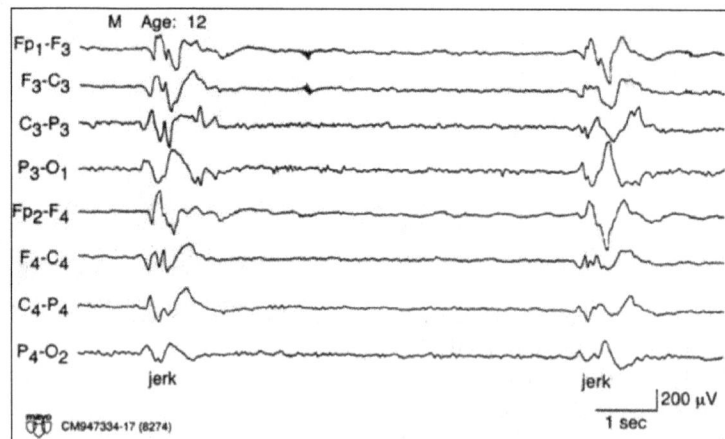

FIGURE 19: A 12-year-old boy with subacute sclerosis panencephalitis. Note high voltage, polyphasic sharp-and slow-wave complexes, lasting from 0.5 to 2 seconds in a pseudoperiodic pattern.

associated with specific EEG patterns, both epileptiform and nonepileptiform. Recognition of these specific EEG patterns can be helpful in identifying the underlying syndrome.

4.3.1. Angelman Syndrome. Angelman syndrome is a neurodevelopmental disorder caused by absence of functional maternally inherited UBE3A gene on chromosome 15q11–q13

[58]. Children have severe developmental delay, poor, or no language acquisition, happy demeanor, stereotypies, and wide-based gait. Epilepsy and EEG abnormalities are seen in 80% of patients [59]. Generalized diffuse slowing with normal sleep patterns is seen. The notched delta pattern (Figure 17) is seen in 73% of patients with Angelman syndrome at a mean age of 5.2 years [60]. Interictal epileptiform abnormalities are focal or multifocal in distribution.

4.3.2. Lissencephaly. Lissencephaly is a severe malformation of cortical development with agyria or pachygyria. Onset of epileptic spasms may be the presenting feature that leads to diagnosis. The background EEG is nonspecific. Three reported EEG patterns are seen in lissencephaly: (1) diffuse greater than $100\,\mu V$ alpha and beta activity in all cortical regions (Figure 18), (2) alternating high amplitude $>300\,\mu V$ bursts of sharp and slow waves followed by short periods of attenuation, and (3) high amplitude spike wave or sharp wave activity, without alpha or beta frequencies or attenuations. Children with anterior agyria-pachygyria with DCX mutation have diffuse moderate amplitude alpha activity, whereas those with posterior predominant cortical abnormality seen in LIS1 mutation tend to have the EEG pattern with bursts of sharp and slow waves with periods of attenuation.

4.3.3. Subacute Sclerosis Panencephalitis. Subacute sclerosis panencephalitis (SSPE) is a postmeasles encephalitis causing a degenerative process in children and adolescents. It is characterized by motor jerks and progressive intellectual deterioration. The typical EEG pattern consists of high voltage, polyphasic sharp- and slow-wave complexes, lasting from 0.5 to 2 seconds in duration and occurring repetitively in a pseudoperiodic fashion (Figure 19). The complexes are usually generalized and bisynchronous but may be asymmetric or occur in a more lateralized or focal fashion. The complexes may occur at irregular intervals initially. As the disease progresses, the complexes occur at regular intervals, typically every 4 to 15 seconds but may range up to 1 to 5 minutes. Stereotyped motor jerks or spasms occur in association with the periodic complexes. The movements may take place simultaneously with, prior to, or following the periodic complexes. The slow-wave complexes occurring in a regular and periodic fashion and having a constant relationship to motor movements make this pattern specific to SSPE [61].

5. Conclusion

When children present with new onset seizures, the long-term outcome is of great concern to parents and clinicians. Knowledge of the EEG findings supportive of specific electroclinical syndromes is important for accurate diagnosis. Classification of epilepsy electroclinical syndromes is essential particularly in epileptic encephalopathy to guide optimal treatments and counsel family regarding expected outcome.

References

[1] J. Aicardi and S. Ohtahara, "Severe neonatal epilepsies with suppression-burst pattern," in *Epileptic Syndromes in Infancy, Childhood and Adolescence,* J. Roger, M. Bureau, C. Dravet, and P. Genton, Eds., pp. 39–50, John Libbey Eurotext, Montrouge, France, 4th edition, 2005.

[2] Y. Yamatogi and S. Ohtahara, "Early-infantile epileptic encephalopathy with suppression-bursts, Ohtahara syndrome; its overview referring to our 16 cases," *Brain and Development,* vol. 24, no. 1, pp. 13–23, 2002.

[3] Y. Yamatogi and S. Ohtahara, "Multiple independent spike foci and epilepsy, with special reference to a new epileptic syndrome of "severe epilepsy with multiple independent spike foci"," *Epilepsy Research,* vol. 70, pp. S96–S104, 2006.

[4] H. Saitsu, M. Kato, T. Mizuguchi et al., "De novo mutations in the gene encoding STXBP1 (MUNC18-1) cause early infantile epileptic encephalopathy," *Nature Genetics,* vol. 40, no. 6, pp. 782–788, 2008.

[5] H. Saitsu, M. Kato, I. Okada et al., "STXBP1 mutations in early infantile epileptic encephalopathy with suppression-burst pattern," *Epilepsia,* vol. 51, no. 12, pp. 2397–2405, 2010.

[6] M. Milh, N. Villeneuve, M. Chouchane et al., "Epileptic and nonepileptic features in patients with early onset epileptic encephalopathy and STXBP1 mutations," *Epilepsia,* vol. 52, no. 10, pp. 1828–1834, 2011.

[7] L. Fusco, C. Pachatz, M. Di Capua, and F. Vigevano, "Video/EEG aspects of early-infantile epileptic encephalopathy with suppression-bursts (Ohtahara syndrome)," *Brain and Development,* vol. 23, no. 7, pp. 708–714, 2001.

[8] S. I. Malik, C. A. Galliani, A. W. Hernandez et al., "Epilepsy surgery for early infantile epileptic encephalopathy (Ohtahara syndrome)," *Journal of Child Neurology,* vol. 2012, 11 pages, 2012.

[9] E. M. Mizrahi and R. R. Clancy, "Neonatal seizures: early-onset seizure syndromes and their consequences for development," *Mental Retardation Developmental Disability Research Reviews,* vol. 6, no. 4, pp. 229–241, 2000.

[10] S. Khan and R. Al Baradie, "Epileptic encephalopathies: an overview," *Epilepsy Research and Treatment,* vol. 2012, Article ID 403592, 8 pages, 2012.

[11] S. Rossi, I. Daniele, P. Bastrenta, M. Mastrangelo, and G. Lista, "Early myoclonic encephalopathy and nonketotic hyperglycinemia," *Pediatric Neurology,* vol. 41, no. 5, pp. 371–374, 2009.

[12] A. Djukic, F. A. Lado, S. Shinnar, and S. L. Moshé, "Are early myoclonic encephalopathy (EME) and the Ohtahara syndrome (EIEE) independent of each other?" *Epilepsy Research,* vol. 70, supplement 1, pp. S68–S76, 2006.

[13] G. Coppola, P. Plouin, C. Chiron, O. Robain, and O. Dulac, "Migrating partial seizures in infancy: a malignant disorder with developmental arrest," *Epilepsia,* vol. 36, no. 10, pp. 1017–1024, 1995.

[14] G. Hmaimess, H. Kadhim, M.-C. Nassogne, C. Bonnier, and K. van Rijckevorsel, "Levetiracetam in a neonate with malignant migrating partial seizures," *Pediatric Neurology,* vol. 34, no. 1, pp. 55–59, 2006.

[15] E. Veneselli, M. V. Perrone, M. Di Rocco, R. Gaggero, and R. Biancheri, "Malignant migrating partial seizures in infancy," *Epilepsy Research,* vol. 46, no. 1, pp. 27–32, 2001.

[16] B. Jocic-Jakubi and L. Lagae, "Malignant migrating partial seizures in Aicardi syndrome," *Developmental Medicine and Child Neurology,* vol. 50, no. 10, pp. 790–792, 2008.

[17] E. H. Lee, M.-S. Yum, M.-H. Jeong, K. Y. Lee, and T.-S. Ko, "A case of malignant migrating partial seizures in infancy as a continuum of infantile epileptic encephalopathy," *Brain and Development,* vol. 34, no. 9, pp. 768–772, 2012.

[18] J. K. Bedoyan, R. A. Kumar, J. Sudi et al., "Duplication 16p11.2 in a child with infantile seizure disorder," *American Journal of Medical Genetics A,* vol. 152, no. 6, pp. 1567–1574, 2010.

[19] D. Carranza Rojo, L. Hamiwka, J. M. McMahon et al., "De novo SCN1A mutations in migrating partial seizures of infancy," *Neurology,* vol. 77, no. 4, pp. 380–383, 2011.

[20] E. R. Freilich, J. M. Jones, W. D. Gaillard et al., "Novel SCN1A mutation in a proband with malignant migrating partial seizures of infancy," *Archives of Neurology*, vol. 68, no. 5, pp. 665–671, 2011.

[21] G. Barcia, M. R. Fleming, A. Deligniere et al., "De novo gain-of-function KCNT1 channel mutations cause malignant migrating partial seizures of infancy," *Nature Genetics*, vol. 44, no. 11, pp. 1255–1259, 2012.

[22] A. Poduri, S. S. Chopra, E. G. Neilan et al., "Homozygous PLCB1 deletion associated with malignant migrating partial seizures in infancy," *Epilepsia*, vol. 53, no. 8, pp. e146–e150, 2012.

[23] G. Coppola, "Malignant migrating partial seizures in infancy: an epilepsy syndrome of unknown etiology," *Epilepsia*, vol. 50, no. 5, pp. 49–51, 2009.

[24] R. H. Caraballo, E. Fontana, F. Darra et al., "Migrating focal seizures in infancy: analysis of the electroclinical patterns in 17 patients," *Journal of Child Neurology*, vol. 23, no. 5, pp. 497–506, 2008.

[25] J. W. Wheless, P. A. Gibson, K. L. Rosbeck et al., "Infantile spasms (West syndrome): update and resources for pediatricians and providers to share with parents," *BMC Pediatrics*, vol. 12, no. 1, pp. 108–116, 2012.

[26] K. M. Klein, S. C. Yendle, A. S. Harvey et al., "A distinctive seizure type in patients with Cdkl5 mutations: hypermotor-tonic-spasms sequence," *Neurology*, vol. 76, no. 16, pp. 1436–1438, 2011.

[27] U. Kramer, W. C. Sue, and M. A. Mikati, "Hypsarrhythmia: frequency of variant patterns and correlation with etiology and outcome," *Neurology*, vol. 48, no. 1, pp. 197–203, 1997.

[28] E. Wyllie, *Wyllie's Treatment of Epilepsy: Principles and Practice*, E. Wyllie, Philadelphia, Pa, USA, 5th edition, 2011.

[29] E. Wyllie, D. K. Lachhwani, A. Gupta et al., "Successful surgery for epilepsy due to early brain lesions despite generalized EEG findings," *Neurology*, vol. 69, no. 4, pp. 389–397, 2007.

[30] M.-S. Yum, T.-S. Ko, J. K. Lee, S. Hong, D. S. Kim, and J. Kim, "Surgical treatment for localization-related infantile spasms: excellent long-term outcomes," *Clinical Neurology and Neurosurgery*, vol. 113, no. 3, pp. 213–217, 2011.

[31] N. Bahi-Buisson, A. Kaminska, N. Boddaert et al., "The three stages of epilepsy in patients with CDKL5 mutations," *Epilepsia*, vol. 49, no. 6, pp. 1027–1037, 2008.

[32] J. Jahn, A. Caliebe, S. von Spiczak et al., "CDKL5 mutations as a cause of severe epilepsy in infancy: clinical and electroencephalographic long-term course in 4 patients," *Journal of Child Neurology*, vol. 28, no. 7, pp. 937–941, 2012.

[33] H. Philippi, G. Wohlrab, U. Bettendorf et al., "Electroencephalographic evolution of hypsarrhythmia: toward an early treatment option," *Epilepsia*, vol. 49, no. 11, pp. 1859–1864, 2008.

[34] A. Arzimanoglou, "Dravet syndrome: from electroclinical characteristics to molecular biology," *Epilepsia*, vol. 50, supplement 8, pp. 3–9, 2009.

[35] C. B. Catarino, J. Y. W. Liu, I. Liagkouras et al., "Dravet syndrome as epileptic encephalopathy: evidence from long-term course and neuropathology," *Brain*, vol. 134, no. 10, pp. 2982–3010, 2011.

[36] J. V. Skluzacek, K. P. Watts, O. Parsy, B. Wical, and P. Camfield, "Dravet syndrome and parent associations: the IDEA League experience with comorbid conditions, mortality, management, adaptation, and grief," *Epilepsia*, vol. 52, supplement 2, pp. 95–101, 2011.

[37] M. Sakauchi, H. Oguni, I. Kato et al., "Retrospective multi-institutional study of the prevalence of early death in Dravet syndrome," *Epilepsia*, vol. 52, no. 6, pp. 1144–1149, 2011.

[38] M. Bureau and B. D. Bernardina, "Electroencephalographic characteristics of Dravet syndrome," *Epilepsia*, vol. 52, no. 2, pp. 13–23, 2011.

[39] M. Akiyama, K. Kobayashi, H. Yoshinaga, and Y. Ohtsuka, "A long-term follow-up study of Dravet syndrome up to adulthood," *Epilepsia*, vol. 51, no. 6, pp. 1043–1052, 2010.

[40] Y. Tsuda, H. Oguni, M. Sakauchi et al., "An electroclinical study of absence seizures in Dravet syndrome," *Epilepsy Research*, vol. 103, no. 1, pp. 88–96, 2013.

[41] K. Nickels and E. Wirrell, "Electrical status epilepticus in sleep," *Seminars in Pediatric Neurology*, vol. 15, no. 2, pp. 50–60, 2008.

[42] A. Beaumanoir and W. Blume, "The Lennox-Gastaut syndrome," in *Epileptic Syndromes in Infancy, Childhood and Adolescence*, J. Roger, M. Bureau, C. Dravet, and P. Genton, Eds., pp. 125–148, John Libbey Eurotext, Montrouge, France, 4th edition, 2005.

[43] A. Arzimanoglou, J. French, W. T. Blume et al., "Lennox-Gastaut syndrome: a consensus approach on diagnosis, assessment, management, and trial methodology," *The Lancet Neurology*, vol. 8, no. 1, pp. 82–93, 2009.

[44] O. N. Markand, "Lennox-Gastaut syndrome (childhood epileptic encephalopathy)," *Journal of Clinical Neurophysiology*, vol. 20, no. 6, pp. 426–441, 2003.

[45] R. A. Hrachovy and J. D. Frost Jr., "The EEG in selected generalized seizures," *Journal of Clinical Neurophysiology*, vol. 23, no. 4, pp. 312–332, 2006.

[46] E. Ferlazzo, M. Nikanorova, D. Italiano et al., "Lennox-Gastaut syndrome in adulthood: clinical and EEG features," *Epilepsy Research*, vol. 89, no. 2-3, pp. 271–277, 2010.

[47] Y. Ohtsuka, R. Amano, M. Mizukawa, and S. Ohtahara, "Long-term prognosis of the Lennox-Gastaut syndrome," *Japanese Journal of Psychiatry and Neurology*, vol. 44, no. 2, pp. 257–264, 1990.

[48] K. Yagi, "Evolution of Lennox-Gastaut syndrome: a long-term longitudinal study," *Epilepsia*, vol. 37, supplement 3, pp. 48–51, 1996.

[49] H. Oguni, Y. Fukuyama, T. Tanaka et al., "Myoclonic-astatic epilepsy of early childhood—clinical and EEG analysis of myoclonic-astatic seizures, and discussions on the nosology of the syndrome," *Brain and Development*, vol. 23, no. 7, pp. 757–764, 2001.

[50] S. A. Kelley and E. H. Kossoff, "Doose syndrome (myoclonic-astatic epilepsy): 40 years of progress," *Developmental Medicine and Child Neurology*, vol. 52, no. 11, pp. 988–993, 2010.

[51] L. F. M. de Siqueira, "Progressive myoclonic epilepsies: review of clinical, molecular and therapeutic aspects," *Journal of Neurology*, vol. 257, no. 10, pp. 1612–1619, 2010.

[52] M. Mastrangelo, A. Celato, and V. Leuzzi, "A diagnostic algorithm for the evaluation of early onset genetic-metabolic epileptic encephalopathies," *European Journal of Paediatric Neurology*, vol. 16, no. 2, pp. 179–191, 2012.

[53] M. F. Hunter, H. Peters, R. Salemi, D. Thorburn, and M. T. MacKay, "Alpers syndrome with mutations in POLG: clinical and investigative features," *Pediatric Neurology*, vol. 45, no. 5, pp. 311–318, 2011.

[54] N. I. Wolf, S. Rahman, B. Schmitt et al., "Status epilepticus in children with Alpers' disease caused by POLG1 mutations: EEG and MRI features," *Epilepsia*, vol. 50, no. 6, pp. 1596–1607, 2009.

[55] I. Rapin, "Myoclonus in neuronal storage and Lafora diseases," *Advances in Neurology*, vol. 43, pp. 65–85, 1986.

[56] C. G. Bien and I. E. Scheffer, "Autoantibodies and epilepsy," *Epilepsia*, vol. 52, no. 3, pp. 18–22, 2011.

[57] S. E. Schmitt, K. Pargeon, E. S. Frechette et al., "Extreme delta brush: a unique EEG pattern in adults with anti-NMDA receptor encephalitis," *Neurology*, vol. 79, no. 11, pp. 1094–1100, 2012.

[58] T. Sahoo, S. U. Peters, N. S. Madduri et al., "Microarray based comparative genomic hybridization testing in deletion bearing patients with Angelman syndrome: genotype-phenotype correlations," *Journal of Medical Genetics*, vol. 43, no. 6, pp. 512–516, 2006.

[59] C. A. Williams, H. Angelman, J. Clayton-Smith et al., "Angelman syndrome: consensus for diagnostic criteria," *American Journal of Medical Genetics*, vol. 56, no. 2, pp. 237–238, 1995.

[60] K. D. Valente, J. Q. Andrade, R. M. Grossmann et al., "Angelman syndrome: difficulties in EEG pattern recognition and possible misinterpretations," *Epilepsia*, vol. 44, no. 8, pp. 1051–1063, 2003.

[61] O. N. Markand and J. G. Panszi, "The electroencephalogram in subacute sclerosing panencephalitis," *Archives of Neurology*, vol. 32, no. 11, pp. 719–726, 1975.

7

A Clinical-EEG Study of Sleepiness and Psychological Symptoms in Pharmacoresistant Epilepsy Patients Treated with Lacosamide

Filippo S. Giorgi,[1] **Chiara Pizzanelli,**[1] **Veronica Pelliccia,**[1] **Elisa Di Coscio,**[1] **Michelangelo Maestri,**[2] **Melania Guida,**[1] **Elena Iacopini,**[1] **Alfonso Iudice,**[1] **and Enrica Bonanni**[1]

[1] *Neurology Unit and Epilepsy Center, Department of Neuroscience, A.O.U.P and Department of Clinical and Experimental Medicine of the University of Pisa, Via Roma 67, 56126 Pisa, Italy*
[2] *Sleep & Epilepsy Center, Neurocenter of the Civic Hospital (EOC) of Lugano, Via Tesserete 46, 6900 Lugano, Switzerland*

Correspondence should be addressed to Filippo S. Giorgi; giorgifs@gmail.com

Academic Editor: Andrea Romigi

Our aim was to evaluate the EEG and clinical modifications induced by the new antiepileptic drug lacosamide (LCM) in patients with epilepsy. We evaluated 10 patients affected by focal pharmacoresistant epilepsy in which LCM (mean 250 mg/day) was added to the preexisting antiepileptic therapy, which was left unmodified. Morning waking EEG recording was performed before ($t0$) and at 6 months ($t1$) after starting LCM. At $t0$ and $t1$, patients were also administered questionnaires evaluating mood, anxiety, sleep, sleepiness, and fatigue (Beck Depression Inventory; State-Trait Anxiety Inventory Y1 and Y2; Pittsburgh Sleep Quality Index; Epworth Sleepiness Scale; Fatigue Severity Scale). We performed a quantitative analysis of EEG interictal abnormalities and background EEG power spectrum analysis. LCM as an add-on did not significantly affect anxiety, depression, sleepiness, sleep quality, and fatigue scales. Similarly, adding LCM to preexisting therapy did not modify significantly patient EEGs in terms of absolute power, relative power, mean frequency, and interictal abnormalities occurrence. In conclusion, in this small cohort of patients, we confirmed that LCM as an add-on does not affect subjective parameters which play a role, among others, in therapy tolerability, and our clinical impression was further supported by evaluation of EEG spectral analysis.

1. Introduction

Epilepsy is one of the most common neurological disorders, affecting up to two percent of the population worldwide. Many patients show recurrent seizures despite treatment with appropriate antiepileptic drugs (AEDs') [1, 2], and many experience AEDs side effects. In the last decades, new AEDs have been developed with the aim of balancing, as far as possible, significant efficacy with good tolerability.

Among them, Lacosamide (LCM) has been recently authorized in Italy and worldwide as a new add-on AED for the treatment of pharmacoresistant focal epilepsy.

Side effects of classical AEDs often involve cognitive functions, mood, and behavior to varying degrees, and this is the case also for newer AEDs (see, for instance, [3–5]). Unfortunately, a clear evaluation of these types of side effects in the single patient is often difficult because of the subjectivity of such complaints. This assessment is even harder in patients undergoing AED polytherapy.

It has been proposed by several authors the usefulness of a quantitative analysis on EEG in patients undergoing treatment with drugs acting on the CNS (for a review, see for instance, [6]), in this setting, abnormalities of EEG power spectrum have been interpreted as an objective measure of cognitive slowing/impairment (see, for instance, [7–9]). Furthermore, in the last decades, questionnaires specifically evaluating mood, anxiety trait, sleepiness, fatigue, and sleep quality have been developed.

The aims of the present study were (i) to analyze the effects of LCM on EEG in terms of EEG background spectra and interictal activity and (ii) to further evaluate LCM effects by using subjective questionnaires addressing depression (Beck Depression Inventory-BDI), anxiety (State-Trait Anxiety Inventory-STAI), sleep quality (Pittsburgh Sleep Quality Index-PSQI), sleepiness (Epworth Sleepiness Scale-ESS,) and fatigue (Fatigue Severity Scale-FSS).

2. Materials and Methods

2.1. Patients and Study Design. Ten patients affected by focal epilepsy (6 males and 4 females, mean age 48.2 ± 14.8 years) were included in this study. The mean age at epilepsy onset was 13.5 ± 7.9 years. Five patients were affected by focal symptomatic epilepsy, and five were affected by probably focal symptomatic epilepsy. In Table 1, we reported a detailed description of etiologies, electroclinical features, and concomitant AEDs, as well as comorbidities.

The design of this study is a prospective open-label pragmatic one. We selected ten consecutive adult outpatients from our tertiary University Epilepsy Center who were fulfilling the following criteria: (a) being affected by partial focal epilepsy, not caused by a progressive etiology; (b) having experienced in the previous three months at least 12 seizures (not less than 2 for each single month); (c) having been treated with more than one appropriate AED, at adequate dose regimen; and (d) being screened for any kind of AV Block by at least a routine EKG.

Recruited Patients were submitted to video-EEG recording and clinical evaluation on the day before (*t*0) and at 6 months (*t*1) after beginning LCM.

LCM was administered to all of the enrolled patients at a starting dose of 50 mg/day, followed by biweekly 50 mg/day dose increase, up to each patient's maintenance dose on the basis of clinical response and tolerability (mean final daily dosage of 250 ± 81.6 mg/die). The remaining AED therapy was left unmodified throughout the study: in 9 patients, this included AEDs acting on voltage-gated Na+ channels (Table 1). Neurological examination and blood tests, including AED plasma levels, were monitored at *t*0 and *t*1; during these same visits, patients were administered the subjective questionnaires that were selected also based on previous studies in epilepsy patients [10–12] and are detailed below.

Starting at six months before *t*0, patients were asked to collect a detailed seizure diary, which were collected by the examiner at *t*1.

As shown in Table 2, there was a seizure reduction of 33.3% at *t*1 versus *t*0. In particular, 7/10 patients showed a seizure reduction at *t*1; in one, there was a slight seizure increase; four patients showed a seizure reduction ≥50%, and one of them was seizure-free at *t*1. When comparing raw seizure number at *t*1 versus *t*0, P was 0.068.

2.2. EEG Procedures. Each patient was admitted at our Sleep-Epilepsy Center for video-EEG monitoring session at *t*0 and *t*1 (see above).

Participants were instructed to follow their usual daily routine, meals, and caffeine consumption and to refrain from alcohol intake for 24 h before starting the recording. The EEG recordings were performed through a 32-channel cable

video-telemetry system. Nineteen collodion-applied scalp-electrodes were placed according to the 10–20 system; chin electromyogram, electrocardiogram, and electrooculogram signals were recorded via additional skin surface electrodes. Electrode impedance was maintained below 5 kΩ. Filters were set at 0.1 and 30 Hz, and signal was notch filtered. Two additional electrodes were placed at mastoid level; for spectral analysis, only O1-mastoidal and O2-mastoidal traces were considered. All the EEG recordings were carried out with the same type of digital EEG equipment (BElite, EBNeuro, Florence), and data were acquired with a 258 bit sampling rate and stored on the PC hard disk for offline evaluation.

The EEG was recorded in a silent room of the University Sleep Center, during constant monitoring by an EEG technician.

The recording periods included (a) a night recording (polysomnography-PSG) from 9 p.m. to 7 a.m. of the following day (not shown) and (b) a routine video-EEG wake recording from 8 to 9.30 a.m. after the end of PSG.

On the morning 1.5 h video EEG recording, we performed an analysis of interictal epileptiform abnormalities (IIA) and power spectrum analysis of background activity.

In detail, we performed the following analysis of EEG data.

2.2.1. Interictal Abnormalities (IIA) Analysis. IIA occurrence was analyzed visually by two independent observers which were blinded, for each patient, as to whether they were scoring a *t*0 or *t*1 EEG tracing. The total number of IIA occurring during the 8–9.30 A.M. wake-EEG was recorded and converted to $n/10'$.

2.2.2. Power Spectrum Analysis. Epoch selection for qEEG analysis was performed offline on waking EEG recording obtained from 8 to 9.30 A.M. We selected randomly, and blindly to patient number and treatment, EEG periods lacking ictal and/or interictal abnormalities, movements artifacts, eye blinking, muscle activity or drowsiness signs. On these EEG parts, we used the fast Fourier transform (FFT), considering 2 minutes of EEG signal, automatically segmented by software into 2.56 s epochs. Analysis was performed for each frequency band: delta [1–4 Hz]; theta [4–8 Hz]; alpha [8–12 Hz], and beta [12–30 Hz].

Measures derived from FFT included (i) absolute power; (ii) percent relative power, and (iii) mean frequency.

We chose to analyze mainly the frequency in occipital derivation according to widely accepted criteria [6]. Moreover, the analysis of occipital recording allows the best identification of alpha activity, and recordings are devoid of artifacts observed in more anterior leads. To minimize statistical problems associated with multiple variables, results from the O1 and O2 leads were averaged for analysis.

2.3. Subjective Questionnaire. In order to evaluate the wake-sleep symptoms and psychological well-being of the patients included in this study, five scales were administered before and after 6 months of LCM therapy.

2.3.1. Beck Depression Index. BDI is a small questionnaire examining 21 symptom areas with a total score ranging from 0 to 63 proportionally to depression severity [13].

2.3.2. The State-Trait Anxiety Inventory. STAI is a brief self-administered questionnaire for the assessment of state and trait anxiety in adults and is composed of a State anxiety scale (STAI Y-1) and a Trait anxiety scale (STAI Y-2), consisting of 20 statements each [14].

2.3.3. Epworth Sleepiness Scale. ESS is the subjective scale that is generally considered as the gold standard for the evaluation of daytime sleepiness [15]. It evaluates individual degree of drowsiness in eight common daily conditions, has been validated in Italian [16], and is widely used in epilepsy [17]. It is generally accepted a cutoff of 10 as normal value [18].

2.3.4. The Pittsburgh Sleep Quality Index. PSQI is an instrument used to measure the quality and patterns of sleep in adults assessing seven domains self-rated by the subject [19] and already used also in epilepsy patients [20]. A global score of 5 or more reveals a poor quality of sleep and is considered as the cutoff from normal to pathological values.

2.3.5. The 9-Item Fatigue Severity Scale. (FSS) is one of the most commonly used self-report questionnaires to measure fatigue [21] with value ranging from 1 (strong disagreement with the statement) to 7 (strong agreement). A cut-off of 4 is generally considered [22].

2.4. Statistical Analysis. For IIAs, absolute power spectrum (for each frequency band), relative power spectrum (for each frequency band), mean alpha frequency, and seizure frequency, a Student's *t*-test analysis for paired data was applied to compare *t*1 and *t*0 data.

For scales (STAI, BDI, ESS, FSS, and PSQI), the score comparisons between *t*1 and *t*0 were performed by the Wilcoxon signed-rank test.

For all of the analyses, the null hypothesis was rejected when $P < 0.05$.

3. Results

3.1. Adverse Effects of LCM. LCM was not discontinued in any of the patients. Five patients complained mild drowsiness, and one patient experienced sleepiness, but these effects were transient and improved right after slowing the titration schedule. Blood levels of concomitant AEDs were not significantly affected by LCM administration (not shown).

3.2. Effects of LCM on EEG IIAs (Table 2). As shown in Table 2, in all but two patients we observed either a decrease or a lack of effect of LCM on IIAs. Patient 1 already at baseline showed a significantly higher IIA number (22.2) than the remaining ones (1.72 ± 0.65), and at *t*1, there was 14% increase in its occurrence. With the exception of these two patients, in all of the remaining ones there was no effect or a slight

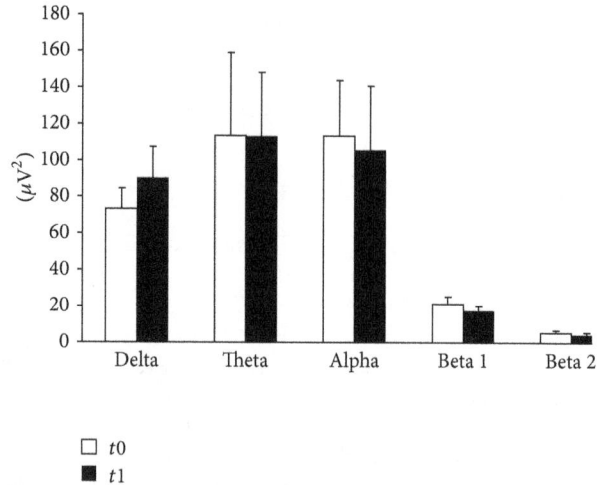

FIGURE 1: Power spectrum analysis of EEG. Patients were assessed at *t*0 and after 6 months (*t*1). The graph shows absolute power (μV^2) calculated on O2-Ref EEG traces. qEEG analysis was performed offline on waking EEG recording obtained from 8 to 9.30 A.M., randomly selecting EEG periods lacking ictal and/or interictal abnormalities, movements artifacts, eye blinking, muscle activity or drowsiness signs. On these EEG parts, we used the fast Fourier transform (FFT), considering 2 minutes of EEG signal, automatically segmented by software into 2.56 s epochs. Analysis was performed for each frequency band: delta [1–4 Hz]; theta [4–8 Hz]; alpha [8–12 Hz], and beta [12–30 Hz]. None of these bands were significantly affected by LCM treatment.

decrease in IIAs occurrence. The mean IIAs % change at *t*1 was −19.3% versus baseline.

3.3. Effects of LCM on qEEG (Table 3 and Figure 1). Concerning qEEG, LCM did not significantly affect the absolute power density for any of the frequency intervals evaluated (Figure 1, Table 3), apart from a slight, nonsignificant increase in delta frequency representation. Similarly, alpha mean frequency was not affected by LCM administration, as well as the mean frequency of the remaining bands (Table 3).

PSG data concerning the night before EEG recording were analyzed in detail and are part of a separate multicenter study (in preparation); in any case, all PSG recordings showed a total sleep time longer than 6 hours, which is considered necessary for a proper evaluation of sleepiness in international guidelines [23], and no statistical differences were found between *t*0 and *t*1 for the variables of sleep continuity (i.e. sleep efficiency, total sleep time).

3.4. Psychological Effects (Tables 4 and 5). We did not observe any significant changes in BDI scores. Nevertheless, in four patients with intermediate BDI scores, we observed an improvement at *t*1 (patients 1, 2, 4 and 7). In patient #6 presenting a high BDI score at *t*0 (22), we did not observe any changes at *t*1.

Similarly, in the STAI scales the scores remained stable throughout the observation period.

TABLE 1: Demography.

Patients	Age	Age at onset (yr)	Epileptic syndrome	Seizure type	AEDs before-LCM
No. 1	45	11	Symptomatic temporal lobe epilepsy (posttraumatic)	Focal limbic seizures, SG	OXC 900 mg/die; LEV 3 g/die; VPA 1,5 g/die; LTG 200 mg/die; TPM 600 mg/die; VNS
No. 2	34	13	Symptomatic temporal lobe epilepsy (postradiotherapy calcification)	Focal limbic seizures, SG	OXC 1200 mg/die; LTG 300 mg/die; LEV 3 g/die; VNS
No. 3	34	18	Probably symptomatic temporal lobe epilepsy	Focal limbic seizures, rarely SG	LEV 3,5 g/die; ZNS 200 mg/die; TPM 600 mg/die; CBZ 1600 mg/die
No. 4	76	16	Probably symptomatic frontal lobe epilepsy	Focal seizures	CBZ CR 1200 mg/die; PB 50 mg/die; LTG 200 mg/die; ZNS 450 mg/die
No. 5	43	13	Probably symptomatic temporal lobe epilepsy	Focal limbic seizures	OXC 1800 mg/die; LEV 3 g/die
No. 6	59	6	Probably symptomatic temporal lobe epilepsy	Focal limbic seizures	ZNS 100 mg/die; LEV 1 g × 3/die; OXC 600 mg × 3/die
No. 7	55	10	Symptomatic temporal lobe epilepsy (left HS)	Focal limbic seizures	LEV 2 g/die; OXC 2100 mg/die; TPM 300 mg/die
No. 8	51	25	Symptomatic temporooccipital epilepsy (right retrotrigonal lesion)	Focal limbic seizures	LEV 1 g × 3/die; CBZ 600 + 400 + 600; ZNS 200 mg/die
No. 9	26	1	Symptomatic frontal lobe epilepsy (calcifications of falx cerebri)	Nocturnal frontal seizures	CBZ 1200 mg/die; TPM 450 mg/die
No. 10	59	27	Probably symptomatic temporal lobe epilepsy	Focal limbic seizures	TPM 350 mg/die

HS: hippocampal sclerosis; SG: secondarily generalized; CBZ: carbamazepine; LEV: levetiracetam; LTG: lamotrigine; OXC: oxcarbazepine; TPM: topiramate; VNS: vagus nerve stimulation; VPA: valproic acid; ZNS: zonisamide.

TABLE 2: Interictal EEG abnormalities and seizures frequency after LCM.

Patient	IIAs/10 min $t0$	IIAs/10 min $t1$	% variation IIAs in $(t1 - t0)$	Seizures/month $t0$	Seizures/month $t1$	% variation seizure in frequency $(t1 - t0)$
No. 1	22,22	25,77	+14	15,16	7,66	−50
No. 2	2,44	1,55	−37	4,66	0	−100
No. 3	1,44	0,77	−45	4	3,16	−21
No. 4	0,33	0,22	−34	22,16	9,16	−59
No. 5	0,88	1	+12	10,16	7,16	−30
No. 6	0,44	0,44	0	3,83	4,33	+12
No. 7	0,77	0,55	−29	4,33	4,33	0
No. 8	0,66	0,44	−34	9,83	7	−29
No. 9	6,66	6,44	−4	54,16	24,16	−56
No. 10	1,88	1,22	−36	3,66	3,66	0
Pooled	3,77 ± 2,13	3,84 ± 2,50	−19,3	13,19 ± 4,94	7,06 ± 2,07	−33,3

Values in bottom row concerning columns 2, 3, 4, and 6 are expressed as mean ± S.E.M.
IIAS: interictal EEG abnormalities.

At baseline, excessive daytime sleepiness (ESS score ≥10) was reported by two patients. Six months after LCM therapy, two other patients had pathological scores at ESS. However, no patients reported severe daytime sleepiness, that is, ESS > 14, and when measuring the group mean values, no statistical differences were observed. Also, FSS showed no differences between $t1$ and $t0$, even if it was higher than normal ranges in both conditions. Concerning PSQI, the percentage of "good sleepers" (i.e., with a score <5) was 50% at $t0$ and 80% at $t1$.

Table 5 shows mean values for each PSQI subitem at $t0$ and $t1$.

4. Discussion

In this small cohort of pharmacoresistant focal epilepsy patients, we investigated the effects of LCM in terms of EEG and psychological effects. We showed that LCM does

TABLE 3: Power spectrum analysis of EEG.

	Delta			Theta			Alpha			Beta 1			Beta 2		
	t0	t1	P	t0	t1	P	t0	t1	P	t0	t1	P	t0	t1	P
Absolute power (μV^2)															
Median	67,145	85,195		53,5	79,395		91,52	70,635		16,125	15,61		4,165	2,92	
Mean	73,0263	89,97	0,42	113,5075	112,9513	0,99	113,3288	105,4775	0,86	21,1188	17,4675	0,47	5,6913	4,3488	0,47
S.E.M.	11,4714	17,2173		45,4567	34,8912		30,1147	34,9935		4,2976	2,4071		1,4159	1,1695	
Relative power															
Median	25,31	28,68		20,15	26,995		31,595	28,37		7,075	5,96		1,415	1,07	
Mean	26,0737	29,2212	0,61	28,2462	30,2275	0,81	33,6137	31,845	0,82	7,9887	6,3487	0,49	2,4275	1,6562	0,45
S.E.M.	4,2267	4,3531		7,0544	4,6986		5,388	5,1308		2,08	1,0074		0,8032	0,5687	
Mean frequency (Hz)															
Median	1,59	1,645		6,22	6,365		9,12	9,07		14,13	13,955		19,9	19,93	
Mean	1,61	1,6113	0,99	6,2087	6,2763	0,74	9,3	9,2113	0,73	14,1525	13,9425	0,12	20,0525	20,0525	0,99
S.E.M.	0,0582	0,0826		0,1541	0,1204		0,18	0,1813		0,0999	0,0816		0,1304	0,1237	

TABLE 4: Psychological effects of lacosamide.

	Score at t0 (mean ± S.D.)	Score at t1 (mean ± S.D.)	P
PSQI	4,4 ± 1,6	3,7 ± 1,3	0.23
ESS	7,7 ± 1,8	8,3 ± 2,4	0.25
FSS	40,4 ± 12,1	36,7 ± 13,5	0.26
BDI	12,1 ± 5,1	9,9 ± 4,4	0.07
STAI Y1	41,1 ± 7,6	39,1 ± 5,9	0.08
STAI Y2	43,7 ± 10,1	42,2 ± 10,9	0.15

Statistical analysis was performed by means of Wilcoxon signed-rank nonparametric test.

BDI: Beck Depression Inventory; ESS: Epworth Sleepiness Scale; FSS: Fatigue Severity Scale; PSQI: Pittsburgh Sleep Quality Index; STAI Y1: S-anxiety scale of the State-Trait Anxiety Inventory form Y; and STAI Y2: T-anxiety scale of the State-Trait Anxiety Inventory form Y.

TABLE 5: Effects of lacosamide on the different subitems of Pittsburgh sleep quality index.

	Score at t0 (mean ± S.D.)	Score at t1 (mean ± S.D.)	P
C1 subjective sleep quality	0,9 ± 0,6	0,7 ± 0,5	0.5
C2 sleep latency	0,4 ± 0,5	0,3 ± 0,5	0.68
C3 sleep duration	0,8 ± 0,4	0,8 ± 0,4	1
C4 sleep efficiency	0,6 ± 0,5	0,5 ± 0,5	0.9
C5 sleep disturbances	1,2 ± 0,8	0,9 ± 0,7	0.34
C6 use of sleeping medication	0,2 ± 0,4	0,3 ± 0,5	0.59
C7 daytime dysfunction	0,3 ± 0,5	0,2 ± 0,4	0.68

Statistical analysis was performed by means of Wilcoxon signed-rank nonparametric test.

not affect significantly EEG background in terms of power spectra, nor does it worsen depressive or anxiety traits, as well as subjective indices of sleepiness, fatigue, and sleep quality in this type of patients. Furthermore, LCM did not affect IIAs occurrence significantly, despite its efficacy on seizures.

We chose a prolonged observation period (6 months from t0 to t1) in order to allow (a) a prolonged slow titration of the LCM; and (b) a complete stabilization of the effects of the drug on both EEG and clinical conditions.

The effect of LCM was much lower on IIAs than toward seizures and not remarkable. This is not surprising, since previous studies failed to show a parallelism between seizure and IIAs frequency concerning other AEDs, such as carbamazepine [24] and gabapentin [25] in focal epilepsy. Incidentally, an elegant experimental study performed in amygdala kindled cats confirmed the lack of an effect of carbamazepine on spike occurrence, despite a significant effect on seizures [26]. Conversely, topiramate [27] and lamotrigine [28] have been shown to reduce IIAs incidence and spreading, in parallel with seizure occurrence. The lack of a correlation between IIAs reduction and seizure frequency we observed in our study might be due to the pharmacodynamic effects of LCM itself. However, further experimental studies would be needed to address this hypothesis.

When deciding to add a new AED in pharmacoresistant epilepsy patients, the main concern of the prescribing physician is to get the maximum efficacy with the lowest incidence of side effects. Among the main complaints of pharmacoresistant epilepsy patients in terms of AED tolerability, there are drowsiness, confusion, and dizziness, as well as mood changes and anxiety.

The low incidence of CNS side effects after LCM we found in our study, as well as the complete lack of dropout during follow up, might be due to the design of our study indeed; in fact, the titration of LCM was shaped on patients' tolerability and efficacy, and the long follow-up period (6 months) allows a full stabilization of the appropriate drug regimen.

Several authors have proposed that EEG background correlates with the degree of alertness and of cognitive performances (for a detailed review, see [29]); even though such a link is indirect and difficult to quantify, many investigators agree on a solid correlation of slowing of alpha mean frequency with cognitive impairment (see, for instance, the reviews by [30, 31]). We could not show any significant reduction of alpha activity at t1 versus t0 nor an increase in the representation of slower frequencies (i.e. delta and theta ones). This is in agreement with the lack of subjective significant complaints reported by our group of patients, both in terms of drowsiness, and in terms of increased cognitive impairment, as compared with baseline. Potentially, the EEG derivations we used (occipital ones) for spectral evaluation are mainly suitable for alpha band analysis, as compared with lower frequency bands, while for slower bands the analysis of additional derivations might be preferable, and this might be a limitation of our study. However, nevertheless we chose to focus on occipital derivations since these are the only ones used also in many similar studies in which significant EEG modifications were observed during AEDs treatment (e.g., [7–9]), while data assessing also other derivations in these types of studies are more sparse and difficult to compare with each other.

Previous studies assessing power spectral analysis in epileptic patients were performed in focal epilepsy populations, either drug free [31] or during AED monotherapy [7, 9, 32–34] or polytherapy [35]. Further, AEDs effects on EEG background have been evaluated also in healthy volunteers [8, 36].

In our study, we did not find, for anyone of the frequency band tested, a difference between $t0$ and $t1$, with this being in line with the effect of other AEDs, such as phenobarbital, lamotrigine, and valproic acid [28, 33, 35]. Conversely, previous studies in patients treated with the sodium-channel blocking AEDs CBZ and OXC showed a decrease of alpha mean frequency [7, 24, 33]. Thus, our findings suggest that the enhancing effects of LCM on voltage-gated sodium channels slow inactivation affects neocortical rhythm in a different manner as compared with the effect of fast-inactivation enhancement. The lack of any significant effect we observed on qEEG might have been due to the fact that already at baseline EEG background was significantly affected both by the underlying disease and by the concomitant AEDs. However, indeed our aim was not to compare our data with those of a control population (since our subjects were not healthy volunteers taking LCM) but to show, if any, the existence of a worsening potential effect of LCM on EEG background in the particular population of patients who are affected by pharmacoresistant epilepsy. Furthermore, we found mean variability in the different frequency bands similar to those observed by other authors in AED monotherapy (see for instance [7, 33, 34]).

AEDs bear, to varying degrees, psychological effects including effects on mood and anxiety [3, 37, 38]; furthermore, it has been shown that the incidence of such adverse effects increases in parallel with the number of ongoing AEDs [3]. In this study, patients were administered with BDI to address depressive features, which is a well-validated scale that has been used extensively in such populations before [10, 39]; this scale was not significantly affected by adding LCM. Anxiety is another one of the commonest complaints in patients undergoing antiepileptic therapy (see [3, 5]); we showed that STAI questionnaires, which explore anxiety trait and state and have been validated in several populations affected by chronic neurological illnesses [39–41], are not modified by LCM add-on. However, it should be noted

that both depressive and anxiety features at $t0$ were slightly elevated in our patients as compared to control populations from our lab historical data (not shown). This might affect the finding of no effect of LCM add-on on these measures. However, as said, the aim of this study was to assess, indeed, the additional effect of LCM on a category of patients already bearing a burden of potential side effects of different drugs and of the disease itself as well.

Concerning sleep-wake cycle, our study shows that subjective standardized scales did not highlight significant changes when LCM was added to previous therapies. As concerns sleepiness, in the registration studies, LCM showed a risk of sleepiness as a side effect (3.1% when considering differences towards placebo), which is lower than other new AEDs (see as a review, [42]). An exhaustive discussion about subjective evaluation of sleep, sleepiness, and fatigue in pharmacoresistant epilepsy patients is complex and far beyond the aim of this study; it is worth noting that the ESS and PSQI scores in our patients are within normal range, while FSS showed higher levels of fatigue than usually reported in general population, but without statistically significant changes during LCM therapy.

A discrepancy between objective and subjective evaluation of sleep and sleepiness in epilepsy has been suggested, and we could hypothesize that single patients could underestimate the degree of these disturbances, since these could be chronic symptoms, and subjects could be more focused on seizure frequency and on daytime fatigue. Moreover, the subjective differentiation between sleepiness and fatigue is complex and not completely understood ([43]).

Thus, a study using objective standardized methods (i.e. polysomnography and multiple sleep latency test) to evaluate sleep and sleepiness would be necessary to further understand the impact of LCM on these aspects.

5. Conclusions

In this study, we observed that our clinical impression of tolerability of LCM as an add-on was further significantly supported by objective EEG measures and by semiquantitative analysis of effects on sleepiness, mood, and anxiety, even though therapy tolerability as a whole is due also to many aspects not specifically evaluated in this paper.

We are aware that this study was not randomized in design and the patients were under previous AEDs. However, since we compared the chronic effects of LCM versus each patient's own baseline and throughout an observation period of 6 months, this makes our findings interesting, since they reflect closely a typical clinical setting of patients taking LCM.

Acknowledgments

The authors gratefully acknowledge Mr. Fabio Cignoni and Miss Rossella Buscemi from the Neurology Unit of the Department of Neurosciences of A.O.U.P., Pisa, for their skillful assistance in EEG recording and analysis.

References

[1] P. Kwan, A. Arzimanoglou, A. T. Berg et al., "Definition of drug resistant epilepsy: consensus proposal by the ad hoc Task Force of the ILAE Commission on Therapeutic Strategies," *Epilepsia*, vol. 51, no. 6, pp. 1069–1077, 2010.

[2] P. Kwan, S. C. Schachter, and M. J. Brodie, "Current concepts: drug-resistant epilepsy," *The New England Journal of Medicine*, vol. 365, no. 10, pp. 919–926, 2011.

[3] A. B. Ettinger, "Psychotropic effects of antiepileptic drugs," *Neurology*, vol. 67, no. 11, pp. 1916–1925, 2006.

[4] B. Schmitz, "Effects of antiepileptic drugs on mood and behavior," *Epilepsia*, vol. 47, no. 2, pp. 28–33, 2006.

[5] G. Zaccara, P. F. Gangemi, and M. Cincotta, "Central nervous system adverse effects of new antiepileptic drugs. A meta-analysis of placebo-controlled studies," *Seizure*, vol. 17, no. 5, pp. 405–421, 2008.

[6] B. Saletu, P. Anderer, G. M. Saletu-Zyhlarz, O. Arnold, and R. D. Pascual-Marqui, "Classification and evaluation of the pharmacodynamics of psychotropic drugs by single-lead pharmaco-EEG, EEG mapping and tomography (LORETA)," *Methods and Findings in Experimental and Clinical Pharmacology*, vol. 24, pp. 97–120, 2002.

[7] J. D. Frost Jr., R. A. Hrachovy, D. G. Glaze, and G. M. Rettig, "Alpha rhythm slowing during initiation of carbamazepine therapy: implications for future cognitive performance," *Journal of Clinical Neurophysiology*, vol. 12, no. 1, pp. 57–63, 1995.

[8] M. C. Salinsky, L. M. Binder, B. S. Oken, D. Storzbach, C. R. Aron, and C. B. Dodrill, "Effects of gabapentin and carbamazepine on the EEG and cognition in healthy volunteers," *Epilepsia*, vol. 43, no. 5, pp. 482–490, 2002.

[9] M. C. Salinsky, B. S. Oken, D. Storzbach, and C. B. Dodrill, "Assessment of CNS effects of antiepileptic drugs by using quantitative EEG measures," *Epilepsia*, vol. 44, no. 8, pp. 1042–1050, 2003.

[10] P. Karzmark, P. Zeifert, and J. Barry, "Measurement of depression in epilepsy," *Epilepsy and Behavior*, vol. 2, no. 2, pp. 124–128, 2001.

[11] D. Kalogjera-Sackellares and J. C. Sackellares, "Improvement in depression associated with partial epilepsy in patients treated with lamotrigine," *Epilepsy and Behavior*, vol. 3, no. 6, pp. 510–516, 2002.

[12] V. K. Kimiskidis, N. I. Triantafyllou, E. Kararizou et al., "Depression and anxiety in epilepsy: the association with demographic and seizure-related variables," *Annals of General Psychiatry*, vol. 6, article 28, 2007.

[13] A. T. Beck, R. A. Steer, and G. K. Brown, *Manual for the Beck Depression Inventory*, Psychological Corporation, San Antonio, Tex, USA, 1996.

[14] C. D. Spielberger, R. L. Gorsuch, P. R. Lushene, P. R. Vagg, and G. A. Jacobs, *Manual for the State-Trait Anxiety Inventory*, Consulting Psychologists Press, Palo Alto, Calif, USA, 1983.

[15] M. W. Johns, "A new method for measuring daytime sleepiness: the Epworth sleepiness scale," *Sleep*, vol. 14, no. 6, pp. 540–545, 1991.

[16] L. Vignatelli, G. Plazzi, A. Barbato et al., "GINSEN (Gruppo Italiano Narcolessia Studio Epidemiologico Nazionale), "Italian version of the Epworth sleepiness scale: external validity," *Neurological Sciences*, vol. 23, no. 6, pp. 295–300, 2003.

[17] A. S. Giorelli, G. S. D. M. L. Neves, M. Venturi, I. M. Pontes, A. Valois, and M. D. M. Gomes, "Excessive daytime sleepiness in patients with epilepsy: a subjective evaluation," *Epilepsy and Behavior*, vol. 21, no. 4, pp. 449–452, 2011.

[18] M. W. Johns, "Sleepiness in different situations measured by the Epworth Sleepiness Scale," *Sleep*, vol. 17, no. 8, pp. 703–710, 1994.

[19] D. J. Buysse, C. F. Reynolds III, T. H. Monk, S. R. Berman, and D. J. Kupfer, "The Pittsburgh Sleep Quality Index: a new instrument for psychiatric practice and research," *Psychiatry Research*, vol. 28, no. 2, pp. 193–213, 1989.

[20] A. Romigi, F. Izzi, F. Placidi et al., "Effects of zonisamide as add-on therapy on sleep-wake cycle in focal epilepsy: a polysomnographic study," *Epilepsy & Behaviour*, vol. 26, no. 2, pp. 170–174, 2013.

[21] L. B. Krupp, N. G. LaRocca, J. Muir-Nash, and A. D. Steinberg, "The fatigue severity scale. Application to patients with multiple sclerosis and systemic lupus erythematosus," *Archives of Neurology*, vol. 46, no. 10, pp. 1121–1123, 1989.

[22] P. O. Valko, C. L. Bassetti, K. E. Bloch, U. Held, and C. R. Baumann, "Validation of the fatigue severity scale in a Swiss cohort," *Sleep*, vol. 31, no. 11, pp. 1601–1607, 2008.

[23] M. R. Littner, C. Kushida, M. Wise et al., "Practice parameters for clinical use of the multiple sleep latency test and the maintenance of wakefulness test," *Sleep*, vol. 28, no. 1, pp. 113–121, 2005.

[24] M. G. Marciani, G. L. Gigli, F. Stefanini et al., "Effect of carbamazepine on EEG background activity and on interictal epileptiform abnormalities in focal epilepsy," *International Journal of Neuroscience*, vol. 70, no. 1-2, pp. 107–116, 1993.

[25] D. Mattia, F. Spanedda, M. A. Bassetti, A. Romigi, F. Placidi, and M. G. Marciani, "Gabapentin as add-on therapy in focal epilepsy: a computerized EEG study," *Clinical Neurophysiology*, vol. 111, no. 2, pp. 311–317, 2000.

[26] G. L. Gigli and J. Gotman, "Effects of seizures and carbamazepine on interictal spiking in amygdala kindled cats," *Epilepsy Research*, vol. 8, no. 3, pp. 204–212, 1991.

[27] F. Placidi, M. Tombini, A. Romigi et al., "Topiramate: effect on EEG interictal abnormalities and background activity in patients affected by focal epilepsy," *Epilepsy Research*, vol. 58, no. 1, pp. 43–52, 2004.

[28] M. G. Marciani, F. Spanedda, M. A. Bassetti et al., "Effect of lamotrigine on EEG paroxysmal abnormalities and background activity: a computerized analysis," *British Journal of Clinical Pharmacology*, vol. 42, no. 5, pp. 621–627, 1996.

[29] W. Klimesch, "EEG alpha and theta oscillations reflect cognitive and memory performance: a review and analysis," *Brain Research Reviews*, vol. 29, no. 2-3, pp. 169–195, 1999.

[30] E. Basar and M. Schurmann, "Brain functioning: integrative models," in *Brain Function and OsillationsIntegrative Brain Function. Neurophysiology and Cognitive Processes*, E. Basar, Ed., vol. 2, pp. 393–406, Springer, Berlin, Germany, 1999.

[31] M. E. Drake, H. Padamadan, and S. A. Newell, "Interictal quantitative EEG in epilepsy," *Seizure*, vol. 7, no. 1, pp. 39–42, 1998.

[32] W. G. Sannita, L. Gervasio, and P. Zagnoni, "Quantitative EEG effects and plasma concentration of sodium valproate: acute and long-term administration to epileptic patients," *Neuropsychobiology*, vol. 22, no. 4, pp. 231–235, 1989.

[33] B. Clemens, A. Ménes, P. Piros et al., "Quantitative EEG effects of carbamazepine, oxcarbazepine, valproate, lamotrigine, and possible clinical relevance of the findings," *Epilepsy Research*, vol. 70, no. 2-3, pp. 190–199, 2006.

[34] M. Y. Neufeld, E. Kogan, V. Chistik, and A. D. Korczyn, "Comparison of the effects of vigabatrin, lamotrigine, and topiramate on quantitative EEGs in patients with epilepsy," *Clinical Neuropharmacology*, vol. 22, no. 2, pp. 80–86, 1999.

[35] G. K. Herkes, T. D. Lagerlund, F. W. Sharbrough, and M. J. Eadie, "Effects of antiepileptic drug treatment on the background frequency of EEGs in epileptic patients," *Journal of Clinical Neurophysiology*, vol. 10, no. 2, pp. 210–216, 1993.

[36] K. J. Meador, D. W. Loring, O. L. Abney et al., "Effects of carbamazepine and phenytoin on EEG and memory in healthy adults," *Epilepsia*, vol. 34, no. 1, pp. 153–157, 1993.

[37] M. Mula and F. Monaco, "Antiepileptic drugs and psychopathology of epilepsy: an update," *Epileptic Disorders*, vol. 11, no. 1, pp. 1–9, 2009.

[38] F. G. Gilliam and J. M. Santos, "Adverse psychiatric effects of antiepileptic drugs," *Epilepsy Research*, vol. 68, no. 1, pp. 67–69, 2006.

[39] A. R. Giovagnoli and G. Avanzini, "Quality of life and memory performance in patients with temporal lobe epilepsy," *Acta Neurologica Scandinavica*, vol. 101, no. 5, pp. 295–300, 2000.

[40] A. R. Giovagnoli, A. M. Da Silva, A. Federico, and F. Cornelio, "On the personal facets of quality of life in chronic neurological disorders," *Behavioural Neurology*, vol. 21, no. 3-4, pp. 155–163, 2009.

[41] F. Kowacs, M. P. Socal, S. C. Ziomkowski et al., "Symptoms of depression and anxiety, and screening for mental disorders in migrainous patients," *Cephalalgia*, vol. 23, no. 2, pp. 79–89, 2003.

[42] G. Zaccara, P. F. Gangemi, and M. Cincotta, "Central nervous system adverse effects of new antiepileptic drugs. A meta-analysis of placebo-controlled studies," *Seizure*, vol. 17, no. 5, pp. 405–421, 2008.

[43] A. Shahid, J. Shen, and C. M. Shapiro, "Measurements of sleepiness and fatigue," *Journal of Psychosomatic Research*, vol. 69, no. 1, pp. 81–89, 2010.

8

Delays and Factors Related to Cessation of Generalized Convulsive Status Epilepticus

Leena Kämppi,[1] Jaakko Ritvanen,[1] Harri Mustonen,[2] and Seppo Soinila[3]

[1]*Clinical Neurosciences, Neurology, University of Helsinki and Helsinki University Hospital, 00029 Helsinki, Finland*
[2]*Department of Surgery, Helsinki University Central Hospital, 00029 Helsinki, Finland*
[3]*Division of Clinical Neurosciences/General Neurology, Department of Neurology, Turku University Hospital, University of Turku, 20521 Turku, Finland*

Correspondence should be addressed to Leena Kämppi; leena.ritvanen@helsinki.fi

Academic Editor: József Janszky

Introduction. This study was designed to identify the delays and factors related to and predicting the cessation of generalized convulsive SE (GCSE). *Methods.* This retrospective study includes 70 consecutive patients (>16 years) diagnosed with GCSE and treated in the emergency department of a tertiary hospital over 2 years. We defined cessation of SE stepwise using clinical seizure freedom, achievement of burst-suppression, and return of consciousness as endpoints and calculated delays for these cessation markers. In addition 10 treatment delay parameters and 7 prognostic and GCSE episode related factors were defined. Multiple statistical analyses were performed on their relation to cessation markers. *Results.* Onset-to-second-stage-medication ($p = 0.027$), onset-to-burst-suppression ($p = 0.005$), and onset-to-clinical-seizure-freedom ($p = 0.035$) delays correlated with the onset-to-consciousness delay. We detected no correlation between age, epilepsy, STESS, prestatus period, type of SE onset, effect of the first medication, and cessation of SE. *Conclusion.* Our study demonstrates that rapid administration of second-stage medication and early obtainment of clinical seizure freedom and burst-suppression predict early return of consciousness, an unambiguous marker for the end of SE. We propose that delays in treatment chain may be more significant determinants of SE cessation than the previously established outcome predictors. Thus, streamlining the treatment chain is advocated.

1. Introduction

Status epilepticus (SE) is a common and life-threatening condition, which requires urgent medical attention. The incidence of SE ranges from 10 to 20 per 100 000 [1] and generalized convulsive SE (GCSE) is by far the most common subtype. SE causes permanent brain damage especially in the hippocampal area [2] and permanently lowers seizure threshold predisposing to epilepsy [3]. Prolonged seizures respond poorly to treatment due to GABA-receptor trafficking occurring along the progressive SE episode [4].

Mortality of SE varies greatly (1.9%–40.0%) in published series [1]. Predictors of a poor outcome include age, structural brain lesion, prolonged seizure, acute symptomatic convulsions, and certain EEG findings during and after SE [5–7]. SE may require treatment in intensive care unit (ICU), which also increases mortality through treatment complications [5, 8]. Both brain damage and mortality are affected by longevity of the seizure and mortality increases greatly after 30 minutes of seizing [9]. In a pediatric study, every minute of ongoing seizure elevated the risk for a seizure prolongation over 60 minutes by five percent [10]. Permanent damage in SE is time-dependent, and seizure duration is the only prognostic factor that can be affected by rapid treatment [11].

It has been recently shown that delays in the treatment of SE are unacceptably long [12]. The effect of treatment delay on prognosis of SE is controversial and subject to debate in the literature. Most studies have focussed on the relation between first-stage medication and outcome, indicated by mortality, patient's condition at discharge and its return to baseline, or by clinical scales. Some studies found that a treatment delay has a clear impact on prognosis; the longer the delay, the worse the outcome [6, 13–15]. A few studies suggested that the treatment delay per se plays an important role on the prognosis besides the etiology [16–18]. Still there are opposite results suggesting that a long treatment delay does not correlate with higher mortality [19–22], and consequently the prognosis of SE is mainly determined by its biological background [23] and affected by its refractoriness [22]. This controversy may partly be explained by the recent observation that, regardless of the adequately started prehospital initial treatment, the delays in consecutive parts of the treatment chain were far from optimal [24].

Treatment of SE is guided by two international guidelines [25, 26]. Adherence to treatment protocol, quality of treatment, and management within the recommended time frames seem to have a significant impact on the prognosis of SE [27–29]. Still a recently published study suggested that treatment latency and adherence to protocol were not related to outcome of SE [30].

SE is a very dynamic process with diagnostic challenges, several treatment stages, and potential misinterpretations over the whole management process. Systematic analysis of the factors related to different parts of the treatment chain is needed to draw definite conclusions on the impact of the delays on prognosis. Our newly published study focussed on factors related to delays in the pre-hospital management of SE [24]. To our knowledge, there are no published studies investigating systematically the factors relating to the cessation of SE.

This study was designed to identify the delays and factors related to markers for cessation of GCSE and particularly to identify factors predicting the return of consciousness after GCSE. We also aim at validation of the stepwise definition for the cessation of SE, published earlier [12].

2. Methods

2.1. Study Design and Setting. This is a retrospective cohort study performed in Helsinki University Central Hospital (HUCH), a tertiary hospital serving a population of 1.4 million. HUCH provides neurological emergency service 24 h a day for the hospital district. The local Emergency Medical Service (EMS) has been instructed to transport patients with GCSE primarily to HUCH Emergency Department (ED). This study conforms to the Finnish legislation concerning medical research and the permission was granted by the HUCH Department of Neurology.

2.2. Selection of Participants. This study material includes consecutive adult patients (over 16 years of age) diagnosed with generalized convulsive status epilepticus (GCSE) and treated in the HUCH ED over a two-year period from January 2002 till December 2003.

The patients were identified in the HUCH electronic patient database by the ICD-10 code G41 (SE), yielding a total of 87 patients. Established SE was defined as continuous seizures lasting over 30 minutes, several recurrent seizures without returning consciousness, or occurrence of more than four seizures within any one hour irrespective of return of consciousness in between. Patients not meeting these criteria were excluded, despite having the SE diagnosis in their records, resulting in a total of 82 patients. The seizure description was collected from original medical records for all these

patients. Patients having a convulsive seizure at any point of the SE period were considered as having convulsive SE (CSE). Patients with impaired consciousness, either primarily or secondarily, were considered as having generalized SE (GSE). Altogether 70 patients met the criteria for GCSE and were included in this study.

2.3. Data Collection. A trained medical doctor collected the data from the original medical records on a standard form designed for this study. The records consisted of notes made by nurses and doctors of EMS, health care centers, regional hospitals, and HUCH ED, ICU, or neurological ward. Ambiguous data were evaluated in collaboration with the research team and if the consensus concerning the original coding rules changed, the data in question were recollected. The electronic database was created using MS Access for data recording. The information of patient identification was removed before further analyses. The Weighted Accuracy Score L_{WAS} and the Data Availability (DA) were calculated for all time parameters, using the method developed for evaluation of retrospective delay materials [12]. L_{WAS} refers to the deviation of the time parameters from the absolute accuracy in the medical records. The data on delays were based on events with exact time points documented in the medical records, whenever possible. For events not accurately documented, clinically grounded estimation of the event time was based on time frames with exact documented time points at each end.

2.4. Measures. Demographic data, medical history of the cases, etiologic and predisposing factors of GCSE and patients' condition at HUCH discharge are presented in Online Table 1 in Supplementary Material available online at http://dx.doi.org/10.1155/2015/591279. Mortality was calculated over HUCH admission period. No postdischarge follow-up was performed in this study.

We defined and calculated 13 parameters for delay in the management of GCSE. All delays were counted from the onset of GCSE. The time parameters and the median delays are presented in Table 1.

We defined 7 grouping variables (prognostic factors and GCSE episode parameters) for subgroup analysis. The variables are presented in Table 2.

Cases with events missing, for example, no burst-suppression (BS) and events happening during prestatus period, or with unknown data were excluded from the final analysis. The missing data information is presented in Online Table 2.

The onset of GCSE was defined as the beginning of the first seizure, fulfilling the criteria for established GCSE. Initial treatment was defined as the first given antiepileptic drug (AED), which was not necessarily the first-stage medication. Alarm delay refers to the primary alarm, in this case the delay in calling the ambulance.

Onset-to-first-convulsion-end refers to the time between the onset of GCSE and the end of the first clinical convulsion. The second-stage medication included i.v. fosphenytoin or valproate, and the third-stage medication included anesthesia with intravenous (i.v.) propofol, thiopental, or midazolam.

TABLE 1: Delay parameters and the delays in the management of GCSE.

Variable	N	%	Time Median	Time Mean	MIN	MAX	DA %	L_{WAS}
All Cases	70	100						
Delays in the treatment								
Onset-to-initial-treatment	67	95.7	30 min	57 min	0 min	8 h 5 min	97.0	1.8
Onset-to-alarm	60	85.7	36 min	2 h 27 min	0 min	57 h 44 min	93.3	1.5
Onset-to-first-convulsion-end	70	100	51 min	2 h 13 min	1 min	63 h 40 min	97.1	1.8
Onset-to-diagnosis	70	100	1 h 48 min	4 h	6 min	60 h 6 min	97.1	1.5
Onset-to-second-stage-medication	67	95.7	2 h 40 min	4 h 49 min	30 min	61 h 54 min	98.5	1.6
Onset-to-anesthesia	62	88.6	2 h 38 min	5 h 43 min	0 min	66 h 20 min	98.4	1.5
Onset-to-first-ED	61	87.1	2 h 2 min	3 h 31 min	0 min	58 h 29 min	98.4	1.5
Onset-to-tertiary-hospital (HUCH)	70	100	2 h 25 min	1 h 25 min	37 min	277 h 40 min	98.6	1.5
Onset-to-EEG	57	81.4	21 h 52 min	33 h	2 h 30 min	142 h	94.7	1.5
Onset-to-EEG-monitoring	42	60.0	11 h 10 min	15 h 45 min	2 h 30 min	82 h 14 min	97.6	1.5
Delays in the markers for cessation of GCSE								
Onset-to-burst-suppression	30	42.9	14 h 42 min	25 h 20 min	5 h 5 min	137 h 50 min	100.0	1.5
Onset-to-clinical-seizure-freedom	70	100	5 h 15 min	31 h 5 min	26 min	533 h 15 min	98.6	1.6
Onset-to-consciousness	61	87.1	42 h 45 min	66 h 5 min	2 h 40 min	444 h 40 min	96.7	1.4

TABLE 2: Grouping variables (prognostic factors and GCSE episode parameters) for the subgroup analysis.

Variable	N	%
All	70	100
Age under 65		
Yes	51	72.9
No	19	27.1
Epilepsy		
Yes	46	65.7
No	23	32.9
Unknown	1	1.4
STESS		
2	35	50.0
3	16	22.9
4	10	14.3
5	9	12.9
Prestatus period		
Yes	14	20.0
No	56	80.0
SE onset		
Continuous	45	64.3
Intermittent	25	35.7
Effect of the first medication		
Yes	17	24.3
No	39	55.7
Spontaneous cessation	11	15.7
Refractoriness		
Non-RSE	8	11.4
RSE	30	42.9
SRSE	32	45.7

Induction was considered as the exact time point of anesthesia. First ED was defined as the first emergency department the patient was transported to. Tertiary hospital always refers to HUCH ED.

We defined the markers for cessation of GCSE with three separate parameters for the treatment response [12]: BS, clinical seizure freedom and return of consciousness. BS refers to the beginning of the first BS sequence during this SE. Clinical seizure freedom refers to the end of the last clinical convulsion and return of consciousness refers to the time point, when the patient no longer presented altered mental status.

Age of 65 years was selected as the classification basis for age as a grouping variable. Only patients with previously diagnosed epilepsy were considered as having epilepsy. Status Epilepticus Severity Score (STESS) [21] was calculated for all patients. Seizures occurring no more than 48 h prior to GCSE onset were referred to as the prestatus period seizures. Seizures lasting clinically at least 30 min were defined as continuous. All other types of seizures were considered as intermittent. The patient was considered to respond to the initial treatment, if the seizure stopped within 10 min after i.v. administration or 20 min after rectal administration of the first medication, with no other simultaneous AEDs. Patients failing to respond to the first or second-stage treatment were considered as having refractory SE (RSE). SE continuing or recurring 24 h or more after the onset of anesthesia was considered as super-refractory SE (SRSE).

2.5. Statistics. The results are expressed as mean/median and range/interquartile range (IQR) or as number of patients and percentage. The normality of variables was tested with the Kolmogorov-Smirnov test. For the nonnormal data, the Spearman's correlation coefficient and, for normally distributed data, the Pearson's correlation coefficient were calculated to find correlation between continuous variables. Bootstrap resampling (1000 samples) was used to calculate the bias corrected percentile confidence intervals for correlation coefficients. Statistical significance of the differences in

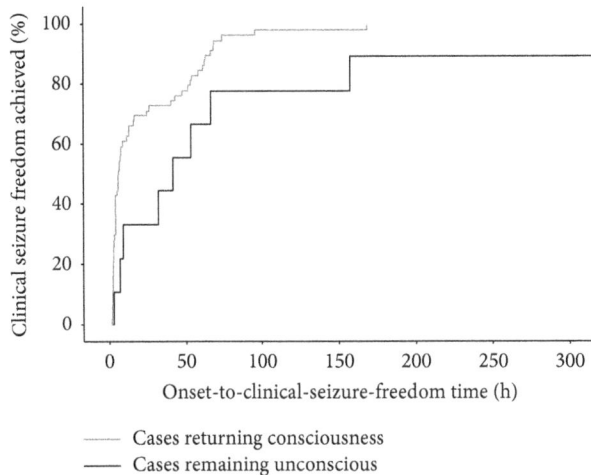

FIGURE 1: Kaplan-Meier curve showing the difference of the onset-to-clinical-seizure-freedom time between patients returning consciousness and remaining unconscious.

variables between independent samples was tested with the nonparametric Wilcoxon-Mann–Whitney test. Differences in categorical variables were examined using the Fisher's exact test. The Kaplan-Meier analysis with the log-rank test was used to analyze time to event data. Linear regression analysis with bootstrap resampling (5000 samples) was used to model delays in treatment response. Statistical analyses were executed using the SPSS software (version 22.0, SPSS, IBM Corp. USA). Statistical significance was defined as $p < 0.05$ and two tailed tests were used.

3. Results

The total-time-correlations, that is, correlations between the onset-to-event and onset-to-treatment-response delays, that is, markers for the cessation of SE, are shown in Table 3(a). Since this method includes cumulative delays in the total time from onset to treatment response and therefore may represent inherent correlations, we also calculated the chronological correlations, that is, correlations between the onset-to-event and event-to-treatment-response delays, shown in Table 3(b). Correlation significances given below are based on chronological correlation.

Regardless of the method of calculation, the delays in giving the second-stage medication ($p = 0.027$), obtaining the BS ($p = 0.005$) and achieving the clinical seizure freedom ($p = 0.035$) correlate significantly with the delay in returning of consciousness (Table 3(b)). 76.7% of the BSs were registered with EEG-monitoring before full scale EEG. Therefore, the statistically significant negative correlation between full scale EEG delay and BS delay is clinically insignificant.

Clinical seizure freedom delay among patients regaining consciousness ($N = 60$, median 3.67 h, 95% CI = 1.64–5.69 h, and DA = 98%, $L_{WAS} = 1.58$) was significantly ($p = 0.022$) shorter than that among patients remaining unconscious ($N = 9$, median 41.17 h, 95% CI 14.87–67.46 h, DA = 100%, and $L_{WAS} = 1.67$) (Figure 1).

The difference in BS delay between patients regaining consciousness ($N = 22$, median 12.0 h, 95% CI 9.32–14.68 h, DA = 95%, and $L_{WAS} = 1.5$) and those remaining unconscious ($N = 8$, median 18.0 h, 95% CI 8.16–27.84 h, DA = 100%, and $L_{WAS} = 1.5$) did not reach statistical significance ($p = 0.398$).

Out of the 70 GCSE cases, 30 cases (42.9%) obtained BS and 40 cases (57.1%) did not. 42 cases (60.0%) of all cases had EEG-monitoring and 30 cases (71.4%) of them obtained BS. In the BS-group eight cases (26.7%) remained unconscious, whereas in the non-BS-group one case (2.5%) remained unconscious, the difference being statistically significant ($p = 0.004$). In the BS-group 23 cases (76.7%) and in the non-BS-group nine cases (22.5%) fulfilled the criteria of SRSE, the difference being statistically significant ($p < 0.001$). The non-BS-group contained all the non-RSE cases of the study material (8/70). Furthermore, in the BS-group all 30 cases were anesthetized with propofol, 20.0% of these cases had multiple anesthetics and 36.7% had several anesthesia periods, the median total anesthesia time being 59 hours 12 minutes (DA = 100%, $L_{WAS} = 1.48$). In the non-BS group all RSE and SRSE cases (32) were anesthetized with only one anesthetic propofol. Four cases (12.5%) had several anesthesia periods, the median total anesthesia time being 20 hours 20 minutes (DA = 97%, $L_{WAS} = 1.48$).

Regression analysis was performed to reveal the correlation of clinical variables with the delays in treatment response. The time parameters having significant effect on the delays of clinical seizure freedom or return of consciousness are shown in Table 4. Regression analysis was not performed on BS delays due to low number of patients ($N = 30$).

Univariate analysis of the factors related to markers for cessation of GCSE is shown in Online Table 3. SRSE cases have significantly longer delays in achieving clinical seizure freedom and returning consciousness than non-SRSE cases ($p < 0.001$).

Univariate analysis of the factors related to return of consciousness is presented in Online Table 4. No significant relations were found, although the non-SRSE cases tended to regain consciousness more likely than the SRSE cases ($p = 0.070$).

In pooled STESS groups 0–2, 42.7% of the cases, and in pooled STESS groups 3–6, 48.6% of the cases presented SRSE. When STESS groups were pooled 0–3 and 4–6, the proportion of cases presenting SRSE was 47.1% and 42.1%, respectively.

4. Discussion

This is to our knowledge the first study analysing systematically the delays and factors related to cessation of GCSE. We found that the earlier the clinical seizure freedom is achieved, the earlier and more likely the consciousness returns. Delay of clinical seizure freedom is significantly affected by several delays in the preceding treatment chain. Short delays in giving the second-stage medication and obtaining BS also correlate with early return of consciousness. Surprisingly, several previously reported prognostic factors, such as age, epilepsy, or STESS and the response to initial treatment are related neither

TABLE 3: (a) Total-time-correlations: correlations between the onset-to-event and onset-to-treatment-response delays, that is, markers for cessation of SE. (b) Chronological correlations: correlations between the onset-to-event delays and event-to-treatment-response delays, that is, markers for cessation of SE.

(a)

Variable	Onset-to-burst-suppression					Onset-to-clinical-seizure-freedom					Onset-to-consciousness				
	N	Coefficient	95% CI (min)	95% CI (max)	p value	N	Coefficient	95% CI (min)	95% CI (max)	p value	N	Coefficient	95% CI (min)	95% CI (max)	p value
Onset-to-initial-treatment	28	0.127	−0.299	0.519	0.520	65	0.054	−0.181	0.289	0.668	56	0.017	−0.213	0.254	0.902
Onset-to-first-convulsion-end	29	0.303	−0.093	0.640	0.110	68	0.122	−0.122	0.363	0.321	58	0.107	−0.166	0.367	0.425
Onset-to-alarm	22	0.467	0.036	0.791	**0.029**	55	0.300	−0.004	0.558	**0.026**	47	0.010	−0.256	0.288	0.946
Onset-to-diagnosis	29	0.415	0.040	0.691	**0.025**	68	0.371	0.120	0.587	**0.002**	59	0.136	−0.111	0.390	0.304
Onset-to-second-stage-medication	30	0.337	−0.080	0.660	0.069	66	0.334	0.087	0.535	**0.006**	56	0.402	0.165	0.610	**0.002**
Onset-to-anesthesia	30	0.510	0.132	0.765	**0.004**	61	0.382	0.098	0.619	**0.002**	51	0.088	−0.175	0.353	0.540
Onset-to-first-ED	23	0.500	0.091	0.781	**0.015**	60	0.260	0.019	0.503	**0.045**	52	0.212	−0.740	0.476	0.131
Onset-to-tertiary-hospital (HUCH)	30	0.538	0.177	0.780	**0.002**	69	0.334	0.081	0.559	**0.005**	59	0.207	−0.550	0.448	0.116
Onset-to-EEG	26	0.099	−0.324	0.496	0.632	54	0.470	0.197	0.688	**<0.001**	46	0.327	0.037	0.568	**0.027**
Onset-to-EEG-monitoring	30	0.775	0.503	0.929	**<0.001**	41	0.413	0.096	0.677	**0.007**	31	0.239	−0.135	0.542	0.194
Onset-to-burst-suppression						30	0.558	0.165	0.857	**0.001**	21	0.527	0.071	0.815	**0.014**
Onset-to-clinical-seizure-freedom											59	0.739	0.576	0.850	**<0.001**

(b)

Variable	Event-to-burst-suppression					Event-to-clinical-seizure freedom					Event-to-consciousness				
Onset-to-event	N	Coefficient	95% CI (min)	95% CI (max)	p value	N	Coefficient	95% CI (min)	95% CI (max)	p value	N	Coefficient	95% CI (min)	95% CI (max)	p value
Onset-to-initial-treatment	28	0.005	−0.421	0.412	0.981	65	−0.095	−0.344	0.156	0.453	56	−0.012	−0.237	0.205	0.928
Onset-to-first-convulsion-end	29	0.109	−0.282	0.474	0.573	68	−0.112	−0.360	0.136	0.362	58	0.085	−0.173	0.322	0.528
Onset-to-alarm	22	0.303	−0.176	0.666	0.171	55	0.020	−0.253	0.295	0.883	47	−0.087	−0.364	0.223	0.563
Onset-to-diagnosis	29	0.169	−0.198	0.497	0.382	68	−0.069	−0.321	0.226	0.574	59	0.037	−0.267	0.322	0.783
Onset-to-second-stage-medication	30	0.057	−0.345	0.421	0.765	66	−0.046	−0.323	0.265	0.713	56	0.295	0.039	0.534	**0.027**
Onset-to-anesthesia	30	−0.152	−0.488	0.175	0.424	61	−0.057	−0.333	0.211	0.662	51	0.025	−0.251	0.330	0.859
Onset-to-first-ED	23	0.343	−0.062	0.732	0.109	60	−0.022	−0.296	0.271	0.870	52	0.101	−0.195	0.385	0.477
Onset-to-tertiary-hospital (HUCH)	30	0.113	−0.247	0.498	0.552	69	−0.037	−0.285	0.195	0.761	59	0.068	−0.220	0.338	0.610
Onset-to-EEG	26	−0.753	−0.914	−0.473	**<0.001**	54	−0.198	−0.475	0.081	0.152	46	−0.162	−0.420	0.116	0.283
Onset-to-EEG-monitoring	30	−0.183	−0.579	0.278	0.332	41	−0.051	−0.386	0.279	0.752	31	0.101	−0.311	0.459	0.588
Onset-to-burst-suppression						30	0.031	−0.359	0.443	0.872	21	0.584	0.058	0.863	**0.005***
Onset-to-clinical-seizure-freedom											59	0.275	−0.036	0.563	**0.035**

Spearman's rho.
*Pearson's rho.

TABLE 4: The regression analysis of the effect of the chronological delay components on markers for cessation on GCSE.

Variable	TIME (h)	95% CI min	95% CI max	p
Onset-to-clinical-seizure-freedom				
Intercept	9.0	−1.4	23.6	0.082
Onset-to-initial-treatment	7.8	−1.6	13.2	0.008
Initial-treatment-to-diagnosis	2.3	0.2	4.2	**0.016**
Intercept	8.2	−5.6	31.3	0.273
Onset-to-initial-treatment	6.6	−2.8	11.6	0.035
Initial-treatment-to-second-stage-medication	3.0	0.4	4.8	**0.021**
Onset-to-consciousness				
Intercept	38.1	14.8	73.4	0.008
Onset-to-initial-treatment	0.4	−15.2	8.1	0.935
Initial-treatment-to-second-stage-medication	9.7	3.9	15.8	**0.002**

to the probability nor the delay of returning consciousness. The present results suggest that the cessation of the GCSE might be more likely related to the delays in the treatment than to the known prognostic factors of SE outcome.

The risk for reporting bias is present in every retrospective study. We controlled the risk by evaluating the adequacy of the data with Data Accuracy (L_{WAS}) and Data Availability (DA) scores using the method published recently [12]. The scores in this study indicate that the accuracy and coverage of patient data recordings seem to be on an adequate level. We included only patients with GCSE in this study to assure the uniformity of our material.

Although the patient material was collected in 2002-2003 in one tertiary hospital and is relatively small, it is comparable to more recent materials since the treatment recommendations have not markedly changed during the past decade. The increased assortment of intravenously administered second-stage medications in the past years does not affect the interpretation of our results. In this study fosphenytoin was almost exclusively administered as the second-stage medication, providing a relatively homogeneous material. At the time of collection of the material the EEG-monitoring availability was insufficient. Still, the criteria for monitoring and the interpretation of the results have not changed. Direct comparison of the present results to previously published studies should be carried out with caution, since return of consciousness is not widely used in the literature as the marker for cessation of SE. Furthermore, definition of the duration of SE varies considerably among previously published studies. The most commonly used endpoint has been outcome, that is, mortality and/or condition at discharge.

4.1. Relation of Delays to Cessation of SE. The exact endpoint of SE is conceptually problematic and varies even in the few previous studies that have clearly defined the endpoint. Cessation of GCSE is defined by Rantsch et al. as the end of the convulsion [22]. Absence of clinical seizure as the only marker seems insufficient since 48% of the seizures continue as electrographic SE [31]. Others have used a combination of last clinical seizure and last continuous electrografic seizure

as the criteria without any specific time frames [32, 33]. Mayer et al. used additional time frame criteria, requiring the patient to be seizure free for at least 72 h after the last clinical or electrographic seizure [34]. SE is a dynamic process, and therefore we have suggested a stepwise definition for cessation of SE, including time points of clinical seizure freedom, obtaining BS and return of consciousness [12]. This definition was used in the present study, since return of consciousness is the only reliable clinical marker for the end of GCSE.

Recent evidence indicates that the median delay in giving the second-stage medication and the third-stage medication is nearly the same [12, 24]. The second-stage medication delay resulted mostly from lack of refrigerator in the ambulance required for fosphenytoin storage [12], and in some cases from failure in choosing an adequately specialized hospital for treatment [24]. Two studies have combined fosphenytoin with traditional first-stage treatment given out of hospital [29, 35]. One of them [29] included doctor-led medical emergency teams and the authors found that patients receiving first long-acting AED according to the protocol (fosphenytoin or lorazepam) were 19.9 times more likely to obtain seizure termination ($p < 0.0001$) [29]. In the present study, the delay in giving the second-stage medication showed a significant correlation with the delay in returning consciousness. These results together strongly suggest that the second-stage medication should be available already in EMS units and be administered together with the first-stage medication, provided that adequate physician evaluation of the patient can be obtained to assure the correct diagnosis and the patient safety.

The evidence for the utility of BS as a goal in the treatment of GCSE is scarce and no prospective studies are available. The effect of BS on the prognosis of GCSE patients is controversial [36]. Jaitly et al. found that the presence of BS, regardless of SE etiology or the medication administered, was a sign of a grave prognosis [37]. In another study seizure control without suppression of electric activity to BS or isoelectric level predicted good functional recovery [38]. A few studies have reported that BS had no effect on treatment response or on prognosis [32, 39]. Claassen et al. suggested that BS correlates with favourable treatment response, but still its significance in predicting permanent absence of seizures, mortality, or clinical recovery was questioned [40]. Usefulness of BS as the goal of SE treatment has been advocated based on evidence that the depth of EEG suppression correlates with favourable outcome [41]. Nevertheless, maintenance of BS for at least 24 h is recommended by the European guideline [25], although, as the American guideline states, the EEG endpoint of treatment is controversial, and there are no data indicating as for what duration of treatment is sufficient to obtain permanent seizure termination [26].

In our material the risk of remaining unconscious was significantly higher among patients achieving BS than among patients not treated to BS. The BS-group contained a significantly higher proportion of SRSE cases than the non-BS group. The BS-group also needed more often several anesthetizing agents and repeated anesthesia periods during the total anesthesia time of nearly 40 h longer than that of the non-BS-group. We also showed that the SRSE cases remained unconscious more likely than the non-SRSE cases. We propose that it is not the BS itself that increases the risk of remaining unconscious. Rather, the GCSE of the patients requiring anesthesia to BS seems to be more aggressive than that of the non-BS-group.

No previous studies have focused on the association of BS to the ending of the GCSE or to return of consciousness. We found a significant correlation between early obtainment of BS and early return of consciousness. In our study, the delays in achieving BS did not reach the time frames recommended in the guidelines, reflecting the clinical reality. At least the anesthesia-to-BS delay could be dramatically shortened with an accurate management protocol, as shown in two prospective studies [42, 43]. Since nearly half of our patients seemed to benefit from early BS, the question remains, whether the third-stage treatment given up to BS level in recommended time frames would increase the proportion of patients returning of consciousness also among severe GCSE cases. In parallel, one previous study has speculated that possibly treatment delay is critical for extremely severe SE episodes, although not for all types of SE [20].

We found a significant correlation between early clinical seizure freedom and early return of consciousness. These results are in accordance with the previous literature showing the impact of seizure freedom on prognosis. Claassen et al. found that the delayed seizure control has a negative effect on the efficacy of treatment and that it increases mortality [40]. It has also been stated that the longer the duration of SE the worse the prognosis, particularly after 1-2 h of continuous seizures. It has been claimed that this relation may be lost, if SE lasts over 10 h [36]. However, in our material the mean delay of clinical seizure freedom, although being over 31 h, still correlated with the return of consciousness and thus predicted the cessation of GCSE.

To our surprise onset-to-initial-treatment time, onset-to-diagnosis time, and onset-to-anesthesia time did not correlate to markers for cessation of GCSE. There are no other studies on the effect of diagnosis- and anesthesia-related delays on duration of GCSE in adult patients. There is evidence from a pediatric study suggesting that prehospital diazepam shortens the duration of SE [44]. On the other hand, we have previously shown that short initial treatment delay per se does not lead to a better treatment response delay, unless the whole prehospital treatment chain functions optimally [24].

Regression analysis showed that prolonged time between initial treatment and second-stage treatment predicts a delayed clinical seizure freedom and return of consciousness. Also the time between initial treatment and diagnosis may affect the delay to clinical seizure freedom. Thus, it is feasible that a failure or slow-up in any single delay component may ravage the benefits acquired by optimal action of the earlier phases of the treatment chain.

4.2. Relation of Prognostic Factors to Cessation of GCSE. Prognostic factors of SE have been studied in detail, and in most reports the main focus has been on outcome, defined as mortality or clinical status at discharge. To our knowledge, there are no studies on the relation of prognostic factors to cessation of GCSE.

There is a consensus in literature that old age, defined in most studies as the age over 65 years, correlates with worse outcome [21, 36, 45–50]. Significance of age is partly based on pediatric studies, in which age was the major determinant of prognosis, in contrast to adult SE [36]. Prehospital delays in adults do not differ significantly between age groups, when the cutoff point is set at 65 years [24]. In the present study, we did not find any correlation between age and markers for cessation of GCSE. Neither were differences in probability of returning consciousness found between age groups. Our results thus support the previous conclusion that higher mortality of old SE patients may be due to higher frequency of treatment complications [16, 22]. A rational conclusion is that quickly administered second-stage medication should improve the prognosis of GCSE in elderly patients by lessening the need for ICU treatment.

The SE episodes in epilepsy-related cases are commonly thought to be easier to treat, and their outcome is in most studies found to be better than that of patients presenting acute symptomatic seizures [7, 21, 33]. The absence of previous seizures implicates that acute symptomatic seizure as such may be used as a prognostic marker [21]. The delays in the treatment of SE patients with known epilepsy in the prehospital management are shorter than those of the nonepileptic patients. Moreover, epilepsy patients are more likely to be triaged directly to tertiary hospital, diagnosed with SE and anesthetized earlier than nonepileptic patients [24]. Surprisingly, this advantage of shorter delays does not seem to be beneficial to epilepsy patients, suggested by our finding that previously diagnosed epilepsy does not predict faster cessation of GCSE or higher likelihood of returning consciousness.

STESS is an internally and externally validated tool for systematic evaluation of the outcome of SE patients and may be used to recognize the patients who need aggressive treatment [21, 51]. Its scoring criteria include established variables, which all are proven to affect the outcome [21]. However, the cutoff-point for poor outcome is subject to debate [21, 22, 51]. We found no correlation between STESS points and markers for cessation of GCSE with any cutoff. Nor did any STESS point cutoff predict return of consciousness.

This is in line with the present observation that two of the STESS variables, age and previous epilepsy diagnosis, lacked correlation with cessation of SE. Taken together, the cessation of GCSE may be more dependent on the management of GCSE than the initial severity of SE.

As can be expected by definition, SRSE cases showed longer delays of clinical seizure freedom and return of consciousness than RSE and non-RSE cases. Interestingly, the delay of obtaining BS did not predict development of SRSE.

4.3. Relation of Other Factors to Cessation of GCSE. In our material, the response to first line treatment neither correlated with any of the markers for cessation of GCSE nor predicted return of consciousness. This may be due to the fact that our material included relatively large number of RSE cases, possibly because SE cases successfully treated with first-stage medication were not referred to the tertiary hospital. A recent study reported that the efficacy of the first-stage treatment does not affect the duration of SE [52], while another study presented an opposite result [35].

Pre-SE period, that is, occurrence of recurring convulsive seizures preceding the actual SE, is a newly introduced concept [12], the significance of which has not yet been established. In the present study, pre-SE period did not correlate with the delay in cessation of SE. We did not find any significant correlation between the type of SE onset and return of consciousness.

5. Conclusions

We conclude that early administration of second-stage medication, early cessation of clinical seizures, and early obtainment of BS predict early return of consciousness, which is an unambiguous marker for the cessation of SE. The present retrospective study suggests that delays in treatment chain may be more significant determinants of SE cessation than the previously established outcome predictors. The correlations presented here serve as validation for the use of stepwise definition of the end of SE and speak for consideration of BS as the target of the third-stage treatment. The delays should also be considered in planning protocols, particularly in matching of patient groups, in prospective SE studies.

Disclosure

The authors confirm that they have read the Journal's position on issues involved in ethical publication and affirm that this report is consistent with those guidelines.

Conflict of Interests

The authors declare that there is no conflict of interests regarding the publication of this paper.

Authors' Contribution

Leena Kämppi and Jaakko Ritvanen made an equal contribution to the paper.

Acknowledgments

This study has been financially supported by Epilepsy Research Foundation in Finland and Maire Taponen Foundation (financial support granted to Leena Kämppi).

References

[1] F. Rosenow, H. M. Hamer, and S. Knake, "The epidemiology of convulsive and nonconvulsive status epilepticus," *Epilepsia*, vol. 48, no. 8, pp. 82–84, 2007.

[2] C. M. DeGiorgio, U. Tomiyasu, P. S. Gott, and D. M. Treiman, "Hippocampal pyramidal cell loss in human status epilepticus," *Epilepsia*, vol. 33, no. 1, pp. 23–27, 1992.

[3] N. B. Fountain, "Status epilepticus: risk factors and complications," *Epilepsia*, vol. 41, supplement 2, pp. S23–S30, 2000.

[4] D. E. Naylor, H. Liu, and C. G. Wasterlain, "Trafficking of $GABA_A$ receptors, loss of inhibition, and a mechanism for pharmacoresistance in status epilepticus," *The Journal of Neuroscience*, vol. 25, no. 34, pp. 7724–7733, 2005.

[5] J. Claassen, J. K. Lokin, B.-F. M. Fitzsimmons, F. A. Mendelsohn, and S. A. Mayer, "Predictors of functional disability and mortality after status epilepticus," *Neurology*, vol. 58, no. 1, pp. 139–142, 2002.

[6] K. Agan, N. Afsar, I. Midi, O. Us, S. Aktan, and C. Aykut-Bingol, "Predictors of refractoriness in a Turkish status epilepticus data bank," *Epilepsy and Behavior*, vol. 14, no. 4, pp. 651–654, 2009.

[7] R. Sutter, P. W. Kaplan, and S. Rüegg, "Outcome predictors for status epilepticus—what really counts," *Nature Reviews Neurology*, vol. 9, no. 9, pp. 525–534, 2013.

[8] R. Sutter, S. Tschudin-Sutter, L. Grize et al., "Associations between infections and clinical outcome parameters in status epilepticus: a retrospective 5-year cohort study," *Epilepsia*, vol. 53, no. 9, pp. 1489–1497, 2012.

[9] S. Legriel, B. Mourvillier, N. Bele et al., "Outcomes in 140 critically ill patients with status epilepticus," *Intensive Care Medicine*, vol. 34, no. 3, pp. 476–480, 2008.

[10] R. F. Chin, B. G. Neville, C. Peckham, A. Wade, H. Bedford, and R. C. Scott, "Treatment of community-onset, childhood convulsive status epilepticus: a prospective, population-based study," *The Lancet Neurology*, vol. 7, no. 8, pp. 696–703, 2008.

[11] S. Legriel, E. Azoulay, M. Resche-Rigon et al., "Functional outcome after convulsive status epilepticus," *Critical Care Medicine*, vol. 38, no. 12, pp. 2295–2303, 2010.

[12] L. Kämppi, H. Mustonen, and S. Soinila, "Analysis of the delay components in the treatment of status epilepticus," *Neurocritical Care*, vol. 19, no. 1, pp. 10–18, 2013.

[13] M. J. Aminoff and R. P. Simon, "Status epilepticus. Causes, clinical features and consequences in 98 patients," *The American Journal of Medicine*, vol. 69, no. 5, pp. 657–666, 1980.

[14] A. Sagduyu, S. Tarlaci, and H. Sirin, "Generalized tonic-clonic status epilepticus: causes, treatment, complications and predictors of case fatality," *Journal of Neurology*, vol. 245, no. 10, pp. 640–646, 1998.

[15] J. Hillman, K. Lehtimäki, J. Peltola, and S. Liimatainen, "Clinical significance of treatment delay in status epilepticus," *International Journal of Emergency Medicine*, vol. 6, no. 1, article 6, 2013.

[16] F. B. Scholtes, W. O. Renier, and H. Meinardi, "Generalized convulsive status epilepticus: causes, therapy, and outcome in 346 patients," *Epilepsia*, vol. 35, no. 5, pp. 1104–1112, 1994.

[17] R. Silbergleit, V. Durkalski, D. Lowenstein et al., "Intramuscular versus intravenous therapy for prehospital status epilepticus," *The New England Journal of Medicine*, vol. 366, no. 7, pp. 591–600, 2012.

[18] E. H. Kossoff, "A shot in the arm for prehospital status epilepticus: the rampart study," *Epilepsy Currents*, vol. 12, no. 3, pp. 103–104, 2012.

[19] K. B. Krishnamurthy and F. W. Drislane, "Relapse and survival after barbiturate anesthetic treatment of refractory status epilepticus," *Epilepsia*, vol. 37, no. 9, pp. 863–867, 1996.

[20] A. O. Rossetti, S. Hurwitz, G. Logroscino, and E. B. Bromfield, "Prognosis of status epilepticus: role of aetiology, age, and consciousness impairment at presentation," *Journal of Neurology, Neurosurgery & Psychiatry*, vol. 77, no. 5, pp. 611–615, 2006.

[21] A. O. Rossetti, G. Logroscino, T. A. Milligan, C. Michaelides, C. Ruffieux, and E. B. Bromfield, "Status Epilepticus Severity Score (STESS): a tool to orient early treatment strategy," *Journal of Neurology*, vol. 255, no. 10, pp. 1561–1566, 2008.

[22] K. Rantsch, U. Walter, M. Wittstock, R. Benecke, and J. Rösche, "Treatment and course of different subtypes of status epilepticus," *Epilepsy Research*, vol. 107, no. 1-2, pp. 156–162, 2013.

[23] A. O. Rossetti and D. H. Lowenstein, "Management of refractory status epilepticus in adults: still more questions than answers," *The Lancet Neurology*, vol. 10, no. 10, pp. 922–930, 2011.

[24] L. Kämppi, H. Mustonen, and S. Soinila, "Factors related to delays in pre-hospital management of status epilepticus," *Neurocritical Care*, vol. 22, pp. 93–104, 2015.

[25] H. Meierkord, P. Boon, B. Engelsen et al., "EFNS guideline on the management of status epilepticus in adults," *European Journal of Neurology*, vol. 17, no. 3, pp. 348–355, 2010.

[26] G. M. Brophy, R. Bell, J. Claassen et al., "Guidelines for the evaluation and management of status epilepticus," *Neurocritical Care*, vol. 17, no. 1, pp. 3–23, 2012.

[27] T. Muayqil, B. H. Rowe, and S. N. Ahmed, "Treatment adherence and outcomes in the management of convulsive status epilepticus in the emergency room," *Epileptic Disorders*, vol. 9, no. 1, pp. 43–50, 2007.

[28] L. Vignatelli, R. Rinaldi, E. Baldin et al., "Impact of treatment on the short-term prognosis of status epilepticus in two population-based cohorts," *Journal of Neurology*, vol. 255, no. 2, pp. 197–204, 2008.

[29] A. Aranda, G. Foucart, J. L. Ducassé, S. Grolleau, A. McGonigal, and L. Valton, "Generalized convulsive status epilepticus management in adults: a cohort study with evaluation of professional practice," *Epilepsia*, vol. 51, no. 10, pp. 2159–2167, 2010.

[30] A. O. Rossetti, V. Alvarez, J.-M. Januel, and B. Burnand, "Treatment deviating from guidelines does not influence status epilepticus prognosis," *Journal of Neurology*, vol. 260, no. 2, pp. 421–428, 2013.

[31] R. J. DeLorenzo, E. J. Waterhouse, A. R. Towne et al., "Persistent nonconvulsive status epilepticus after the control of convulsive status epilepticus," *Epilepsia*, vol. 39, no. 8, pp. 833–840, 1998.

[32] A. O. Rossetti, G. Logroscino, and E. B. Bromfield, "Refractory status epilepticus: effect of treatment aggressiveness on prognosis," *Archives of Neurology*, vol. 62, no. 11, pp. 1698–1702, 2005.

[33] F. W. Drislane, A. S. Blum, M. R. Lopez, S. Gautam, and D. L. Schomer, "Duration on refractory status epilepticus and outcome: loss of prognostic utility after several hours," *Epilepsia*, vol. 50, pp. 1566–1571, 2009.

[34] S. A. Mayer, J. Claassen, J. Lokin, F. Mendelsohn, L. J. Dennis, and B.-F. Fitzsimmons, "Refractory status epilepticus: frequency, risk factors, and impact on outcome," *Archives of Neurology*, vol. 59, no. 2, pp. 205–210, 2002.

[35] B. Ozdilek, I. Midi, K. Agan, and C. A. Bingol, "Episodes of status epilepticus in young adults: etiologic factors, subtypes, and outcomes," *Epilepsy & Behavior*, vol. 27, no. 2, pp. 351–354, 2013.

[36] A. Neligan and S. D. Shorvon, "Prognostic factors, morbidity and mortality in tonic-clonic status epilepticus: a review," *Epilepsy Research*, vol. 93, no. 1, pp. 1–10, 2011.

[37] R. Jaitly, J. A. Sgro, A. R. Towne, D. Ko, and R. J. DeLorenzo, "Prognostic value of EEG monitoring after status epilepticus: a prospective adult study," *Journal of Clinical Neurophysiology*, vol. 14, no. 4, pp. 326–334, 1997.

[38] S. E. Hocker, J. W. Britton, J. N. Mandrekar, E. F. M. Wijdicks, and A. A. Rabinstein, "Predictors of outcome in refractory status epilepticus," *JAMA Neurology*, vol. 70, no. 1, pp. 72–77, 2013.

[39] G. K. Bergey, "Refractory status epilepticus: is EEG burst suppression an appropriate treatment target during drug-induced coma? What is the Holy Grail?" *Epilepsy Currents*, vol. 6, no. 4, pp. 119–120, 2006.

[40] J. Claassen, L. J. Hirsch, R. G. Emerson, and S. A. Mayer, "Treatment of refractory status epilepticus with pentobarbital, propofol, or midazolam: a systematic review," *Epilepsia*, vol. 43, no. 2, pp. 146–153, 2002.

[41] K. B. Krishnamurthy and F. W. Drislane, "Depth of EEG suppression and outcome in barbiturate anesthetic treatment for refractory status epilepticus," *Epilepsia*, vol. 40, no. 6, pp. 759–762, 1999.

[42] I. Parviainen, A. Uusaro, R. Kälviäinen, E. Kaukanen, E. Mervaala, and E. Ruokonen, "High-dose thiopental in the treatment of refractory status epilepticus in intensive care unit," *Neurology*, vol. 59, no. 8, pp. 1249–1251, 2002.

[43] I. Parviainen, R. Kälviäinen, and E. Ruokonen, "Propofol and barbiturates for the anesthesia of refractory convulsive status epilepticus: pros and cons," *Neurological Research*, vol. 29, no. 7, pp. 667–671, 2007.

[44] B. K. Alldredge, D. Pharm, D. B. Wall, and D. M. Ferriero, "Effect of prehospital treatment on the outcome of status epilepticus in children," *Pediatric Neurology*, vol. 12, no. 3, pp. 213–216, 1995.

[45] A. R. Towne, J. M. Pellock, D. Ko, and R. J. DeLorenzo, "Determinants of mortality in status epilepticus," *Epilepsia*, vol. 35, no. 1, pp. 27–34, 1994.

[46] D. C. Hesdorffer, G. Logroscino, G. Cascino, J. F. Annegers, and W. A. Hauser, "Incidence of status epilepticus in Rochester, Minnesota, 1965–1984," *Neurology*, vol. 50, no. 3, pp. 735–741, 1998.

[47] D. H. Lowenstein, "Status epilepticus: an overview of the clinical problem," *Epilepsia*, vol. 40, no. 1, pp. S3–S8, 1999.

[48] Y. W. Wu, D. W. Shek, P. A. Garcia, S. Zhao, and S. C. Johnston, "Incidence and mortality of generalized convulsive status epilepticus in California," *Neurology*, vol. 58, no. 7, pp. 1070–1076, 2002.

[49] S. Legriel, E. Azoulay, M. Resche-Rigon et al., "Functional outcome after convulsive status epilepticus," *Critical Care Medicine*, vol. 38, no. 12, pp. 2295–2303, 2010.

[50] A. O. Rossetti, G. Logroscino, and E. B. Bromfield, "A clinical score for prognosis of status epilepticus in adults," *Neurology*, vol. 66, no. 11, pp. 1736–1738, 2006.

[51] R. Sutter, P. W. Kaplan, and S. Rüegg, "Independent external validation of the status epilepticus severity score," *Critical Care Medicine*, vol. 41, no. 12, pp. e475–e479, 2013.

[52] J. Kalita, P. P. Nair, and U. K. Misra, "A clinical, radiological and outcome study of status epilepticus from India," *Journal of Neurology*, vol. 257, no. 2, pp. 224–229, 2010.

9

The Relationship between Self-Efficacy and Psychosocial Care in Adolescents with Epilepsy

Masoomeh Akbarbegloo,[1,2] **Leila Valizadeh,**[3]
Vahid Zamanzadeh,[4] **and Faranak Jabarzadeh**[5]

[1]*Department of Pediatric Nursing, Faculty of Nursing and Midwifery, Urmia University of Medical Sciences, Urmia 51389 47977, Iran*
[2]*Tabriz University of Medical Sciences, Tabriz 51389 47977, Iran*
[3]*Department of Pediatric Nursing, Faculty of Nursing and Midwifery, Tabriz University of Medical Sciences, Tabriz 51389 47977, Iran*
[4]*Department of Medical Surgical Nursing, Faculty of Nursing and Midwifery, Tabriz University of Medical Sciences,*
 Tabriz 51389 47977, Iran
[5]*Department of Medical Surgical Nursing, Student Research Committee, Faculty of Nursing and Midwifery,*
 Tabriz University of Medical Sciences, Tabriz 51389 47977, Iran

Correspondence should be addressed to Leila Valizadeh; valizadehl@tbzmed.ac.ir

Academic Editor: Luigi Maria Specchio

Introduction. Studies about epilepsy are more associated with physiological aspects and drug therapy and far too little attention has been paid to psychological and social care, especially in teens. Hence, the present study aimed to assess relationship between self-efficacy and psychosocial care in adolescents with epilepsy. *Methods.* A cross-sectional association study was conducted on 74 consecutive adolescents aged 10 to 18 years with general attacks of epilepsy referred to Pediatric Neurology Clinics affiliated with the Tabriz University of Medical Sciences in 2013. Data were collected by interview using multisegment tools including demographic characteristics, self-efficacy scaling in children with epilepsy, and reporting tools for children psychosocial care. *Results.* Our study showed a significant association of self-efficacy with "information received" ($P < 0.02$) and also with "need for information or support" ($P < 0.01$) as well as "concerns and fears" ($P < 0.01$). The comments of doctor or nurse were directly associated with higher self-efficacy and patients' information needs were inversely associated with higher self-efficacy. *Conclusion.* For adolescents with epilepsy, providing educational materials such as pamphlets and booklets, designing especial websites, and setting especial meetings with and without parents separately are recommended. Scheduling psychosocial supports and collecting more information about this disorder for adolescents will be helpful.

1. Introduction

Epilepsy influences all physical, psychological, and social aspects of affected individuals [1]. In Iran, 4.2 per 1000 school-age children suffered from epilepsy and about 56% of them belong to children and adolescents groups [2]. Caring of patients with epilepsy requires attention to all aspects of the illness as well as to teamwork between physicians, nurses, psychologists, 2 social workers, and other professionals [1]. In this regard, nurses can have effective advising and educating roles [3]. If one receives appropriate and timely caring services, the appearance of epilepsy related complications will perhaps be reduced or prevented [4].

children and adolescents with epilepsy have a multiplicity of physical, emotional, and cognitive concerns that could be addressed by a nurse in the outpatient clinic [5]. In total, comprehensive cares are recommended in epilepsy [6]. Moreover, the goal of treatment in health psychology is to change individuals' behaviors in a way that influences their response to a disease or illness. It is widely recognized that knowledge alone is not sufficient to change health behavior [7]. There is evidence that chronic disease self-management is influenced by an individual's beliefs about health, including self-efficacy [8]. Self-efficacy is a person's belief in his/her ability to successfully organize, control his/her health habit, and achieve valuable health outcomes. It is one aspect of individual motivation [7, 9]. The results of the studies on chronic disorders have shown that the individuals with high self-efficacy are more successful in management of self-care responsibilities, drug use, avoidance of stimuli, symptoms of disease, and control of health status [9–11]. So, self-efficacy is an effective factor on patients' ability to control the disease, coping with illness and drug control of epilepsy [12].

The needs in epileptic patients are widely varied including health protection needs (identifying different therapeutic and historical aspects of disease), barriers and safety (assessing disease-related risks such as possible risks of bathing time and also disease effects on the presence in the community), quality of care (quality of environment, the ability to manage the treatment, and the ability to perform life-saving drugs), specialized facilities (training, hosing, behavioral and psychological supports, and searching some diagnostic services such as MRI and EEG), and familial needs (emergency services, education, training, and support). The assessment by a nurse at the outpatient clinics could identify individual goals, specific concerns, and proper strategies to treat. It can be performed by interviewing, grading scales, and self-reporting questionnaires [5]. Conflict between the normal desire of the adolescent for independence and autonomy and the parental desire to maintain control is accentuated by the presence of epilepsy [13]. In addition, adolescence is associated with significant changes in mental, physical (pubertal), social, and psychological (identity, self-determination) aspects. Adolescents with chronic illnesses are at risk of various crises. The patients should be faced with complex evolutionary feature of this period and also stress induced by serious and prolonged treatment schedule. In adolescence, there is an effort to achieve independence, while these patients are conflicted because of compulsory reliance, surrendering, and loss of the sense of control. So, it is much harder to deal with illness for adolescents [13]. Improving self-efficacy might provide the foundation for long-term behavior change among adolescents with epilepsy by improving self-care skills which can lead to better control on disease. On the other hand, self-efficacy is an assurance that person can do a complementary behavior to achieve his desired goal [7]. For improving the self-efficacy, educating people about self-care is essential [14, 15]. One of the main factors affecting the outcome in patients with epilepsy is social cares. It has been demonstrated that the community support is not available for the social development of young people with epilepsy and thus they are susceptible to be picked on by others [6]. Also, patients with epilepsy are needed to assess social performance because they are more prone to social problems. One of the other factors that have important consequences for children with epilepsy is receiving information. If the patients have enough information about various aspects of the illness, returning to the normal living state like other people is possible [4]. In this regard, an important aspect of caring for children with epilepsy is educating people about the disease and providing emotional support for children and their family members [1]. The studies performed in western countries have shown that a large percentage of children with epilepsy felt the lack of information about their disease causing more concerns [16, 17]. Parents want to provide information to reduce the concerns of school, seizure, and the future of their children. Since the patient's needs can vary of the views of professionals and patients, and the evaluation of patient is critical in the planning of critical care processes [5]. Psychosocial cares include satisfaction of the total amount of information, attitudes of clinic staff, spending a time with the staff, and the comfort of being in contact with the staff [6]. Due to the changes in today's health care, this caring is increasingly presented ambulatory and evaluation of training, education, counseling, and support services run along with the evaluation and treatment of neurological and psychological assessments [5]. It should be noted that appropriate caring in an outpatient setting can also increase the self-efficacy of adolescents with chronic illnesses and this is because the expected positive correlation between self-efficacy and psychosocial care of adolescents suffered epilepsy with general attacks. Moreover, an extensive literature review did not result in finding research studies on the relationship between these two variables. Thus, the aim of this study was to investigate the relationship between self-efficacy and psychosocial care in outpatient clinics for adolescents with epilepsy.

2. Methods

A cross-sectional association study was conducted on 74 consecutive adolescents aged 10 to 18 years with general attacks of epilepsy referred to Pediatric Neurology Clinics affiliated with the Tabriz University of Medical Sciences in 2013, within 6 months. This clinic is the main place for presenting neurology subspecialty cares to children in East Azerbaijan province. Inclusion criteria were using antiepileptic drugs and being with no history of concomitant physical impairments or mental retardation. The researchers obtained "baseline personal and social information" and administered the "Seizure Self-Efficacy Scale for Children (SSES-C)" and the "Child Report of Psychosocial Care."

Seizure Self-Efficacy Scale for Children (SSES-C) was developed by Caplin et al. and used for assessing self-efficacy in children with epilepsy including some questions on confidence and belief in the patient ability to care as well as manage epilepsy. This tool is a 15-item scale that measures the degree of self-efficacy related to the management of the seizure disorder. Children rate each statement on a 5-point scale of 1 (*I'm very unsure I can do that*) to 5 (*I'm very sure I can do that*). The final score ranged between 15 and 75 with a higher score reflecting greater self-efficacy. Support for reliability and validity has been found [18].

Child Report of Psychosocial Care was firstly designed by Austin et al. including three parts. (a) The first part consisted of 6 items about receiving some information on illness by children that was expected to be provided by physician or nurse. Children rate each statement on a 3-point scale of 1 (less than what I wanted) to 3 (more than what I wanted) and the final score ranged between 6 and 18 with a higher score reflecting more information received by child. (b) The second part included 6 items in child's feelings about the occurrence of epileptic seizures and is based on 5-likert scaling from 1 (never) to 5 (more often). The total score of this statement ranged from 6 to 30 with a higher score reflecting more concern regarding epileptic attacks. (c) The third part included 8 items related to assessing the needs of children with epilepsy answered by "yes" or "no" with the final score ranging from 0 to 8 [16].

The original version of the questionnaire was translated from English to Persian; the accuracy of the translation was assessed by an expert in English language and literature. Then, the content validity of the questionnaire was determined through a panel of experts and also the reliability of the questionnaire was assessed by Cronbach's alpha coefficient through a study on a sample of 15 children. Cronbach's alpha coefficient was obtained: 0.85 for SSES-C, and also 0.81, 0.72, and 0.81 for the first, second, and third parts of the questionnaire for assessing child report of psychosocial cares, respectively.

The study was first approved by the Regional Committee for Medical Research Ethic at the Tabriz University of Medical Sciences. The two researchers conducted the study by referring to the clinic where eligible children for the study were selected. The details of the study were explained to the children and their parents and the written informed consent was obtained from all parents. Then, the data were gathered by personal interviews with all children. For statistical analysis, SPSS software (version 13.0) was employed. The mean ± SD or number (percentages) was used for describing children characteristics and also the level of self-efficacy and psychosocial cares. Association between self-efficacy and the level of receiving psychosocial cares was examined by Pearson's correlation test.

3. Results

Eligible participants consisted of 74 children (40 girls and 34 boys) with ages 10 to 18 years (M = 12.72, SD = 2). The mean age of seizure onset was 7.48 years (SD = 3.4). Most participants (40%) had primary school education and 45% had secondary school education. The remainders were currently studying in high school. Positive epileptic history was in family of 27 percent. The major caregiver (93.2%) was both the mother and the father.

Most of the patients (76.7%) suffered mild epilepsy, 12.3% had moderate epilepsy, and others had severe epilepsy. The large majority of children (72.2%) had only one type of seizure (generalized tonic/colonic). With regard to the response to treatment, 21.9% of seizures were partially controlled, 6.8% were uncontrolled, and others were completely controlled. 21.65% of children had their epilepsy controlled with monotherapy and others required polypharmacy.

3.1. Self-Efficacy. The answers of adolescents to each option of self-efficacy questionnaire are presented in Table 1. As shown in this table, the highest level of reported self-efficacy was related to the item of "If there are problems about epilepsy, I can talk with my parents" (63.1%) and the lowest level was related to "When I am in school, I can predict and control my epilepsy" (11%). The mean score of self-efficacy was 45.4 ± 9.0 (95% CI: 43.3–47.4) totally.

3.2. Psychosocial Caring. Assessment of questions about receiving information from health personnel (doctors or nurses) showed that the mean score of this item was 10.0 ± 2.8 (95% CI: 9.4–10.7). More than half of the patients reported that received explanation was less than what they expected by doctor or nurse in all items except item "The doctors and nurses told me how the medicine worked" (Table 2).

3.3. Feelings and Concerns about Seizures. Assessment of questions in feelings and concerns about seizures and epileptic attacks obtained a mean score of 22.2 ± 5.7 (95% CI: 20.8–23.5) in this item. The highest concerns were related to "telling the state of seizure to others" (31.3%) and "avoid doing the things that the friends do due to attacks" (22.5%) (Table 3).

3.4. Educational Needs. Assessment of the questions on psychosocial cares in the part of educational needs indicated that the mean score of subjects was 6.1 ± 2.1 (95% CI: 5.6–6.6). As summarized in Table 4, adolescents felt the need to get more information.

The study of association between self-efficacy and three dimensions of psychosocial caring using Pearson's correlation test showed that the score of self-efficacy in adolescents was directly associated with receiving more information and inversely associated with feelings and concerns about seizures and educational needs (Table 5). On the other hand, by raising awareness of epilepsy, reducing negative feelings about epilepsy, and reducing educational needs of adolescents, their self-efficacy on controlling epilepsy can be effectively increased.

4. Discussion

Appropriate management of chronic disorders is directly associated with professional supports, proper outpatient cares, and the patient's belief system. Perceived self-efficacy has become an important and useful construct in psychology because it is related to the willingness and the ability of people to engage in various behavioral challenges including preventive and disease management behaviors [19]. Individuals who provide social support experience less depression, heightened self-esteem and self-efficacy, and improved quality of life, even after adjusting for baseline health status and socioeconomic status [20]. Therefore, the present study attempted to determine the association between self-efficacy and the level of psychosocial cares in teenagers with epilepsy in a pediatrics neurology outpatient clinic. In this study, self-efficacy was significantly associated with explanations of health personnel, concerns about epilepsy state, and also educational needs so that higher level of information given by the physician as well as lower needing information was related to higher self-efficacy. In fact, by increasing the level of information, self-efficacy was increased in parallel. In order to increase motivation following the increase of efficacy, Bandura believed that people with high self-efficacy are more motivated and do more attempts to overcome the challenges of life [21, 22]. With regard to the attempt to increase social support following the increase of self-efficacy, Videbeck thought that those with high self-efficacy

TABLE 1: Self-efficacy in epileptic patients aged 10 to 18 years.

SSES-C	No answer	Not at all	Nearly sure	Doubtfully	Partially sure	Pretty sure
I can talk with my parents about problems of epilepsy	1	4 (5.5)	3 (4.1)	5 (6.8)	15 (20.5)	46 (63.1)
I can stop myself from doing things that will aggravate epilepsy	1	6 (8.2)	6 (8.2)	7 (9.6)	12 (16.4)	42 (57.6)
I can do things the doctor said to control epilepsy	1	2 (2.7)	4 (5.5)	6 (8.2)	20 (27.4)	41 (56.2)
I can check the status of my seizures by avoiding the things that make it worse	1	2 (2.7)	8 (11.0)	4 (5.5)	23 (31.5)	36 (49.3)
I can talk with the doctor or nurse when you have questions about epilepsy	1	9 (12.4)	3 (4.1)	6 (8.2)	20 (27.4)	35 (47.9)
I can control my seizures by selecting appropriate activities	0	5 (6.8)	5 (6.8)	11 (14.8)	20 (27.0)	33 (44.6)
I can control my epilepsy so can participate easily in school-related activities	0	0 (0.0)	6 (8.2)	4 (5.5)	28 (38.4)	35 (47.9)
I can control my epilepsy situation by refraining from doing things that make it worse	0	3 (4.1)	7 (9.6)	6 (8.2)	22 (30.2)	35 (47.9)
I can control my epileptic condition because I can handle all the problems that it creates epilepsy	0	2 (2.8)	5 (6.8)	13 (17.8)	24 (32.9)	29 (39.7)
I can control my seizures despite some troubling issues in my family	1	14 (19.2)	9 (12.3)	12 (16.4)	24 (32.9)	14 (19.2)
I can predict and control their epilepsy when I'm at school	4	40 (57.2)	5 (7.1)	8 (11.4)	6 (8.6)	11 (15.7)
I can control my seizures even when I am angry or sad	1	29 (39.2)	6 (8.2)	9 (12.3)	18 (24.7)	11 (15.1)

TABLE 2: Child report of psychosocial care subscale 1 (patient received explanation from doctor or nurse).

Psychosocial care subscale 1	Less than I wanted (percent)	Just as much as I wanted (percent)	More than I wanted (percent)
The doctors and nurses told me what to do if I felt an attack coming on.	53 (71.6%)	16 (21.6%)	5 (6.8%)
The doctors and nurses talked to me about my fears and worries about my seizure condition.	51 (68.9%)	20 (27%)	3 (4.1%)
The doctors and nurses told me about possible problems or side effects with the medicine.	49 (67.1%)	21 (28.8%)	3 (4.1%)
I have had a chance to ask questions about my seizure condition.	46 (62.2%)	24 (32.4%)	4 (5.4%)
The doctors and nurses explained my seizure condition to me.	45 (60.8%)	23 (31.1%)	6 (8.1%)
The doctors and nurses told me things I can and can not do because of seizures.	39 (54.2%)	24 (33.3%)	9 (12.5%)
The doctors and nurses told me how the medicine worked.	36 (48.6%)	31 (41.9%)	7 (9.5%)

are seeking support from others [23]. Pajares also believed that people with low self-efficacy refrain from discussing complex issues and problems and thus are unable to achieve their goals, select introspection rather than remedy the problem, and focus on their weaknesses and barriers when dealing with stress, and in total they are lodged in the problem and suffered depression. In contrast, those with high self-efficacy used some challenge to solve it when faced with problems and do not perceive it as a threat [24]. Studies

have indicated that more confidence in ability to perform self-care behaviors can lead to more tendency to perform the desired behaviors [25, 26]. Adams et al. believed that psychosocial problems should be identified and early shown. Giving simple and reliable information is very helpful to cope with the feelings of inferiority and shyness [27]. In a study by Baker et al. in England to assess the psychosocial effects of epilepsy in adolescents, it was indicated that repeated seizures are associated with lower self-efficacy and also tonic-colonic

TABLE 3: Child report of psychosocial care subscale 2 (feelings and concerns about seizures).

Psychosocial care subscale 2	Never (percent)	Not often (percent)	Sometimes (percent)	Often (percent)	Very often (percent)
How often do you worry about telling others about your seizure condition?	29 (39.2%)	11 (14.9%)	6 (8.1%)	5 (6.8%)	23 (31%)
How often do you avoid doing something with your friends because of fear about having a seizure attack?	29 (40.8%)	11 (15.5%)	11 (15.5%)	4 (5.6%)	16 (22.6%)
How often do you worry about having another seizure attack?	37 (50%)	8 (10.8%)	14 (18.9%)	2 (2.7%)	13 (17.6%)
How often are you worried about what others will say about your seizure condition?	38 (51.4%)	10 (13.5%)	11 (14.9%)	2 (2.7%)	13 (17.6%)
How often do you worry about being sick because of the seizure condition?	36 (48.6%)	13 (17.6%)	8 (10.8%)	5 (6.8%)	12 (16.2%)
How often do you worry about hurting yourself because of a seizure attack?	36 (48.6%)	19 (25.7%)	10 (13.5%)	3 (4.1%)	6 (8.1%)

TABLE 4: Child report of psychosocial care subscale 3 (educational needs).

Psychosocial care subscale 3 (ranked)	Yes number (percent)	No number (percent)
More information about any activities or things you can or cannot do because of seizures?	68 (91.9%)	6 (8.1%)
More information about keeping safe during a seizure? miss = 1 (1.4%)	65 (89%)	8 (11%)
More information about how to handle future seizures?	62 (83.8%)	12 (16.2%)
More information about your seizure condition?	60 (81.1%)	14 (18.9%)
More information about possible causes of your seizure condition?	60 (81.8%)	14 (18.2%)
More information about your medication?	59 (79.7%)	15 (20.3%)
To talk to someone about how to handle seizures at school?	41 (55.4%)	33 (44.6%)
To talk to someone about how your seizure condition might affect your future?	40 (54.1%)	34 (45.9%)

TABLE 5: Association between psychosocial cares and self-efficacy in adolescents with epilepsy.

Variable	Pearson's coefficient	P value
Self-efficacy/comments on physician or nurse	0.25	0.022
Self-efficacy/concern about epilepsy state	−0.27	0.016
Self-efficacy/educational needing	−0.31	0.006

seizure was associated with appearance of depression [28]. In another study by Frizzell and colleagues, it was shown that holding training sessions in epilepsy syndrome and epilepsy effects on lifestyle resulted in the increase of knowledge and self-efficacy in adolescents compared with before intervention. They also indicated, by educational intervention, even without psychological approaches, achieving increased level of psychological functioning [29]. In another study by Zamnzadeh et al., following educational sessions in diabetics, the rate of self-efficacy in part of managing psychosocial aspects was significantly increased [30]. Baker et al. also showed that lower knowledge was in line with lower self-efficacy as well as higher level of depression [28]. Talking with physicians and participating in decision-making is

an aspect of communication that contribute to tend from asking the questions to action. Sense of satisfaction of caregivers and getting support cause a sense of competence and self-efficacy, leading to better control of epilepsy [12]. Although availability can be helpful, developing confidence is based more on verbal emphasis and encouragements [21]. Creating an environment where patients feel comfortable to discuss issues related to living with epilepsy and also supplying and providing supportive statements and sentences that respect the individual's ability to manage are important in the creation of trust. In addition, the nurses and doctors often emphasize their previous attempts at self-management, including the administration of drugs, creation of a safe environment, and centrally monitored seizures [31]. The results of the study by DiIorio et al. have shown that providers should consider social and emotional aspects of epilepsy that involve in providing confidence for the daily management of epilepsy [31].

5. Conclusion

The strong expressed need for information about handling future seizures and the need to talk about strategies for dealing with seizures that occur at school indicate that these might be areas to include in an intervention that aimed at enhancing self-efficacy [32].

Conflict of Interests

The authors declare that there is no conflict of interests regarding the publication of this paper.

Acknowledgments

This study was supported by Pediatric Health Research Center of the Tabriz University of Medical Sciences. The authors honorably thank the respectable authorities and also all participants and their families to participate in this survey. This project was approved and funded by the Tabriz University of Medical Sciences.

References

[1] L. M. Bernard, *Current Management in Child Neurology*, Walsworth Printing Company, 4th edition, 2009.

[2] S. A. Masoud and E. Kochaki, "Surveying the family attitude of a patients with epilepsy hospitalized in Shahid Beheshti Hospital in Kashan, 1378-79," *KAUMS Journal (FEYZ)*, vol. 8, no. 1, pp. 79–86, 2004 (Persian).

[3] C. Hayes, "Clinical skills: practical guide for managing adults with epilepsy," *British Journal of Nursing*, vol. 13, no. 7, pp. 380–387, 2004.

[4] P. Kalantary, *Effect of self care education on knowledge level and attitudes of child 6–14 years old with epilepsy and their parents reffered to neurology clinics [Dissertation]*, Tehran University of Medical Sciences, Tehran, Iran, 1994 (Persian).

[5] J. Engel, T. A. Pedley, J. Aicardi, S. Moshé, and M. A. Dichter, *Epilepsy: A Comprehensive Textbook*, Lippincott Williams & Wilkins, Philadelphia, Pa, USA, 2nd edition, 2008.

[6] A. B. Ettinger and A. M. Kanner, *Psychiatric Issues in Epilepsy [Electronic Resource]: A Practical Guide to Diagnosis and Treatment*, Wolters Kluwer Health/Lippincott Williams & Wilkins, 2007.

[7] A. Bandura, "Social cognitive theory: an agentic perspective," *Annual Review of Psychology*, vol. 52, pp. 1–26, 2001.

[8] B. E. Rahimian, *Effects of Sociostructural determinants and participative decision making in diabetes self-management: consideration in moderator role of patient's beliefs system [Dissertation]*, Tehran University of Medical Sciences, University of Tehran, Tehran, Iran, 2010 (Persian).

[9] R. Marks, J. P. Allegrante, and K. Lorig, "A review and synthesis of research evidence for self-efficacy-enhancing interventions for reducing chronic disability: implications for health education practice (part I)," *Health Promotion Practice*, vol. 6, no. 1, pp. 37–43, 2005.

[10] N. C. Gyurcsik, P. A. Estabrooks, and M. J. Frahm-Templar, "Exercise-related goals and self-efficacy as correlates of aquatic exercise in individuals with arthritis," *Arthritis Care and Research*, vol. 49, no. 3, pp. 306–313, 2003.

[11] K. R. Lorig and H. R. Holman, "Self-management education: history, definition, outcomes, and mechanisms," *Annals of Behavioral Medicine*, vol. 26, no. 1, pp. 1–7, 2003.

[12] M. D. Landover, "Living well with epilepsy II," in *Proceedings of the National Conference on Public Health and Epilepsy*, p. 18, 2004.

[13] D. L. Wong and M. J. Hockenberry, *Nursing Care of Infants and Children*, Mosby Elservier, 8th edition, 2007.

[14] T. Bodenheimer, K. Lorig, H. Holman, and K. Grumbach, "Patient self-management of chronic disease in primary care," *Journal of the American Medical Association*, vol. 288, no. 19, pp. 2469–2475, 2002.

[15] C. L. Grus, C. Lopez-Hernandez, A. Delamater et al., "Parental self-efficacy and morbidity in pediatric asthma," *Journal of Asthma*, vol. 38, no. 1, pp. 99–106, 2001.

[16] J. K. Austin, G. Dunn, D. Huster, and D. Rose, "Development of scales to measure psychosocial care needs of children with seizures and their parents," *The Journal of Neuroscience Nursing*, vol. 30, no. 3, pp. 155–160, 1998.

[17] A. McNelis, B. Musick, J. K. Austin, D. Dunn, and K. Creasy, "Psychosocial care needs of children with new-onset seizures," *Journal of Neuroscience Nursing*, vol. 30, no. 3, pp. 161–165, 1998.

[18] D. Caplin, J. K. Austin, D. W. Dunn, J. Shen, and S. Perkins, "Development of a self-efficacy scale for children and adolescents with epilepsy," *Children's Health Care*, vol. 31, no. 4, pp. 295–309, 2002.

[19] C.-C. Lin and S. E. Ward, "Perceived self-efficacy and outcome expectancies in coping with chronic low back pain," *Research in Nursing and Health*, vol. 19, no. 4, pp. 299–310, 1996.

[20] M. A. Musick and J. Wilson, "Volunteering and depression: the role of psychological and social resources in different age groups," *Social Science and Medicine*, vol. 56, no. 2, pp. 259–269, 2003.

[21] A. Bandura, *Self-Efficacy: The Exercise of Control*, Worth Publishers, New York, NY, USA, 1st edition, 1997.

[22] E. A. Skarbeck, *Psychosocial Predicttors of Self-Care Behaviors in Type 2 Diabetes Mellitus Patients: Analysis of Social Suport, Self-Efficacy and Depression*, Texas Tech University, Lubbock, Tex, USA, 2006.

[23] S. L. Videbeck, *Psychiatric Mental Health Nursing*, Lippincott Williams & Wilkins, Philadelphia, Pa, USA, 2001.

[24] F. Pajares, *Self-Beliefs and School Success: Self-Efficacy, Self-Concept and School Achievement*, Ablex Publishing, London, UK, 2001.

[25] L. K. Wen, M. D. Shepherd, and M. L. Parchman, "Family support, diet, and exercise among older Mexican Americans with type 2 diabetes," *Diabetes Educator*, vol. 30, no. 6, pp. 980–993, 2004.

[26] H. Bernal, S. Woolley, J. J. Schensul, and J. K. Dickinson, "Correlates of self-efficacy in diabetes self-care among hispanic adults with diabetes," *Diabetes Educator*, vol. 26, no. 4, pp. 673–680, 2000.

[27] R. D. Adams, *Principles of Neurology*, MC Graw-Hill, New York, NY, USA, 1997.

[28] G. A. Baker, S. Spector, Y. McGrath, and H. Soteriou, "Impact of epilepsy in adolescence: a UK controlled study," *Epilepsy & Behavior*, vol. 6, no. 4, pp. 556–562, 2005.

[29] C. K. Frizzell, A. M. Connolly, E. Beavis, J. A. Lawson, and A. M. Bye, "Personalised epilepsy education intervention for adolescents and impact on knowledge acquisition and psychosocial function," *Journal of Paediatrics and Child Health*, vol. 47, no. 5, pp. 271–275, 2011.

[30] V. Zamnzadeh, A. Seyedrasoli, and Jabarzade, "Impact of education powerment program in psychosocial aspect in diabetics," *Nusing and Midwifery Journal*, vol. 11, pp. 25–32, 2008 (Persian).

[31] C. DiIorio, P. O. Shafer, R. Letz, T. R. Henry, D. L. Schomer, and K. Yeager, "Behavioral, social, and affective factors associated

with self-efficacy for self-management among people with epilepsy," *Epilepsy and Behavior*, vol. 9, no. 1, pp. 158–163, 2006.

[32] J. K. Austin, D. W. Dunn, S. M. Perkins, and J. Shen, "Youth with epilepsy: development of a model of children's attitudes toward their condition," *Children's Health Care*, vol. 35, no. 2, pp. 123–140, 2006.

10

Semantic Processing Impairment in Patients with Temporal Lobe Epilepsy

Amanda G. Jaimes-Bautista,[1,2] **Mario Rodríguez-Camacho,**[1]
Iris E. Martínez-Juárez,[3] **and Yaneth Rodríguez-Agudelo**[2]

[1]*Proyecto de Neurociencias, Facultad de Estudios Superiores Iztacala, Universidad Nacional Autónoma de México, 54090 Ciudad de México, MEX, Mexico*
[2]*Departamento de Neuropsicología, Instituto Nacional de Neurología y Neurocirugía, 14269 Ciudad de México, DF, Mexico*
[3]*Clínica de Epilepsia, Instituto Nacional de Neurología y Neurocirugía, 14269 Ciudad de México, DF, Mexico*

Correspondence should be addressed to Mario Rodríguez-Camacho; marcizta@gmail.com

Academic Editor: József Janszky

The impairment in episodic memory system is the best-known cognitive deficit in patients with temporal lobe epilepsy (TLE). Recent studies have shown evidence of semantic disorders, but they have been less studied than episodic memory. The semantic dysfunction in TLE has various cognitive manifestations, such as the presence of language disorders characterized by defects in naming, verbal fluency, or remote semantic information retrieval, which affects the ability of patients to interact with their surroundings. This paper is a review of recent research about the consequences of TLE on semantic processing, considering neuropsychological, electrophysiological, and neuroimaging findings, as well as the functional role of the hippocampus in semantic processing. The evidence from these studies shows disturbance of semantic memory in patients with TLE and supports the theory of declarative memory of the hippocampus. Functional neuroimaging studies show an inefficient compensatory functional reorganization of semantic networks and electrophysiological studies show a lack of N400 effect that could indicate that the deficit in semantic processing in patients with TLE could be due to a failure in the mechanisms of automatic access to lexicon.

1. Introduction

Temporal lobe epilepsy (TLE) constitutes 80% of focal epilepsies and is the most frequent form in adults [1, 2]. Mesial TLE with hippocampal sclerosis is an epileptic syndrome very resistant to pharmacologic treatment [3], and approximately 50% of patients with this form of epilepsy present drug resistance, so it has been considered both a medical and a social problem [4].

Patients with TLE show great heterogeneity in clinical and cognitive characteristics. It is known that these patients are at significant risk for cognitive impairment and behavioral abnormalities [5–7]. Impairment of the memory system constitutes the most common cognitive deficit in TLE; around 70% of patients have problems in episodic memory, associated with the presence of hippocampal sclerosis [8, 9].

Neuropsychological studies have reported alterations in episodic memory with profiles of lateralization of selecting deficits in the verbal memory of patients with left TLE and in the visual memory of patients with right TLE [10–18]. It is interesting that recent research has also found impairment in the semantic memory of patients with TLE [19–24]; however, there are still few reports that have explored these alterations in detail.

Semantic memory is important because it contains the knowledge that allows individuals to communicate, represent, and mentally operate situations, objects, and relations with the world, which otherwise are not available to the senses. It allows the identification of events and use of general knowledge that forms the basis of our knowledge of the world [25]. The impairment of this kind of memory is manifested by difficulties in naming and concept definition and by poor understanding of oral or written language, and it can also impact other cognitive functions [26].

The main objective of this paper is to review recent research regarding the consequences of TLE on semantic memory, considering neuropsychological, electrophysiological, and neuroimaging findings. Taking into consideration the important relation between the hippocampus and TLE, an additional objective is to analyze the role of this cerebral structure in the semantic processing.

The literature included in this review was published between 2000 and 2014 for neuroimaging and electrophysiological studies and between 1990 and 2014 for neuropsychological studies. The search was made in PubMed using as key words: temporal lobe epilepsy, hippocampus, semantic memory and semantic processing, event related potentials, and N400 component and functional magnetic resonance imaging.

2. Semantic Memory

Memory is an active cognitive process that involves the acquisition, storage, and retrieval of information. Acquisition is achieved through coding, which is the initial process by which physical information is transformed into a mental representation. Coding takes various forms that depend on the characteristics of the stimulus; it is carried out from the level of processing of physical and sensory traits to the most abstract and semantic of information [27]. Storage is the ability to accumulate and maintain previously registered information for a period of time. Retrieval implies access, search, and extraction of information held in different kinds of storage [28].

Semantic memory is integrated by knowledge acquired about the world, including word meanings, kinds of information, events, and ideas. It represents organized mental knowledge about words and other verbal symbols, their meanings, and referents, about relations around them, and about the rules, formulas, and/or algorithm for the manipulation of these symbols, concepts, and relations. Therefore, it is the memory necessary for language [29].

2.1. Searching for the Neuroanatomy of Semantic Memory. Studies of patients with amnesia reported the following neuroanatomical structures related to memory: anterior and medial part of the temporal lobe, prefrontal region, portions of the limbic system including the hippocampal gyrus and uncus, thalamic nuclei, and mammillary bodies [30].

Squire et al. in 2004 [31] suggested that the medial temporal lobe includes a system of anatomically related subcortical structures that are critical for declarative memory; these structures along with the neocortex operate to establish and maintain long-term memory. Subcortical structures system is constituted by the hippocampal region (CA1–3 fields, dentate gyrus, and subicular complex), the adjacent perirhinal cortex, the entorhinal cortex, and parahippocampal cortex. Actually Squire et al. (1993) [32] proposed that the semantic memory depends on the integrity of the hippocampus and the neuroanatomical structures related to it, such as the medial temporal lobe and diencephalon.

The anterior temporal lobe has also been related to semantic memory; however, the role of this structure is unclear because patients with focal damage have deficiencies in recognizing and naming people that are famous or familiar, suggesting that this area might store specific semantic information; nonetheless, epileptic patients with lobectomy in this area do not show significant alterations in semantic memory [33].

Recent functional magnetic resonance image (fMRI) studies have added some more specific information on the matter. The anterior inferior and medial temporal gyrus, the anterior fusiform gyrus, and the upper anterior temporal sulcus were activated in normal subjects performing semantic tasks. It was proposed that such structures are importantly linked to semantic memory [34, 35]. Medial temporal gyrus integrates auditory and visual information and the anterior ventral surface produces transmodals (i.e., more integrated and abstract forms of objects), representing a core structure for the formation of coherent concepts.

Binder and Desai [36] proposed a neuroanatomical model of semantic memory based on data from fMRI of healthy participants and subjects with impaired memory. This model related the cortices of specific modality with the temporoparietal supramodal cortices which store more abstract representations of knowledge of data and the prefrontal cortex that controls the activation and selects behavior directed towards a goal. On the other hand, the posterior cingulate gyrus and the precuneus may function as an interface between the semantic network and the hippocampal memory system, which could help to codify significant events in episodic memory.

In summary, clinical data show different structures involved in semantic memory, among which are the temporoparietal cortex, left anterolateral temporal cortex, the medial and inferior temporal gyrus, fusiform gyrus, the amygdala, ventromedial frontal cortex, perirhinal cortex, and inferior frontal cortex. These structures have been related to semantic memory because different brain lesions that result in impaired memory provide evidence as which brain areas are related to different types of memory, but since the lesions are not circumscribed, it is difficult to determine whether a specific deficit is the result of a lesion to a specific structure [37].

2.2. The Hippocampus and Its Relation with Semantic Memory. The functional role of the hippocampus in semantic processing is currently under debate and there are two points of view about it.

On one side, the *episodic theory* of the hippocampus suggests that it plays a selective role in episodic memory but contributes very little or nothing to semantic memory [38]. The main evidence that supports this position comes from the cognitive description of a group of patients with development amnesia, who during their first years of life acquire damage to the hippocampus (secondary to perinatal hypoxic-ischaemic) and as a consequence, they exhibit impaired episodic memory with intact or spare semantic memory [39, 40].

On the other side, the *declarative theory* suggests that the hippocampus, together with the entorhinal, perirhinal, and parahippocampal cortices, contributes to both episodic memory and semantic memory [41]. This position is based on evidence from cognitive results in patients with amnesia due to acquired pathologies at adulthood in which the lesion of the mesial temporal cortex produced impairment in both types of memory [42–45]. In addition research with functional neuroimaging in healthy subjects has described hippocampal activation during retrieval of various kinds of semantic knowledge, such as retrieval of elements of semantic categories [46], semantic decisions [47, 48], historic events [49], and famous people [50, 51].

Until now, research has suggested that in the adult brain the hippocampus plays an important role in both episodic memory and semantic memory, since both are significantly impaired following even discrete damage limited to the hippocampus. When the damage is sustained at an early age, such as development amnesia, it is possible that there is a certain functional reorganization in the damaged temporal lobe [41].

3. Semantic Memory and Temporal Lobe Epilepsy

From the case of patient H.M. published by Scoville and Milner [52], the study of TLE has contributed importantly to knowledge about the neurocognition of human memory.

3.1. Neuropsychological Studies. Memory is the most studied cognitive process and one where more abnormalities have consistently been found in patients with TLE.

Regarding semantic memory, the majority of the studies in patients with TLE have analyzed their performance in verbal fluency and naming tasks, finding that those patients with seizures in the dominant temporal lobe for language (generally left) show deficits characterized by naming failures and poor verbal fluency [19, 22, 24, 53–55].

The effect of mesial TLE on semantic verbal fluency has been found to depend greatly on the interaction between hippocampal sclerosis (HS) and the laterality of the epileptic focus. Gleissner and Elger [21] compared the performance of TLE patients based on the type of lesion (HS versus extrahippocampal lesions such as tumors or arteriovenous malformations) and the laterality of the focus. They found that verbal fluency was impaired regardless of the laterality of the focus in patients with TLE and HS, unlike patients with other types of lesions. Patients with left TLE had deficits independent of the type of lesion, while only patients with right TLE along with HS exhibited deficits. Based on these results, the authors concluded that the hippocampus plays an important role in the retrieval of semantic knowledge; however, independently of the presence of HS, damage to the dominant hemisphere for language is sufficient to affect verbal fluency.

Only two neuropsychological studies have evaluated the semantic system extensively, through the use of a greater number of tests, including both verbal and nonverbal stimuli, and exploring the relation between abnormalities and the laterality of the epileptic focus. Both Giovagnoli et al. [20] and Messas et al. [23] demonstrated deficits in semantic memory

in patients with TLE; however, the former reported that only patients with left TLE had deficits in retrieving both verbal and nonverbal semantic information [20] while the latter found that patients with either left or right TLE had deficits in the semantic system, although the most pronounced and extensive problems were in patients with left TLE [23].

Studies have also been carried out to explore the semantic aspect of remote memory of patients with TLE [56–59]. In these studies questions about events of public knowledge corresponding to a specific period and related to politics, sports, scandals, social events, or catastrophes were made; photos of famous people faces that had to be recognized and identified (e.g., to give the name, occupation, or say if they were alive or dead) were displayed.

The results of these studies were that patients with TLE had problems retrieving names, a reduction in conceptual knowledge regarding famous people, and failures both in spontaneous evocation and recognition of events. Specifically, patients with left TLE had a poor performance compared to patients with right TLE in the information retrieval about public events and exhibit a selective impairment characterized by a temporal gradient, with poor naming of faces from the most recent periods compared to distant ones. Patients with right TLE showed impairment in the recognition, identification, and naming of famous faces [56–59].

Neuropsychological studies have offered sufficient evidence of the presence of impairment in semantic memory in patients with TLE and it seems that lateralized lesions in the temporal lobe have differential effects on the retrieval of semantic information. However, it is important to consider that the majority of the tests used to assess this type of memory also require the participation of other cognitive processes such as attention and executive functions, which are also altered in these patients [60–64]. Therefore, there is a possibility that semantic dysfunction in TLE may be secondary to deficits in other cognitive processes [20].

3.2. Event-Related Potentials (ERP) Studies. ERPs allow an online observation of the cognitive processes that generate the observed behavior by reflecting changes in cerebral electrical activity that keep a specific temporal relationship with the physical stimuli and the cognitive processes that provoke them.

ERPs greatest advantage is a real-time assessment (in milliseconds) of electrical activity and cognitive processes in the brain, offering high-resolution information concerning chronology and sequence of cognitive processes. They also allow distinguishing in which stage of information processing an alteration can be found [65].

Study through ERP of patients with TLE candidates for surgical treatment offers a unique opportunity to know the electrophysiological correlates of cognitive processes. In these patients the electrodes can be placed directly on relevant structures for language or memory and so correlate deficits of ERP in paradigms associated with these processes.

Therefore, more studies through intracranial records have been carried out than noninvasive studies; however, the majority has focused on episodic memory [66–70].

In spite of the advantages this kind of study offers, there are also some problems. On one hand, the results are limited to plausible epileptogenic areas, so anatomic coverage restriction limits the information about other areas. On the other hand, invasive records are only used in patients undergoing a temporal lobectomy procedure, so the data obtained cannot be contrasted with healthy people that serve as a parameter of normality, restricting the generalization of findings.

The scarce noninvasive studies corroborate the effect of TLE on semantic processing. Olichney et al. [71] carried out a research to investigate if impairment in the N400, ERP component related to semantic processing, was related to the laterality of the epileptic focus. They used a crossmodal semantic categorization task; with the auditory presentation of sentences followed by target words presented visually, 50% were congruent and 50% were incongruent regarding the previously presented category (e.g., a type of wood, cedar/pancake). Patients with right TLE showed an increase in the amplitude of N400 for incongruent words compared with congruent (N400 effect). In contrast, patients with left TLE did not show this N400 effect.

The results of this study suggest that semantic processing is sensitive to left temporal dysfunction; however, the question remains open as to whether the absence of the N400 effect may be associated with deficits in access and retrieval of semantic information or with the attentional processes necessary to carry out the semantic categorization task.

Miyamoto et al. [72] investigated the mechanism of semantic priming (facilitation effect of the processing of semantically related words) in patients with TLE and a control group of healthy participants through a visual task of category matching. Each trial of the task was composed of a warning sign, a prime (first word), and a target (second word). Two conditions were presented according to the semantic relationship between the prime and the target: (1) match condition (both stimuli belonged to the same category, such as sparrow-bird) or (2) mismatch condition, where the target and the prime belonged to different semantic categories (such as dragonfly-fish). Data were analyzed at the behavioral level (reaction time and percentage of errors) and at the electrophysiological level through the amplitude of N400, contingent negative variation (CNV), and late positive component (LPC), the two latter being related to different demands on attention processing.

The behavioral results showed that patients with TLE had a nonsignificant tendency to present more prolonged reaction times and a greater percentage of errors for both conditions compared to the control group; nevertheless, both groups had shorter reaction times in the related condition compared with the nonrelated, revealing a behavioral semantic priming effect. Regarding electrophysiological data, a reduction was found in the amplitude of N400 component for both conditions (match and mismatch) in patients compared with the control group, in addition to an absence of the N400 effect (lack of increase in amplitude in mismatch compared with match condition). On the other hand, there was no intergroup difference in the amplitude of CNV and LPC components. The authors concluded that the reduced amplitude of N400

for both conditions in the patients suggested the presence of an alteration in generators of this component (located in the left temporal pole). They stated that failures in semantic processing can be located at the level of access and automatic activation of semantic information and that deficits cannot be attributed to attention disorders given that the CNV and LPC components did not show abnormality.

Jaimes-Bautista et al. [73] presented preliminary results that corroborated these findings. They carried out a study to determine if semantic impairment in TLE was related to deficit in automatic activation of semantic networks or to failures in strategies for information retrieval. A lexical decision tasks were used, manipulating the interstimuli interval (ISI) to generate automatic and controlled semantic priming. The results showed that TLE patients did not present the N400 effect associated with semantic priming, for both the automatic and controlled conditions. This study showed that semantic processing impairment in patients with TLE is related to deficiencies in the automatic activation mechanisms, and in addition, it seems that patients do not benefit from the use of strategies for retrieval of information.

Although the studies with noninvasive ERP in patients with TLE are scarce, they show potential to reveal the underlying mechanisms involved in the semantic memory processes impairment in these patients.

3.3. Functional Magnetic Resonance Images (fMRI) Studies. In TLE, electrical hyperexcitability is spread within the temporal medial/limbic network, which includes the hippocampus, amygdala, entorhinal cortex, lateral temporal cortex, and extratemporal components such as the medial thalamus and inferior frontal lobes. These anatomical structures operate together to culminate in the eventual expression of seizures [74]. Various regions that form part of this network are also directly involved in semantic processing.

The results of researches into semantic processing in TLE through fMRI, using tasks of semantic decision (SDT), lexical decision (LDT), and verbal fluency (VFT), have demonstrated that patterns of cerebral activation in patients with TLE differ significantly from those of healthy subjects.

Köylü et al. [75] investigated the impact of mesial TLE on the network of frontal and temporal structures involved in semantic memory. They used auditory SDT that consisted of deciding if the objects presented could be found in a supermarket and judging their cost. Patients with TLE with either right or left epileptic focus had a lower percentage of correct answers compared to a control group of healthy participants. The results showed that the networks involved in semantic processing of patients differed significantly from the control group and, in addition, they showed a pattern of activation dependent on the side of the epileptic focus. Therefore, for the control group the pattern of activation included the bilateral frontal and temporal areas, with left predominance; in patients with left TLE activation was predominant in right frontal, bilateral temporal, and basal ganglia regions, and in patients with right TLE the pattern of activation showed a posterior network including temporal and parietal regions (lateral and mesial), with left predominance, as well as occipital regions, but without including frontal or subcortical areas.

These data show that both epileptic activity originating in the temporal lobe and the side of epileptic focus were associated with an alteration in the underlying neuronal circuits in semantic processing; in addition, not only the cortical but also subcortical structures appear to participate in semantic processing in TLE, particularly in the left hemisphere.

Bartha et al. [76] analyzed the contribution of hippocampal formation to semantic processing through the same SDT used by Köylü et al. [75]. During the task, both the control group and patients with TLE showed activation of bilateral hippocampal formation with left predominance. However, there were significant differences in the pattern of activation between groups. Patients with left TLE showed reduction in activation of the bilateral hippocampal formation compared with the control group and less activation of the right side compared with the right TLE group. Patients with right TLE activated the right hippocampal formation to a lesser degree but compared with the control group they showed an increase in left activation. The authors noted that the decrease in activation of the ipsilateral hippocampal formation in patients with left and right TLE was related to the reduction in hippocampus volume.

These results suggest that semantic processing is related to the bilateral functioning of the hippocampus and, while patients with right TLE appear to achieve compensation of the impairment through greater work by the contralateral hippocampus, patients with left TLE do not achieve the same kind of functional reorganization.

The above findings have been replicated in similar studies with different semantic tasks. Bonelli et al. [77] investigated the relation between the naming process and the integrity of semantic networks in patients with TLE through a VFT. In the control group and in patients with right TLE, activation of the left hippocampus during the VFT correlated positively with performance on naming task. In left TLE patients, the correlation was found with the activation of the left medial and inferior frontal cortex (and to a lesser degree, the right), which suggests compensatory strategies to support the naming process. In addition, they observed that a poor naming ability was parallel to the lack of left hippocampal activation.

It is then possible that the previously mentioned cerebral areas are recruited when the hippocampus does not function correctly, as in hippocampal sclerosis. In this way, the difficulties in the naming processes in patients with left TLE could be explained by the participation of a compensatory network in the frontal lobe, which turns out to be less functional.

Using an LDT (in which participants must decide if the stimulus presented is a word or not), Jensen et al. [78] also analyzed if the presence of hippocampal sclerosis in patients with left TLE related to the efficiency of semantic processing and the associated cerebral activation. Patients with hippocampal sclerosis showed significantly longer reaction times than the control group. Neuroimaging data revealed greater activation in the inferior and medial frontal gyrus and the precuneus bilaterally during the LDT in the control group; the group of patients without hippocampal sclerosis showed

greater activation only in the left medial temporal gyrus, while the group with hippocampal sclerosis showed greater activation in various regions, such as the superior and medial temporal cortex, precuneus and left cingulated gyrus, and right medial temporal and supramarginal cortex.

These results again corroborate that when the hippocampal sclerosis is in the left temporal lobe, various cerebral structures are recruited but they do not achieve sufficient compensation, so deficient semantic processing is presented.

Studies with tractography have shown that TLE is associated with impairment in the integrity of the frontotemporal connections, describing a reduction in the structural connections in the epileptogenic hemisphere and a possible increase in compensatory connections in the unaffected contralateral hemisphere [79, 80]. Therefore, deficiency in frontotemporal connectivity may affect function in this part of the semantic memory network.

Neuroimaging studies suggest the possibility that the morphofunctional bases that give rise to semantic impairment in TLE may be hippocampal sclerosis or the epileptic activity in course and its propagation to other temporal and frontal regions.

4. Conclusions

The objective of this paper was to present an updated review of research regarding the consequences of TLE on semantic memory and to analyze the role of the hippocampus in semantic processing.

Each of the methods reviewed contribute to approaching the subject from different levels of analysis, allowing a complementary vision. Neuropsychology offers a general view concerning semantic deficits at the behavioral level, while the ERP reveal specific data about the stage in which information processing is impaired and neuroimaging studies allow knowing the cerebral structures involved in semantic dysfunction.

Neuropsychological and functional neuroimaging studies have investigated the effect of alteration of the hippocampus and the laterality of epileptic focus on semantic processing. The results show that the hippocampus has an important participation in semantic processing, supporting the theory of declarative memory of the hippocampus. It has also been demonstrated that when the lesion in the temporal lobe is in the dominant hemisphere for language functioning, semantic processing is altered independently of the type of lesion (i.e., hippocampal sclerosis, tumors, or arteriovenous malformations).

Additionally, studies with fMRI show that TLE is associated with deficits in the functional organization of cortical networks involved in semantic processing, likely caused by morphological changes inherent to chronic TLE, such as hippocampal sclerosis. Therefore, during semantic tasks, TLE relates to a pattern of activation that is different from the normal, probably due to a compensatory functional reorganization that includes various cerebral structures, that nevertheless is less functional.

In spite of the aforementioned findings, the underlying mechanisms of semantic processing impairment in TLE are still not completely understood; that is, it is still not clear if it is due to failures in accessing and retrieving information from semantic storage or even degradation of such information. Some studies have suggested the possibility that semantic deficit may be secondary to alterations in other cognitive processes, since the majority of the experimental tasks and neuropsychological tests used to evaluate semantic memory require the participation of other processes such as attention and executive functions, which are also affected by this disease.

Studies through ERPs have offered data that allow resolution of this question. The specific finding of reduction in the amplitude of the N400 component and the lack of N400 effect, added to the fact that ERP components that reflect other cognitive processes are not affected, seems to indicate that the deficits are directly related to access and retrieval of information from semantic storage. Nevertheless, ERP studies on the effect of TLE on semantic memory are scarce and it is necessary to develop more research in this area.

Future studies with the methods currently available to neuroscience may approach aspects such as the following: if semantic impairment is exclusively linguistic or is also presented at nonlinguistic level and if it is related to the laterality of epileptic focus.

Another important issue to analyze is the effect of various clinical variables such as age at onset, chronicity, frequency of seizures, and antiepileptic drugs on semantic processing.

These aspects, among other questions, would be of great utility in the development of knowledge of semantic impairment in TLE, as well as of the cerebral structures and mechanisms involved in the semantic memory functioning.

On the other hand, greater knowledge of the memory impairments in TLE patients will allow implementing more specific programs for cognitive rehabilitation for these patients.

TLE, compared with other kinds of pathologies such as dementia, traumatic brain injury, and cerebral vascular disease, allows the study of a younger clinical population with known and more easily identifiable lesion. For this reason, patients with TLE, especially those with hippocampal sclerosis, offer a unique clinical scenario to study the consequences that mesial temporal lobe damage may have on memory systems. In this way, TLE continues to serve as an important model for understanding the cerebral bases of memory.

Conflict of Interests

The authors declare that there is no conflict of interests regarding the publication of this paper.

Acknowledgment

This study is supported by CONACYT project 240856 "Electrophysiological Study of Semantic Priming in Patients with Temporal Lobe Epilepsy and in Parkinson Disease."

References

[1] G. D. Cascino, "Use of routine and video electroencephalography," *Neurologic Clinics*, vol. 19, no. 2, pp. 271–287, 2001.

[2] G. D. Cascino, "When drugs and surgery don't work," *Epilepsia*, vol. 49, supplement 9, pp. S79–S84, 2008.

[3] J. Engel Jr., "Mesial temporal lobe epilepsy: what have we learned?" *Neuroscientist*, vol. 7, no. 4, pp. 340–352, 2001.

[4] C. Panayiotopoulos, *A Clinical Guide to Epileptic Syndromes and their Treatment*, Springer, London, UK, 2nd edition, 2007.

[5] S. Baxendale, D. Heaney, P. J. Thompson, and J. S. Duncan, "Cognitive consequences of childhood-onset temporal lobe epilepsy across the adult lifespan," *Neurology*, vol. 75, no. 8, pp. 705–711, 2010.

[6] C. E. Elger, C. Helmstaedter, and M. Kurthen, "Chronic epilepsy and cognition," *The Lancet Neurology*, vol. 3, no. 11, pp. 663–672, 2004.

[7] C. M. Marques, L. O. S. F. Caboclo, T. I. da Silva et al., "Cognitive decline in temporal lobe epilepsy due to unilateral hippocampal sclerosis," *Epilepsy and Behavior*, vol. 10, no. 3, pp. 477–485, 2007.

[8] C. Helmstaedter and E. Kockelmann, "Cognitive outcomes in patients with chronic temporal lobe epilepsy," *Epilepsia*, vol. 47, supplement 2, pp. S96–S98, 2006.

[9] Ç. Özkara, L. Hanoglu, C. Keskinkiliç et al., "Memory in patients with drug-responsive mesial temporal lobe epilepsy and hippocampal sclerosis," *Epilepsia*, vol. 45, no. 11, pp. 1392–1396, 2004.

[10] L. H. Castro, L. C. A. M. Silva, C. C. Adda et al., "Low prevalence but high specificity of material-specific memory impairment in epilepsy associated with hippocampal sclerosis," *Epilepsia*, vol. 54, no. 10, pp. 1735–1742, 2013.

[11] A. R. Giovagnoli and G. Avanzini, "Learning and memory impairment in patients with temporal lobe epilepsy: relation to the presence, type, and location of brain lesion," *Epilepsia*, vol. 40, no. 7, pp. 904–911, 1999.

[12] C. Helmstaedter, "Effects of chronic epilepsy on declarative memory systems," *Progress in Brain Research*, vol. 135, pp. 439–453, 2002.

[13] B. P. Hermann, A. R. Wyler, E. T. Richey, and J. M. Rea, "Memory function and verbal learning ability in patients with complex partial seizures of temporal lobe origin," *Epilepsia*, vol. 28, no. 5, pp. 547–554, 1987.

[14] R. F. Allegri, M. Drake, and A. Thompson, "Neuropsychological findings in patients with middle temporal lobe epilepsy," *Revista de Neurologia*, vol. 29, no. 12, pp. 1160–1163, 1999.

[15] S. Oddo, P. Solís, D. Consalvo et al., "Mesial temporal lobe epilepsy and hippocampal sclerosis: cognitive function assessment in Hispanic patients," *Epilepsy & Behavior*, vol. 4, no. 6, pp. 717–722, 2003.

[16] L. M. Selwa, "Disturbances of learning and memory in temporal lobe epilepsy," in *Psychological Disturbances in Epilepsy*, J. C. Sackellares and S. Berent, Eds., pp. 109–120, Butterworth-Heinemann, Boston, Mass, USA, 1996.

[17] P. J. Thompson and R. Corcoran, "Everyday memory failures in people with epilepsy," *Epilepsia*, vol. 33, supplement 6, pp. S18–S20, 1992.

[18] I. V. Viskontas, M. P. McAndrews, and M. Moscovitch, "Remote episodic memory deficits in patients with unilateral temporal lobe epilepsy and excisions," *The Journal of Neuroscience*, vol. 20, no. 15, pp. 5853–5857, 2000.

[19] B. D. Bell, B. P. Hermann, A. R. Woodard et al., "Object naming and semantic knowledge in temporal lobe epilepsy," *Neuropsychology*, vol. 15, no. 4, pp. 434–443, 2001.

[20] A. R. Giovagnoli, A. Erbetta, F. Villani, and G. Avanzini, "Semantic memory in partial epilepsy: verbal and non-verbal deficits and neuroanatomical relationships," *Neuropsychologia*, vol. 43, no. 10, pp. 1482–1492, 2005.

[21] U. Gleissner and C. E. Elger, "The hippocampal contribution to verbal fluency in patients with temporal lobe epilepsy," *Cortex*, vol. 37, no. 1, pp. 55–63, 2001.

[22] C. Lomlomdjian, P. Solis, N. Medel, and S. Kochen, "A study of word finding difficulties in Spanish speakers with temporal lobe epilepsy," *Epilepsy Research*, vol. 97, no. 1-2, pp. 37–44, 2011.

[23] C. S. Messas, L. L. Mansur, and L. H. M. Castro, "Semantic memory impairment in temporal lobe epilepsy associated with hippocampal sclerosis," *Epilepsy and Behavior*, vol. 12, no. 2, pp. 311–316, 2008.

[24] B. N'Kaoua, V. Lespinet, A. Barsse, A. Rougier, and B. Claverie, "Exploration of hemispheric specialization and lexico-semantic processing in unilateral temporal lobe epilepsy with verbal fluency tasks," *Neuropsychologia*, vol. 39, no. 6, pp. 635–642, 2001.

[25] E. Tulving, "Episodic memory: from mind to brain," *Annual Review of Psychology*, vol. 53, pp. 1–25, 2002.

[26] S. Mårdh, K. Nägga, and S. Samuelsson, "A longitudinal study of semantic memory impairment in patients with Alzheimer's disease," *Cortex*, vol. 49, no. 2, pp. 528–533, 2013.

[27] A. Baddeley, "The psychology of memory," in *Handbook of Memory Disorders*, A. Baddeley, B. Wilson, and M. Kopelman, Eds., pp. 3–17, John Wiley & Sons, Chichester, UK, 2nd edition, 2002.

[28] A. Baddeley, "What is memory?" in *Memory*, A. Baddeley, M. Eysenck, and M. Anderson, Eds., pp. 1–18, Psychology Press, New York, NY, USA, 2009.

[29] E. Tulving, "Episodic and semantic memory," in *Organization of Memory*, E. Tulving and W. Donaldson, Eds., pp. 381–402, Academic Press, New York, NY, USA, 1972.

[30] H. Schmolck, E. A. Kensinger, S. Corkin, and L. R. Squire, "Semantic knowledge in patient H.M. and other patients with bilateral medial and lateral temporal lobe lesions," *Hippocampus*, vol. 12, no. 4, pp. 520–533, 2002.

[31] L. R. Squire, C. E. L. Stark, and R. E. Clark, "The medial temporal lobe," *Annual Review of Neuroscience*, vol. 27, pp. 279–306, 2004.

[32] L. R. Squire, B. Knowlton, and G. Musen, "The structure and organization of memory," *Annual Review of Psychology*, vol. 44, no. 1, pp. 453–495, 1993.

[33] W. K. Simmons and A. Martin, "The anterior temporal lobes and the functional architecture of semantic memory," *Journal of the International Neuropsychological Society*, vol. 15, no. 5, pp. 645–649, 2009.

[34] R. Binney, K. Embleton, E. Jefferies, G. Parker, and M. Lambon-Ralph, "The ventral and inferotemporal aspects of the anterior temporal lobe are crucial in semantic memory: evidence from a novel direct comparison of distortion-corrected fMRI, rTMS and semantic dementia," *Cerebral Cortex*, vol. 20, no. 11, pp. 2728–2738, 2010.

[35] M. Visser, E. Jefferies, K. V. Embleton, and M. A. L. Ralph, "Both the middle temporal gyrus and the ventral anterior temporal area are crucial for multimodal semantic processing: distortion-corrected fMRI evidence for a double gradient of information convergence in the temporal lobes," *Journal of Cognitive Neuroscience*, vol. 24, no. 8, pp. 1766–1778, 2012.

[36] J. R. Binder and R. H. Desai, "The neurobiology of semantic memory," *Trends in Cognitive Sciences*, vol. 15, no. 11, pp. 527–536, 2011.

[37] J. D. E. Gabrieli, "Cognitive neuroscience of human memory," *Annual Review of Psychology*, vol. 49, pp. 87–115, 1998.

[38] E. Tulving and H. J. Markowitsch, "Episodic and declarative memory: role of the hippocampus," *Hippocampus*, vol. 8, no. 3, pp. 198–204, 1998.

[39] F. Vargha-Khadem, D. G. Gadian, K. E. Watkins, A. Connelly, W. Van Paesschen, and M. Mishkin, "Differential effects of early hippocampal pathology on episodic and semantic memory," *Science*, vol. 277, no. 5324, pp. 376–380, 1997.

[40] C. Bindschaedler, C. Peter-Favre, P. Maeder, T. Hirsbrunner, and S. Clarke, "Growing up with bilateral hippocampal atrophy: from childhood to teenage," *Cortex*, vol. 47, no. 8, pp. 931–944, 2011.

[41] W. A. Suzuki, "Declarative versus episodic: two theories put to the test," *Neuron*, vol. 38, no. 1, pp. 5–7, 2003.

[42] P. J. Bayley, R. O. Hopkins, and L. R. Squire, "Successful recollection of remote autobiographical memories by amnesic patients with medial temporal lobe lesions," *Neuron*, vol. 38, no. 1, pp. 135–144, 2003.

[43] M. de Haan, M. Mishkin, T. Baldeweg, and F. Vargha-Khadem, "Human memory development and its dysfunction after early hippocampal injury," *Trends in Neurosciences*, vol. 29, no. 7, pp. 374–381, 2006.

[44] J. R. Manns and L. R. Squire, "The medial temporal lobe and memory for facts and events," in *Handbook of Memory Disorders*, A. Baddeley, M. Kopelman, and B. Wilson, Eds., pp. 81–100, John Wiley and Sons, New York, NY, USA, 2002.

[45] J. R. Manns, R. O. Hopkins, and L. R. Squire, "Semantic memory and the human hippocampus," *Neuron*, vol. 38, no. 1, pp. 127–133, 2003.

[46] L. Ryan, C. Cox, S. M. Hayes, and L. Nadel, "Hippocampal activation during episodic and semantic memory retrieval: comparing category production and category cued recall," *Neuropsychologia*, vol. 46, no. 8, pp. 2109–2121, 2008.

[47] L. Bartha, C. Brenneis, M. Schocke et al., "Medial temporal lobe activation during semantic language processing: fMRI findings in healthy left- and right-handers," *Cognitive Brain Research*, vol. 17, no. 2, pp. 339–346, 2003.

[48] K. Henke, C. R. A. Mondadori, V. Treyer, R. M. Nitsch, A. Buck, and C. Hock, "Nonconscious formation and reactivation of semantic associations by way of the medial temporal lobe," *Neuropsychologia*, vol. 41, no. 8, pp. 863–876, 2003.

[49] E. A. Maguire and C. J. Mummery, "Differential modulation of a common memory retrieval network revealed by positron emission tomography," *Hippocampus*, vol. 9, no. 1, pp. 54–61, 1999.

[50] F. A. Bernard, E. T. Bullmore, K. S. Graham, S. A. Thompson, J. R. Hodges, and P. C. Fletcher, "The hippocampal region is involved in successful recognition of both remote and recent famous faces," *NeuroImage*, vol. 22, no. 4, pp. 1704–1714, 2004.

[51] K. Douville, J. L. Woodard, M. Seidenberg et al., "Medial temporal lobe activity for recognition of recent and remote famous names: an event-related fMRI study," *Neuropsychologia*, vol. 43, no. 5, pp. 693–703, 2005.

[52] W. B. Scoville and B. Milner, "Loss of recent memory after bilateral hippocampal lesions," *Journal of Neurology, Neurosurgery, and Psychiatry*, vol. 20, no. 1, pp. 11–21, 1957.

[53] R. M. Busch, J. S. Chapin, J. S. Haut, M. F. Dulay, R. I. Naugle, and I. Najm, "Word-finding difficulties confound performance on verbal cognitive measures in adults with intractable left temporal lobe epilepsy," *Epilepsia*, vol. 54, no. 3, pp. e37–e40, 2013.

[54] R. C. Martin, D. W. Loring, K. J. Meador, and G. P. Lee, "The effects of lateralized temporal lobe dysfunction on normal and semantic word fluency," *Neuropsychologia*, vol. 28, no. 8, pp. 823–829, 1990.

[55] A. I. Tröster, V. Warmflash, I. Osorio, A. M. Paolo, L. J. Alexander, and W. B. Barr, "The roles of semantic networks and search efficiency in verbal fluency performance in intractable temporal lobe epilepsy," *Epilepsy Research*, vol. 21, no. 1, pp. 19–26, 1995.

[56] T. Benke, E. Kuen, M. Schwarz, and G. Walser, "Proper name retrieval in temporal lobe epilepsy: naming of famous faces and landmarks," *Epilepsy and Behavior*, vol. 27, no. 2, pp. 371–377, 2013.

[57] G. Glosser, A. E. Salvucci, and N. D. Chiaravalloti, "Naming and recognizing famous faces in temporal lobe epilepsy," *Neurology*, vol. 61, no. 1, pp. 81–86, 2003.

[58] M. Seidenberg, R. Griffith, D. Sabsevitz et al., "Recognition and identification of famous faces in patients with unilateral temporal lobe epilepsy," *Neuropsychologia*, vol. 40, no. 4, pp. 446–456, 2002.

[59] V. Voltzenlogel, O. Després, J.-P. Vignal, B. J. Steinhoff, P. Kehrli, and L. Manning, "Remote memory in temporal lobe epilepsy," *Epilepsia*, vol. 47, no. 8, pp. 1329–1336, 2006.

[60] R. Corcoran and D. Upton, "A role for the hippocampus in card sorting?" *Cortex*, vol. 29, no. 2, pp. 293–304, 1993.

[61] D. L. Drane, G. P. Lee, H. Cech et al., "Structured cueing on a semantic fluency task differentiates patients with temporal versus frontal lobe seizure onset," *Epilepsy and Behavior*, vol. 9, no. 2, pp. 339–344, 2006.

[62] B. P. Hermann, A. R. Wyler, and E. T. Richey, "Wisconsin card sorting test performance in patients with complex partial seizures of temporal-lobe origin," *Journal of Clinical and Experimental Neuropsychology*, vol. 10, no. 4, pp. 467–476, 1988.

[63] C.-H. Kim, S.-A. Lee, H.-J. Yoo, J.-K. Kang, and J.-K. Lee, "Executive performance on the Wisconsin card sorting test in mesial temporal lobe epilepsy," *European Neurology*, vol. 57, no. 1, pp. 39–46, 2007.

[64] M. Keiski, D. Fuerst, A. Shah, J. Shah, and G. Watson, "Executive functions in temporal lobe epilepsy: relationship to disease variables," in *Proceedings of the 60th American Epilepsy Society Meeting*, San Diego, Calif, USA, December 2006.

[65] M. Rodriguez-Camacho, B. Prieto, and J. Bernal, "Potenciales relacionados con eventos (PRE): aspectos basicos y conceptuales," in *Metodos en Neurociencias Cognoscitivas*, J. Silva, Ed., pp. 41–67, Manual Moderno, Mexico City, Mexico, 2011, (Spanish).

[66] G. Fernández, P. Klaver, J. Fell, T. Grunwald, and C. E. Elger, "Human declarative memory formation: segregating rhinal and hippocampal contributions," *Hippocampus*, vol. 12, no. 4, pp. 514–519, 2002.

[67] E. Ludowig, P. Trautner, M. Kurthen et al., "Intracranially recorded memory-related potentials reveal higher posterior than anterior hippocampal involvement in verbal encoding and retrieval," *Journal of Cognitive Neuroscience*, vol. 20, no. 5, pp. 841–851, 2008.

[68] P. Meyer, A. Mecklinger, T. Grunwald, J. Fell, C. E. Elger, and A. D. Friederici, "Language processing within the human medial temporal lobe," *Hippocampus*, vol. 15, no. 4, pp. 451–459, 2005.

[69] G. A. Ojemann, J. Schoenfield-McNeill, and D. Corina, "Different neurons in different regions of human temporal lobe distinguish correct from incorrect identification or memory," *Neuropsychologia*, vol. 42, no. 10, pp. 1383–1393, 2004.

[70] M. Vannucci, T. Dietl, N. Pezer et al., "Hippocampal function and visual object processing in temporal lobe epilepsy," *NeuroReport*, vol. 14, no. 11, pp. 1489–1492, 2003.

[71] J. M. Olichney, B. R. Riggins, D. G. Hillert et al., "Reduced sensitivity of the N400 and late positive component to semantic congruity and word repetition in left temporal lobe epilepsy," *Clinical EEG Electroencephalography*, vol. 33, no. 3, pp. 111–118, 2002.

[72] T. Miyamoto, J. I. Katayama, M. Kohsaka, and T. Koyama, "Disturbance of sematic processing in temporal lobe epilepsy demonstrated with scalp ERPs," *Seizure*, vol. 9, no. 8, pp. 572–579, 2000.

[73] A. Jaimes-Bautista, M. Rodriguez-Camacho, Y. Rodriguez-Agudelo, and I. Martinez-Juarez, "Estudio del procesamiento lexico-semantico en la epilepsia del lobulo temporal mediante potenciales relacionados con eventos," in *LVII Congreso Nacional de Ciencias Fisiologicas*, Oaxaca, Mexico, August-September 2014, (Spanish).

[74] S. S. Spencer, "Neural networks in human epilepsy: evidence of and implications for treatment," *Epilepsia*, vol. 43, no. 3, pp. 219–227, 2002.

[75] B. Köylü, E. Trinka, A. Ischebeck et al., "Neural correlates of verbal semantic memory in patients with temporal lobe epilepsy," *Epilepsy Research*, vol. 72, no. 2-3, pp. 178–191, 2006.

[76] L. Bartha, P. Mariën, C. Brenneis et al., "Hippocampal formation involvement in a language-activation task in patients with mesial temporal lobe epilepsy," *Epilepsia*, vol. 46, no. 11, pp. 1754–1763, 2005.

[77] S. B. Bonelli, R. Powell, P. J. Thompson et al., "Hippocampal activation correlates with visual confrontation naming: fMRI findings in controls and patients with temporal lobe epilepsy," *Epilepsy Research*, vol. 95, no. 3, pp. 246–254, 2011.

[78] E. J. Jensen, I. S. Hargreaves, P. M. Pexman, A. Bass, B. G. Goodyear, and P. Federico, "Abnormalities of lexical and semantic processing in left temporal lobe epilepsy: an fMRI study," *Epilepsia*, vol. 52, no. 11, pp. 2013–2021, 2011.

[79] J. J. Lin, J. D. Riley, J. Juranek, and S. C. Cramer, "Vulnerability of the frontal-temporal connections in temporal lobe epilepsy," *Epilepsy Research*, vol. 82, no. 2-3, pp. 162–170, 2008.

[80] H. W. R. Powell, G. J. M. Parker, D. C. Alexander et al., "Abnormalities of language networks in temporal lobe epilepsy," *NeuroImage*, vol. 36, no. 1, pp. 209–221, 2007.

Highights in the History of Epilepsy: The Last 200 Years

Emmanouil Magiorkinis,[1] **Aristidis Diamantis,**[1]
Kalliopi Sidiropoulou,[1] **and Christos Panteliadis**[2]

[1] *Office for the Study of Hellenic Naval Medicine, Naval Hospital of Athens, Deinokratous 70, 11527 Athens, Greece*
[2] *Division of Paediatric Neurology and Developmental Medicine, Aristotle University of Thessaloniki, AHEPA Hospital,*
   Stilp Kiriakidi 1, 54634 Thessaloniki, Greece

Correspondence should be addressed to Emmanouil Magiorkinis; emmanouil.magiorkinis@gmail.com

Academic Editor: Giangennaro Coppola

The purpose of this study was to present the evolution of views on epilepsy as a disease and symptom during the 19th and the 20th century. A thorough study of texts, medical books, and reports along with a review of the available literature in PubMed was undertaken. The 19th century is marked by the works of the French medical school and of John Hughlings Jackson who set the research on epilepsy on a solid scientific basis. During the 20th century, the invention of EEG, the advance in neurosurgery, the discovery of antiepileptic drugs, and the delineation of underlying pathophysiological mechanisms, were the most significant advances in the field of research in epilepsy. Among the most prestigious physicians connected with epilepsy one can pinpoint the work of Henry Gastaut, Wilder Penfield, and Herbert Jasper. The most recent advances in the field of epilepsy include the development of advanced imaging techniques, the development of microsurgery, and the research on the connection between genetic factors and epileptic seizures.

1. Introduction

The history of epilepsy is intermingled with the history of human existence; the first reports on epilepsy can be traced back to the Assyrian texts, almost 2,000 B.C. [1]. Multiple references to epilepsy can be found in the ancient texts of all civilizations, most importantly in the ancient Greek medical texts of the Hippocratic collection. For example, Hippocrates in his book *On Sacred Disease* described the first neurosurgery procedure referring that craniotomy should be performed at the opposite side of the brain of the seizures, in order to spare patients from "phlegma" that caused the disease [2]. However, it was not until the 18th and 19th century, when medicine made important advances and research on epilepsy was emancipated from religious superstitions such as the fact that epilepsy was a divine punishment or possession [3, 4]. At the beginning of the 18th century, the view that epilepsy was an idiopathic disease deriving from brain and other inner organs prevailed. One should mention the important work in this field by William Culen (1710–1790) and Samuel A. Tissot whose work set the base of modern epileptology describing accurately various types of epilepsies.

2. Anatomy and Physiology of Epilepsy

2.1. Evolution of Thoughts around the Pathophysiology and Causes of Epilepsy. At the beginning of the 19th century, physicians from the French medical school started to publish their research in the field of epileptology; famous French physicians published their works on epilepsy such as Maisonneuve (1745–1826) [5], Calmeil (1798–1895) [6], and Jean-Etienne Dominique Esquirol (1772–1840). Maisonneuve stressed the importance for hospitalization of epileptic patients, categorized epilepsy into idiopathic and sympathetic and described the so-called sensitive aura of sympathetic epilepsy. Esquirol distinguished between petit and grand mal and along with his pupils Bouchet and Cazauvieilh studied systematically insanity and epilepsy conducting clinical and postmortem studies [3].

During the second half of the 19th century, medicine focused on the delineation of pathophysiology of epilepsy and the topographic localization of epileptic seizures. Important works on epileptogenesis, aetiology, and taxonomy of epilepsy were published by prestigious physicians such as Théodore Herpin (1799–1865) in 1852 and 1867, Louis

Jean François Delasiauve (1804–1893) in 1854, John Russell Reynolds (1828–1896) in 1861, and in 1881 by Sir William Richard Gowers (1845–1915). Regarding the delineation of the epileptic mechanisms, the proof that epilepsy derives from the brain came from the work of physiologist Fritsch (1838–1927) and psychiatrist Hitzig (1838–1907); in their paper entitled "*On the Electric Excitability of the Cerebrum*" they presented experiments in which they provoked seizures by electric stimulation in the brain cortex of dogs [7]. The work, however, of John Hughling Jackson (1835–1911) (Figure 1), set the scientific base of epileptology [3]. Jackson studied epilepsy on pathological and anatomical basis. His *Study of Convulsions* was the culmination of his research stressing the existence of localised lesions on cortex involved in epileptic convulsions. In 1873, Jackson gave the following definition for epilepsy: "Epilepsy is the name for occasional, sudden, excessive, rapid and local discharges of grey matter" [3].

Epileptology, based on the work of Jackson and other eminent doctors of the 19th century, such as John Simon (1816–1904), John Russell Reynolds (1828–1896), Samuel Wilks, William Richard Gowers (1845–1915), Adolf Kussmaul (1822–1902), and Adolf Tenner, expanded and made important steps towards the elucidation of the pathophysiology of the disease and in the field of therapeutics [3].

At the beginning of the 20th century, Santiago Ramón y Cajal (1852–1934), a Spanish pathologist, histologist, and neuroscientist, made important advances in the field of the microscopic structure of the brain and the nervous system. He was the first to describe the structure of neurons and synapses, a hallmark finding in the history of neurology. His findings were the culmination of efforts which began in 1887, when he started employing the Golgi staining in the study of the nervous system. As a reward of his efforts, Cajal, in 1906, received the Nobel Prize [8].

In 1907, Gowers published his famous book *The Borderlands of Epilepsy* [9] focusing on faints, vagal and vasovagal attacks, migraine, vertigo, and some sleep symptoms, especially narcolepsy. In 1914, Dale (1875–1968) identified acetylcholine [10], the first neurotransmitter, a discovery confirmed later in 1921 by Loewi (1873–1961) who initially named it *Vagusstoff*, since it was released by the vagus nerve [11–13].

During the 1920s, Lennox (1884–1960) and Cobb (1887–1968) focused on the effects of starvation, ketogenic diet, and altered cerebral oxygen in seizures and published their first monograph entitled "*Epilepsy from the Standpoint of Physiology and Treatment*" [14]. In 1922, Cobb and Lennox published another monograph entitled "*Epilepsy and Related Disorders*" (1928) [15] and an important paper summarizing their research entitled "*The Relation of Certain Physicochemical Processes to Epileptiform Seizures*" (1929) [16]. Lennox and Cobb focused on the effects of various stimuli to the generation of epileptic convulsions such as starvation, ketogenic diet, and lack of oxygen, most of them with negative results.

During the 1940s, important discoveries were made in the field of psychomotor epilepsy. Klüver (1897–1979), a German-American psychologist, and Bucy (1904–1992), an American neuropathologist, well known for the discovery of the

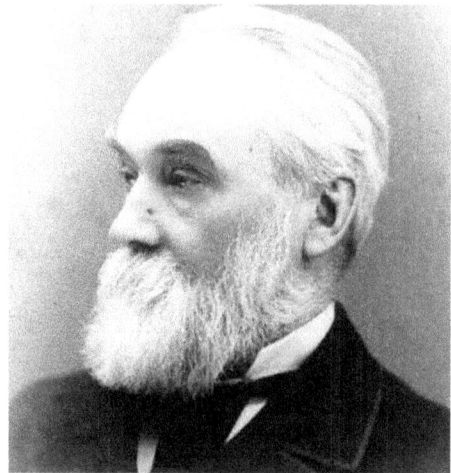

FIGURE 1: John Hughlings Jackson (1835–1911) (adopted by public domain at http://www.denstoredanske.dk/).

Klüver-Bucy syndrome, showed that changes in the behavior of monkeys could be associated with temporal lobe lesions [17]. In 1941, Jasper (1906–1999) and Kershmann proved that the temporal lobe is the site of origin of psychomotor seizures [18]. At the same period, Moruzzi (1910–1986) and Magoun (1907–1991) discovered the reticular formation in the brain [19]. Magoun continued his research with Lindsley (1907–2003) and Starzl (1926-) identifying various neural pathways within the brain and pointing out the important role in alert wakefulness as a background for sensory perception, higher intellectual activity, voluntary movements, and behaviors [20, 21]. Dawson in 1947 recorded the responses from the human scalp in response to somatosensory stimuli (somatosensory evoked potential) [22], whereas in 1949 Roberts (1920-) and Frankel discovered γ-aminobutyric acid (GABA) [23].

Important advances were made in the field of neuroscience and in the physiology of synapses by Eccles (1903–1997), Kandel (1929-), Spencer (1931–1977), Speckmann (1939-), Purpura, Meldrum, and others [24–38].

James Kiffin Penry (1929–1996), in 1969, published important treatises such as the series *Basic Mechanisms of the Epilepsies* and afterwards *Antiepileptic Drugs, Neurosurgical Management of the Epilepsies, Complex Partial Seizures, and their Treatment*, and *Antiepileptic Drugs Mechanisms of Action and Advances in Epileptology*. In the same year Gastaut managed to organize a meeting in Marseilles attended by 120 members of ILAE and a preliminary classification of epilepsies was presented to a commission on terminology of epilepsy. The General Assembly of the ILAE accepted the first publication of clinical and electroencephalographic classification of epileptic seizures [39, 40].

Dreifuss (1926–1997) worked on video-monitoring of absence seizures and helped in the classification of various epileptic conditions [41]. Prince et al. made the first studies of cellular phenomena of epileptic events in the human cortex [42–44]. Meldrum et al. proved that the assumption connecting brain damage from seizures as a result of hypoxia is wrong [45–47]; he demonstrated that the excessive excitatory activity is responsible for the brain cellular loss.

During the last two decades, various changes regarding the epileptic brain damage were also studied, such as the mossy fiber sprouting and synaptic reorganization [48–51].

2.2. The Electrophysiology of Epilepsy and the EEG. The first reference regarding the association of electric stimuli and brain activity came from the work of Fritsch (1838–1927) and Hitzig (1938–1907), who managed to cause convulsion to dogs by applying electric stimuli on the animals' cortex. Five years later, in 1875, Caton (1842–1926) examined the electrical activity of nerve-muscle preparations and explored the possibility whether similar changes in electrical potential occurred in the brain [52]. A few years later, in 1890, Beck from Cracau in the pages of Zentrallblatt for Physiologie argued the case for the priority of the electrical activity of the brain, after electrical stimulation in the brain of dogs and rabbits [53]. In 1912, Kaufman (1877–1951), a Russian physiologist, noticed the electric changes in the brain during experimentally induced seizures, associating epileptic attacks with abnormal electric discharges [54] (EEG). In the same year, Pravdich-Neminsky (1879–1952), a Ukrainian physiologist, published the first animal EEG and the evoked potential of the mammalian (dog) [55].

Two years later, Cybulski (1854–1919), a Polish physiologist and pioneer in electroencephalography, in cooperation with Jelenska-Macieszyna [56], published the first photographs of electroencephalography recording action potentials at a dog with focal epilepsy.

Important discoveries in the fields of electroencephalography were made during the 1920s and 1930s. In 1929, Berger (1873–1941), a German neurologist, reported his findings on human brain waves [57], five years after his initial recording of the first human electroencephalogram. His results brought controversy and scepticism within the scientific community, but he was neither rejected nor ignored; his results were confirmed later by Adrian (1899–1977) and Matthews [58]. In 1932, Berger reported sequential postictal EEG changes after a generalized tonicoclonic seizure, and in 1933 he published the first example of interictal changes and a minor epileptic seizure with 3/s rhythmic waves in the EEG [59, 60]. In the next few years until 1939, Berger made important observations on patients and on healthy subjects. His work on epileptic EEG was completed by Frederic Andrews Gibbs (1903–1992), an American neurologist, and Erna Leonhardt-Gibbs (1904–1987), technician and wife of Frederic, who, in collaboration with Lennox, established the correlation between EEG findings and epileptic convulsions [61–63]; Lennox and Gibbs published in 1941 their monumental monograph "*Atlas of Electroencephalography,*" in which they included also mechanical and mathematical analysis of electroencephalograms [64].

An important and influential figure in the field of EEG whose work was intensified during the 1950s was Henri Jean Pascal Gastaut (1915–1995) (Figure 2). After his graduation in 1945 from the University of Marseilles, Gastaut worked at the laboratory of William Grey Walter (1910–1977) in Bristol learning the basics of EEG and discovered photic stimulation as an EEG seizure activator. In 1949, he went

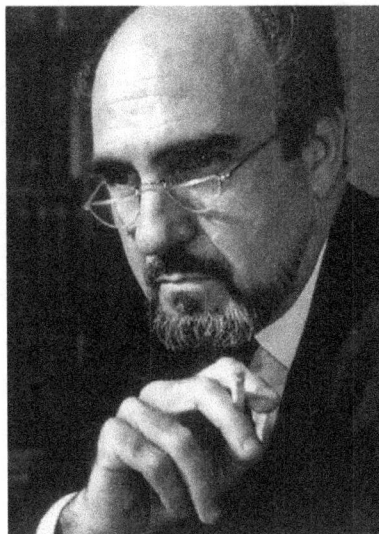

FIGURE 2: Henri Jean Pascal Gastaut (1915–1995) (adopted by public domain at http://www.lennox-gastaut.de/Krankheitsbild.112.0.html).

to the Montreal Neurological Institute (MNI) with Wilder Penfield (1891–1976), famous Canadian neurosurgeon, and Herbert Jasper (Figure 3) (1906–1999), a Canadian psychologist, physiologist, anatomist, chemist, and neurologist who established in 1939 an EEG laboratory and studied the role of thalamic reticular structures in the genesis of metrazol-induced generalized paroxysmal EEG discharges and developed the concept of centrencephalic seizures [65]. After his return to Marseilles, Gastaut founded the International EEG Federation and, in 1953, became the Head of the Marseilles Hospital Neurobiological Laboratories establishing a school of neurology that dominated for the next decades. In 1958, he participated in the foundation of the Toul Ar C'hoat Center in Brittany for the education of epileptic children, whereas two years later he created the Saint Paul Center for epileptic children and, in 1961, the INSERM Neurobiology Research Unit. His contribution in the study of epileptology was monumental; with his wife, Yvette, he defined five major human EEG patterns (lambda waves, pi rhythm, mu rhythm, rolandic spikes, and posterior theta rhythm) [66, 67]. He also described two syndromes under his name: Gastaut syndrome, a type of photosensitive epilepsy [68], and the Lennox-Gastaut syndrome (severe childhood encephalopathy) with onset in childhood with myoclonic seizures at night, head nodding, and drop attacks particularly prominent [69, 70]. He also studied photic and other self-induced seizures, startle epilepsy, HHE syndrome, and benign partial epilepsy of childhood with occipital spike-waves [68, 71–75].

During the 1960s, important EEG studies were conducted in animals mainly by Prince and his research team demonstrating the spikes and waves associated with synchronous paroxysmal depolarizing bursts occurring in cortical neurons [76–79] and the spike-wave complex [80]. In 1968, Falconer recognized the importance of hippocampal sclerosis in temporal lobe epilepsy [81].

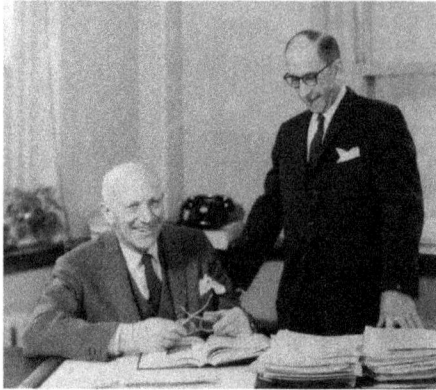

FIGURE 3: Wilder Penfield (1891–1976) on the right and Herbert Jasper (1906–1999) on the left (adopted by public domain at http://baillement.com/lettres/penfield.html).

2.3. The Patch-Clamp Technique. An important development in the field of neuroscience was that of Neher (1944-), who invented the patch-clamp method to measure the flow of current through single-ion channels [82]. Neher and Sakmann developed the patch-clamp technique for which in 1992 they received the Nobel Prize [83]. Using the patch-clump technique, the various ion channels were able to be studied and, thus, the role of calcium channels was clarified in epilepsy [84].

3. Therapy of Epilepsy

3.1. The Evolution of Antiepileptic Surgery. The first surgical procedures on epileptic patients were performed during the 19th century; Heyman in 1831 was the first one to perform a surgery to an epileptic patient due to a brain abscess. Surgical excision was performed on November 25, 1884, by Dr. Godlee in the National Hospital of London. In 1880, Wilhelm Sommer (1852–1900), German neurologist and psychiatrist, described precisely Ammon's horn lesions and epileptic manifestations part with sensible occurrence. Both Theodor Kocher (1841–1917), a Swiss surgeon from Bern, Nobelist, and pioneer in epileptic surgery, and Harvey Cushing (1869–1939), father of modern neurological surgery, in Baltimore dealt with posttraumatic epileptic disorders especially with patients displaying high endocranial pressure [85, 86]. In 1886, Horsley (1875–1916) excised an epileptogenic posttraumatic cortical scar at the National Hospital of London in a 23-year-old man under general anesthesia and discussed his choice of anesthesia: *"I have not employed ether in operations on man, fearing that it would tend to cause cerebral excitement; chloroform, of course, producing on the contrary, well-marked depression."* [87]. In Germany, Krause (1857–1937) and Foerster (1873–1941) refined Horsley's technique [88, 89].

At the beginning of the 20th century, Dandy (1886–1946) introduced hemispherectomy as a neurosurgical procedure in 1923 [90]. However it was not until the 1930s than important advances were made in epileptic surgery. The notion of operating the epileptogenic focus was introduced

by Gibbs and Lennox in 1938 [91]. The introduction of EEG into epilepsy surgery was important in the development of surgical techniques.

Penfield along with Jasper and Theodore Brown Rasmussen (1910–2002) in the Neurologic Center of University of Montreal also contributed importantly to the evolution of the surgery of epilepsy [92, 93]. Penfield applied the Foerster method for removing epileptogenic lesions on an epilepsy patient. After founding the Montreal Neurological Institute (MNI), in 1934, in collaboration with Jasper, he invented the *Montreal procedure* for the surgical treatment of epilepsy. According to the Montreal procedure, through the administration of local anesthetic, the surgeon removes part of the skull to expose brain tissue and, by the use of probes, the conscious patient describes to the surgeon his/her feelings so that the surgeon can identify the exact location of seizure activity. Then the surgeon proceeds in the removal of brain tissue in this location reducing the side effects of surgery [94]. Through his operations, Penfield was able to identify various brain centers and to create maps of the sensory and motor cortices of the brain. Research in MNI focused also on other areas of epileptology such as neurochemistry, oncology, and brain angiology. Penfield perfected and established his surgical procedures as a treatment of choice in intractable epilepsy, especially of neocortical regions [94–96]. In 1954, Penfield published with Jasper one of the greatest classics in neurology, *Epilepsy and the Functional Anatomy of the Human Brain* [93].

Around the same period, van Wagenen and Herren (1897–1961), Chief of Neurosurgery at the University of Rochester Medical Center (URMC), performed and perfected the procedure of callosotomy [97]. Bailey (1892–1973), an American neuropathologist, neurosurgeon, and psychiatrist, known for his work on brain oncology, was the first to attempt temporal lobectomies for psychomotor seizures and the first to use electrocorticography for intraoperative localization [98]. One should also mention the method of hemispherectomy introduced by McKenzie (1892–1964) [99] and Krynauw in 1950 [100].

Bailey and Gibbs in 1951 employed the EEG as a guide to perform temporal lobe surgery [98], whereas, in 1953, Falconer, a neurosurgeon from New Zealand, in London, introduced the en bloc anterior temporal lobe resection and the term mesial temporal sclerosis [101]. The work of Margerison and Corsellis led to the term of hippocampal sclerosis [102], a pathological entity which was initially described almost 80 years earlier by Sommer in 1880 [103]. Niemeyer, in 1958, suggested a more selective procedure of resection of the mesiobasal limbic structure [104], a technique which was later on abandoned.

The next important step in the field of antiepileptic surgery was done by Tailarach and his team. In 1957, Tailarach (1911–2007) published his stereotactic atlas, a work that changed the future of epilepsy neurosurgery the next decade [105]; Marcel David adopting Tailarach's views supported the creation of an operating room in which stereotactic surgery would take place. Within this operating room teleradiography would take place and the use of parallel X-ray beams would avoid distortions of skull, vessels, ventricles, and the frame and grids used for guiding the placement of intracranial electrodes. The first stereotactic surgery operating room was opened in Sainte-Anne in 1959 [106]. Tailarach's team obtained two members, Alain Bonis and Gabor Szikla. In 1962, the term stereoelectroencephalography (SEEG) was introduced by Talairach and Jean Bancaud (1921–1993). Their method brought a revolution in the surgery of epilepsy, since it allowed investigative presurgical and therapeutic surgical phases to be completely dissociated. Tailarach and Bancaud employing their technique showed that lesional and irritative zones had a variable topographic relationship within the epileptogenic zone [14]. Tailarach's method allowed the individualization of epileptic surgery for each patient [18, 19].

During the 1960s, Bogen and Vogel reintroduced the procedure of callosotomy [107] as a procedure for certain cases of pharmacoresistant epilepsy with severe atonic akinetic seizures. In 1961, White published a comprehensive review on the surgical procedure of hemispherectomy summarizing the results of 269 published cases [108] in the treatment of infantile-type hemiplegia and seizures. In 1969, Morell and Hanbrey introduced "multiple subpial transection" (MST) for nonresectable epileptic foci [108].

At the beginning of the 1980s, in the field of antiepileptic surgery, MTLE suggested selective amygdalohippocampectomy (AHE) with the trans-Sylvian approach, replacing the anterior temporal lobe resection [109]. The advent of modern diagnostic techniques such as MRI, PET, and SPECT (single photon emission tomography), ^{31}P and ^{1}H-MR spectroscopy, and MEG (magnetoencephalography) revolutionized epileptic surgery, as well. The application of microsurgery led to selective operations with less complications; such procedures include "selective amygdalohippocampectomy" [109], the innovation of older ones, anterior callosotomy, subtotal functional hemispherectomy, and extended multilobar resections, and the introduction of new operative techniques such as multiple subpial transection [109] and gamma knife.

3.2. Drug Therapy. As far as therapies and the neurophysiology of epilepsy are concerned, much were already known during the second half of 19th century. Treatment of epilepsy till that time mostly consisted of herbal and chemical substances. In 1857, Sir Locock (1799–1875) discovered the anticonvulsant and sedative traits of potassium bromide and began treating his patients. From that point, potassium bromide became a choice treatment for humans with epileptic seizures and nervous disorders until the 1912 discovery of phenobarbital [110].

In 1912, Hauptmann (1881–1948), a German physician, introduced phenobarbital in the therapy of epilepsy, one of the first antiepileptic drugs [111]. Phenobarbital was brought to market by the drug company Bayer using the brand Luminal. Hauptmann administered Luminal to his epilepsy patients as a tranquilizer and discovered that their epileptic attacks were susceptible to the drug. The introduction of animal models in the study of the anticonvulsant properties of various substances will contribute to the development of new antiepileptic drugs.

The next drug introduced in the therapy of epilepsy was phenytoin in 1938. Although phenytoin was already known from 1908 and was synthesized by Heinrich Biltz (1865–1943), there was no interest for that drug since it did not have any sedative properties. Merritt (1902–1979), an eminent academic neurologist, along with Putnam (1894–1975), discovered, in 1938, the anticonvulsant properties of phenytoin (Dilantin) and its effect on the control of epileptic seizures publishing their results in a series of papers [112–115]. Phenytoin became the first-line medication for the prevention of partial and tonic-clonic seizures and for acute cases of epilepsies or status epilepticus, giving an alternative therapeutic choice for patients not responding to bromides or barbiturates. In 1946, a new antiepileptic drug was added in the quiver of antiepileptic therapy, trimethadione; it was reported by Richards and Everett to prevent pentylenetetrazol-induced seizures and to be effective especially in absence seizures [116].

During the 1950s, new drugs came up such as carbamazepine in 1953 [117], primidone in 1954, ethosuximide in 1958 by Vossen [118], sodium valproate in 1963 by Meunier et al. [119], and sultiame. Buchtal and Svensmark were the first ones in 1960 to measure the levels of the antiepileptic drugs in the blood [120]. Although carbamazepine and valproate were available in Europe during the 1960s, no other drug was licensed in the USA. The development of carbamazepine was based on the neuroleptic drug chlorpromazine from Firma Rhône-Poulenc in Lyon. Jean Pierre (1907–1987) and Pierre Deniker (1917–1998), French psychiatrists, used chlorpromazine in Centre Hospitalier Sainte Anne in Paris to treat patients with schizophrenia. However, research on neuroleptic drugs continued in Geigy labs; carbamazepine was synthesized by Schindler and Blattner (1921-?) at J. R. Geigy AG, Basel, Switzerland, 1953, in the course of development of another antidepressant drug imipramine [117]. Initial animal screening showed that carbamazepine was effective against trigeminal neuralgia, which was confirmed by clinical trials [121]. Antiepileptic effects were reported in 1963 and 1964 [122, 123]. It was used as an anticonvulsant drug in the UK since 1965 and has been approved in the USA since 1974. The reason for the delay of approval in the USA was due to reports of aplastic anemia caused by the drug [124]. Ethosuximide was first introduced in clinical practice in the early 1950s for the therapy of absence "petit mal."

In 1967, valproate came up as a new promising antiepileptic drug. Valproate was initially synthesized in 1881 by Beverly Burton in the USA and was initially employed as an organic solvent [125]; his research on valproate begun in Würzburg, Germany. The anticonvulsant properties of valproate were reported by Pierre Eymard, who worked at Firma Berthier laboratories in Grenoble, and it was first released as antiepileptic drug in France in 1967 [126] after the publication of preclinical studies by Carraz et al. in 1964. During 1970, it received license to other European countries, but in the USA it was not licensed before 1978.

In 1970, Penry and Cereghino were employed in designing clinical trials for antiepileptic drugs (AEDs). Harvey Kupferberg joined their team and together they developed a methodology for measuring the blood-levels of albutoin, an experimental drug which was proved to be ineffective in epilepsy. The first edition of *Antiepileptic Drugs* came forth as a result of their research efforts in 1972 [127]. Carbamazepine was the first drug to be licensed by the FDA based on the results of clinical trials. Pippenger (1939-) developed methods for measuring blood-levels of AEDs [128]. Other antiepileptic drugs introduced during the 1970s were clobazam (1,5-benzodiazepine) (1970), clonazepam (1,4-benzodiazepine) (1970), and piracetam.

The last decade newer antiepileptic drugs such as vigabatrin (1989), lamotrigine (1990), oxcarbazepine (1990), gabapentin (1993), felbamate (1993), topiramate (1995), tiagabine (1998), zonisamide (1989 in Japan and 2000 in the USA), levetiracetam (2000), stiripentol (2002), pregabalin (2004), rufinamide (2004), lacosamide (2008), eslicarbazepine (2009), and perampanel (2012) were used. FDA ended clinical use of felbamate in 1994 due to its association with complications. The newer generation antiepileptic drugs including vigabatrin, felbamate, gabapentin, lamotrigine, tiagabine, topiramate, levetiracetam, oxcarbazepine, zonisamide, pregabalin, rufinamide, and lacosamide have improved tolerability and safety compared to their older counterparts. Stiripentol, pregabalin, rufinamide, lacosamide, eslicarbazepine, and perampanel are licensed for adjunctive use only. The research in antiepileptic drugs is an active field and many drugs are currently under development in clinical trials including eslicarbazepine acetate, brivaracetam, and retigabine.

In phase III clinical trials (which used eslicarbazepine doses of 400, 800, and 1200 mg/day), eslicarbazepine was well tolerated, with the most common AEs reported to include dizziness, headache, and somnolence [129–132]. Two large-scale, phase III clinical trials have been conducted for retigabine. In both studies, AEs leading to discontinuation included dizziness, somnolence, headache, and fatigue [133–136].

3.3. The Idea of Ketogenic Diet. Ketogenic diet was used for the first time in the treatment of epilepsy in 1911 by the French physicians Guelpa and Marie. It was introduced as a diet full of fats and low in proteins and carbohydrates and managed to treat 20 children and adults with epilepsy reporting decrease in the number of seizures [137]. However, fasting and other diets were employed for the treatment of epilepsy since the Hippocratic era [138].

In 1922, Hugh Conklin, an osteopathic physician from Michigan, applied this diet to epileptic patients with encouraging results. Conklin believed that epilepsy was due to toxins that damage the brain and so he obliged his patients to a strict diet. In his papers, he wrote, *"I restrict from my patients any kind of food except of water for as long as their physical condition allows it."* Conklin had a personal interest in ketogenic diet, since by this way he tried to cure his nephew, who suffered from drug-resistant epilepsy. Several papers have been published about the usefulness of ketogenic diet and the indications that will lead to the beginning of such a treatment [139, 140]. Further studies were published by Talbot [141], Helmholz [142], Lennox [143], and Bridge and Iob [144].

Charles Howland, a wealth New York lawyer, funded his brother John Howland to search whether there was a scientific basis for the success of the starvation treatment by which his epileptic son was treated [145, 146]. Dr. John Howland, Professor of paediatrics, John Hopkins Hospital, used this funding to create the first laboratory at the Harriet Lane Home for Invalid Children. John Howland Memorial Fund was established at John Hopkins Hospital and supported the research on the ketogenic diet [147]. Although multiple investigations have been performed, the anticonvulsive mechanisms of ketogenic diet remain unexplained. In the years to follow, many authors published articles with positive or negative results. Then, this therapy was forgotten for many years, since progress in pharmaceutical therapy was in the foreground. In the last 20–30 years, KD experienced a revival, especially in the Anglo-American world where it is established as a treatment option for therapy-resistant infantile epilepsy. Livingston [148], Hopkins and Lynch [149, 150], and Huttenlocher [151] were the advocates of this direction. The multitude of side effects and procedural problems however reduced the initial euphoria. Only as recently as 1996, the *Institute Charlie* (the institute was named by a father of a child with epilepsy which was treated with *KD*) educated the public about the benefit of KD, organized seminars and training courses, and published a book entitled *The Epilepsy Diet Treatment: An Introduction to the Ketogenic Diet.* More recently new versions of ketogenic diet such as the modified Atkins diet have been employed successfully for the treatment of children and adults with refractory epilepsy [152, 153] and are especially recommended in cases of pharmacologically intractable epilepsy.

3.4. The Technique of Vagus Nerve Stimulation. An important advance in epilepsy treatment was the development of the technique of vagus nerve stimulation (VNS), especially for patients experiencing serious adverse effects of antiepileptic drugs. VNS involves implantation of a programmable signal generator (neurocybernetic prosthesis NCP) in the chest cavity, and the stimulating electrodes carry electrical signals from the generator to the left vagus nerve [154].

3.5. Complimentary Treatments for Epilepsy. During the last two decades a series of alternative or complimentary therapies have emerged in the therapy of epilepsy. These include relaxation therapies such as massage, aromatherapy, reflexology and chiropractic therapy, holistic therapies such as herbal medicine (St. John's Wort, evening primrose oil), homeopathy, Ayurvedic medicine, and traditional Chinese medicine (herbal remedies plus acupuncture), traditional and psychological therapies such as autogenic training, neurofeedback, and other psychological therapies, and music therapy. Although some of those therapies seem to have an effect, most of them are considered as complementary therapies and more studies are needed in order to establish their therapeutic effect and their usefulness in everyday clinical practice [155]. Recent studies have pinpointed the use of cannabidiol and medical marijuana for the treatment of epilepsy [156].

4. The Evolution of Thoughts around Epilepsy: Society and Science Cooperate for the Good of Epileptic Patients

Just before the turn of the twentieth century, in 1898, William Pryor Letchworth (1823–1910), a businessman devoted to charities, and Frederick Peterson (1859–1938), an eminent American neurologist and Professor of neurology, Columbia University, organized the first National Association for the Study of Epilepsy and the Care and Treatment of Epileptics in the USA and the Craig Colony in Sonyea, the first comprehensive public epilepsy center, along with other eminent physicians such as Roswell Park (1852–1914), Professor of surgery, University of Buffalo Medical School, and a surgeon, Buffalo General Hospital, William P. Spratling (1863–1915), American neurologist, known for his studies in epilepsy, and Frederick Munson [157, 158]. William Spartling introduced for the first time the term "epileptologist" for a physician specializing in epilepsy.

During World War I, Pearce Bailey organised the systematic examination of military recruits creating a database with epidemiological data on epilepsy. The same year is considered to be the founding year of the American Epilepsy Society (AES) in commemoration of a joint meeting focusing on epilepsy organised by the Association for the Research in Nervous and Mental Disease (ARNMD) and the American League Against Epilepsy (ALAE). The proceedings of this meeting recapitulated the state of the art on epilepsy research and stimulated further research [159]. The first president of AES was Dr. Charles Dair Aring (1904–1998), a renowned American neurologist and pioneer in medical education in the USA.

The beginning of the 1950s was marked by the establishment by the US congress and the American Academy of Neurology of the National Institute of Neurological Diseases and Blindness (NINDB), now known as the National Institute of Neurological Disorders and Stroke. The main purpose of this institute was to study and treat the neurological and psychiatric casualties of World War II under the direction of Bailey. Bailey recruited in his team Maitland Baldwin (1918–1970), a famous American neurosurgeon, as the Chief of surgical neurology, Bethesda, Donald Bayley Tower (1919–2007), in 1953, as the Chief of the section on clinical neurochemistry, and Cosimo Ajmone-Marsan (1918–2004), as the Head of the electroencephalography branch in 1954. As a result of their cooperation, a treatise on temporal lobe epilepsy was published [160].

During the 1960s, in 1961, the International Bureau for Epilepsy (IBE) was established as an organisation of laypersons and professionals interested in the medical and non-medical aspects of epilepsy (http://www.ibe-epilepsy.org). In 1962, the US Public Health Service Surgeon General created the Neurological and Sensory Disease Control Program (NSDCP) supporting research on epilepsy in various ways. In 1965, Anthony Joseph Celebrezze (1941–2003), Secretary of the Department of Health, Education, and Welfare, organized a meeting for the expansion of epilepsy research and services. As a result of it, in 1966, Surgeon General William Stewart (1921–2008) created the Surgeon General's Public Health Service Advisory Committee on the Epilepsies, whereas, in 1969, the Society for Neuroscience was established. Stewart created two subcommittees: one with David Daily entitled *Service Training Subcommittee* with Terrance Capistrant and James Cereghino as Executive Secretaries and a second one with Arthur Ward entitled *Research Training Subcommittee* with William Caveness and J. Kiffin Penry as Executive Secretaries [65].

In 1970, a classification of epilepsies was proposed by the International League Against Epilepsy [161]. This classification was revised several times through the last decades, in order to clarify terms and meanings and to avoid any confusion towards the understanding of epilepsy. In 1975, the US Commission for the Control of Epilepsy and its Consequences was established under the direction of Dr. Richard H. Masland and Dr. David Daly, creating a plan for nation-wide action on epilepsy.

During the last two decades, epileptics are being evaluated psychologically and socially and, before 1990, quality of life tools were developed. In 1981, the International League Against Epilepsy (ILAE) published the first classification of epilepsies which were discussed extensively and revised in 1989 [162–164]; the classification and terminology for epileptic seizures and syndromes provided a fundamental instrument for diagnosing, organizing, and differentiating the epilepsies.

During the 1990s, the decade of the brain, WHO in collaboration with ILAE and IBE launched the Global Campaign Against Epilepsy in 1997, in order to bring epilepsy out of the shadows and to further improve diagnosis, treatment, prevention and social acceptability. In 1993, the ILAE defined fever seizures as the seizures occurring in childhood after the age of 1 month, usually between 3 months and 6 years old, associated with a febrile illness, not caused by an infection of central nervous system (CNS), without previous neonatal or unprovoked seizure, and not meeting criteria for other acute symptomatic seizures [165]. In 2001, the ILAE Task Force on Classification and Terminology under Engel proposed a diagnostic scheme for people with epileptic seizures and with epilepsy [166] which was also supported in 2006 by the ILAE Classification Core Group [167]. ILAE's classification of epilepsies and convulsive disorders was extensively discussed and new classification was suggested but not implemented since 2010 when ILAE published a new classification [168, 169].

5. The Contribution of Imaging Techniques in the Diagnosis of Epilepsy

After the end of World War I, Dandy (1886–1946), an American neurosurgeon, described in 1918 and 1919, pneumoventriculography and pneumoencephalography [170–172], the first imaging techniques of the brain with the use of X-rays. For his discovery, he was nominated by Hans Christian Jacobaeus for the Nobel Prize in 1933. In the field of imaging, it was not until 1972 when computerized tomography (CT) was invented by the British engineer Godfrey

Hounsfield (1919–2004), EMI Laboratories, UK, and by the South African physicist Allan MacLeod Cormack (1924–1998), Tufts University, Massachusetts [173]. The use of ^{18}F-fluorodeoxyglucose for determination of local cerebral localization began in 1977 [174, 175].

During the last decades great steps have been taken to the diagnostic approach of epilepsy by the use of neuroimaging. Techniques as magnetic resonance tomography (MRI), SPECT, and PET contributed to the diagnosis of pathological areas of the brain, such as tumors, cortical/subcortical dysgeneses, inflammation, strokes, vascular dysplasia, and posttraumatic insult. Newer imaging techniques in the diagnosis of epilepsy include functional MRI [176] (fMRI), clinical proton MR spectroscopy [177], and magnetoencephalography (MEG) [178].

6. Genetics in Epilepsy

The first connection between heredity and epilepsy was made in 1903 by Lundborg (1868–1943), a Swedish physician, notorious for his views on eugenics and racial hygiene, who published his research on the genetics of progressive myoclonic epilepsy first described by Heinrich Unverricht in 1891 (1853–1912) [179]; his analysis was pioneering since he was able to trace back the disease in the family since the 18th century. In that way, Lundborg was also a pioneer in the study of human genetics.

The concept of eugenics became an issue in the control of epilepsy during the 1930s; in 1936, the American Neurological Association Committee for the Investigation of Eugenical Sterilization published a report [180] stating that sterilization of epileptics should be voluntary and conducted under supervision and only with patient consent.

The most important evolution, however, in the field of the genetics of epilepsy, took place during the last twenty years; in 1989, Leppert was the first to identify the link between chromosome 20 and idiopathic human epilepsy syndrome in a family with benign familial neonatal convulsions [181]. Epilepsy still remains a field of active research, occupying different medical specialties. The growing evidence on the connection between various genes and epilepsies is the cutting edge of modern epilepsy research, and in the next decades new exciting discoveries are going to change epileptology [182]. Recently, in 2011, Engel published the identification of reliable biomarkers which would greatly facilitate differential diagnosis, eliminate the current trial-and-error approach to pharmacotherapy, facilitate presurgical evaluation, and greatly improve the cost-effectiveness of drug discovery and clinical trials of agents designed to treat, prevent, and cure epilepsy [167].

7. Conclusions

The fascinating history of epilepsy is connected with the history of humanity; early reports on epilepsy go back to the ancient Assyrian and Babylonian texts, scanning a period of almost 4,000 years. The first hallmark in the history of epilepsy is the Hippocratic texts which set in doubt the divine origin of the disease. Major advances in the understanding of epilepsy came much later, during the 18th and 19th century; theories on epilepsy during this period are formulated on a solid scientific basis and epileptics are for the first time treated as patients and not as lunatics or possessed. During this period, experimental studies were conducted and advances made in the pathology of the disease and the connection of epilepsy with various psychiatric symptoms. The work of John Hughlings Jackson was preceded by a plethora of studies by Dutch, German, English, and French physicians who evolved scientific thought and performed thorough studies on epilepsy. The advent of the 20th century led to the in-depth understanding of the mechanisms of the disease, the development of effective drugs, and neuroimaging methods. Last but not least, one should mention the important advances in the molecular biology of the disease and the connection of various genes with various forms of epilepsy.

Conflict of Interests

The authors declare that there is no conflict of interests regarding the publication of this paper.

References

[1] E. Magiorkinis, K. Sidiropoulou, and A. Diamantis, "Hallmarks in the history of epilepsy: epilepsy in antiquity," *Epilepsy and Behavior*, vol. 17, no. 1, pp. 103–108, 2010.

[2] Hippocrates, *The Sacred Disease*, vol. 2, Loeb Classical Library and Harvard University Press, London, UK, 1965, translated by W. H. S. Jones.

[3] K. Sidiropoulou, A. Diamantis, and E. Magiorkinis, "Hallmarks in 18th- and 19th-century epilepsy research," *Epilepsy and Behavior*, vol. 18, no. 3, pp. 151–161, 2010.

[4] A. Diamantis, K. Sidiropoulou, and E. Magiorkinis, "Epilepsy during the middle ages, the renaissance and the enlightenment," *Journal of Neurology*, vol. 257, no. 5, pp. 691–698, 2010.

[5] J. G. F. Maisonneuve, *Recherches et observations sur l'épilepsie, presentées a L'École de médecine de Paris*, Paris, France, 1803.

[6] L. F. Calmeil, *De l' epilepsie etudiee sous le rapport de son siege et de son influence sur la production de l' alienation mentale [Thesis]*, Imprimerie de Didot le jeune, Paris, France, 1824.

[7] G. Fritsch and E. Hitzig, "Ueber die elektrische Erregbarkeit des Grosshirns," *Archiv für Anatomie, Physiologie und Wissenschaftliche Medicin*, vol. 37, pp. 300–332, 1870.

[8] V. S. Wong and S. Y. Tan, "Santiago ramón y cajal (1852–1934): pride of petilla," *Singapore Medical Journal*, vol. 51, no. 9, pp. 683–684, 2010.

[9] W. R. Gowers, *The Borderland Of Epilepsy: Faints, Vagal Attacks, Vertigo, Migraine, Sleep Symptoms, and Their Treatment*, P. Blakiston's Son & Co, Philadelphia, Pa, USA, 1903.

[10] H. H. Dale, "The action of certain esters and ethers of choline and their relation to muscarine," *Journal of Pharmacology and Experimental Therapeutics*, vol. 6, pp. 147–190, 1914.

[11] O. Loewi, "Über humorale übertragbarkeit der herznervenwirkung," *Pflügers Archiv: European Journal of Physiology*, vol. 189, pp. 239–242, 1921.

[12] O. Loewi, "Über humorale Übertragbarkeit der Herznervenwirkung. II. Mitteilung," *Pflügers Archiv für die Gesamte Physiologie des Menschen und der Tiere*, vol. 193, pp. 201–213, 1921.

[13] O. Loewi and E. Navratil, "Über humorale Übertragbarkeit der Herznervenwirkung: X. Mitteilung. Über das Schicksal des Vagusstoffs," *Pflüger's Archiv für die Gesamte Physiologie*, vol. 214, no. 1, pp. 678–688, 1926.

[14] W. Lennox and S. Cobb, *Epilepsy from the Standpoint of Physiology and Treatment. Medicine Monograph XIV*, Williams and Wilkins, Baltimore, Maryland, USA, 1928.

[15] W. Lennox and S. Cobb, *Epilepsy*, Wiiliams & Wilkins, Baltimore, Md, USA, 1928.

[16] W. Lennox and S. Cobb, "The relation of certain physicochemical processes to epileptiform seizures," *The American Journal of Psychiatry*, vol. 85, pp. 837–847, 1929.

[17] H. Klüver and P. C. Bucy, "Preliminary analysis of functions of the temporal lobes in monkeys," *Journal of Neuropsychiatry and Clinical Neurosciences*, vol. 9, no. 4, pp. 606–620, 1997.

[18] H. Jasper and J. Kershmann, "Electroencepahlografic classification of the epilepsies," *Archives of Neurology & Psychiatry*, vol. 45, no. 6, pp. 903–943, 1941.

[19] G. Moruzzi and H. W. Magoun, "Brain stem reticular formation and activation of the EEG," *Electroencephalography and Clinical Neurophysiology*, vol. 1, no. 1–4, pp. 455–473, 1949.

[20] D. B. Lindsley, J. W. Bowden, and H. W. Magoun, "Effect upon the EEG of acute injury to the brain stem activating system," *Electroencephalography and Clinical Neurophysiology*, vol. 1, no. 1–4, pp. 475–486, 1949.

[21] T. E. Starzl, C. W. Taylor, and H. W. Magoun, "Ascending conduction in reticular activating system, with special reference to the diencephalon," *Journal of Neurophysiology*, vol. 14, no. 6, pp. 461–477, 1951.

[22] G. D. Dawson, "Investigations on a patient subject to myoclonic seizures after sensory," *Journal of Neurology, Neurosurgery, and Psychiatry*, vol. 10, no. 4, pp. 141–162, 1947.

[23] E. Roberts and S. Frankel, "Gamma-Aminobutyric acid in brain: its formation from glutamic acid," *The Journal of Biological Chemistry*, vol. 187, no. 1, pp. 55–63, 1950.

[24] J. C. Eccles, R. Schmidt, and W. D. Willis, "Pharmacological studies on presynaptic inhibition," *The Journal of physiology*, vol. 168, pp. 500–530, 1963.

[25] J. C. Eccles, *The Physiology of Synapses*, Springer, Berlin, Germany, 1964.

[26] E. R. Kandel and W. A. Spencer, "Electrophysiological properties of an archicortical neuron," *Annals of the New York Academy of Sciences*, vol. 94, pp. 570–603, 1961.

[27] E. R. Kandel and L. Tauc, "Mechanism of prolonged heterosynaptic facilitation," *Nature*, vol. 202, no. 4928, pp. 145–147, 1964.

[28] E. R. Kandel and L. Tauc, "Anomalous rectification in the metacerebral giant cells and its consequences for synaptic transmission," *Journal of Physiology*, vol. 183, no. 2, pp. 287–304, 1966.

[29] E. J. Speckmann and H. Caspers, "Shifts of cortical standing potential in hypoxia and asphyxia," *Electroencephalography and Clinical Neurophysiology*, vol. 23, no. 4, p. 379, 1967.

[30] E. Speckman and H. Caspers, "Shifts in the cortical potentials during changes in the ventilation rate," *Pflugers Archiv*, vol. 310, pp. 235–250, 1969.

[31] D. P. Purpura, "Analysis of axodendritic synaptic organizations in immature cerebral cortex," *Annals of the New York Academy of Sciences*, vol. 94, pp. 604–654, 1961.

[32] D. P. Purpura, "Functional organization of neurons," *Annals of the New York Academy of Sciences*, vol. 109, pp. 505–535, 1963.

[33] D. P. Purpura and H. Waelsch, "Brain reflexes," *Science*, vol. 143, no. 3606, pp. 598–604, 1964.

[34] E. M. Housepian and D. P. Purpura, "Electrophysiological studies of subcortical-cortical relations in man," *Electroencephalography and Clinical Neurophysiology*, vol. 15, no. 1, pp. 20–28, 1963.

[35] J. B. Brierley, A. W. Brown, B. J. Excell, and B. S. Meldrum, "Alterations in somatosensory evoked potentials and cerebral cortical damage produced by profound arterial hypotension in the Rhesus monkey," *Journal of Physiology*, vol. 196, no. 2, pp. 113P–114P, 1968.

[36] B. S. Meldrum and J. B. Brierley, "Brain damage in the rhesus monkey resulting from profound arterial hypotension. II. Changes in the spontaneous and evoked electrical activity of the neocortex," *Brain Research*, vol. 13, no. 1, pp. 101–118, 1969.

[37] J. B. Brierley, A. W. Brown, B. J. Excell, and B. S. Meldrum, "Brain damage in the rhesus monkey resulting from profound arterial hypotension. I. Its nature, distribution and general physiological correlates," *Brain Research*, vol. 13, no. 1, pp. 68–100, 1969.

[38] J. B. Brierley, B. S. Meldrum, and A. W. Brown, "The threshold and neuropathology of cerebral "anoxic ischemic" cell change," *Archives of Neurology*, vol. 29, no. 6, pp. 367–374, 1973.

[39] H. Gastaut, "Classification of the epilepsies. Proposal for an international classification," *Epilepsia*, vol. 10, pp. 14–21, 1969.

[40] H. Gastaut, "Clinical and electroencephalographical classification of epileptic seizures," *Epilepsia*, vol. 10, pp. 2–13, 1969.

[41] J. K. Penry, R. J. Porter, and F. E. Dreifuss, "Simultaneous recording of absence seizures with video tape and electroencephalography. A study of 374 seizures in 48 patients," *Brain*, vol. 98, no. 3, pp. 427–440, 1975.

[42] P. A. Schwartzkroin and D. A. Prince, "Cellular and field potential properties of epileptogenic hippocampal slices," *Brain Research*, vol. 147, no. 1, pp. 117–130, 1978.

[43] R. K. S. Wong and D. A. Prince, "Participation of calcium spikes during intrinsic burst firing in hippocampal neurons," *Brain Research*, vol. 159, no. 2, pp. 385–390, 1978.

[44] R. K. S. Wong and D. A. Prince, "Afterpotential generation in hippocampal pyramidal cells," *Journal of Neurophysiology*, vol. 45, no. 1, pp. 86–97, 1981.

[45] B. S. Meldrum and R. W. Horton, "Cerebral functional effects of 2-deoxy D-glucose and 3-O-methylglucose in rhesus monkeys," *Electroencephalography and Clinical Neurophysiology*, vol. 35, no. 1, pp. 59–66, 1973.

[46] B. S. Meldrum and R. W. Horton, "Physiology of status epilepticus in primates," *Archives of Neurology*, vol. 28, no. 1, pp. 1–9, 1973.

[47] B. S. Meldrum, R. A. Vigourous, and J. B. Brierley, "Systemic factors and epileptic brain damage: prolonged seizures in paralyzed, artificially ventilated baboons," *Archives of Neurology*, vol. 29, no. 2, pp. 82–87, 1973.

[48] C. R. Houser, J. E. Miyashiro, B. E. Swartz, G. O. Walsh, J. R. Rich, and A. V. Delgado-Escueta, "Altered patterns of dynorphin immunoreactivity suggest mossy fiber reorganization in human hippocampal epilepsy," *Journal of Neuroscience*, vol. 10, no. 1, pp. 267–282, 1990.

[49] T. Sutula, H. Xiao-Xian, J. Cavazos, and G. Scott, "Synaptic reorganization in the hippocampus induced by abnormal functional activity," *Science*, vol. 239, no. 4844, pp. 1147–1150, 1988.

[50] T. Sutula, G. Cascino, J. Cavazos, I. Parada, and L. Ramirez, "Mossy fiber synaptic reorganization in the epileptic human

temporal lobe," *Annals of Neurology*, vol. 26, no. 3, pp. 321–330, 1989.

[51] D. L. Tauck and J. V. Nadler, "Evidence of functional mossy fiber sprouting in hippocampal formation of kainic acid-treated rats," *Journal of Neuroscience*, vol. 5, no. 4, pp. 1016–1022, 1985.

[52] R. Caton, "The electric currents of the brain," *British Medical Journal*, vol. 2, p. 278, 1875.

[53] A. Beck, "Die Bestimmung der Localisationder Gehirn-und Rückenmarksfunctionen vermittelst der elektrischen Ersch einungen," *Zentralblatt für Physiologie*, vol. 4, pp. 473–476, 1890.

[54] P. Kaufman, "Electric phenomena in cerebral cortex," *Obz Psichiatr Nev Eksp Psikhol*, vol. 7–9, p. 403, 1912.

[55] V. Pravdich-Neminsky, "Ein Versuch der Registrierung der elektrischen Gehirnerscheinungen," *Zentralblatt für Physiologie*, vol. 27, pp. 951–960, 1913.

[56] N. Cybulski and X. Jelenska-Macieszyna, "Action currents of the cerebral cortex," *Bulletin of the Academy of Science Krakov*, pp. 776–781, 1914.

[57] H. Berger, "Über das Elektrenkephalogramm des Menschen," *Archiv für Psychiatrie und Nervenkrankheiten*, vol. 87, no. 1, pp. 527–570, 1929.

[58] E. D. Adrian and B. H. C. Matthews, "The berger rhythm: potential changes from the occipital lobes in man," *Brain*, vol. 57, no. 4, pp. 355–385, 1934.

[59] H. Berger, "Uber das Elektroenzephalogram des Menschen," *Archiv fur Psychiatrie und Nervenkrankheiten*, vol. 97, pp. 6–26, 1932.

[60] H. Berger, "Uber das Elektroenzephalogram des Menschen," *Archiv für Psychiatrie und Nervenkrankheiten*, vol. 100, pp. 301–320, 1933.

[61] F. Gibbs, H. Davis, and W. Lennox, "The electroencephalogram in epilepsy and in conditions of impaired consciousness," *Archives of Neurology and Psychiatry*, vol. 34, no. 6, pp. 1133–1148, 1935.

[62] F. Gibbs, W. Lennox, and E. Gibbs, "The electroencephalogram in diagnosis and in localization of epileptic seizures," *Archives of Neurology & Psychiatry*, vol. 36, no. 6, pp. 1225–1235, 1936.

[63] F. A. Gibbs, E. L. Gibbs, and W. G. Lennox, "Epilepsy: a paroxysmal cerebral dysrhythmia," *Brain*, vol. 60, no. 4, pp. 377–388, 1937.

[64] F. A. Gibbs and E. Gibbs, *Atlas of Electroencephalography*, Boston City Hospital, Oxford, UK, 1941.

[65] J. J. Cereghino, "The major advances in epilepsy in the 20th century and what we can expect (hope for) in the future," *Epilepsia*, vol. 50, no. 3, pp. 351–357, 2009.

[66] R. Naquet, "Henri gastaut (1915–1995)," *Electroencephalography and Clinical Neurophysiology*, vol. 98, no. 4, pp. 231–235, 1996.

[67] R. Naquet, "Tribute to Henri Gastaut (1915–1995)," *Neurophysiologie Clinique*, vol. 26, no. 3, pp. 170–176, 1996.

[68] H. Gastaut, "L'épilepsie photogénique," *La Revue du Praticien*, vol. 1, pp. 105–109, 1951.

[69] F. A. Gibbs, E. L. Gibbs, and W. G. Lennox, "Influence of blood sugar level on the wave and spike formation in petit mal epilepsy," *Archives of Neurology and Psychiatry*, vol. 41, pp. 1111–1116, 1939.

[70] H. Gastaut, M. Vigoroux, C. Trevisan et al., "Le syndrome "hémiconvulsion-hémiplégie-épilepsie (syndrome HHE)," *Revue Neurologique*, vol. 97, pp. 37–52, 1957.

[71] H. Gastaut and J. Corriol, "Preliminary notes on a new procedure especially effective in intermittent luminous stimulation," *Revue Neurologique*, vol. 83, no. 6, pp. 583–585, 1950.

[72] H. Gastaut, H. Terzian, R. Naquet, and K. Luschnat, "Correlations between automatism in temporal crises and electroencephalographic phenomena which accompany them," *Revue Neurologique*, vol. 86, no. 6, pp. 678–682, 1952.

[73] H. Gastaut and Y. Gastaut, "Electroencephalographic and clinical study of anoxic convulsions in children. Their location within the group of infantile convulsions and their differenciation from epilepsy," *Electroencephalography and Clinical Neurophysiology*, vol. 10, no. 4, pp. 607–620, 1958.

[74] K. Andermann, S. Berman, P. M. Cooke et al., "Self-induced epilepsy. A collection of self-induced epilepsy cases compared with some other photoconvulsive cases," *Archives of Neurology*, vol. 6, pp. 49–65, 1962.

[75] H. Gastaut, F. Poirier, H. Payan, G. Salamon, M. Toga, and M. Vigouroux, "H.H.E. syndrome hemiconvulsions, hemiplegia, epilepsy," *Epilepsia*, vol. 1, no. 1–5, pp. 418–447, 1959.

[76] H. Matsumoto and C. A. Marsan, "Cortical cellular phenomena in experimental epilepsy: ictal manifestations," *Experimental Neurology*, vol. 9, no. 4, pp. 305–326, 1964.

[77] H. Matsumoto and C. A. Marsan, "Cortical cellular phenomena in experimental epilepsy: interictal manifestations," *Experimental Neurology*, vol. 9, no. 4, pp. 286–304, 1964.

[78] D. A. Prince and K. J. Futamachi, "Intracellular recordings in chronic focal epilepsy," *Brain Research*, vol. 11, no. 3, pp. 681–684, 1968.

[79] D. A. Prince, "The depolarization shift in "epileptic" neurons," *Experimental Neurology*, vol. 21, no. 4, pp. 467–485, 1968.

[80] D. A. Prince, "Inhibition in "epileptic" neurons," *Experimental Neurology*, vol. 21, no. 3, pp. 307–321, 1968.

[81] M. A. Falconer, "The significance of mesial temporal sclerosis (Ammon's horn sclerosis) in epilepsy," *Guy's Hospital Reports*, vol. 117, no. 1, pp. 1–12, 1968.

[82] E. Neher, B. Sakmann, and J. H. Steinbach, "The extracellular patch clamp: a method for resolving currents through individual open channels in biological membranes," *Pflügers Archiv European Journal of Physiology*, vol. 375, no. 2, pp. 219–228, 1978.

[83] E. Neher, B. Sakmann, and J. H. Steinbach, "The extracellular patch clamp: a method for resolving currents through individual open channels in biological membranes," *Pflugers Archiv European Journal of Physiology*, vol. 375, no. 2, pp. 219–228, 1978.

[84] A. Stefani, F. Spadoni, and G. Bernardi, "Voltage-activated calcium channels: targets of antiepileptic drug therapy?" *Epilepsia*, vol. 38, no. 9, pp. 959–965, 1997.

[85] D. M. Long, "Harvey cushing at johns hopkins," *Neurosurgery*, vol. 45, no. 5, pp. 983–989, 1999.

[86] G. Hildebrandt, W. Surbeck, and M. N. Stienen, "Emil Theodor Kocher: the first Swiss neurosurgeon," *Acta Neurochirurgica*, vol. 154, no. 6, pp. 1105–1115, 2012.

[87] S. V. Horsley, "Brain surgery," *British Medical Journal*, vol. 2, pp. 670–675, 1886.

[88] F. Krause, *Surgery of the Brain and Spinal Cord-Based on Personal Experiences*, vol. 3, Rebman, New York, NY, USA, 1912.

[89] O. Foerster, "Zur operativen Behandlung der Epilepsie," *Deutsche Zeitschrift für Nervenheilkunde*, vol. 89, no. 1–3, pp. 137–147, 1926.

[90] W. E. Dandy, "Removal of right cerebral hemisphere for certain tumors with hemiplegia," *The Journal of the American Medical Association*, vol. 90, pp. 823–825, 1928.

[91] B. P. Hermann and J. L. Stone, "A historical review of the epilepsy surgery program at the University of Illinois Medical Center:

the contributions of Bailey, Gibbs, and Collaborators to the refinement of anterior temporal lobectomy," *Journal of Epilepsy*, vol. 2, no. 3, pp. 155–163, 1989.

[92] W. Penfield and H. H. Jasper, "Heighest level seizures," *Research Publications-Association for Research in Nervous and Mental Disease*, vol. 26, p. 252, 1947.

[93] W. Penfield and H. Jasper, *Epilepsy and the Functional Anatomy of the Human Brain*, Little, Brown, Boston, Mass, USA, 1954.

[94] W. Penfield and H. Steelman, "The treatment of focal epilepsy by cortical excision," *Annals of Surgery*, vol. 126, no. 5, pp. 740–762, 1947.

[95] W. Penfield and H. Flanigin, "Surgical therapy of temporal lobe seizures," *A. M. A. Archives of Neurology and Psychiatry*, vol. 64, no. 4, pp. 491–500, 1950.

[96] W. Penfield and M. Baldwin, "Temporal lobe seizures and the technic of subtotal temporal lobectomy," *Annals of surgery*, vol. 136, no. 4, pp. 625–634, 1952.

[97] W. P. van Wagenen and R. Y. Herren, "Surgical division of commisural pathways in the corpus callosum. Relation to spread of an epileptic attack," *Archives of Neurology & Psychiatry*, vol. 44, pp. 740–759, 1940.

[98] P. Bailey and F. A. Gibbs, "The surgical treatment of psychomotor epilepsy," *The Journal of the American Medical Association*, vol. 145, no. 6, pp. 365–370, 1951.

[99] K. G. Mckenzie, "The present status of a patient who had the right cerebral hemisphere removed," *Proceedings of the American Medical Association*, vol. 111, p. 168, 1938.

[100] R. A. Krynauw, "Infantile hemiplegia treated by removing one cerebral hemisphere," *Journal of Neurology, Neurosurgery & Psychiatry*, vol. 13, no. 4, pp. 243–267, 1950.

[101] M. A. Falconer, D. A. Pond, A. Meyer et al., "Temporal lobe epilepsy with personality and behaviour disorders caused by an unusual calcifying lesion; report of two cases in children relieved by temporal lobectomy," *Journal of Neurology, Neurosurgery & Psychiatry*, vol. 16, no. 4, pp. 234–244, 1953.

[102] J. H. Margerison and J. A. N. Corsellis, "Epilepsy and the temporal lobes: a clinical, electroencephalographic and neuropathological study of the brain in epilepsy, with particular reference to the temporal lobes," *Brain*, vol. 89, no. 3, pp. 499–530, 1966.

[103] W. Sommer, "Erkrankung des Ammonshorns als aetiologisches Moment der Epilepsie," *Archiv für Psychiatrie und Nervenkrankheiten*, vol. 10, no. 3, pp. 631–675, 1880.

[104] P. Niemeyer, "The transventricular amygdalohippocampectomy," in *Temporal Lobe Epilepsy*, M. Baldwin and P. Bailey, Eds., pp. 565–581, Raven Press, 1958.

[105] J. Tailarach, M. David, P. Tournoux et al., *Atlas d'Anatomie Stéréotactique des Noyaux Gris Centraux*, Masson, Paris, France, 1957.

[106] P. Chauvel, *Contributions of Jean Tailarach and Jean Bancaud to Epilepsy Surgery*, Lippincott Williams & Wilkins, Philadelphia, Pa, USA, 2001.

[107] J. E. Bogen and P. J. Vogel, "Treatment of Generalized Seizures by Cerebral Commissurotomy," *Surgical Forum*, vol. 14, pp. 431–433, 1963.

[108] H. H. White, "Cerebral hemispherectomy in the treatment of infantile hemiplegia; review of the literature and report of two cases," *Confinia Neurologica*, vol. 21, pp. 1–50, 1961.

[109] H. G. Wieser and M. G. Yasargil, "Selective amygdalohippocampectomy as a surgical treatment of mesiobasal limbic epilepsy," *Surgical Neurology*, vol. 17, no. 6, pp. 445–457, 1982.

[110] C. Locock, "Analysis of fifty-two cases of epilepsy observed by the author," *The Lancet*, vol. 70, pp. 527–529, 1857.

[111] A. Hauptmann, "Luminal bei Epilepsie," *Munchen Med Wochenschr*, vol. 59, pp. 1907–1909, 1912.

[112] H. Merrit and T. Putnam, "A new series of anticonvulsant drugs tested by experiments in animals," *Archives of Neurology & Psychiatry*, vol. 39, no. 5, pp. 1003–1015, 1938.

[113] H. Merrit and T. Putnam, "Sodium diphenyl hydantoinate in the treatment of convulsive disorders," *JAMA*, vol. 111, no. 12, pp. 1068–1073, 1938.

[114] H. Merrit and T. Putnam, "Sodium diphenyl hydantoinate in the treatment of convulsive seizures. Toxic symptoms and their prevention," *Archives of Neurology & Psychiatry*, vol. 42, no. 6, pp. 1053–1058, 1939.

[115] H. Merrit and T. Putnam, "Further experiences with the use of sodium diphenyl hydantoinate in the treatment of convulsive disorders," *American Journal of Psychiatry*, vol. 96, no. 5, pp. 1023–1027, 1940.

[116] R. K. Richards and G. M. Everett, "Tridione: a new anticonvulsant drug," *The Journal of Laboratory and Clinical Medicine*, vol. 31, no. 12, pp. 1330–1336, 1946.

[117] W. Schindler and H. Blattner, "Über derivative des iminodibenzyls Iminostilben-Derivative," *Helvetica Chimica Acta*, vol. 44, no. 3, pp. 562–753, 1961.

[118] R. Vossen, "Uber die antikonvulsive Wirking von Succinimiden," *Deutsche Medizinische Wochenschrift*, vol. 83, pp. 1227–1230, 1958.

[119] H. Meunier, G. Carraz, Y. Meunier et al., "Propriétés pharmacodynamiques de l'acide n-dipropylacetique," *Therapie*, vol. 18, pp. 435–438, 1963.

[120] F. Buchtal and O. Svensmark, "Aspects of the pharmacology of phenytoin (dilantin) and phenobarbital relevant to their dosage in the treatment of epilepsy," *Epilepsia*, vol. 1, pp. 373–384, 1960.

[121] S. Blom, "Trigeminal neuralgia: its treatment with a new anticonvulsant drug (G-32883)," *The Lancet*, vol. 1, no. 7234, pp. 839–840, 1962.

[122] M. Bonduelle, P. Bouygues, B. Jolivet et al., "Automatisms of long duration and epileptic fugues in adults," *Annales Médico-Psychologiques*, vol. 122, pp. 169–174, 1964.

[123] M. Lorge, "Klinische Erfahrungen mit einem neuen Antiepilepticum, Tegretol (G 32 883) mit besonderer Wirkung auf die epileptische Wesenveränderung," *Schweizerische Medizinische Wochenschrift*, vol. 93, pp. 1042–1047, 1963.

[124] E. J. Fertig and R. H. Mattson, "Mattson: carbamazepine," in *Epilepsy: A Comprehensive Textbook*, J. Engel and T. A. Pedley, Eds., pp. 1543–1556, Lippincott Williams & Wilkins, Philadelphia, Pa, USA, 2007.

[125] S. D. Shorvon, "Drug treatment of epilepsy in the century of the ILAE: the second 50 years, 1959–2009," *Epilepsia*, vol. 50, supplement 3, pp. 93–130, 2009.

[126] P. J. Loiseau, "Clinical experience with new antiepileptic drugs: antiepileptic drugs in Europe," *Epilepsia*, vol. 40, no. 6, pp. S3–S8, 1999.

[127] D. M. Woodbury, J. K. Penry, and R. P. Schmidt, *Antiepileptic Drugs*, Raven Press, New York, NY, USA, 1972.

[128] M. J. Painter, C. Pippenger, H. MacDonald, and W. Pitlick, "Phenobarbital and diphenylhydantoin levels in neonates with seizures," *Journal of Pediatrics*, vol. 92, no. 2, pp. 315–319, 1978.

[129] C. Elger, P. Halász, J. Maia, L. Almeida, and P. Soares-Da-Silva, "Efficacy and safety of eslicarbazepine acetate as adjunctive

treatment in adults with refractory partial-onset seizures: a randomized, double-blind, placebo-controlled, parallel-group phase III study," *Epilepsia*, vol. 50, no. 3, pp. 454–463, 2009.

[130] A. Hufnagel, E. Ben-Menachem, A. A. Gabbai, A. Falcão, L. Almeida, and P. Soares-da-Silva, "Long-term safety and efficacy of eslicarbazepine acetate as adjunctive therapy in the treatment of partial-onset seizures in adults with epilepsy: results of a 1-year open-label extension study," *Epilepsy Research*, vol. 103, no. 2-3, pp. 262–269, 2013.

[131] A. Gil-Nagel, C. Elger, E. Ben-Menachem et al., "Efficacy and safety of eslicarbazepine acetate as add-on treatment in patients with focal-onset seizures: integrated analysis of pooled data from double-blind phase III clinical studies," *Epilepsia*, vol. 54, no. 1, pp. 98–107, 2013.

[132] A. Gil-Nagel, J. Lopes-Lima, L. Almeida, J. Maia, and P. Soares-Da-Silva, "Efficacy and safety of 800 and 1200 mg eslicarbazepine acetate as adjunctive treatment in adults with refractory partial-onset seizures," *Acta Neurologica Scandinavica*, vol. 120, no. 5, pp. 281–287, 2009.

[133] M. J. Brodie, H. Lerche, A. Gil-Nagel et al., "Efficacy and safety of adjunctive ezogabine (retigabine) in refractory partial epilepsy," *Neurology*, vol. 75, no. 20, pp. 1817–1824, 2010.

[134] M. J. Brodie, J. A. French, S. A. Mcdonald et al., "Adjunctive use of ezogabine/retigabine with either traditional sodium channel blocking antiepileptic drugs (AEDs) or AEDs with other mechanisms of action: evaluation of efficacy and tolerability," *Epilepsy Research*, vol. 108, no. 5, pp. 989–994, 2014.

[135] V. Biton, A. Gil-Nagel, M. J. Brodie, S. E. Derossett, and V. Nohria, "Safety and tolerability of different titration rates of retigabine (ezogabine) in patients with partial-onset seizures," *Epilepsy Research*, vol. 107, no. 1-2, pp. 138–145, 2013.

[136] A. Gil-Nagel, M. J. Brodie, R. Leroy et al., "Safety and efficacy of ezogabine (retigabine) in adults with refractory partial-onset seizures: interim results from two ongoing open-label studies," *Epilepsy Research*, vol. 102, no. 1-2, pp. 117–121, 2012.

[137] G. Guelpa and A. Marie, "La lutte contrel epilepsie parlade's intoxication et par la re education alimentaire," *Revue de Therapie Medico-Chirurgicale*, vol. 18, pp. 8–13, 1911.

[138] Hippocrates, J. Chadwick, and W. N. Mann, Eds., *The Sacred Disease*, Blackwell, 1950.

[139] M. G. Peterman, "The ketogenic diet in epilepsy," *The Journal of the American Medical Association*, vol. 84, no. 26, pp. 1979–1983, 1925.

[140] P. R. Huttenlocher, A. J. Wilbourn, and J. M. Signore, "Medium-chain triglycerides as a therapy for intractable childhood epilepsy," *Neurology*, vol. 21, no. 11, pp. 1097–1103, 1971.

[141] F. B. Talbot, "The ketogenic diet in epilepsy," *Bulletin of the New York Academy of Medicine*, vol. 4, pp. 401–408, 1927.

[142] H. F. Helmholz, "The treatment of epilepsy in childhood: five years' experience with the ketogenic diet," *The Journal of the American Medical Association*, vol. 88, pp. 218–225, 1927.

[143] W. G. Lennox, "Ketogenic diet in the treatment of epilepsy," *The New England Journal of Medicine*, vol. 199, pp. 74–75, 1928.

[144] E. M. Bridge and L. V. Iob, "The mechanism of the ketogenic diet in epilepsy," *Bull Johns Hopkins Hosp*, vol. 48, pp. 373–389, 1931.

[145] H. W. Welch, F. J. Goodnow, S. Flexner et al., "Memorial meeting for Dr. John Howland," *Bulletin of the Johns Hopkins Hospital*, vol. 41, pp. 311–321, 1927.

[146] T. D. Swink, E. P. Vining, and J. M. Freeman, "The ketogenic diet: 1997," *Advances in Pediatrics*, vol. 44, pp. 297–329, 1997.

[147] L. Wilkins, "Epilepsy in childhood. III. Results with the ketogenic diet," *The Journal of Pediatrics*, vol. 10, no. 3, pp. 341–357, 1937.

[148] S. Livingston, "The ketogenic diet in the treatment of epilepsy in children," *Postgraduate Medicine*, vol. 10, no. 4, pp. 333–336, 1951.

[149] I. J. Hopkins and B. C. Lynch, "Use of ketogenic diet in epilepsy in childhood," *Australian Paediatric Journal*, vol. 6, no. 1, pp. 25–29, 1970.

[150] I. J. Hopkins and B. C. Lynch, "Use of the ketogenic diet in epilepsy in childhood," *Proceedings of the Australian Association of Neurologists*, vol. 7, pp. 25–30, 1970.

[151] P. R. Huttenlocher, "Ketonemia and seizures: metabolic and anticonvulsant effects of two ketogenic diets in childhood epilepsy," *Pediatric Research*, vol. 10, no. 5, pp. 536–540, 1976.

[152] E. H. Kossoff, B. J. Henry, and M. C. Cervenka, "Transitioning pediatric patients receiving ketogenic diets for epilepsy into adulthood," *Seizure*, vol. 22, no. 6, pp. 487–489, 2013.

[153] M. M. Vaccarezza, M. V. Toma, J. D. R. Guevara et al., "Treatment of refractory epilepsy with the modified Atkins diet," *Archivos Argentinos de Pediatria*, vol. 112, no. 4, pp. 348–351, 2014.

[154] S. C. Schachter and C. B. Saper, "Vagus nerve stimulation," *Epilepsia*, vol. 39, no. 7, pp. 677–686, 1998.

[155] V. Ricotti and N. Delanty, "Use of complementary and alternative medicine in epilepsy," *Current Neurology and Neuroscience Reports*, vol. 6, no. 4, pp. 347–353, 2006.

[156] G. Mathern, A. Nehlig, and M. Sperling, "Cannabidiol and medical marijuana for the treatment of epilepsy," *Epilepsia*, vol. 55, no. 6, pp. 781–782, 2014.

[157] W. Letchworth, "Transactions of the National Association for the Study for the of Epilepsy at the Annual Meeting Held in Washington, DC, USA, May 14th and 15th, 1901," CE Brinkworth, Buffalo, New York, 1901.

[158] E. J. Fine, D. L. Fine, L. Sentz, and E. D. Soria, "Contributions of the founders of Craig Colony to epileptology and public care of epileptics: 1890–1915," *Journal of the History of the Neurosciences*, vol. 4, no. 2, pp. 77–100, 1995.

[159] Association for Research in Nervous and Mental Disease, Ed., *Epilepsy: Proceedings of the Association Held Jointly with the International League Against Epilepsy*, Williams & Wilkins, 1946.

[160] M. Baldwin and P. Bailey, *Temporal Lobe Epilepsy*, Charles C. Thomas, Springfield, Ill, USA, 1958.

[161] J. K. Merlis, "Proposal for an international classification of the epilepsies," *Epilepsia*, vol. 11, no. 1, pp. 114–119, 1970.

[162] F. E. Dreifuss, J. Bancaud, and O. Henriksen, "Proposal for revised clinical and electroencephalographic classification of epileptic seizures," *Epilepsia*, vol. 22, no. 4, pp. 489–501, 1981.

[163] "Proposal for revised classification of epilepsies and epileptic syndromes. Commission on classification and terminology of the international league against epilepsy," *Epilepsia*, vol. 30, no. 4, pp. 389–399, 1989.

[164] F. E. Dreifuss, M. Martinez-Lage, and J. Roger, "Proposal for classification of epilepsies and epileptic syndromes," *Epilepsia*, vol. 26, no. 3, pp. 268–278, 1985.

[165] "Guidelines for epidemiologic studies on epilepsy. Commission on Epidemiology and Prognosis, International League Against Epilepsy," *Epilepsia*, vol. 34, no. 4, pp. 592–596, 1993.

[166] Jr. Engel J., "Classification of epileptic disorders," *Epilepsia*, vol. 42, no. 3, p. 316, 2001.

[167] J. Engel Jr., "Report of the ILAE classification core group," *Epilepsia*, vol. 47, no. 9, pp. 1558–1568, 2006.

[168] A. T. Berg, S. F. Berkovic, M. J. Brodie et al., "Revised terminology and concepts for organization of seizures and epilepsies: report of the ILAE Commission on Classification and Terminology, 2005–2009," *Epilepsia*, vol. 51, no. 4, pp. 676–685, 2010.

[169] A. T. Berg and I. E. Scheffer, "New concepts in classification of the epilepsies: entering the 21st century," *Epilepsia*, vol. 52, no. 6, pp. 1058–1062, 2011.

[170] W. E. Dandy, "Ventriculography following the injection of air into the cerebral ventricles," *American Journal of Roentgenology*, vol. 68, no. 1, pp. 5–11, 1918.

[171] W. E. Dandy, "Ventriculography following the injection of air into the cerebral ventricles," *The American Journal of Roentgenology*, vol. 6, pp. 26–36, 1919.

[172] W. E. Dandy, "Rontgenography of the brain after the injection of air into the spinal canal," *Annals of Surgery*, vol. 70, no. 4, pp. 397–403, 1919.

[173] G. W. Friedland and B. D. Thurber, "The birth of CT," *American Journal of Roentgenology*, vol. 168, no. 6, p. 1622, 1996.

[174] M. Reivich, D. Kuhl, and A. Wolf, "Measurement of local cerebral glucose metabolism in man with 18F-2-fluoro-2-deoxy-d-glucose," *Acta Neurologica Scandinavica*, vol. 64, pp. 190–191, 1977.

[175] M. Reivich, D. Kuhl, A. Wolf et al., "The [18F]fluorodeoxy-glucose method for the measurement of local cerebral glucose utilization in man," *Circulation Research*, vol. 44, no. 1, pp. 127–137, 1979.

[176] J. S. Duncan and J. de Tisi, "MRI in the diagnosis and management of epileptomas," *Epilepsia*, vol. 54, supplement 9, pp. 40–43, 2013.

[177] G. Oz, J. R. Alger, P. B. Barker et al., "Clinical proton MR spectroscopy in central nervous system disorders," *Radiology*, vol. 270, no. 3, pp. 658–679, 2014.

[178] H. Kim, C. K. Chung, and H. Hwang, "Magnetoencephalography in pediatric epilepsy," *Korean Journal of Pediatrics*, vol. 56, no. 10, pp. 431–438, 2013.

[179] H. Lundborg, *Die progressive Myoklonus-Epilepsy (Unverricht's Myoklonie)*, Almqvist & Wiksell, Uppsala, Sweden, 1903.

[180] A. Myerson, J. Ayer, T. Putnam et al., *Eugenical sterilization- a reorientation of the problem. By the Committee of the American Neurological Association for the Investigation of Eugenical Sterilzation*, Macmillan, New York, NY, USA, 1936.

[181] M. Leppert, V. E. Anderson, T. Quattlebaum et al., "Benign familial neonatal convulsions linked to genetic markers on chromosome 20," *Nature*, vol. 337, no. 6208, pp. 647–648, 1989.

[182] S. Baulac and M. Baulac, "Advances on the genetics of Mendelian idiopathic epilepsies," *Clinics in Laboratory Medicine*, vol. 30, no. 4, pp. 911–929, 2010.

12

Neuromodulation Therapy with Vagus Nerve Stimulation for Intractable Epilepsy: A 2-Year Efficacy Analysis Study in Patients under 12 Years of Age

Suresh Gurbani,[1,2] Sirichai Chayasirisobhon,[1] Leslie Cahan,[1] SooHo Choi,[1] Bruce Enos,[1] Jane Hwang,[1] Meei Lin,[1] and Jeffrey Schweitzer[1]

[1]Comprehensive Epilepsy Program, Southern California Permacothe Medical Group, CA, USA
[2]Department of Neurology, Kaiser Permacothe Medical Center, Suite No. 208, 3460 E. La Palma Avenue, Anaheim, CA 92806, USA

Correspondence should be addressed to Suresh Gurbani; suresh.g.gurbani@kp.org

Academic Editor: József Janszky

To study the efficacy of vagus nerve stimulation (VNS) therapy as an adjunctive treatment for intractable epilepsy in patients under 12 years of age, we analyzed 2-year postimplant data of 35 consecutive patients. Of the 35 patients, 18 (51.4%) at 6 months, 18 (51.4%) at 12 months, and 21 (60.1%) at 24 months showed ≥50% reduction in seizure frequency (responders). Although incremental seizure freedom was noted, no patient remained seizure-free throughout the 3 study periods. Partial response (≥50% seizure reduction in 2 or less study periods) was seen in 8 (22.9%) patients. Twelve patients (34.3%) were nonresponders. Out of 29 patients with primary generalized epilepsy, 20 (68.9%) and, out of 6 patients with focal epilepsy, 3 (50%) had ≥50% seizure control in at least one study period. No major complications or side effects requiring discontinuation of VNS therapy were encountered. We conclude that (1) patients with intractable primary generalized epilepsy respond better to VNS therapy, (2) cumulative effect of neuromodulation with improving responder rate to seizure freedom with continuation of VNS therapy is noted, and (3) VNS therapy is safe and is well tolerated in children receiving implant under 12 years of age.

1. Introduction

Neuromodulation therapies are nonpharmacotherapeutic options for patients with drug resistant epilepsy who are not candidates for resective epilepsy surgery. In 1997, the US Food and Drug Administration (FDA) approved vagus nerve stimulation (VNS) implant as adjunctive therapy for reducing the frequency of seizures in patients >12 years of age with partial-onset seizures refractory to antiepileptic drugs (AEDs) [1].

Initial studies with randomized controlled trials reporting on the efficacy of VNS involved rather short follow-up duration (3 months to 3.5 months) and ≥50% seizure reduction ranged from 23.4% to 39% of the patients [2–5]. Since 1999, several studies have reported long-term follow-up ranging from 6 months to 10 years with ≥50% seizure reduction observed in 35% to 63.8% of the patients [6–22].

Literature search identified 16 studies regarding the efficacy of VNS in children [17, 18, 23–36]. However, most of these studies did not truly reflect the efficacy of VNS therapy in children <12 years old as they included older patients as well. Ten of the 16 studies included subjects through 18 years of age, and one each included subjects up to 19, 20, 21, and 25 years of age. One study of 11 patients with tuberous sclerosis had a mean age of 14 years with a range from 2 to 35 years [23]. In this study, we report long-term (2 years) observation on the efficacy and the safety of VNS in epileptic patients <12 years of age.

2. Methods

Ours is a prospectively collected data analysis retrospective study. All patients with epilepsy being treated at our center maintain daily seizure diary which is entered in the electronic database during follow-up visits. All patients with recalcitrant epilepsy undergo long-term video EEG monitoring and neuroimaging studies including MRI brain examination and are presented at Kaiser multidisciplinary epilepsy surgery case conference to discuss alternate nonpharmacotherapeutic treatment options. A total of 160 patients with drug resistant epilepsy (failed at least 3 AEDs at adequate doses appropriate for the type of epilepsy) who were not candidates for resective surgery received VNS implant from September 1998 to December 2011, 35 of whom were <12 years of age at the time of implant. VNS device from Cyberonics was implanted by our neurosurgeons who had received the required training.

To allow wound healing, the VNS implant was not activated until one week postoperatively. Output current was gradually increased in 0.25 mA increments once per week at six weekly visits, then at six subsequent biweekly visits, and then at each of three monthly visits to the clinic. After an informed decision by the parents, type of VNS cycling (standard versus rapid) and parameters were selected by the treating pediatric epileptologist. For standard cycling, the signal on-time was ≥30 seconds and signal off-time ranged from 3 to 5 minutes. For rapid cycling, signal on-time was ≤21 seconds and signal off-time ranged from 0.2 to 1.8 minutes. Rapid cycling was initiated with the parameters of 7 seconds on-time and 0.2 minutes off-time. Output current was adjusted depending on the patient's tolerance to the electrical stimulation and seizure control. Maximum output current used was 3.0 mA for rapid cycling and 3.5 mA for standard cycling. Ongoing AED regimen (dosing regimen and if needed AED) was adjusted as clinically warranted.

The efficacy of VNS therapy was analyzed by comparing the mean seizure frequency (prior 8-week period) at baseline (at VNS implant) to that at 6-month, 12-month, and 24-month postimplant study points. We defined the efficacy of VNS therapy as follows: (1) responders: ≥50% reduction of seizures in all three study periods, (2) partial responders: ≥50% reduction of seizures in 2 or less study periods, and (3) nonresponders: <50% response and/or worsening seizure control in all 3 study periods. Efficacy of standard versus rapid cycling therapy parameters was also studied. We analyzed the efficacy of VNS therapy according to the type of epilepsies as well. We also assessed for postoperative adverse events, side effects, and tolerability of both the surgical implantation procedure and the VNS device.

3. Results

Thirty-five patients (23 males, 12 females) with age ranging from 5 years to 12 years (mean age, 7.79 ± 2.65 years) met the selection criteria. Clinical characteristics for the patients at baseline are summarized in Table 1. Mean age of onset of epilepsy was 1.25 ± 1.55 years. Mean duration of epilepsy before the VNS implant was 6.67 ± 2.95 years. Mean number of AEDs at baseline was 2.5. Mean output current setting was 1.9 ± 0.7 mA at 6 months, 2.3 ± 0.7 mA at 12 months, and 2.5 ± 0.7 mA at 24 months. Of the 35 patients, 18 (51.4%) at 6

TABLE 1: Clinical data of patients at baseline.

(A) Epilepsy and seizure types	
Generalized tonic-clonic	9 patients
Absence atypical	5 patients
Tonic	3 patients
Myoclonic	1 patient
Atonic	1 patient
Focal with secondary generalized tonic-clonic	4 patients
Focal with dyscognitive features	2 patients
Mixed	10 patients
(B) Etiology	
Lennox-Gastaut syndrome	13 patients
Postencephalitis	5 patients
Cortical dysgenesis	4 patients
Postanoxic encephalopathy	3 patients
Idiopathic	3 patients
Tuberous sclerosis	3 patients
Chromosomal abnormality	2 patients
Stroke	2 patients

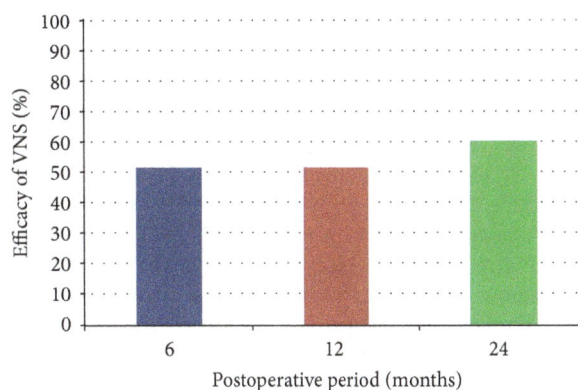

FIGURE 1: Efficacy of VNS (≥50% reduction in seizure frequency) at 3 study periods.

months, 18 (51.4%) at 12 months, and 21 (60.1%) at 24 months showed ≥50% reduction in seizure frequency (Figure 1).

Although, among the responders, a complete (100%) seizure control was seen in 4 of 18 patients (22.2%) at 6-month, 5 of 18 patients (27.8%) at 12-month, and 7 of 21 patients (33.3%) at 24-month follow-up period, no single patient remained seizure-free throughout the 3 study periods. A total of 15 (42.9%) patients had ≥50% reduction in seizure frequency in all three periods and a partial response was seen in 8 (22.8%) more patients. Twelve patients (34.3%) showed no clinically significant benefit in all three periods (Table 2).

For the 22 patients who were treated with rapid cycle of VNS, the output current ranged from 0.75 mA to 3 mA and pulse width from 125 microseconds to 250 microseconds, with signal on-time set at 7 seconds to 14 seconds and signal off-time ranging from 0.5 minutes to 1.1 minutes. Seizure frequency reduction of ≥50% was seen in 11 of 22 patients (50%) at 6-month, 11 of 22 patients (50%) at 12-month, and

TABLE 2: The efficacy of VNS with ≥50% reduction of seizures for all patients at 6 months, 12 months, and 24 months.

Study period	Number of patients	Percent
At 6 months, 12 months, and 24 months	15	42.9
At 6 months	2	5.7
At 6 months and 24 months	1	2.8
At 12 months and 24 months	3	8.6
At 24 months	2	5.7
No response	12	34.3

12 of 22 patients (54.5%) at 24-month follow-up period. The remaining 13 patients were treated with the standard cycle of VNS with output current ranging from 0.75 mA to 3.5 mA and pulse width from 250 microseconds to 500 microseconds, with signal on-time of 30 seconds and signal off-time from 3 minutes to 5 minutes. Seizure frequency reduction of ≥50% was seen in 7 of 13 patients (53.8%) at 6-month, 6 of 13 patients (46.2%) at 12-month, and 9 of 13 patients (69.2%) at 24-month follow-up period.

The efficacy of VNS according to the etiologies of epilepsy is shown in Table 3 and according to the seizure types in Table 4. During the study period 25 patients had a single type of seizures, 6 patients had 2 types of seizures, and 4 patients had 3 types of seizures. Out of 35 patients, 29 (82.9%) had primary generalized epilepsy and 6 (17.1%) had focal epilepsy. Twenty patients (68.9%) with primary generalized epilepsy and 3 patients (50%) with focal epilepsy had ≥50% reduction in seizure frequency. Best responders were patients with primary generalized epilepsy with tonic-clonic seizures followed by primary generalized epilepsy with atypical absence seizures.

Cough and pharyngeal paresthesia commonly occurred during initial application or ramming up of output current. These adverse events were successfully managed by adjusting the parameters. No side effects necessitating discontinuation of VNS therapy were encountered.

4. Discussion

VNS therapy has been approved as adjunctive treatment for drug resistant focal epilepsy in patients >12 years of age [1]. However, as drug resistant epilepsies in pediatric population are also an unconquered challenge despite availability of second and third generation AEDs and as the epilepsy treatment goal remains seizure freedom, VNS therapy has been used in patients <12 years of age as well. Many researchers have reported the efficacy of VNS for treatment of epilepsy in children [17, 18, 23–36]. Among these 16 studies, ten studies included subjects through 18 years of age, and one each included subjects up to 19, 20, 21, and 25 years of age. One study of 11 patients with tuberous sclerosis had a mean age of 14 years with a range from 2 to 35 years [23]. Our study reports the efficacy and safety of VNS therapy in a group of 35 epileptic patients <12 years of age.

Similar to the observations of prior VNS studies, with increasing duration of VNS therapy, a trend towards improving responder rate and seizure freedom was noted in our study as well [37–39]. The exact mechanism for the improving efficacy of VNS with increasing duration of therapy is not fully understood. Chronic therapeutic response to VNS therapy is highly correlated with bilateral thalamic increases in synaptic activity [40]. During chronic VNS therapy, brain excitatory amino acid neurotransmitter levels are reduced and inhibitory neurotransmitter levels are increased but no direct relationship to seizure control has been noted [40].

Optimal parameter settings for VNS therapy are not yet well defined. In current study, both rapid and standard cycle settings of VNS parameters were used. Patients who were treated with rapid cycling showed ≥50% reduction of seizure frequency in all three periods while those treated with standard cycling showed ≥50% reduction of seizure at 6-month and 24-month periods. Both rapid cycling and standard cycling demonstrated the cumulative seizure response to VNS therapy at 24-month period. The comparison of the efficacy between rapid cycling and standard cycling was not conclusive. Our previous study in 39 patients (age ranging from 5 to 72 years) demonstrated a trend towards greater seizure frequency reduction in patients with rapid cycle than standard cycle parameters. It also showed that when compared to adult patients, the response to rapid cycle in pediatric patients was greater [41]. However, a 2-year follow-up study has reported greater overall seizure frequency reduction with the standard cycle than the rapid cycle [12]. Other studies did not show any difference in responder rate with either cycle [24, 29]. More research with larger population is recommended to study this further.

In our study, VNS therapy was effective in both focal epilepsy and some types of generalized epilepsy. VNS therapy has been reported to be effective in patients with Lennox-Gastaut syndrome [27, 29, 30] and tuberous sclerosis complex [36, 37]. In our study, VNS therapy was effective in achieving ≥50% reduction in seizure in patients with Lennox-Gastaut syndrome, encephalitis, cortical dysgenesis, perinatal encephalopathy, and tuberous sclerosis complex. Best responders were patients with primary generalized epilepsy with tonic-clonic seizures followed by primary generalized epilepsy with atypical absence seizures. Small sample size did not permit statistical analysis by seizure types and etiologies.

Our patients tolerated the VNS implantation well. There was no serious wound infection requiring explantation. No major complications or side effects requiring discontinuation of VNS therapy occurred during the 2-year study period.

Patients included in this study were offered VNS as an adjunctive treatment modality to ongoing antiepilepsy medication regimen and not after failing most available antiepilepsy medications. Therefore, change in the dosing regimen and, if needed, in the antiepilepsy medications used (which is a limitation of this study) was done per the choice of the treating physician. As many more AED choices (second and third generation AEDs) are available now, with a small study subject size it was not possible to comment on synergism of any specific AED mechanism of action being responsible for the seizure control noted after VNS implant.

TABLE 3: The efficacy of VNS with ≥50% reduction of seizures according to the etiologies of epilepsy.

Etiology (patients)	Responders	Partial responders	Nonresponders
Lennox-Gastaut syndrome (13)	38.5%	23.0%	38.5%
Postencephalitis (5)	20.0%	40.0%	40.0%
Cortical dysgenesis (4)	75.0%	0%	25.0%
Postanoxic encephalopathy (3)	33.3%	0%	66.7%
Perinatal encephalopathy (3)	66.7%	0%	33.3%
Tuberous sclerosis (3)	50.0%	50.0%	0%
Chromosomal abnormality (2)	50.0%	0%	50.0%
Stroke (2)	50.0%	50.0%	0%

TABLE 4: Number of patients with ≥50% reduction of seizures according to the seizure types during 3 study periods.

Seizure type (# at baseline)	6 months	12 months	24 months
Generalized tonic-clonic (16)	10	11	11
Absence atypical (8)	6	5	5
Tonic (8)	4	4	4
Myoclonic (4)	3	1	0
Atonic (5)	2	3	2
Focal with generalized tonic-clonic (4)	0	2	2
Focal with dyscognitive features (2)	1	1	1

Many studies have reported lack of improvement in responder rate after failing 2 appropriate AEDs [1]. All the patients in the current study had failed at least 3 AEDs in adequate doses appropriate for the type of epilepsy before VNS therapy was initiated. Therefore, it can be safely assumed that in these patients maximum response to AEDs had already been attained and reduction in seizure frequency noted after the implant can be attributed to the VNS therapy. On the other hand, the patient's desire to decrease the dose and reduce the number of AEDs after VNS implantation may have resulted in a negative impact on the responder rate.

In conclusion, neuromodulation with VNS therapy can be used successfully as an adjunctive treatment for patients <12 years of age with both focal and generalized drug resistant epilepsies.

The cumulative seizure response to VNS therapy necessitates long-term efficacy analysis studies. Due to availability of third generation AEDs it is unethical to design a prospective double blind research study with unchanged AED regimen to further define the findings of this study. Therefore, our retrospective data analysis study has limited but definite scientific contribution.

Conflict of Interests

The authors declare that there is no conflict of interests regarding the publication of this paper.

References

[1] Cyberonics, *VNS Therapy Products Manuals and Safety Alerts: Part1—Introduction—Indications, Warnings and Precautions*, Cyberonics, Houston, Tex, USA, 2012.

[2] M. C. Salinsky, B. M. Uthman, R. K. Ristanovic, J. F. Wernicke, and W. B. Tarver, "Vagus nerve stimulation for the treatment of medically intractable seizures: results of a 1-year open-extension trial," *Archives of Neurology*, vol. 53, no. 11, pp. 1176–1180, 1996.

[3] G. W. Hornig, J. V. Murphy, G. Schallert, and C. Tilton, "Left vagus nerve stimulation in children with refractory epilepsy: an update," *Southern Medical Journal*, vol. 90, no. 5, pp. 484–488, 1997.

[4] J. V. Murphy, G. Hornig, and G. Schallert, "Left vagal nerve stimulation in children with refractory epilepsy: preliminary observations," *Archives of Neurology*, vol. 52, no. 9, pp. 886–889, 1995.

[5] E. Ben-Menachem, R. Mañon-Espaillat, R. Ristanovic et al., "Vagus nerve stimulation for treatment of partial seizures: 1. A controlled study of effect on seizures. First International Vagus Nerve Stimulation Study Group," *Epilepsia*, vol. 35, no. 3, pp. 616–626, 1994.

[6] C. M. DeGiorgio, S. C. Schachter, A. Handforth et al., "Prospective long-term study of vagus nerve stimulation for the treatment of refractory seizures," *Epilepsia*, vol. 41, no. 9, pp. 1195–1200, 2000.

[7] M. Frost, J. Gates, S. L. Helmers et al., "Vagus nerve stimulation in children with refractory seizures associated with Lennox-Gastaut syndrome," *Epilepsia*, vol. 42, no. 9, pp. 1148–1152, 2001.

[8] S. Chayasirisobhon, W. V. Chayasirisobhon, S. Koulouris, and S. Gurbani, "Vagus nerve stimulation in drug-resistant epilepsy," *Acta Neurologica Taiwanica*, vol. 12, pp. 123–129, 2003.

[9] D. R. Labar, "Antiepileptic drug use during the first 12 months of vagus nerve stimulation therapy: a registry study," *Neurology*, vol. 59, no. 6, supplement 4, pp. S38–S43, 2002.

[10] A. P. Amar, C. M. DeGiorgio, W. B. Tarver, and M. L. Apuzzo, "Long-term multicenter experience with vagus nerve stimulation for intractable partial seizures: results of the XE5 trial," *Stereotactic and Functional Neurosurgery*, vol. 73, no. 1–4, pp. 104–108, 1999.

[11] E. Ben-Menachem, K. Hellström, C. Waldton, and L. E. Augustinsson, "Evaluation of refractory epilepsy treated with vagus nerve stimulation for up to 5 years," *Neurology*, vol. 52, no. 6, pp. 1265–1267, 1999.

[12] J. Scherrmann, C. Hoppe, T. Kral, J. Schramm, and C. E. Elger, "Vagus nerve stimulation: clinical experience in a large patient

series," *Journal of Clinical Neurophysiology*, vol. 18, no. 5, pp. 408–414, 2001.

[13] J. V. Murphy, R. Torkelson, I. Dowler, S. Simon, and S. Hudson, "Vagal nerve stimulation in refractory epilepsy: the first 100 patients receiving vagal nerve stimulation at a pediatric epilepsy center," *Archives of Pediatrics and Adolescent Medicine*, vol. 157, no. 6, pp. 560–564, 2003.

[14] B. M. Uthman, A. M. Reichl, J. C. Dean et al., "Effectiveness of vagus nerve stimulation in epilepsy patients: a 12-year observation," *Neurology*, vol. 63, no. 6, pp. 1124–1126, 2004.

[15] K. Vonck, V. Thadani, K. Gilbert et al., "Vagus nerve stimulation for refractory epilepsy: a transatlantic experience," *Journal of Clinical Neurophysiology*, vol. 21, no. 4, pp. 283–289, 2004.

[16] D. Labar, "Vagus nerve stimulation for 1 year in 269 patients on unchanged antiepileptic drugs," *Seizure*, vol. 13, no. 6, pp. 392–398, 2004.

[17] A. V. Alexopoulos, P. Kotagal, T. Loddenkemper, J. Hammel, and W. E. Bingaman, "Long-term results with vagus nerve stimulation in children with pharmacoresistant epilepsy," *Seizure*, vol. 15, no. 7, pp. 491–503, 2006.

[18] M. Benifla, J. T. Rutka, W. Logan, and E. J. Donner, "Vagal nerve stimulation for refractory epilepsy in children: indications and experience at the Hospital for Sick Children," *Child's Nervous System*, vol. 22, no. 8, pp. 1018–1026, 2006.

[19] V. De Herdt, P. Boon, B. Ceulemans et al., "Vagus nerve stimulation for refractory epilepsy: a Belgian multicenter study," *European Journal of Paediatric Neurology*, vol. 11, no. 5, pp. 261–269, 2007.

[20] A. P. Amar, M. L. Apuzzo, and C. Y. Liu, "Vagus nerve stimulation therapy after failed cranial surgery for intractable epilepsy: results from the vagus nerve stimulation therapy patient outcome registry," *Neurosurgery*, vol. 62, supplement 2, pp. 506–513, 2008.

[21] R. E. Elliott, A. Morsi, S. P. Kalhorn et al., "Vagus nerve stimulation in 436 consecutive patients with treatment-resistant epilepsy: long-term outcomes and predictors of response," *Epilepsy and Behavior*, vol. 20, no. 1, pp. 57–63, 2011.

[22] R. E. Elliott, A. Morsi, O. Tanweer et al., "Efficacy of vagus nerve stimulation over time: review of 65 consecutive patients with treatment-resistant epilepsy treated with VNS >10 years," *Epilepsy & Behavior*, vol. 20, no. 3, pp. 478–483, 2011.

[23] N. Zamponi, C. Petrelli, C. Passamonti, R. Moavero, and P. Curatolo, "Vagus nerve stimulation for refractory epilepsy in tuberous sclerosis," *Pediatric Neurology*, vol. 43, no. 1, pp. 29–34, 2010.

[24] T. Hallböök, J. Lundgren, K. Stjernqvist, G. Blennow, L.-G. Strömblad, and I. Rosén, "Vagus nerve stimulation in 15 children with therapy resistant epilepsy; its impact on cognition, quality of life, behaviour and mood," *Seizure*, vol. 14, no. 7, pp. 504–513, 2005.

[25] H. C. Kang, Y. S. Hwang, D. S. Kim, and H. D. Kim, "Vagus nerve stimulation in pediatric intractable epilepsy: a Korean bicentric study," in *Advances in Functional and Reparative Neurosurgery*, vol. 99 of *Acta Neurochirurgica Supplementum*, pp. 93–96, Springer, Vienna, Austria, 2006.

[26] E. Rossignol, A. Lortie, T. Thomas et al., "Vagus nerve stimulation in pediatric epileptic syndromes," *Seizure*, vol. 18, no. 1, pp. 34–37, 2009.

[27] A. Shahwan, C. Bailey, W. Maxiner, and A. S. Harvey, "Vagus nerve stimulation for refractory epilepsy in children: more to VNS than seizure frequency reduction," *Epilepsia*, vol. 50, no. 5, pp. 1220–1228, 2009.

[28] N. Zamponi, C. Passamonti, E. Cesaroni, R. Trignani, and F. Rychlicki, "Effectiveness of vagal nerve stimulation (VNS) in patients with drop-attacks and different epileptic syndromes," *Seizure*, vol. 20, no. 6, pp. 468–474, 2011.

[29] E. M. S. Sherman, M. B. Connolly, D. J. Slick, K. L. Eyrl, P. Steinbok, and K. Farrell, "Quality of life and seizure outcome after vagus nerve stimulation in children with intractable epilepsy," *Journal of Child Neurology*, vol. 23, no. 9, pp. 991–998, 2008.

[30] G. Colicchio, D. Policicchio, G. Barbati et al., "Vagal nerve stimulation for drug-resistant epilepsies in different age, aetiology and duration," *Child's Nervous System*, vol. 26, no. 6, pp. 811–819, 2010.

[31] B. Majkowska-Zwolińska, P. Zwoliński, M. Roszkowski, and K. Drabik, "Long-term results of vagus nerve stimulation in children and adolescents with drug-resistant epilepsy," *Child's Nervous System*, vol. 28, no. 4, pp. 621–628, 2012.

[32] M. Wheeler, V. De Herdt, K. Vonck et al., "Efficacy of vagus nerve stimulation for refractory epilepsy among patient subgroups: a re-analysis using the Engel classification," *Seizure*, vol. 20, no. 4, pp. 331–335, 2011.

[33] R. E. Elliott, S. D. Rodgers, L. Bassani et al., "Vagus nerve stimulation for children with treatment-resistant epilepsy: a consecutive series of 141 cases," *Journal of Neurosurgery: Pediatrics*, vol. 7, no. 5, pp. 491–500, 2011.

[34] E. A. Pastrana, S. Estronza, and I. J. Sosa, "Vagus nerve stimulation for intractable seizures in children: the university of Puerto Rico experience," *Puerto Rico Health Sciences Journal*, vol. 30, no. 3, pp. 128–131, 2011.

[35] D. Parain, M. J. Penniello, P. Berquen, T. Delangre, C. Billard, and J. V. Murphy, "Vagal nerve stimulation in tuberous sclerosis complex patients," *Pediatric Neurology*, vol. 25, no. 3, pp. 213–216, 2001.

[36] N. Zamponi, C. Passamonti, S. Cappanera, and C. Petrelli, "Clinical course of young patients with Dravet syndrome after vagal nerve stimulation," *European Journal of Paediatric Neurology*, vol. 15, no. 1, pp. 8–14, 2011.

[37] D. R. Labar, "Antiepileptic drug use during the first 12 months of vagus nerve stimulation therapy: a registration study," *Neurology*, vol. 59, pp. 538–543, 2002.

[38] E. García-Navarrete, C. V. Torres, I. Gallego, M. Navas, J. Pastor, and R. G. Sola, "Long-term results of vagal nerve stimulation for adults with medication-resistant epilepsy who have been on unchanged antiepileptic medication," *Seizure*, vol. 22, no. 1, pp. 9–13, 2013.

[39] S. Chayasirisobhon, L. Cahan, S. H. Choi et al., "Efficacy of neuromodulation therapy with vagus nerve stimulator in patients with drug-resistant epilepsy on unchanged antiepileptic medication regimen for 24 months following the implant," *Journal of Neurology & Neurophysiology*, vol. 6, pp. 1–4, 2015.

[40] T. R. Henry, "Anatomical, experimental, and mechanistic investigations," in *Vagus Nerve Stimulation*, S. C. Schachter and D. Schmidt, Eds., pp. 1–29, Martin Dunitz, London, UK, 2001.

[41] S. G. Gurbani, M. Mittal, N. Gurbani, S. Koulouris, S. Choi, and S. Chayasirisobhon, "Efficacy of rapid cycling of vagus nerve stimulation in pharmaco-resistant epilepsy," *Neurology Asia*, vol. 9, supplement 1, p. 131, 2004.

13

Epidemiology of Acute Symptomatic Seizures among Adult Medical Admissions

Paul Osemeke Nwani,[1]
Maduaburochukwu Cosmas Nwosu,[2] **and Monica Nonyelum Nwosu**[3]

[1]*Clinical Pharmacology and Therapeutics Unit/Neurology Unit, Department of Medicine,*
 Nnamdi Azikiwe University Teaching Hospital, PMB 5025, Nnewi 435101, Anambra State, Nigeria
[2]*Neurology Unit, Department of Medicine, Nnamdi Azikiwe University Teaching Hospital, PMB 5025,*
 Nnewi 435101, Anambra State, Nigeria
[3]*Gastroenterology Unit, Department of Medicine, Nnamdi Azikiwe University Teaching Hospital, PMB 5025,*
 Nnewi 435101, Anambra State, Nigeria

Correspondence should be addressed to Paul Osemeke Nwani; paul.nwani@yahoo.com

Academic Editor: Morten I. Lossius

Acute symptomatic seizures are seizures occurring in close temporal relationship with an acute central nervous system (CNS) insult. The objective of the study was to determine the frequency of presentation and etiological risk factors of acute symptomatic seizures among adult medical admissions. It was a two-year retrospective study of the medical files of adults patients admitted with acute symptomatic seizures as the first presenting event. There were 94 cases of acute symptomatic seizures accounting for 5.2% (95% CI: 4.17–6.23) of the 1,802 medical admissions during the period under review. There were 49 (52.1%) males and 45 (47.9%) females aged between 18 years and 84 years. The etiological risk factors of acute symptomatic seizures were infections in 36.2% ($n = 34$) of cases, stroke in 29.8% ($n = 28$), metabolic in 12.8% ($n = 12$), toxic in 10.6% ($n = 10$), and other causes in 10.6% ($n = 10$). Infective causes were more among those below fifty years while stroke was more in those aged fifty years and above. CNS infections and stroke were the prominent causes of acute symptomatic seizures. This is an evidence of the "double tragedy" facing developing countries, the unresolved threat of infectious diseases on one hand and the increasing impact of noncommunicable diseases on the other one.

1. Introduction

Acute symptomatic seizures are clinical seizures occurring in close temporal relationship with an acute central nervous system (CNS) insult, which may be metabolic, toxic, structural, infectious, or inflammatory [1]. Such seizures are considered to be an acute manifestation of the insult and may not recur when the underlying cause has been removed or the acute phase has elapsed [2].

Acute symptomatic seizures represent about 40% of all cases of afebrile seizures in developed countries and more than half in some geographic areas, for example, where cysticercosis is endemic [2, 3]. Acute symptomatic seizures are more frequent among males and in the extremes of age (youngest age class and in the elderly) [2]. The causes of acute symptomatic seizures in developed countries may differ from the causes in developing countries [4]. The commonest causes among adults in developed nations include traumatic brain injury, stroke, medication, or alcohol withdrawal, brain tumors, and metabolic insult [2, 5].

Treatment of acute symptomatic seizures requires the simultaneous treatment of the underlying aetiology and the use of anticonvulsant drugs [6]. The anticonvulsants preferred for the treatment of acute symptomatic seizures are those available for intravenous use, such as benzodiazepines, fosphenytoin or phenytoin, valproate, levetiracetam, and phenobarbital [6]. Acute symptomatic seizures are an undisputable risk factor for epilepsy [2].

When seizures complicate acute neurological disorders, they add an additional layer of complexity to patient management [4]. The knowledge of the etiologic risk factors of acute symptomatic seizures in third-world countries will invariably contribute to the effort aimed at preventing and managing medical conditions frequently complicated by seizures. Currently there is dearth of information on the epidemiology of acute symptomatic seizures among adult medical admissions in Nigeria and Africa in general.

2. Methods

This was a retrospective study of medical records of adults patients admitted with acute symptomatic seizures as the first presenting event at medical wards of the Nnamdi Azikiwe University Teaching Hospital (NAUTH), Nnewi. NAUTH is the largest medical referral centre in Anambra State, Southeast Nigeria. Anambra State occupies an area of 4,844 Km sq. and has a population of 4,182,032 according to the 2006 Nigeria population census. The average attendance of NAUTH has been on the increase since inception of the hospital and currently the average annual attendance is 117,351 patients (103,601 outpatients and 13,750 inpatients) accounting for a 2.8% medical coverage of population of over four million of Anambra State. The current annual adult medical admissions of NAUTH are about 1,992 accounting for 14.5% ($n = 1,992/13,750$) of the entire hospital admissions. Patients from all clinical subspecialties in internal medicine are admitted to the two medical wards of the hospital either from the accident and emergency department or from the medical outpatient clinics.

The medical records of all medical wards admissions from January 2005 to December 2006 were retrieved from the records department of the hospital and reviewed. Those who presented with seizures as a presenting complaint were selected and analysed. Data extracted from the medical record files included demographic data (age and sex), relevant history and clinical examination findings, available investigation results, and diagnosis. All cases of acute symptomatic seizures are reviewed by the neurologists in our centre.

Acute symptomatic seizure was defined as a clinical seizure occurring in close temporal relationship with an acute central nervous system (CNS) insult, which may be metabolic, toxic, structural, infectious, or inflammatory [1].

Seizures were defined as acute symptomatic ones if they occurred within one week of stroke, central nervous system infection, or systemic infection or if they occur in the presence of severe metabolic derangements documented by biochemical abnormalities obtained within the immediate period of the metabolic event. The definitions used for the various etiologic agents are as follows.

Seizures following stroke were defined as acute symptomatic ones if they occurred within seven days of stroke. Stroke was defined as sudden onset focal or global neurological deficit of vascular origin lasting for more than 24 hours or resulting in death. Stroke type was categorized using the World Health Organisation stroke criteria and/or brain CT scan.

Seizures occurring in relation to meningoencephalitis and sepsis in our study were defined as acute symptomatic ones if they occurred within seven days of the events. The diagnosis of meningoencephalitis was based on documentation of fever, headache, alteration in the level of

consciousness and signs of meningism on examination, and a positive cerebrospinal fluid result with or without isolation of pathogen. Sepsis was diagnosed based on documented clinical and laboratory (hematologic indices) evidence of systemic infection in a patient who does not meet the criteria of meningoencephalitis as defined above.

Metabolic causes of seizures were diagnosed based on documentation of appropriate laboratory results obtained within the periods of the seizures and other relevant clinical data. Uremic encephalopathy was diagnosed as cause of seizure based on documentation of azotemia within the periods of the seizures in a patient with relevant clinical history and findings. Hepatic encephalopathy was diagnosed as cause of acute symptomatic seizures if seizures occurred during the period of overt neuropsychiatric symptoms in a patient with history of liver disease.

Acute symptomatic seizures associated with hypertensive encephalopathy were defined as seizures occurring in patients with severe elevation of blood pressure, altered mental status, or evidence of diffuse brain dysfunction with prompt response to antihypertensive therapy.

The cases of acute symptomatic seizures relating to alcohol use were seizures occurring in patients with history of chronic alcohol abuse, presence of alcohol withdrawal symptoms, and seizures within 48 hours of last drink.

The diagnosis of brain space occupying lesions for cases with HIV/AIDS was based on clinical history, examination findings, and/or brain CT scan.

Eleven patients had brain CT scan; of these patents ten were cases of acute symptomatic seizures due to stroke while one was due to HIV infection.

Patients with epilepsy and those below 18 years of age were excluded (patients below 18 years are admitted to the hospital paediatric unit).

Statistical Analysis. Data collected was analysed using Statistical Package for the Social Sciences SPSS version 15 (SPSS Inc., Chicago, IL, USA). Prevalence values with their 95% confidence intervals (95% CI) were calculated. Relevant percentages, frequencies, means and standard deviations, and confidence intervals were calculated. Findings were represented with tables and a figure.

3. Results

There were 94 cases of acute symptomatic seizures accounting for 5.2% (95% CI: 4.17–6.23) of the 1,802 medical admissions during the period under review. There were 49 (52.1%) males and females 45 (47.9%) but the observed difference was not statistically significant $\chi^2 = 7.063$, $p = 0.422$. The patients were aged between 18 and 84 years with a mean age of 51 ± 16 years (males: 49.8 ± 16; females: 53.7 ± 15.7).

The etiological risk factors of acute symptomatic seizures were infections in 36.2% ($n = 34$) of cases, stroke in 29.8% ($n = 28$), metabolic in 12.8% ($n = 12$), and toxic in 10.6% ($n = 10$) (Table 1). The 28 cases of stroke accounted for 24.3% ($n = 28/115$) of all stroke admissions during the period under review while the 34 infectious cases accounted for 18.9% ($n =$

TABLE 1: Classes of etiological risk factors of acute symptomatic seizures.

Disease class	Frequency (n = 94)	Diseases	Frequency (n = 94)	Percentage (%)
Infectious	34 (36.2%)	Meningoencephalitis	13	13.8
		HIV/AIDS*	11	11.7
		Sepsis	7	7.4
		Cerebral malaria	2	2.1
		Cerebral abscess	1	1.1
Stroke	28 (29.8%)	Haemorrhagic stroke	14	14.9
		Ischaemic stroke	9	9.6
		Subarachnoid haemorrhage	5	5.3
Metabolic	17 (18.1%)	Hyperglycaemia	6	6.4
		Hypoglycaemia	5	5.3
		Uraemia	3	3.2
		Hepatic	2	2.1
		Hyponatremia	1	1.1
Toxic	7 (7.4%)	Poisoning**	4	4.3
		Alcohol	3	3.2
Others	8 (8.5%)	Hypertensive encephalopathy	5	5.3
		Uncertain	3	3.2

*HIV/AIDS (encephalopathy: 5, space occupying lesion: 4, and meningoencephalitis: 3), **poisoning (CO poisoning: 1, organophosphate: 1, and unknown medication: 2).

34/201) of cases of infectious diseases admitted during the period.

The group designated "uncertain" did not have sufficient data to be classified into any of the groups as defined above and where indicated as patients living with epilepsy. Two cases of seizures due to brain tumours that presented during the period under review were excluded as acute symptomatic ones since they belong to the group progressive symptomatic according to the proposed ILEA definition as they occur in the context of an evolving clinical condition [1]. There were no documented cases of acute symptomatic seizures caused by inflammation during the period under review.

Figure 1 shows the relative age distribution of the two major etiological risk factors. Infectious causes peaked at 30–49 age group and those aged below 49 years accounted for 70.6% (n = 24/34) of seizures due to infectious causes while stroke peaked at 50–69 age group and those aged 50 years and above accounted for 82.1% (n = 23/28) of cases of seizures due to stroke.

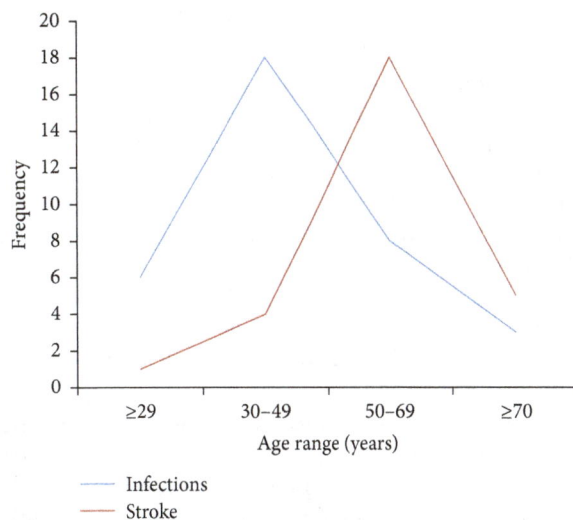

FIGURE 1: Age distribution of the two major causes of acute symptomatic seizures.

4. Discussion

4.1. Prevalence of Acute Symptomatic Seizures. The prevalence of acute symptomatic seizures among medical admissions found in our study was 5.2% (95% CI: 4.17–6.23). This is more than 2.1% reported among neurological intensive care patients in India and 3.5% reported among medical intensive care unit patients in the USA [4, 7]. Though methodological differences and differences in patient selection limited direct comparisons of the results of these previous studies and our study, the higher prevalence found in our study may indicate a high frequency of acute symptomatic seizures among our medical admissions.

There was an insignificant male preponderance of acute symptomatic seizures in our study. The risk of acute symptomatic seizures in males is almost double that of females in population based studies [5]. This sex difference has been attributed to the incidence of underlying risk factors like head trauma rather than any biological phenomenon [5]. Our study was among medical admissions which excluded risk factors like traumatic brain injuries which are commoner in males; this may in part account for the insignificant sex difference we observed.

4.2. Aetiology of Acute Symptomatic Seizures. Infectious causes were the most frequent cause of acute symptomatic seizures in our study accounting for 36.2% (n = 34/94) of cases. This is comparable to 32% (n = 21/66) reported among patients admitted to a neurological intensive care unit in India [4]. Among the infective causes meningoencephalitis accounted for 13.8% (n = 13/94) of acute symptomatic seizures in this present study and this is comparable to the Indian study where meningoencephalitis ranked highest among the infective causes of acute symptomatic seizures. Studies in western nations report higher frequencies of etiologic risk factors like stroke, medication or alcohol withdrawal, brain tumor, and eclampsia among adults while infections are dominant causes of acute symptomatic seizures in newborns and children [5]. The risk of acute symptomatic seizures occurring in patients with acute central nervous system infections is more with encephalitis than meningitis [8, 9]. In our study, the absence of results of appropriate investigational facilities due to their unavailability or high cost in part limited further differentiation of these two entities among those with meningoencephalitis. Sepsis accounted for 7.5% (n = 7/94) of cases of acute symptomatic seizures in this present study. Seizures in these cases may be due to encephalopathy relating to such factors, hemodynamic dysfunction and metabolic derangement in patients with severe infections. Sepsis is a documented frequent cause of encephalopathy [7].

Human immunodeficiency virus (HIV) infection was the etiological risk factor for 11.7% (n = 11/94) of cases of acute symptomatic seizures in our study. Acute symptomatic seizures are common among HIV infected individuals and are present in up to 2% to 20% of cases [10]. Identifiable causes of acute symptomatic seizures in HIV infected individuals in this present study were HIV encephalopathy, meningoencephalitis, and space occupying lesions (SOL) from probable opportunistic infections. This agrees with reported causes of seizures in HIV infected persons like opportunistic infections, systemic illness, drug or alcohol abuse, antiretroviral drug usage, and acquired immunodeficiency syndrome (AIDS) encephalopathy [10].

In our study neurocysticercosis was not among the causes of acute symptomatic seizures. This may indicate a low frequency of neurocysticercosis in our environment or under diagnosis of the condition due to lack of adequate facilities to make the diagnosis. Neurocysticercosis has been rarely reported in Nigeria hospitals studies even with the reports on the high prevalence of cysticercosis in meat in various parts of the country [11–13]. In a prospective study in India, neurocysticercosis ranked the same as meningoencephalitis as infective cause of acute symptomatic seizures [4]. In places where neurocysticercosis is endemic it is the most common cause of epilepsy in developing countries, where it accounts for up to 30% of all seizures [14].

Cerebral malaria which is a common cause of acute febrile seizures in children in developing countries including Nigeria accounted for only 2.1% (n = 2/94) of acute seizures in our study [15]. Cerebral malaria is rare among adults in the tropics and this has been attributed to the development of immunity against malaria under the stable endemic conditions prevailing in the region [16].

Stroke was a common cause of acute symptomatic seizures in our study accounting for 29.8% (n = 28/94) of cases. Acute symptomatic seizures following stroke tend to occur in 2.4% to 6.3% of patients but in our study acute symptomatic seizures were present in 24.3% of cases [17, 18]. This higher frequency of acute symptomatic seizures following stroke found in our study may be related to the poor initial management of the acute stage of stroke and the attendant complications of such managements. Most stroke patients in this part of the country present initially to nonspecialist with little knowledge and inadequate facilities for acute management of stroke and are referred to specialist centres only when complications begin to develop. In a prospective multicentre study most of the seizures following stroke occurred within 2 days and almost half (43%) within 24 hours after the stroke [19]. The frequency of acute symptomatic seizures following stroke is more with haemorrhagic than ischemic stroke as was found in this present study [20].

Metabolic derangements accounted for 18.1% (n = 17/94) of cases of acute symptomatic seizures in this present study. Unlike the India study where hyponatremia accounted for most metabolic derangement hyperglycaemia accounting for 6.4% (n = 6/94) and hypoglycaemia accounting for 5.3% (n = 5/94) were the most frequent metabolic contributors in our study [4]. Such disparities in the metabolic causes of seizures between their study and ours may arise from differences in frequencies of the major primary diagnosis in both series. Also the level of baseline medical care available to the patients before the onset of seizures may be contributory since most of the metabolic causes in our study were due to poor glycaemic control. Hyperglycaemic emergencies are significant causes of endocrine admission and deaths in Nigeria [21]. Among hyperglycaemic comas in diabetes, seizures are more frequently encountered in hyperosmolar hyperglycaemic state than in diabetic ketoacidosis probably due to the anticonvulsant effect of ketosis [22].

In our study poisoning and alcohol related causes were implicated in 4.3% (n = 4/94) and 3.2% (n = 3/94) of cases of acute symptomatic seizures, respectively. Acute symptomatic seizures associated with alcohol intake may occur after alcohol withdrawal (as in our study) or acute intoxication and this can represent as much as one-third of total hospital admissions due to seizures [23]. The names of the implicated medications in two cases were documented as unknown in the record files but the clinical histories were highly suspicious of the medications poisoning. This highlights not too infrequent problem associated with studying drug related problems in developing countries. Due to the low level of literacy the patients have little knowledge of the drugs they are taking. This is further complicated by concealment of drug names from the patients by the prescribers in most private owned medical establishments. The concomitants use of herbal and orthodox medications even further complicates the matter and undermines adequate study of the medications use especially when they are involved in suspected cases of drug toxicity.

4.3. Study Limitations.
This study however had several limitations owning to the retrospective nature of the study

and the frequent problems of poor record keeping associated with such studies. However, notwithstanding these limitations the findings afford a baseline for further studies on this subject in developing nations. The study was among medical admissions and so did not include etiologic risk factors like traumatic brain injuries which are managed primarily by the neurosurgical teams. Cases of acute symptomatic seizures developing in patients admitted without seizures as the first presenting feature were also not captured because of problems of inadequate documentations not infrequent with retrospective studies like this present study. This study was also limited by unavailability of high yield neurologic investigative modalities (like serological test, electroencephalography, viral studies, neuroimaging, and others) that would have enhanced accurate delineation of the differential diagnosis of the causes of acute symptomatic seizures. This is because of the absence of such facilities and for those that are available their high cost limits their use since patients pay out of pocket for medical facilities in the countries.

5. Conclusion

Infections and stroke were the prominent causes of acute symptomatic seizures. This an evidence of the "double tragedy" facing developing countries, the unresolved threat of infectious diseases on one hand and the increasing impact of noncommunicable diseases on the other one. The need for further studies in this area has been made bare given the high frequency of this condition found in this study.

Conflict of Interests

The authors declare that there is no conflict of interests regarding the publication of this paper.

References

[1] E. Beghi, A. Carpio, L. Forsgren et al., "Recommendation for a definition of acute symptomatic seizure," *Epilepsia*, vol. 51, no. 4, pp. 671–675, 2010.

[2] W. A. Hauser and E. Beghi, "First seizure definitions and worldwide incidence and mortality," *Epilepsia*, vol. 49, supplement 1, pp. 8–12, 2008.

[3] D. K. Pal, A. Carpio, and J. W. A. S. Sander, "Neurocysticercosis and epilepsy in developing countries," *Journal of Neurology Neurosurgery and Psychiatry*, vol. 68, no. 2, pp. 137–143, 2000.

[4] J. Narayanan and J. M. K. Murthy, "New-onset acute symptomatic seizure in a neurological intensive care unit," *Neurology India*, vol. 55, no. 2, pp. 136–140, 2007.

[5] J. F. Annegers, W. A. Hauser, J. R.-J. Lee, and W. A. Rocca, "Incidence of acute symptomatic seizures in Rochester, Minnesota, 1935–1984," *Epilepsia*, vol. 36, no. 4, pp. 327–333, 1995.

[6] B. S. Koppel, "Treatment of acute and remote symptomatic seizures," *Current Treatment Options in Neurology*, vol. 11, no. 4, pp. 231–241, 2009.

[7] T. P. Bleck, M. C. Smith, S. J.-C. Pierre-Louis, J. J. Jares, J. Murray, and C. A. Hansen, "Neurologic complications of critical medical illnesses," *Critical Care Medicine*, vol. 21, no. 1, pp. 98–103, 1993.

[8] J. F. Annegers, W. A. Hauser, E. Beghi, A. Nicolosi, and L. T. Kurland, "The risk of unprovoked seizures after encephalitis and meningitis," *Neurology*, vol. 38, no. 9, pp. 1407–1410, 1988.

[9] M. A. Kim, K. M. Park, S. E. Kim, and M. K. Oh, "Acute symptomatic seizures in CNS infection," *European Journal of Neurology*, vol. 15, no. 1, pp. 38–41, 2008.

[10] G. J. Dal Pan, J. C. McArther, and M. J. G. Harrison, "Neurological symptoms in HIV infection," in *AIDS and Nervous System*, J. R. Berger and R. M. Levy, Eds., pp. 141–172, Lippincott-Raven, Philadelphia, Pa, USA, 2nd edition, 1997.

[11] A. O. Ogunrin, "Epilepsy in Nigeria—a review of etiology, epidemiology and management," *Benin Journal of Postgraduate Medicine*, vol. 8, no. 1, pp. 27–51, 2006.

[12] R. P. Weka, E. Ikeh, and J. Kamani, "Seroprevalence of antibodies (IgG) to *Taenia solium* among pig rearers and associated risk factors in Jos metropolis, Nigeria," *Journal of Infection in Developing Countries*, vol. 7, no. 2, pp. 67–72, 2013.

[13] L. P. E. Usip, L. Isaac, E. C. Amadi, E. Utah, and U. Akpaudo, "The occurrence of cysticercosis in cattle and Taeniasis in man in Uyo, capital city of Akwa Ibom State, Nigeria," *Nigerian Journal of Agriculture, Food and Environment*, vol. 7, no. 2, pp. 47–51, 2011.

[14] M. T. Medina, E. Rosas, F. Rubio-Donnadieu, and J. Sotelo, "Neurocysticercosis as the main cause of late-onset epilepsy in Mexico," *Archives of Internal Medicine*, vol. 150, no. 2, pp. 325–327, 1990.

[15] I. O. Oluwayemi, B. J. Brown, O. A. Oyedeji, and M. A. Oluwayemi, "Neurological sequelae in survivors of cerebral malaria," *Pan African Medical Journal*, vol. 15, article 88, 2013.

[16] A. M. Dondorp, "Pathophysiology, clinical presentation and treatment of cerebral malaria," *Neurology Asia*, vol. 10, pp. 67–77, 2005.

[17] C. Lamy, V. Domigo, F. Semah et al., "Early and late seizures after cryptogenic ischemic stroke in young adults," *Neurology*, vol. 60, no. 3, pp. 400–404, 2003.

[18] E. Beghi, R. D'Alessandro, S. Beretta et al., "Incidence and predictors of acute symptomatic seizures after stroke," *Neurology*, vol. 77, no. 20, pp. 1785–1793, 2011.

[19] C. F. Bladin, A. V. Alexandrov, A. Bellavance et al., "Seizures after stroke: a prospective multicenter study," *Archives of Neurology*, vol. 57, no. 11, pp. 1617–1622, 2000.

[20] D. L. Labovitz, W. A. Hauser, and R. L. Sacco, "Prevalence and predictors of early seizure and status epilepticus after first stroke," *Neurology*, vol. 57, no. 2, pp. 200–206, 2001.

[21] A. O. Ogbera, S. Chinenye, A. Onyekwere, and O. Fasanmade, "Prognostic indices of diabetes mortality," *Ethnicity and Disease*, vol. 17, no. 4, pp. 721–725, 2007.

[22] X. Gao, A. S. Wee, and T. G. Nick, "Effect of keto-acidosis on seizure occurrence in diabetic patients," *Journal of the Mississippi State Medical Association*, vol. 46, no. 5, pp. 131–133, 2005.

[23] M. P. Earnest and P. R. Yarnell, "Seizure admissions to a city hospital: the role of alcohol," *Epilepsia*, vol. 17, no. 4, pp. 387–393, 1976.

14

Epilepsy Surgery Series: A Study of 502 Consecutive Patients from a Developing Country

Abdulaziz Alsemari,[1,2] **Faisal Al-Otaibi,**[1] **Salah Baz,**[1] **Ibrahim Althubaiti,**[1] **Hisham Aldhalaan,**[1] **David MacDonald,**[1] **Tareq Abalkhail,**[1] **Miguel E. Fiol,**[3] **Suad Alyamani,**[1] **Aziza Chedrawi,**[1] **Frank Leblanc,**[4] **Andrew Parrent,**[5] **Donald Maclean,**[1] **and John Girvin**[5]

[1] *Department of Neurosciences, King Faisal Specialist Hospital and Research Centre, Riyadh 11211, Saudi Arabia*
[2] *Neurology Section, Department of Neurosciences, King Faisal Specialist Hospital & Research Centre, MBC.76, P.O. Box 3354, Riyadh 11211, Saudi Arabia*
[3] *University of Minnesota Medical Center, Fairview, Epilepsy Care Center, Minnesota, MN 55455, USA*
[4] *University of Calgary, AB, Canada T2N 1N4*
[5] *London Health Science Center, London, ON, Canada N6G 2V4*

Correspondence should be addressed to Abdulaziz Alsemari; alsemari@kfshrc.edu.sa

Academic Editor: József Janszky

Purpose. To review the postoperative seizure outcomes of patients that underwent surgery for epilepsy at King Faisal Specialist Hospital & Research Centre (KFSHRC). *Methods.* A descriptive retrospective study for 502 patients operated on for medically intractable epilepsy between 1998 and 2012. The surgical outcome was measured using the ILAE criteria. *Results.* The epilepsy surgery outcome for temporal lobe epilepsy surgery (ILAE classes 1, 2, and 3) at 12, 36, and 60 months is 79.6%, 74.2%, and 67%, respectively. The favorable 12- and 36-month outcomes for frontal lobe epilepsy surgery are 62% and 52%, respectively. For both parietal and occipital epilepsy lobe surgeries the 12- and 36-month outcomes are 67%. For multilobar epilepsy surgery, the 12- and 36-month outcomes are 65% and 50%, respectively. The 12- and 36-month outcomes for functional hemispherectomy epilepsy surgery are 64.2% and 63%, respectively. According to histopathology diagnosis, mesiotemporal sclerosis (MTS) and benign CNS tumors had the best favorable outcome after surgery at 1 year (77.27% and 84.3%, resp.,) and 3 years (76% and 75%, resp.,). The least favorable seizure-free outcome after 3 years occurred in cases with dual pathology (66.6%). Thirty-four epilepsy patients with normal magnetic resonance imaging (MRI) brain scans were surgically treated. The first- and third-year epilepsy surgery outcome of 17 temporal lobe surgeries were (53%) and (47%) seizure-free, respectively. The first- and third-year epilepsy surgery outcomes of 15 extratemporal epilepsy surgeries were (47%) and (33%) seizure-free. *Conclusion.* The best outcomes are achieved with temporal epilepsy surgery, mesial temporal sclerosis, and benign CNS tumor. The worst outcomes are from multilobar surgery, dual pathology, and normal MRI.

1. Introduction

The incidence of epilepsy in developed countries is currently estimated to be 57 people per 100,000 inhabitants [1], and the prevalence of active epilepsy is between 3 and 8 people per 1,000 citizens [2–4]. The rate for active epilepsy in Saudi Arabia is 6.54 per 1,000 [5]. In Saudi Arabia, epilepsy disorders are common, with a hospital frequency rate of 8 per 1,000. Men were more frequently affected than women, and 60% of the patients were under 10 years of age at the onset of the illness [6].

Seventy to 80% of epilepsy patients can be satisfactorily managed with anticonvulsive medication [7] while 20% to 30% develop medically intractable epilepsy [8]. Epilepsy surgery started in the 19th century, but significant contributions were made to the procedure in the 20th century

[9]. Currently, epilepsy surgery is the standard treatment for patients with refractory epilepsy. The effectiveness of surgery over constant pharmacotherapy for intractable epilepsy has been established in a randomized controlled trial [10]. Results from a controlled trial justified the use of surgery as soon as 2 years after the development of pharmacoresistance [11, 12]. Published evidence showed a significantly better quality of life for the patient, which certainly balances the somewhat minor risks associated with epilepsy surgery [13, 14].

Epilepsy surgery procedures were initiated in Saudi Arabia in 1998. Our first evaluation of these procedures was published in *Epilepsy: a comprehensive textbook* (chapter 296). This study, however, was an early systematic review of epilepsy surgery outcomes and related variables in the comprehensive epilepsy program at a single center (KFSH&RC) in Saudi Arabia. The focus of this current study is to review the postoperative seizure outcomes of patients that underwent epilepsy surgery at our centre over the 14-year period from 1998 to 2012. The clinical semiology, preoperative investigations, histopathological diagnoses, and surgical procedures were identified in the determination of outcomes.

2. Methods

2.1. Study Design. A descriptive retrospective study was conducted using data from the epilepsy registry database of our epilepsy program. The study analyzed all patients operated on between 1998 and 2012. The inclusion criteria for surgical evaluation were as follows: (1) recurrent partial seizures with or without secondary generalized seizures and (2) failure of at least two first-line antiepileptic drugs to control the seizures [15].

2.2. Presurgical Evaluation. The preoperative evaluation includes a neurological examination, MRI video-EEG recording with electrodes placed according to the International 10–20 system, invasive video-EEG recording, a neuropsychological evaluation, a sodium amobarbital test, and nuclear brainscan studies. Once the evaluation is completed, the data are usually discussed in a multidisciplinary patient management conference, which includes epileptologists, neurosurgeons, a neuroradiologist, and a neuropsychologist. A standard epilepsy MRI protocol was used to study all patients (GE 1.5 and 3 T; GE Sigma Excite 1.5 T): sagittal T1 sequences (5 mm slice thickness), coronal FLAIR (5 mm), T2 (3 mm), axial T1, T2, and T2* (5 mm), 3D T1 sequences, and diffusion of 1.6 mm slice thickness. Video-EEG monitoring with intracranial electrode implants was also used prior to surgery. Interictal FDG-PET scan was used to evaluate surgical cases. Neuropsychological evaluation was done using a comprehensive test battery and following clinical diagnostic requirements. In contrast to the inclusion criteria for surgical evaluation (*vide supra*), the selection criteria for epilepsy surgery includes (1) a confirmed diagnosis of epilepsy, (2) the presence of medically intractable or disabling seizures, (3) a concordance of the localization data to a respectable focus, (4) the presence of a nonprogressive underlying disease (except Rasmussen's encephalitis), and (5) high probability that seizure control will significantly improve the patient's quality of life.

2.3. Surgical Procedures. The epilepsy procedures were classified as follows: (1) temporal lobe surgery (it includes the anterior temporal lobe with amygdalohippocampectomies and lesionectomies in anterior, middle temporal lobe, posterior lateral, and basal posterior temporal regions), (2) frontal lobe surgery, (3) parietal lobe surgery, (4) occipital lobe surgery, (5) functional hemispherectomy, (6) multilobar surgery (frontotemporal, temporoparietal, frontoparietal, temporoparietooccipital, parietooccipital, and temporooccipital), (7) anterior 2/3 callostomy, and (8) multiple subpial transaction.

2.4. Postsurgical and Outcome Assessment. Epilepsy surgery outcomes were measured according to the ILAE classification. Seizure-free patients with or without auras and patients with 1–3 seizures per year were considered to have favorable outcomes while more than 3 seizures per year were considered unfavorable (Table 1). Epilepsy surgery outcomes were assessed at 12, 36, and 60 months for temporal lobe surgery and at 12 and 36 months for the other procedures. The outcomes were measured using the parameters of procedure, histopathology (mesial temporal sclerosis, benign CNS tumor, cortical dysplasia, and dual pathology), and normal MRI brain.

2.5. Histopathology. The histopathology results were classified into one of the following nine categories: mesial temporal sclerosis (MTS), cerebral dysgenesis (focal cortical dysplasia and heterotopia), primary CNS tumor, vascular malformation, chronic inflammation (*Rasmussen encephalitis*), gliosis, dual pathology (i.e., the association of two potentially epileptogenic features), non specific and normal.

3. Results

3.1. Patients' Demography and Epilepsy Procedures. A total of 502 patients (296 male, 206 female) underwent surgery for their refractory epilepsy between 1998 and 2012. Out of those 502 patients, 65.3% were adults, and 34.7% were pediatric. The epilepsy surgical procedures included 295 temporal lobe surgeries, 53 frontal lobe surgeries, 16 parietal and occipital lobe surgeries, 64 functional hemispherectomies, 26 multilobar surgeries, 10 corpus callosotomies, and 3 multiple subpial transections and one hypothalamic hamartoma resection. The surgical outcome assessments of 468 patients that completed at least 3 years after surgery were evaluated. The invasive EEG was used in 141 patients (28%). The invasive EEG procedure was performed in patients with intractable epilepsy in whom the clinical analysis, scalp EEG, MRI, PET scan, and neuropsychology failed to lateralize seizure origin confidently.

3.2. Neuroimaging Results. MRI brain scans revealed 202 MTS cases, 78 primary CNS tumors, 66 cerebral cortical dysgenesis, 35 normal MRI, 66 focal atrophy and encephalomalacia, 22 arachnoid and *porencephalic* cysts, 15 vascular malformations, 11 tuberous scleroses, and 7 others. A PET scan was conducted on 398 patients, which showed 358 with

TABLE 1: ILAE classification of surgical outcome with respect to epileptic seizures.

Outcome classification	Definition
1	Completely seizure-free; no auras
2	Only auras; no other seizures
3	One to three seizure days per year; ±auras
4	Four seizure days per year to 50% reduction of baseline seizure days; ±auras
5	Less than 50% reduction of baseline seizure days to 100% increase of baseline seizure days; ±auras
6	More than 100% increase of baseline seizure days; ±auras

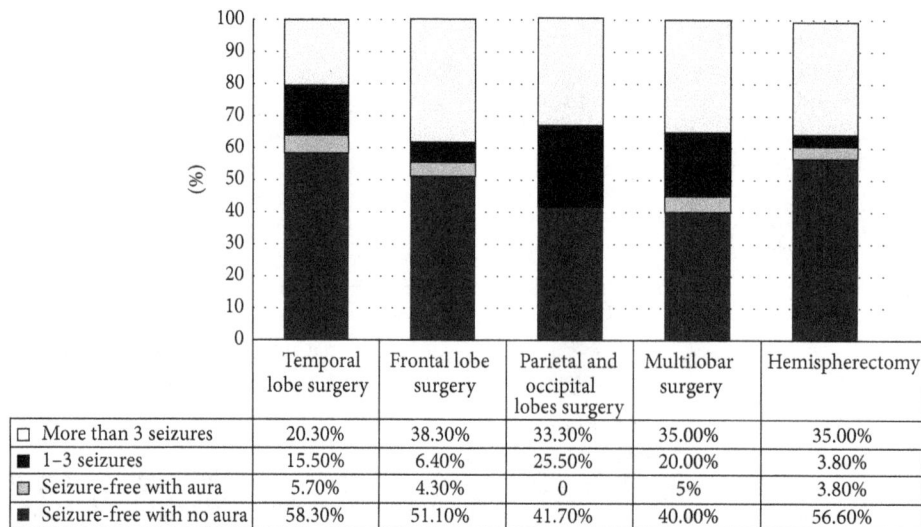

	Temporal lobe surgery	Frontal lobe surgery	Parietal and occipital lobes surgery	Multilobar surgery	Hemispherectomy
☐ More than 3 seizures	20.30%	38.30%	33.30%	35.00%	35.00%
■ 1–3 seizures	15.50%	6.40%	25.50%	20.00%	3.80%
▨ Seizure-free with aura	5.70%	4.30%	0	5%	3.80%
■ Seizure-free with no aura	58.30%	51.10%	41.70%	40.00%	56.60%

FIGURE 1: first-year epilepsy surgery outcome according to procedure.

hypometabolism, 21 with hypermetabolism, and 19 as normal.

3.3. Histopathology Results. The histopathology results showed 11 patients were normal, 203 had MTS, 142 had a cortical dysplasia/heterotopia, 96 had CNS tumors, 11 had encephalomulacia, 11 had chronic inflammations, 12 had vascular malformations, and other 16 (6 nonspecific and 10 cases of callosotomy). Thirty-eight of the histopathology results disclosed a dual pathology, each of which might have contributed to, or been responsible for, the epilepsy.

4. Epilepsy Surgery Outcomes according to Procedure

4.1. Temporal Lobe Surgery. According to the ILAE, the favorable first-year epilepsy surgery outcome for patients following temporal lobe surgery is 79.6%; in our study, 172 patients (58.3%) were seizure-free without auras, 17 (5.7%) were seizure-free with auras, and 46 (15.5%) had 1–3 seizures per year. The favorable outcome for the third year following temporal lobe surgery, according to ILAE criteria, is 74.2%. At this point, our study found 105 patients (53.8%) were seizure-free without auras, 13 patients (6.6%) were seizure-free with auras, and 27 patients (13.8%) had 1–3 seizures per year. According to ILAE, the favorable outcome for the fifth year following temporal lobe surgery was 67%; in our series, 47 patients (47%) were seizure-free without auras, 9 (9%)

were seizure-free with auras, and 11 (11.0%) had 1–3 seizures per year (Figures 1, 2, and 3).

4.2. Frontal Lobe Surgery. The favorable outcome for patients after the first year following epilepsy surgery is 62% according to ILAE criteria. Our study found 24 patients (51.1%) were seizure-free without auras, 2 patients (4.3%) were seizure-free with auras, and 3 patients (6.4%) suffered from 1–3 seizures per year. According to the ILAE, the favorable outcome for the third year following frontal lobe surgery is 52%; in our series, 10 patients (40.0%) were seizure-free without auras, 2 (8%) were seizure-free with auras, and 1 (4.0%) with 1–3 seizures per year (Figures 1 and 2).

4.3. Parietal and Occipital Lobe Surgery. According to the ILAE, the favorable first-year outcome for patients following parietal and occipital surgery is 67%. Our results found 5 patients (41.6%) were seizure-free without auras and 3 patients (25.5%) had 1–3 seizures per year. The favorable outcome in the third year following parietal and occipital surgery is 66.6%; our cases showed 4 patients (44.4%) were seizure-free without auras, 1 (11.1%) was seizure-free with auras, and 1 (11.1%) had 1–3 seizures per year (Figures 1 and 2).

4.4. Multilobar Surgery. The favorable outcome for patients in the first year following multilobar surgery, according to ILAE criteria, is 65%. Our study found 8 patients (40%) were seizure-free without auras, 1 (5%) was seizure-free with auras,

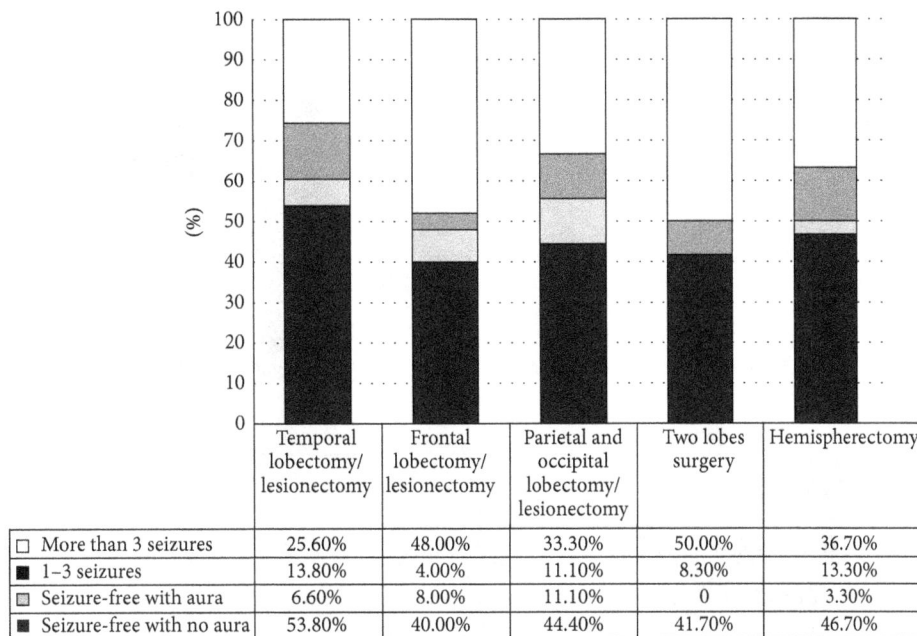

	Temporal lobectomy/ lesionectomy	Frontal lobectomy/ lesionectomy	Parietal and occipital lobectomy/ lesionectomy	Two lobes surgery	Hemispherectomy
☐ More than 3 seizures	25.60%	48.00%	33.30%	50.00%	36.70%
■ 1–3 seizures	13.80%	4.00%	11.10%	8.30%	13.30%
☐ Seizure-free with aura	6.60%	8.00%	11.10%	0	3.30%
■ Seizure-free with no aura	53.80%	40.00%	44.40%	41.70%	46.70%

FIGURE 2: The third-year epilepsy surgery outcome according to procedure.

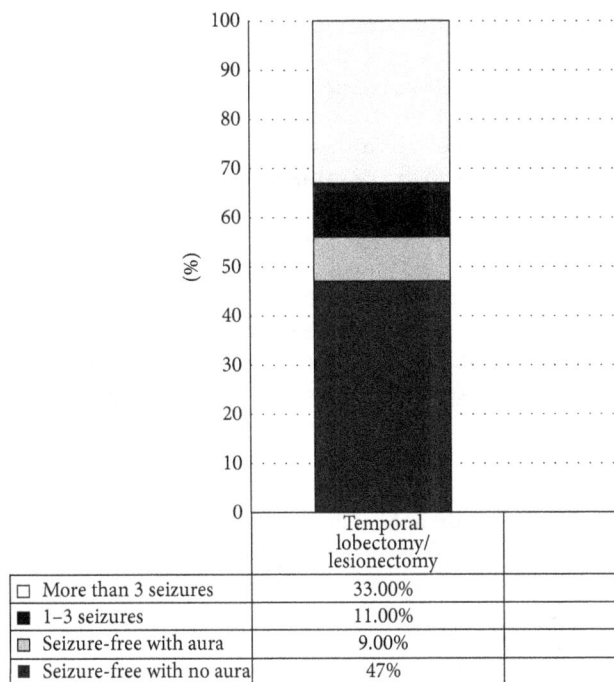

	Temporal lobectomy/ lesionectomy	
☐ More than 3 seizures	33.00%	
■ 1–3 seizures	11.00%	
☐ Seizure-free with aura	9.00%	
■ Seizure-free with no aura	47%	

FIGURE 3: The fifth year epilepsy outcome temporal lobe surgery.

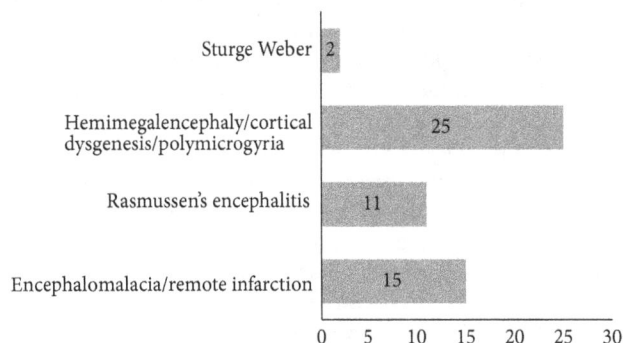

FIGURE 4: The underlying epilepsy disease of functional hemispherectomy cases.

and 4 (20%) had 1–3 seizures per year. According to ILAE, the favorable outcome for the third year following multilobar surgery, according to the ILAE, is 50%; in our cases, we had 5 patients (41.7%) that were seizure-free without auras, and 1 (8.3%) had 1–3 seizures per year (Figures 1 and 2).

4.5. Functional Hemispherectomy. According to ILAE criteria, the favorable outcome for patients in the first year following a hemispherectomy is 64.2%. Our results found 30

patients (56.6%) were seizure-free without auras, 2 (3.8%) were seizure-free with auras, and 2 (3.8%) had 1–3 seizures per year. The favorable outcome for the third year following a hemispherectomy, according to the ILAE, is 63%. Our study found 14 patients (46.7%) were seizure-free without auras, 1 (3.3%) was seizure-free with auras, and 4 (13.3%) had 1–3 seizures per year (Figures 1 and 2).

A total of 53 functional hemispherectomies were performed in our series. The MRI brain diagnosis disclosed 11 cases of Rasmussen encephalitis, 25 of cerebral cortical dysgenesis and hemimegalencephaly, 15 of remote infarction and encephalomalacia (gliosis), and 2 of Sturge Weber disease. Forty-one of the patients were children (Figure 4).

5. Pediatric Epilepsy Surgery Outcome

146 children with refractory epilepsy underwent epilepsy surgery. The favorable first-year epilepsy surgery outcome for

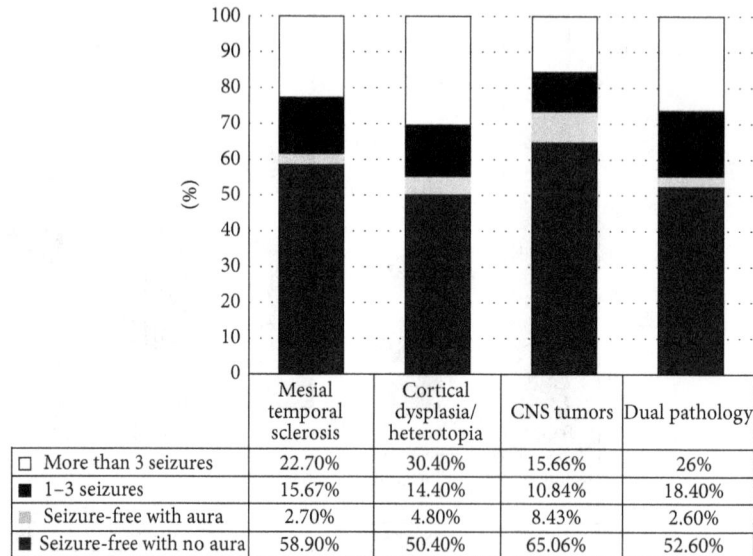

	Mesial temporal sclerosis	Cortical dysplasia/ heterotopia	CNS tumors	Dual pathology
☐ More than 3 seizures	22.70%	30.40%	15.66%	26%
■ 1–3 seizures	15.67%	14.40%	10.84%	18.40%
▨ Seizure-free with aura	2.70%	4.80%	8.43%	2.60%
■ Seizure-free with no aura	58.90%	50.40%	65.06%	52.60%

FIGURE 5: The first-year epilepsy surgery outcome according to histopathology.

temporal lobe surgery according to ILAE criteria is 88.4%, (48 (69.6%) were seizure-free without aura, 2 (2.8%) seizure-free with aura, and 11 (16%) 1–3 seizures per year). The favorable third year for temporal lobe surgery (ILAE) is 72%; (25 (58%) seizure-free without aura, 4 (9%) seizure-free with aura, and 2 (5%) with 1–3 seizures per year). The favorable fifth year for temporal lobe surgery (ILAE) is 71%; (12 (57%) seizure-free without aura, 3 (14%) seizure-free with aura).

The favorable first year epilepsy surgery outcome for frontal lobe surgery according to ILAE criteria is 70% (11 (55%) were seizure-free without aura, 1 (5%) seizure-free with aura, and 2 (10%) 1–3 seizures per year). The favorable third year for frontal lobe surgery (ILAE) is 70% (6 (60%) seizure-free without aura and 1 (10%) seizure-free with aura).

The favorable first-year epilepsy surgery outcome for parietal and occipital lobes surgery according to ILAE criteria is 50% (2 (50%) were seizure-free without aura). Only one case completed three years after surgery and the outcome was seizure-free without aura.

The favorable first-year epilepsy surgery outcome for multilobar surgery according to ILAE criteria is 80%, (3 (60%) were seizure-free without aura and 1 (20%) with 1–3 seizures per year).

The favorable first-year epilepsy surgery outcome for functional hemispherectomy according to ILAE criteria is 60% (22 (55%) were seizure-free without aura, 1 (2.5%) seizure-free with aura, and 1 (2.5%) 1–3 seizures per year). The favorable third-year epilepsy surgery outcome for functional hemispherectomy (ILAE) is 58%; (10 (53%) seizure-free without aura and 1 (5%) 1–3 seizures per year).

6. Epilepsy Surgery Outcome according to Histopathology

6.1. Mesial Temporal Sclerosis. According to the ILAE, the favorable outcome for patients with a histopathology

diagnosis of mesial temporal sclerosis in the first year following epilepsy surgery is 77.27%. In our cases, 109 patients (58.9%) were seizure-free without auras, 5 (2.7%) were seizure-free with auras, and 29 (15.6%) had 1–3 seizures per year. The favorable outcome for patients in the third year following epilepsy surgery with a histopathology diagnosis of mesial temporal sclerosis, according to the ILAE, is 76%. In our cases, we found 68 patients (57%) were seizure-free without auras, 3 (2.0%) were seizure-free with auras, and 20 (17%) had 1–3 seizures per year. The favorable outcome for patients with a histopathology diagnosis of mesial temporal sclerosis in the fifth year following epilepsy surgery, according to ILAE criteria, is 58%. Our series found 21 patients (42%) were seizure-free without auras, 1 (2%) was seizure-free with auras, and 7 (24%) had 1–3 seizures per year (Figures 5 and 6).

6.2. Cortical Dysplasia/Heterotopias. The favorable outcome for patients with a histopathology diagnosis of cortical dysplasia/heterotopias in the first year following epilepsy surgery, according to the ILAE, is 69.6%. Our cases showed 63 patients (50.4%) were seizure-free without auras, 6 (4.8%) were seizure-free with auras, and 18 (14.4%) had 1–3 seizures per year. According to ILAE criteria, the favorable outcome for patients in the third year following epilepsy surgery is 65.48%. In our series, 40 patients (47.6%) were seizure-free without auras, 6 (7.14%) were seizure-free with auras, and 9 (10.7%) suffered from 1–3 seizures per year. According to the ILAE criteria, the favorable outcome for patients in the fifth year following epilepsy surgery is 61.2%. Our study showed 23 patients (47%) were seizure-free without auras, 5 (10.2%) were seizure-free with auras, and 2 (4%) had 1–3 seizures per year (Figures 5 and 6).

6.3. Benign CNS Tumors. According to the ILAE, the favorable outcome for patients with a histopathology diagnosis

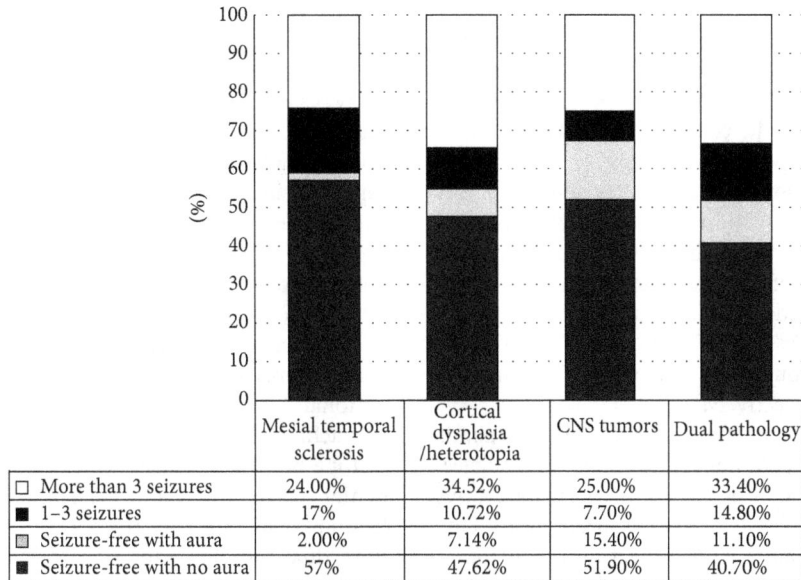

	Mesial temporal sclerosis	Cortical dysplasia /heterotopia	CNS tumors	Dual pathology
☐ More than 3 seizures	24.00%	34.52%	25.00%	33.40%
■ 1–3 seizures	17%	10.72%	7.70%	14.80%
▨ Seizure-free with aura	2.00%	7.14%	15.40%	11.10%
■ Seizure-free with no aura	57%	47.62%	51.90%	40.70%

FIGURE 6: The third-year epilepsy surgery outcome according to histopathology.

of benign CNS tumors in the first year following epilepsy surgery is 84.3%. Our studies showed 54 patients (65.1%) were seizure-free without auras, 7 (8.43%) were seizure-free with auras, and 9 (10.9%) had 1–3 seizures per year. The favorable outcome for patients in the third year following epilepsy surgery, according to the ILAE, is 75%. In our series, we found 27 patients (51.9%) were seizure-free without auras, 8 (15.4%) were seizure-free with auras, and 4 (7.7%) suffered from 1–3 seizures per year. According to the ILAE, the favorable outcome for patients in the fifth year following epilepsy surgery is 66.5%. Our research found 12 patients (44.5%) were seizure-free without auras, 3 (11%) were seizure-free with auras, and 3 (11%) had 1–3 seizures per year (Figures 5 and 6).

6.4. Dual Pathology. The favorable outcome for patients with a histopathology diagnosis of dual pathology in the first year following epilepsy surgery, according to the ILAE, is 73.6%. Our cases showed 20 patients (52.6%) were seizure-free without auras, 1 (2.6%) was seizure-free with auras, and 7 (18.4%) had 1–3 seizures per year. According to the ILAE, the favorable outcome for patients in the third year following epilepsy surgery is 66.6%. In our study, we found 11 patients (40.7%) were seizure-free without auras, 3 (11.1%) were seizure-free with auras, and 4 (14.8%) suffered from 1–3 seizures per year (Figures 5 and 6).

7. Epilepsy Surgery Outcomes in Patients with Normal MRI Scans

Thirty-four epilepsy patients with normal MRI brain scans were surgically treated. Surgical outcomes were assessed in 34 out of 35 patients that were seen one year after surgery. The PET scan result of 24 patients showed hypometabolism. The surgical procedures were 17 temporal lobe surgeries,

12 frontal lobe surgeries, 2 parietal and occipital surgeries, 2 corpus callosotomies, and 1 frontal multiple subpial transaction. The epileptogenic region was identified using the clinical semiology and the invasive intracranial EEG recording. The 12- and 36-month epilepsy surgery outcome of 17 temporal lobe surgeries were (53%) and (47%) seizure-free, respectively. The first- and third-year epilepsy surgery outcomes of 15 extratemporal epilepsy surgeries were (47%) and (33%) seizure-free. The histopathology results were 12 focal cortical dysplasia and heterotopias, 12 sclerosis and gliosis, 2 nonspecific, 5 had normal histopathology results and no histopathology tissues were obtained for 2 corpus callosotomies and 1 frontal multiple subpial transaction.

8. Discussion

This study of the Saudi epilepsy surgery series demonstrated that the epilepsy surgery outcomes in our epilepsy center compare well to those from other countries [16]. In this study, we have reported the outcomes of adults and pediatric epilepsy procedures at 12, 36, and 60 months for temporal lobe surgeries and outcomes at 12 and 36 months for frontal, parietal, occipital, multilobar surgery, and hemispherectomy.

The study included the patients that underwent resective surgery in the epilepsy program of Riyadh's KFSHRC between 1998 and 2012. The postoperative outcome was assessed according to a classification adapted from the ILAE. Seizure-free patients without auras, seizure-free patients with postoperative auras, and patients with fewer than three seizures per year were considered to be favorable outcomes based on the recommendations of the ILAE commission report [17, 18].

The literature showed a significant improvement in seizures with temporal and extratemporal epilepsy surgery in children and adults [19–24]. Significant improvements were established based on short- and long-term followups [25, 26]. The estimates of the likelihood of seizure-freedom after epilepsy surgery are 65% to 80% of lesional temporal lobe epilepsy patients [13]. In our series, the favorable outcomes following surgery for temporal lobe epilepsy patients are 79.6%, 74.2%, and 67% for 12, 36, and 60 months, respectively. These results are similar to the reported long-term followup results for surgery for temporal lobe epilepsy [27].

Various studies have examined the rates and predictors of seizure-freedom after resection for frontal lobe epilepsy. There is significant variability in their results due to patient diversity. Across 1,199 patients in 21 studies, the overall rate of postoperative seizure-freedom for at least 48 months (Engel Class I outcome) was 45.1% [28, 29]. In our series, the ILAE Class I–3 outcomes for frontal lobe epilepsy are 62% and 52% for 12 and 36 months, respectively.

Surgery on the parietal and occipital lobes depends largely on the underlying pathology. Previous studies suggest 20% of nonlesional and 75% of lesional parietal lobe cases may be rendered seizure-free by resective surgery [30]. One of the reports in the literature with respect to the outcomes of occipital lobe epilepsy surgery indicated that 46% became seizure-free and 21% had a significant reduction in seizure frequency [31]. Our experience in occipital and parietal lobe epilepsy surgeries indicated that the ILAE class 1–3 surgical outcomes for both first- and third-year followups are 67%.

A total of 53 functional hemispherectomies were performed in our series. Of the 53 procedures, 11 cases were *Rasmussen encephalitis, 25 were hemimegalencephaly and cerebral cortical dysgenesis, and 15 were encephalomalacia. Forty-one of the 53 patients were children.* ILAE class 1–3 surgical outcomes for the first- and third-year followup are 64% and 63%, respectively. The atypical variable in our series is the high ratio (47%) of the *hemimegalencephaly* and cortical dysgenesis.

Hemimegalencephaly was first described by Sims in 1835 [32]. 15 cases with *hemimegalencephaly that underwent* a functional hemispherectomy were described. Engel class (1a–c) was achieved in 10 out of 15 cases [33]. Another report evaluated 58 children that underwent anatomical, functional, or modified anatomical hemispherectomy for intractable seizures from 1986 to 1995 for seizure control. Seizure control with more than one year of followup revealed a better reduction in seizure frequency in 44 out of 50 (88%). Interestingly, there was no seizure-freedom achievement in this series [34]. Moreover, 23 patients *with Rasmussen encephalitis* underwent surgery [35]. The mean followup was 63.3 months. Eleven patients had total seizure control while 12 individuals persisted with seizures [35].

We did analyze the surgical outcome based on the histopathology diagnosis. CNS and MTS patients had a better outcome than those with cortical dysplasia (CD) or dual pathology at 1 and 3 years after surgery. In the Irish epilepsy surgery experience, MTS patients had a significantly better outcome than those with CD, a CNS tumor, and other pathology groups at 1, 2, and 5 years after surgery [36]. Dual pathology is recognized in the histopathology of epileptic tissues [37, 38]. Our results demonstrated that 7.5% of the total histopathology results had two or more different potentially epileptiform abnormalities. It is remarkable that the least

seizure-free outcome after 3 years did occur in the cases with dual pathology.

In our series, 34 cases of refractory nonlesional focal epilepsy cases have been operated upon with encouraging results, although the number is too small to allow indisputable analysis; however, our results match with some of the reported similar literature. Jayakar et al. studied 102 patients with nonlesional intractable partial epilepsy that underwent excisional surgery. At the 2-year followup, 44 out of 101 patients were seizure-free, and 15 experienced greater than 90% reduction [39].

In conclusion, the epilepsy surgery outcome in our comprehensive epilepsy program is comparable to the international standard. In our series, the most favorable outcomes are achieved with temporal epilepsy surgery procedure, histopathological diagnosis of mesial temporal sclerosis, benign CNS tumor, and cortical dysplasia, while the least favorable outcomes occurred with multilobar surgery procedure, dual pathology, and normal MRI brain patients.

Disclosure

The research protocol has been approved by the research centre's ethics committee.

Conflict of Interests

The authors indicate no potential conflict of interests.

References

[1] N. Senanayake and G. C. Roman, "Epidemiology of epilepsy in developing countries," *Bulletin of the World Health Organization*, vol. 71, no. 2, pp. 247–258, 1993.

[2] V. N. Halatchev, "Epidemiology of epilepsy—recent achievements and future," *Folia medica*, vol. 42, no. 2, pp. 17–22, 2000.

[3] E. Granieri, E. Paolino, M. R. Tola et al., "Epidemiology of epilepsy in the U.S.L. 34, Copparo, Emilia-Romagna," *Revista de Neurología*, vol. 54, no. 4, pp. 245–264, 1984.

[4] W. A. Hauser, "The prevalence and incidence of convulsive disorders in children," *Epilepsia*, vol. 35, supplement 2, pp. S1–S6, 1994.

[5] S. Al Rajeh, A. Awada, O. Bademosi, and A. Ogunniyi, "The prevalence of epilepsy and other seizure disorders in an Arab population: a community-based study," *Seizure*, vol. 10, no. 6, pp. 410–414, 2001.

[6] S. Al-Rajeh, A. Abomelha, A. Awada, O. Bademosi, and H. Ismail, "Epilepsy and other convulsive disorders in Saudi Arabia: a prospective study of 1,000 consecutive cases," *Acta Neurologica Scandinavica*, vol. 82, no. 5, pp. 341–345, 1990.

[7] J. F. Annegers, W. A. Hauser, and L. R. Elveback, "Remission of seizures and relapse in patients with epilepsy," *Epilepsia*, vol. 20, no. 6, pp. 729–737, 1979.

[8] P. Kwan and M. J. Brodie, "Early identification of refractory epilepsy," *The New England Journal of Medicine*, vol. 342, no. 5, pp. 314–319, 2000.

[9] W. Feindel, R. Leblanc, and A. N. de Almeida, "Epilepsy surgery: historical highlights 1909–2009," *Epilepsia*, vol. 50, no. 3, pp. 131–151, 2009.

[10] S. Wiebe, W. T. Blume, J. P. Girvin, and M. Eliasziw, "A randomized, controlled trial of surgery for temporal-lobe epilepsy," *The New England Journal of Medicine*, vol. 345, no. 5, pp. 311–318, 2001.

[11] K. Kingwell, "Epilepsy: surgical therapy should not be considered a last resort for pharmacoresistant epilepsy," *Nature Reviews Neurology*, vol. 8, no. 5, p. 238, 2012.

[12] J. Engel Jr., M. P. McDermott, S. Wiebe et al., "Early surgical therapy for drug-resistant temporal lobe epilepsy: a randomized trial," *Journal of the American Medical Association*, vol. 307, no. 9, pp. 922–930, 2012.

[13] S. S. Spencer, A. T. Berg, B. G. Vickrey et al., "Initial outcomes in the multicenter study of epilepsy surgery," *Neurology*, vol. 61, no. 12, pp. 1680–1685, 2003.

[14] J. Engel Jr., S. Wiebe, J. French et al., "Practice parameter: temporal lobe and localized neocortical resections for epilepsy—report of the quality standards subcommittee of the American Academy of Neurology, in association with the American Epilepsy Society and the American Association of Neurological Surgeons," *Neurology*, vol. 60, no. 4, pp. 538–547, 2003.

[15] C. Baumgartner, M. Brazdil, C. Binnie et al., "Pre-surgical evaluation for epilepsy surgery—European standards: European Federation of Neurological Societies Task Force," *European Journal of Neurology*, vol. 7, no. 1, pp. 119–122, 2000.

[16] "Epilepsy surgery: an evidence summary," *Ontario Health Technology Assessment Series*, vol. 12, no. 17, pp. 1–28, 2012.

[17] H. G. Wieser, W. T. Blume, D. Fish et al., "ILAE Commission Report. Proposal for a new classification of outcome with respect to epileptic seizures following epilepsy surgery," *Epilepsia*, vol. 42, no. 2, pp. 282–286, 2001.

[18] A. J. Durnford, W. Rodgers, F. J. Kirkham et al., "Very good inter-rater reliability of Engel and ILAE epilepsy surgery outcome classifications in a series of 76 patients," *Seizure*, vol. 20, no. 10, pp. 809–812, 2011.

[19] J. Engel Jr., "Update on surgical treatment of the epilepsies: summary of The Second International Palm Desert Conference on the Surgical Treatment of the Epilepsies (1992)," *Neurology*, vol. 43, no. 8, pp. 1612–1617, 1993.

[20] I. Jensen and K. Vaernet, "Temporal lobe epilepsy. Follow up investigation of 74 temporal lobe resected patients," *Acta Neurochirurgica*, vol. 37, no. 3-4, pp. 173–200, 1977.

[21] S. F. Berkovic, A. M. McIntosh, R. M. Kalnins et al., "Preoperative MRI predicts outcome of temporal lobectomy: an actuarial analysis," *Neurology*, vol. 45, no. 7, pp. 1358–1363, 1995.

[22] R. Morace, G. Di Gennaro, A. Picardi et al., "Surgery after intracranial investigation with subdural electrodes in patients with drug-resistant focal epilepsy: outcome and complications," *Neurosurgical Review*, vol. 35, no. 4, pp. 519–526, 2012.

[23] K. M. Aaberg, A. S. Eriksson, J. Ramm-Pettersen, and K. O. Nakken, "Long-term outcome of resective epilepsy surgery in Norwegian children," *Acta Paediatrica*, vol. 101, no. 12, pp. e557–e560, 2012.

[24] A. M. Siegel, "Epilepsy surgery of extratemporal epilepsy," *Therapeutische Umschau*, vol. 58, no. 11, pp. 676–683, 2001.

[25] S. Wiebe, "Epilepsy: outcome patterns in epilepsy surgery—the long-term view," *Nature Reviews Neurology*, vol. 8, no. 3, pp. 123–124, 2012.

[26] A. M. Mcintosh, C. A. Averill, R. M. Kalnins et al., "Long-term seizure outcome and risk factors for recurrence after extra-temporal epilepsy surgery," *Epilepsia*, vol. 53, no. 6, pp. 970–978, 2012.

[27] H. Nakase, K. Tamura, Y. Kim, H. Hirabayashi, T. Sakaki, and T. Hoshida, "Long-term follow-up outcome after surgical treatment for lesional temporal lobe epilepsy," *Neurological Research*, vol. 29, no. 6, pp. 588–593, 2007.

[28] D. J. Englot, D. D. Wang, J. D. Rolston, T. T. Shih, and E. F. Chang, "Rates and predictors of long-term seizure freedom after frontal lobe epilepsy surgery: a systematic review and meta-analysis," *Journal of Neurosurgery*, vol. 116, no. 5, pp. 1042–1048, 2012.

[29] L. E. Jeha, I. Najm, W. Bingaman, D. Dinner, P. Widdess-Walsh, and H. Lüders, "Surgical outcome and prognostic factors of frontal lobe epilepsy surgery," *Brain*, vol. 130, part 2, pp. 574–584, 2007.

[30] A. Olivier and W. Boling Jr., "Surgery of parietal and occipital lobe epilepsy," *Advances in Neurology*, vol. 84, pp. 533–575, 2000.

[31] V. Salanova, F. Andermann, A. Olivier, T. Rasmussen, and L. F. Quesney, "Occipital lobe epilepsy: electroclinical manifestations, electrocorticography, cortical stimulation and outcome in 42 patients treated between 1930 and 1991. Surgery of occipital lobe epilepsy," *Brain*, vol. 115, part 6, pp. 1655–1680, 1992.

[32] J. Sims, "On hypertrophy and atrophy of the brain," *Medico-Chirurgical Transactions*, vol. 19, pp. 315–380, 1835.

[33] C. Di Rocco and A. Iannelli, "Hemimegalencephaly and intractable epilepsy: complications of hemispherectomy and their correlations with the surgical technique: a report on 15 cases," *Pediatric Neurosurgery*, vol. 33, no. 4, pp. 198–207, 2000.

[34] W. J. Peacock, M. C. Wehby-Grant, W. D. Shields et al., "Hemispherectomy for intractable seizures in children: a report of 58 cases," *Child's Nervous System*, vol. 12, no. 7, pp. 376–384, 1996.

[35] V. C. Terra-Bustamante, H. R. MacHado, R. Dos Santos Oliveira et al., "Rasmussen encephalitis: long-term outcome after surgery," *Child's Nervous System*, vol. 25, no. 5, pp. 583–589, 2009.

[36] O. Dunlea, C. P. Doherty, M. Farrell et al., "The Irish epilepsy surgery experience: long-term follow-up," *Seizure*, vol. 19, no. 4, pp. 247–252, 2010.

[37] Y. M. Hart, F. Andermann, Y. Robitaille, K. D. Laxer, T. Rasmussen, and R. Davis, "Double pathology in Rasmussen's syndrome: a window on the etiology?" *Neurology*, vol. 50, no. 3, pp. 731–735, 1998.

[38] K. S. Firlik, P. D. Adelson, and R. L. Hamilton, "Coexistence of a Ganglioglioma and Rasmussen's encephalitis," *Pediatric Neurosurgery*, vol. 30, no. 5, pp. 278–282, 1999.

[39] P. Jayakar, C. Dunoyer, P. Dean et al., "Epilepsy surgery in patients with normal or nonfocal MRI scans: integrative strategies offer long-term seizure relief," *Epilepsia*, vol. 49, no. 5, pp. 758–764, 2008.

15

Cerebral Hemispheric Lateralization Associated with Hippocampal Sclerosis May Affect Interictal Cardiovascular Autonomic Functions in Temporal Lobe Epilepsy

Rokia Ghchime,[1,2,3] Halima Benjelloun,[3] Hajar Kiai,[4] Halima Belaidi,[2] Fatiha Lahjouji,[2] and Reda Ouazzani[1,2]

[1] Physiology Laboratory, Faculty of Medicine and Pharmacy, Mohammed V-Souissi University, 6203 Rabat, Morocco
[2] Department of Clinical Neurophysiology, Hospital of Specialties, Ibn Sina University Hospital, Rabat Institute, 6220 Rabat, Morocco
[3] Unit of Cardiology A, Ibn Sina University Hospital, 10000 Rabat, Morocco
[4] Food Sciences Laboratory, Department of Biology, Faculty of Sciences Semlalia, Prince Moulay Abdellah Avenue, 40090 Marrakesh, Morocco

Correspondence should be addressed to Rokia Ghchime; rokairo@gmail.com

Academic Editor: Louis Lemieux

It is well established that the temporal lobe epilepsy (TLE) is linked to the autonomic nervous system dysfunctions. Seizures alter the function of different systems such as the respiratory, cardiovascular, gastrointestinal, and urogenital systems. The aim of this work was to evaluate the possible factors which may be involved in interictal cardiovascular autonomic function in temporal lobe epilepsy with complex partial seizures, and with particular attention to hippocampal sclerosis. The study was conducted in 30 patients with intractable temporal lobe epilepsy (19 with left hippocampal sclerosis, 11 with right hippocampal sclerosis). All subjects underwent four tests of cardiac autonomic function: heart rate changes in response to deep breathing, heart rate, and blood pressure variations throughout resting activity and during hand grip, mental stress, and orthostatic tests. Our results show that the right cerebral hemisphere predominantly modulates sympathetic activity, while the left cerebral hemisphere mainly modulates parasympathetic activity, which mediated tachycardia and excessive bradycardia counterregulation, both of which might be involved as a mechanism of sudden unexpected death in epilepsy patients (SUDEP).

1. Introduction

Temporal lobe epilepsy (TLE) is well known to be associated with autonomic nervous system dysfunctions [1, 2]. Seizures alter the function of different systems such as the respiratory, gastrointestinal, urogenital, and, most importantly, cardiovascular system [1, 3, 4].

Autonomic cardiovascular functions are mainly regulated by cortical, midbrain, and brainstem areas [5, 6]. The vital cortical area is the insular cortex folding into the inner temporal lobe that is often dysfunctional in TLE. Lesions of the insular cortex are usually associated with abnormalities in heart rate (HR) and blood pressure (BP) regulation as well as with cardiac arrhythmia [7]. In addition, mesiotemporal

structures were reported to be involved in both epileptogenesis and autonomic control in animal models [8]. Besides, several studies also indicate that the insular cortex and temporal lobe are powerful in the control of cardiovascular function in humans [7–10].

Hemispheric centers of autonomic nervous control show distinct modulation activities. For instance, while the right hemisphere modulates the sympathetic cardiovascular activity, the left hemisphere contributes more to the parasympathetic activity. These modulation discrepancies occur in various neurologic disorders, such as intracranial tumors, cerebral trauma, encephalitis, hemorrhagic or ischemic stroke, or epilepsy. In epilepsy patients, signs of autonomic dysfunction occur both interictally and ictally. During seizures, cardiovascular disturbances such as tachy- or bradyarrhythmia are frequent findings, indicating close interactions between epileptogenic brain areas and centers of autonomic control [11–13]. Supraventricular bradycardia has been highly reported in TLE with left HS compared to TLE with right HS and the tachycardia more reported in TLE with right HS compared to TLE with left HS, suggesting an increase of sympathetic cardiac activity caused by the right hemisphere innervations.

On that focus, our study is designed to compare the changes of heart rate (HR) and blood pressure (BP) in two groups of TLE, with right HS and with left HS to investigate the possible factors related to the structural characteristics of TLE, especially cerebral lateralization associated with hippocampal sclerosis.

2. Patients and Methods

2.1. Patients. This study was conducted between 2012 and 2015 at the Department of Clinical Neurophysiology and at the unit of autonomic nervous system (ANS) exploration at the Department of Cardiology A, University Hospital Center (UHC) Ibn Sina, Rabat, Morocco. It was approved by the Ibn Sina ethical committee. A written consent form was obtained from each patient before the tests.

Thirty patients with refractory temporal lobe epilepsy destined to surgery were recruited at the Department of Clinical Neurophysiology for pretreatment and diagnosis protocol, including clinical, neurophysiological, and electrophysiological examinations (video-EEG) as well as MRI and battery of tests for the assessment of cardiac autonomic functions. The study subjects have mesial temporal lobe epilepsy with complex partial seizures according to the classifications of the International League Against Epilepsy, 1981 and 1989. However, patients with lesions other than hippocampal sclerosis on cranial MRI; patients with EEGs within the last 24 hours showing interictal epileptiform discharges; subjects suffering from diseases other than epilepsy that are known to affect the autonomic cardiovascular system (renal failure, diabetes mellitus, and cardiopulmonary disease) were excluded. The following subjects were also expelled from our study: subjects diagnosed for psychiatric illnesses, or those with abuse of alcohol or smoking as well as patients breastfeeding, or in pregnancy [14, 15].

2.2. Methods. All patients underwent an autonomic cardiac function testing which is based on HR and BP responses at rest and after different stimuli. All tests were conducted under standardized conditions. The measurements were carried out in quiet room with an ambient temperature of 22°C between 9 and 12 a.m. Patients were asked to avoid taking any drugs other than their AEDs a week before the tests [16, 17]. The interval between the different tests was standardized so that the following test did not start until the HR and BP had returned to the baseline level after the preceding test. HR and BP responses at rest and after stimulation were recorded under the subsequent conditions: normal breathing, deep breathing, isometric work (hand grip), mental stress, and tilting. ECG was first recorded through the normal breathing. Consecutive RR intervals were measured from the ECG for a period of 5 min and the standard deviation of the intervals was employed as the test variable.

2.2.1. Deep Breathing Test. This test evaluates the autonomic function by measuring the changes of HR in response to controlled breathing [16, 18]. During the test of deep breathing (DB), patients were asked to breathe deeply at frequency of six breaths per minute. The respiratory frequency has an influence on the variation of RR interval on the EKG. The vagal response to the DB is calculated using the following equation:

$$DB = \frac{(RR_{maximal} - RR_{minimal})}{RR_{minimal}} \times 100. \tag{1}$$

$RR_{minimal}$ and $RR_{maximal}$ are intervals obtained at the end of expiration and the end of inspiration, respectively.

2.2.2. Isometric Contraction or Hand Grip Test. During 3 minutes the subject carries out a manual pressure of 50% of the maximum using a dynamometer (Jetter and Scheerer, Germany) with his dominant hand and the maximum voluntary contraction (MVC) was calculated. BP was measured before and after contraction at 1, 2, and 4 min in the contralateral arm.

The muscular contraction involves an increase in BP related to a rise of sympathetic nervous system at the muscular level that is effort- and time-dependent [19, 20]. The peripheral sympathetic nervous response "α" is given by the increase of the BP:

Peripheral sympathetic response "α"

$$= \frac{(BP_{after\ the\ test} - BP_{before\ the\ test})}{BP_{before\ the\ test}} \times 100. \tag{2}$$

2.2.3. Mental Stress Test. The patient performs mental arithmetic calculations by removing the number 7 successively from 200. The result is an augmentation in HR and in BP by activation of the central sympathetic nervous system [21].

In mental stress, the central sympathetic nerves activities "α" were assessed by measuring the changes of BP as follows [19, 20]:

Central sympathetic response "α"

$$= \frac{(BP_{after\ stimulation} - BP_{before\ stimulation})}{BP_{before\ stimulation}} \times 100. \tag{3}$$

The central sympathetic nervous activity "β" was assessed by measuring the changes of HR as follows [19, 20]:

Central sympathetic response "β"

$$= \frac{(HR_{after\ stimulation} - HR_{before\ stimulation})}{HR_{before\ stimulation}} \times 100. \tag{4}$$

TABLE 1: Demographics and resting autonomic parameters of thirty temporal lobe epilepsy patients with hippocampal sclerosis.

Parameters	TLE with left HS ($N = 19$) (mean ± SD)	TLE with right HS ($N = 11$) (mean ± SD)	All patients ($N = 30$) (mean ± SD)	p values
Age (years)	32.47 ± 9.90	32 ± 11.71	32.3 ± 10.40	0.788
Gender (F/M)	14/5	4/7	18/12	0.044
Age of onset of epilepsy (years)	7.37 ± 4.6	8.09 ± 6.8	7.63 ± 5.4	0.682
Duration of illness (years)	25.11 ± 11.75	23.91 ± 11.07	24.67 ± 11.32	0.503
HR (bpm)	63.63 ± 6.78	67.09 ± 9.80	64.90 ± 8.04	0.101
SBP (mm Hg)	109.82 ± 10.27	115.4 ± 11.13	111.87 ±10.76	0.027
DBP (mm Hg)	68.45 ± 12.11	73 ± 7.74	70 ± 10.78	0.057
Frequency seizures	16 ± 13	8 ± 5	12 ± 9	0.003

Values expressed as mean ± SD. p is significant if < 0.05. Student's t-test.
SBP: systolic blood pressure; DBP: diastolic blood pressure; HR: heart rate; HS: hippocampal sclerosis; F: female; M: male.

2.2.4. Orthostatic or Tilt Test. The responses of HR and BP to quick postural change (from standing to supine position) were recorded. Systolic and diastolic BP were measured at rest and immediately after and during standing position. The difference between BP at rest and the lowest BP after standing was calculated [14, 22]. The assessment of peripheral sympathetic response beta is given by the following formula:

Peripheral sympathetic response "β"

$$= \frac{\left(BP_{after\ stimulation} - BP_{before\ stimulation}\right)}{BP_{before\ stimulation}} \times 100. \tag{5}$$

In both orthostatic and mental stress tests, values above 10% correspond to sympathetic hyperactivity; a response equal to 10% is considered normal. However, patients with values below 10% are deficient.

2.3. MR Imaging. Patients underwent a standard MRI protocol that was carried out using a 1.5-T scanner (Philips Intera System). Imaging studies included (1) FLAIR, T1 IR, and T2 weighted hippocampal images, coronal oblique images perpendicular to the long axis of the hippocampus, with a 2 mm slice thickness and no intervening gap and (2) axial T1 and T2 weighted, coronal T2 weighted, and sagittal T1 weighted cranial images with a 5-mm slice thickness and 1.5-mm intervening gap [17, 18, 20].

2.4. EEG. Interictal EEG was recorded several times before the autonomic cardiac function testing, employing a video-EEG monitoring system (Micromed; Treviso, Italy); the electrodes were arranged according to the International 10-20 system. The duration of video-EEG monitoring varied from 2 to 7 days, and at least three habitual seizures were recorded for each patient.

3. Statistics

Data were analyzed using the SPSS software (version 15.0; SPSS Inc., Chicago, IL, USA). The tests selected for the comparisons between the two studied groups, TLE with right hippocampal sclerosis and TLE with left hippocampal sclerosis, were the following: mental stress for the study of alpha and beta central sympathetic nerve activities; the hand grip of 3 min to assess the alpha peripheral sympathetic nerve reactivity; the orthostatic or tilt test of 10 min for the study of beta peripheral sympathetic nerve activity; and the deep breathing test for the study of vagal system. The values are expressed as average ± standard deviation.

The comparison of the results between TLE patients with right hippocampal sclerosis and TLE subjects with left hippocampal sclerosis was carried out by means of Student's t-test for paired samples. A value $p < 0.05$ was considered significant.

4. Results

4.1. Demographic and Clinical Features. Thirty patients were recruited in the Department of Clinical Neurophysiology and then addressed to the Unit of Cardiology A, Ibn Sina University Hospital, for performing cardiovascular autonomic test.

A clinical diagnosis and detailed medical history were carried out with special emphasis on types of AEDs taken, interictal EEG recordings, and cranial and hippocampal MRI. The epilepsy type was classified according to the recommendations of the International League Against Epilepsy (ILAE) [23–25].

The interictal EEG registration including T1 and T2 electrodes (International 10-20 system) showed interictal epileptiform discharges for all studied subjects, with 19 patients having left-sided temporal focal spikes and slow waves on the left in the EEG and 11 patients who had right-sided temporal focal spikes and slow waves on the right in the EEG.

The results of analysis on MRI in TLE patients showed 19 patients with left- and 11 patients with right-sided hippocampal sclerosis. Most of patients were under polytherapy with varying combination of two or three antiepileptic drugs, such as sodium valproate (VPA), carbamazepine (CBZ), lamotrigine (LTG), clobazam (CLB), clonazepam (CZP), and phenobarbital (PB). However, only five patients were taking carbamazepine (CBZ) and clobazam (CLB) as monotherapy.

As can be seen from Table 1, there is no significant difference between subjects with left hippocampal sclerosis

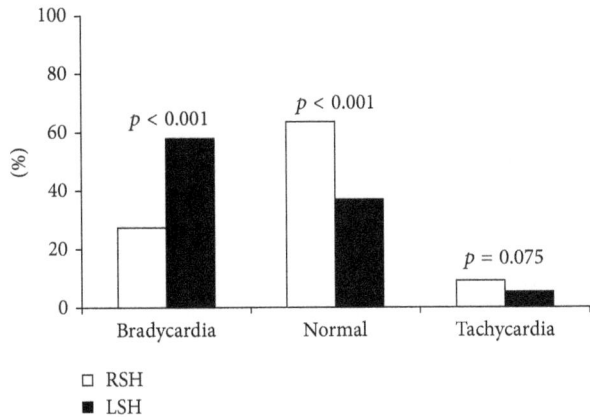

FIGURE 1: Comparison of basal heart rate in TLE with left and right hippocampal sclerosis.

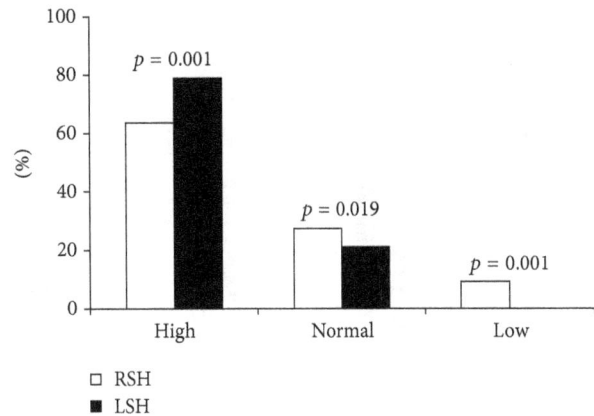

FIGURE 2: Vagal response on deep breathing test in TLE with right and left hippocampal sclerosis.

and patients with right hippocampal sclerosis with respect to age, age of onset, and duration of epilepsy distribution ($p > 0.05$).

Mean basal heart rate (HR) as well as diastolic blood pressure (DBP) did not differ significantly between the two groups. However, the mean basal systolic blood pressure (SBP) differs significantly between patients with left hippocampal sclerosis and patients with right hippocampal sclerosis.

4.2. Basal Heart Rate and Blood Pressure.
Based on the measurement of basal HR variability in the two groups (TLE with left HS and TLE with right HS) at resting, patients are considered bradycardic if their basal HR is less than 60 beats per minute or tachycardic if their basal HR is greater than or equal to 85 beats per minute.

The occurrence of bradycardia is significantly higher ($p < 0.001$) in TLE with left HS (57.9%) than TLE with right HS (27.27%) (Figure 1), while the prevalence of tachycardia was lower in TLE with left HS (5.2%) with respect to TLE with right HS (9.1%), without any significant difference ($p = 0.075$).

The normal values of basal HR are significantly higher ($p < 0.001$) in TLE with right HS (63.63%) compared to TLE with left HS (36.9%) (Figure 1).

4.3. Vagal Response.
The vagal response measured by the deep breathing (DB) test in TLE with right and left hippocampal sclerosis showed a higher parasympathetic activity in TLE patients with left HS (78.9%) than TLE subjects with right HS (63.6%). The difference between the two groups was statistically significant ($p < 0.001$) (Figure 2).

In contrast, a low parasympathetic activity (9.1%) was found in TLE with right HS. However, no case was declared in TLE with left HS. The difference between the two groups was statistically significant ($p = 0.001$). A normal parasympathetic response was higher in TLE with left HS versus right HS. The statistical analysis supports such observation ($p = 0.004$) (Figure 2).

4.4. Peripheral Sympathetic Response Alpha.
The peripheral sympathetic response alpha assessed by the hand grip (HG) test in TLE with right hippocampal sclerosis and TLE with a left hippocampal sclerosis showed a significant elevated peripheral sympathetic response alpha in TLE with right HS (54.5%) compared to TLE with left HS (47.36%) ($p = 0.012$, Figure 3(a)), whereas we noted a deficient but not significant ($p = 0.216$) peripheral sympathetic activity alpha in TLE with right HS (18.2%), as compared to TLE with left HS (15.8%). The normal peripheral sympathetic alpha response is slightly higher in TLE with left HS versus TLE with right HS. The statistical analysis supports such observation ($p = 0.004$) (Figure 3(a)).

4.5. Peripheral Sympathetic Response Beta.
The comparison of the peripheral sympathetic response beta obtained with the orthostatic test (OT) between TLE with right hippocampal sclerosis and TLE with a left hippocampal sclerosis reveals a high peripheral sympathetic beta response in TLE with right HS (72.7%) than TLE with left HS (31.6%). The difference between the two groups was highly significant ($p < 0.001$) (Figure 3(b)). A low peripheral sympathetic beta activity (31.6%) was observed in TLE with left HS. However, there was no noticeable case in TLE with right HS. The difference between the two groups was highly significant ($p < 0.001$). Hence, the normal peripheral sympathetic beta response was found statistically ($p = 0.004$) superior in TLE with left HS (36.8%) with respect to TLE with right HS (27.3%) (Figure 3(b)).

4.6. Central Sympathetic Response Alpha.
The assessment of the central sympathetic response alpha by the mental stress test, in two groups of TLE, showed a similar high central sympathetic alpha response in TLE with right HS (63.64%) and TLE with left HS (63.16%) ($p = 0.783$) (Figure 3(c)). Deficiency of central sympathetic alpha activity was observed in TLE with left HS (21.05%). However, no declared case was observed in TLE with right HS. The difference between the two groups was highly significant ($p < 0.001$). Normal response of the central sympathetic alpha

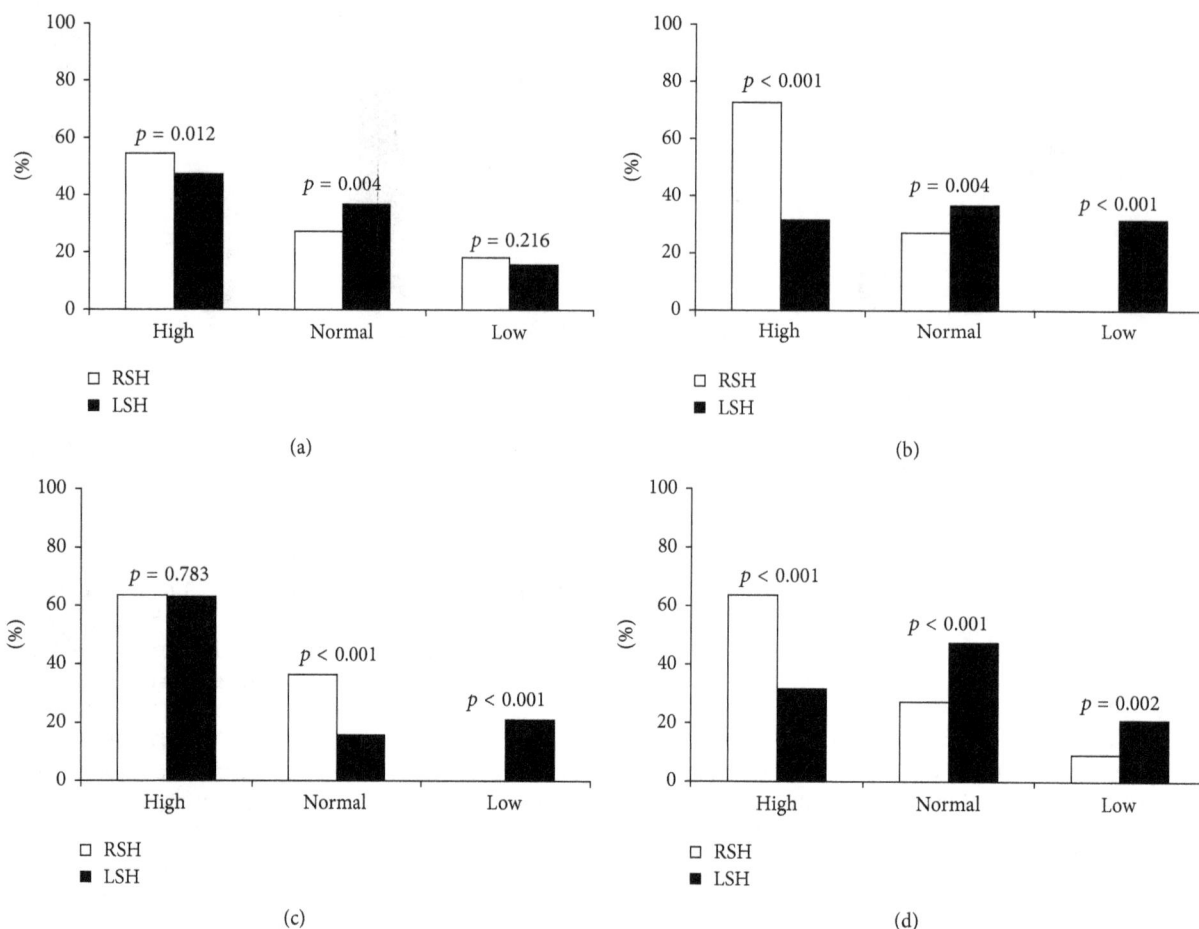

FIGURE 3: (a) Peripheral sympathetic response alpha (alpha SP) obtained on hand grip test, (b) peripheral sympathetic response beta (beta SP) obtained with orthostatic test, (c) central sympathetic response alpha (alpha SC), and (d) central sympathetic response beta (beta SC) obtained during mental stress.

system is significantly higher ($p < 0.001$) in TLE with left HS (36.8%) compared to TLE with right HS (27.3%) (Figure 3(c)).

4.7. Central Sympathetic Response Beta. The central sympathetic response beta evaluated by the mental stress test, in two groups of TLE, showed a highly significant ($p < 0.001$) elevated central sympathetic beta response in TLE with right HS (63.63%) as compared to TLE with left HS (31.59%) (Figure 3(d)). The same observation concerns the deficiency of central sympathetic beta activity, which was significantly important ($p = 0.002$) in TLE with left HS (21.05%) with respect to TLE with right HS (9.1%), while normal response of the central sympathetic beta system was found to be significantly ($p < 0.001$) higher in TLE with left HS (47.36%) in comparison to TLE with right HS (27.27%) (Figure 3(d)).

5. Discussion

Through the present study we brought evidence of an association of hippocampal sclerosis with cerebral lateralization that may cause disturbances in parasympathetic and sympathetic autonomic functions during the interictal period in patients with TLE. According to our finding, we revealed profound changes in HR by means of cardiovascular autonomic tests in two groups of TLE that allowed us to identify cerebral lateralization in cardiac autonomic control. Most patients with left-sided temporal focus associated with left HS showed bradycardia, whereas a tendency to tachycardia has been more observed in patients with right-sided temporal focus associated with right HS. Such observation is still under the significance threshold probably due to the low number of sampled patients.

Such finding could be explained by analyzing the sympathetic and parasympathetic activities of the two groups, showing a highly elevated parasympathetic activity in TLE with left HS compared to TLE with right HS. Moreover, comparison of the sympathetic cardiac response between the two groups demonstrates an increase of peripheral and central sympathetic response alpha and beta in patients with right-sided temporal focus associated with right HS, contrary to those with left-sided temporal focus associated with left HS.

We then suggest a possibility of different contributions between the right and left cerebral hemispheres. The left hemisphere predominantly modulates cardiac parasympathetic tone, by increasing its activity, and consequently provokes bradycardia, while the right hemisphere predominantly modulates cardiac sympathetic tone, by increasing its activity, and accordingly causes tachycardia that fits previous studies [7, 11–13, 25, 26].

In another study of humans, Oppenheimer et al. [8] showed that the electrical stimulation of the insular cortex was responsible for cardiovascular changes. Additional investigation showed that bradycardia was often observed during left insular stimulation, while tachycardia occurred during right insular stimulation [7]. Furthermore, neuroimaging studies, animal studies, and clinical observations propose a hemispheric lateralization of parasympathetic or sympathetic cardiovascular control [7, 11, 12, 27–31]. However, results of diverse investigations are contradictory.

Many studies have demonstrated that the right hemisphere dominates sympathetic cardiovascular activity [7, 11, 12, 27–31]. Critchley et al. [31] reported an association between arousal-induced sympathetically mediated skin conductance responses and activity predominantly localized in the right orbitofrontal cortex and the right anterior insula. A rise in regional blood flow in the right insular over stressful tasks associated with sympathetic activation using positron emission tomography was observed in healthy persons. Though, left insular activation concurred with BP and HR diminution during nonstrenuous tasks [29].

Contrary to the findings in healthy subjects, investigations in patients are more equivocal. Oppenheimer et al. [7] reported on subjects with complex partial seizures rightsided dominance of sympathetic BP and HR modulation by intraoperative electrical insular stimulation. With seizure subjects incurring presurgical assessment, Zamrini et al. [12] noticed a hastening of HR after left hemispheric inactivation during intracarotid amobarbital procedure. Likewise, Yoon et al. [11] stated improved sympathetic HR modulation during left-sided intracarotid amobarbital procedure and inferred that there is right hemispheric lateralization of cardiac sympathetic control. Conversely, other authors observed a decrease of parasympathetic HR modulation after right hemispheric stroke [27, 32]. Robinson et al. [33] stated a change in sympathovagal balance with elevated sympathetic activity after right hemispheric lesions in acute stroke patients. This result sustains the assumption of parasympathetic cardiac modulation in the right hemisphere.

Ansakorpi et al. [34] recently showed by investigating the role of hippocampal sclerosis directly in patients with TLE that cardiovascular autonomic dysfunction tended to be greater in patients with hippocampal sclerosis.

Moreover, the cardioregulatory function is a continuously functioning network widely in the inner temporal lobes with various ascending and descending connections mediated by various biochemical neurotransmitters to other areas of the brain [10, 35]. The experimental and clinical data showed the important role of the insular and limbic structures, such as amygdala, in cerebrogenic cardiovascular disturbances in sudden unexpected death in epilepsy patients (SUDEP) [36].

The anatomic or functional infractions such as a neuronal loss and excessive inhibition may cause interictal hypometabolism. Strong projections from limbic to hypothalamic areas and link of autonomic brainstem nuclei to hippocampus suggest that alterations in hippocampal anatomy and/or physiology may provoke disturbances in the autonomic function in patients with temporal epilepsy [37].

In addition to epilepsy itself, the antiepileptic drugs may alter the cardiovascular system as well as the centrally mediated cardiovascular control system function. An interaction between cardiovascular disturbances and AEDs may also contribute as a mechanism of sudden unexpected death in epileptic patients (SUDEP) [38, 39].

6. Conclusion

The present study is of a crucial importance, since it brought evidence of a central implication in the sudden unexpected death in temporal epileptic patients. Thus, intracranial disorders associated with hemispheric lateralization, such as hippocampal lesions, are strongly linked to disturbed cardiac features causing bradycardia or tachycardia. Nevertheless, several hypotheses related to possible factors affecting interictal autonomic dysfunction in patients with TLE, factors other than the structural abnormality of hippocampal sclerosis, such as refractoriness and chronic nature of epilepsy, epilepsy itself, duration of epilepsy, drug effects, infrequent seizures, were suggested to be related. Thus, further studies are needed to investigate factors affecting autonomic dysfunction in order to understand and prevent SUDEP.

Conflict of Interests

The authors declared that there is no conflict of interests to disclose.

References

[1] R. Freeman and S. C. Schachter, "Autonomic epilepsy," *Seminars in Neurology*, vol. 15, no. 2, pp. 158–166, 1995.

[2] M. J. Hilz, M. Dütsch, and C. Kölsch, "Epilepsy and autonomic dysfunction," *Fortschritte der Neurologie—Psychiatrie*, vol. 67, no. 2, pp. 49–59, 1999.

[3] E. E. Benarroch, "Telencephalic disorders," in *Central Autonomic Network: Functional Organization and Clinical Correlations*, pp. 539–559, Futura Publishing Company, Armonk, NY, USA, 1997.

[4] K. M. Spyer, "Central nervous control of the cardiovascular system," in *Autonomic Failure: A Textbook of Clinical Disorders of the Autonomic Nervous System*, pp. 45–55, Oxford University Press, 1999.

[5] D. F. Cechetto and C. B. Saper, "Role of the cerebral cortex in autonomic function," in *Central Regulation of Autonomic Functions*, pp. 208–223, Oxford University Press, New York, NY, USA, 1990.

[6] D. F. Cechetto, "Neuropathology and cardiovascular regulation," in *The Nervous System and the Heart*, pp. 159–179, Humana Press, Totowa, NJ, USA, 2000.

[7] S. M. Oppenheimer, A. Gelb, J. P. Girvin, and V. C. Hachinski, "Cardiovascular effects of human insular cortex stimulation," *Neurology*, vol. 42, no. 9, pp. 1727–1732, 1992.

[8] S. M. Oppenheimer, J. X. Wilson, C. Guiraudon, and D. F. Cechetto, "Insular cortex stimulation produces lethal cardiac arrhythmias: a mechanism of sudden death?" *Brain Research*, vol. 550, no. 1, pp. 115–121, 1991.

[9] M. A. Epstein, M. R. Sperling, and M. J. O'Connor, "Cardiac rhythm during temporal lobe seizures," *Neurology*, vol. 42, no. 1, pp. 50–53, 1992.

[10] C. Baumgartner, S. Lurger, and F. Leutmezer, "Autonomic symptoms during epileptic seizures," *Epileptic Disorders*, vol. 3, no. 3, pp. 103–116, 2001.

[11] B.-W. Yoon, C. A. Morillo, D. F. Cechetto, and V. Hachinski, "Cerebral hemispheric lateralization in cardiac autonomic control," *Archives of Neurology*, vol. 54, no. 6, pp. 741–744, 1997.

[12] E. Y. Zamrini, K. J. Meador, D. W. Loring et al., "Unilateral cerebral inactivation produces differential left/right heart rate responses," *Neurology*, vol. 40, no. 9, pp. 1408–1411, 1990.

[13] M. J. Hilz, M. Dütsch, K. Perrine, P. K. Nelson, U. Rauhut, and O. Devinsky, "Hemispheric influence on autonomic modulation and baroreflex sensitivity," *Annals of Neurology*, vol. 49, no. 5, pp. 575–584, 2001.

[14] S. Mukherjee, M. Tripathi, P. S. Chandra et al., "Cardiovascular autonomic functions in well-controlled and intractable partial epilepsies," *Epilepsy Research*, vol. 85, no. 2-3, pp. 261–269, 2009.

[15] E. Chroni, V. Sirrou, E. Trachani, G. C. Sakellaropoulos, and P. Polychronopoulos, "Interictal alterations of cardiovagal function in chronic epilepsy," *Epilepsy Research*, vol. 83, no. 2-3, pp. 117–123, 2009.

[16] D. J. Ewing, C. N. Martyn, R. J. Young, and B. F. Clarke, "The value of cardiovascular autonomic function tests: 10 years experience in diabetes," *Diabetes Care*, vol. 8, no. 5, pp. 491–498, 1985.

[17] F. Cendes, F. Andermann, F. Dubeau et al., "Early childhood prolonged febrile convulsions, atrophy and sclerosis of mesial structures, and temporal lobe epilepsy: an MRI volumetric study," *Neurology*, vol. 43, no. 6, pp. 1083–1087, 1993.

[18] F. Cendes, F. Andermann, P. Gloor et al., "Atrophy of mesial structures in patients with temporal lobe epilepsy: cause or consequence of repeated seizures?" *Annals of Neurology*, vol. 34, no. 6, pp. 795–801, 1993.

[19] T. L. Johansen, G. Kambskar, and J. Mehlsen, "Heart rate variability in evaluation of the autonomic nervous system. A review," *Ugeskrift for Læger*, vol. 159, no. 45, pp. 6666–6671, 1997.

[20] E. Koseoglu, S. Kucuk, F. Arman, and A. O. Ersoy, "Factors that affect interictal cardiovascular autonomic dysfunction in temporal lobe epilepsy: role of hippocampal sclerosis," *Epilepsy & Behavior*, vol. 16, no. 4, pp. 617–621, 2009.

[21] P. A. Low, "Laboratory evaluation of autonomic function," in *Clinical Autonomic Disorders: Evaluation and Management*, pp. 179–208, Lippincott-Raven, Philadelphia, Pa, USA, 1997.

[22] J. M. Ravits, "Autonomic nervous system testing," *Muscle & Nerve*, vol. 20, no. 8, pp. 919–937, 1997.

[23] J. Engel Jr., "Report of the ILAE classification core group," *Epilepsia*, vol. 47, no. 9, pp. 1558–1568, 2006.

[24] A. T. Berg, S. F. Berkovic, M. J. Brodie et al., "Revised terminology and concepts for organization of seizures and epilepsies: report of the ILAE Commission on Classification and Terminology, 2005–2009," *Epilepsia*, vol. 51, no. 4, pp. 676–685, 2010.

[25] A. H. Erciyas, K. Topalkara, S. Topaktas, A. Akyüz, and S. Dener, "Supression of cardiac parasympathetic functions in patients with right hemispheric stroke," *European Journal of Neurology*, vol. 6, no. 6, pp. 685–690, 1999.

[26] E. Koseoglu, S. Kucuk, F. Arman, and A. O. Ersoy, "Factors that affect interictal cardiovascular autonomic dysfunction in temporal lobe epilepsy: role of hippocampal sclerosis," *Epilepsy and Behavior*, vol. 16, no. 4, pp. 617–621, 2009.

[27] S. A. Barron, Z. Rogovski, and J. Hemli, "Autonomic consequences of cerebral hemisphere infarction," *Stroke*, vol. 25, no. 1, pp. 113–116, 1994.

[28] I. C. Al-Aweel, K. B. Krishnamurthy, J. M. Hausdorff et al., "Postictal heart rate oscillations in partial epilepsy," *Neurology*, vol. 53, no. 7, pp. 1590–1592, 1999.

[29] H. D. Critchley, D. R. Corfield, M. P. Chandler, C. J. Mathias, and R. J. Dolan, "Cerebral correlates of autonomic cardiovascular arousal: a functional neuroimaging investigation in humans," *The Journal of Physiology*, vol. 523, no. 1, pp. 259–270, 2000.

[30] D. F. Cechetto, "Experimental cerebral ischemic lesions and autonomic and cardiac effects in cats and rats," *Stroke*, vol. 24, no. 12, pp. I6–I9, 1993.

[31] H. D. Critchley, R. Elliott, C. J. Mathias, and R. J. Dolan, "Neural activity relating to generation and representation of galvanic skin conductance responses: a functional magnetic resonance imaging study," *The Journal of Neuroscience*, vol. 20, no. 8, pp. 3033–3040, 2000.

[32] H. K. Naver, C. Blomstrand, and B. G. Wallin, "Reduced heart rate variability after right-sided stroke," *Stroke*, vol. 27, no. 2, pp. 247–251, 1996.

[33] T. G. Robinson, M. James, J. Youde, R. Panerai, and J. Potter, "Cardiac baroreceptor sensitivity is impaired after acute stroke," *Stroke*, vol. 28, no. 9, pp. 1671–1676, 1997.

[34] H. Ansakorpi, J. T. Korpelainen, P. Tanskanen et al., "Cardiovascular regulation and hippocampal sclerosis," *Epilepsia*, vol. 45, no. 8, pp. 933–939, 2004.

[35] L. Nashef, "Sudden unexpected death in epilepsy: terminology and definitions," *Epilepsia*, vol. 38, no. 11, pp. S6–S8, 1997.

[36] R. T. F. Cheung and V. Hachinski, "The insula and cerebrogenic sudden death," *Archives of Neurology*, vol. 57, no. 12, pp. 1685–1688, 2000.

[37] O. Devinsky, K. Perrine, and W. H. Theodore, "Interictal autonomic nervous system function in patients with epilepsy," *Epilepsia*, vol. 35, no. 1, pp. 199–204, 1994.

[38] J. I. T. Isojärvi, H. Ansakorpi, K. Suominen, U. Tolonen, M. Repo, and V. V. Myllylä, "Interictal cardiovascular autonomic responses in patients with epilepsy," *Epilepsia*, vol. 39, no. 4, pp. 420–426, 1998.

[39] T. Tomson, M. Ericson, C. Ihrman, and L. E. Lindblad, "Heart rate variability in patients with epilepsy," *Epilepsy Research*, vol. 30, no. 1, pp. 77–83, 1998.

16

Episodic and Semantic Autobiographical Memory in Temporal Lobe Epilepsy

Claudia P. Múnera,[1,2] **Carolina Lomlomdjian,**[1,2] **Belen Gori,**[1,2] **Verónica Terpiluk,**[1,2] **Nancy Medel,**[1,2] **Patricia Solís,**[1,2,3] **and Silvia Kochen**[1,2,3]

[1]*Epilepsy Center, Neurology Division, Ramos Mejia Hospital, Gral Urquiza 609, C1221ADC Buenos Aires, Argentina*
[2]*Center for Clinical and Experimental Neurosciences, Epilepsy , Cognition and Behavior, Institute of Cell Biology and Neurosciences (IBCN), School of Medicine, UBA-CONICET, 2nd Floor, Paraguay 2155, C1121ABG Buenos Aires, Argentina*
[3]*National Neuroscience Center, Epilepsy Unit, El Cruce Hospital, Avenue Calchaquí 5401, C1888, Florencio Varela, C1073ABA Buenos Aires, Argentina*

Correspondence should be addressed to Claudia P. Múnera; claudia.muneramartinez@gmail.com

Academic Editor: Louis Lemieux

Autobiographical memory (AM) is understood as the retrieval of personal experiences that occurred in specific time and space. To date, there is no consensus on the role of medial temporal lobe structures in AM. Therefore, we investigated AM in medial temporal lobe epilepsy (TLE) patients. Twenty TLE patients candidates for surgical treatment, 10 right (RTLE) and 10 left (LTLE), and 20 healthy controls were examined with a version of the Autobiographical Interview adapted to Spanish language. Episodic and semantic AM were analyzed during five life periods through two conditions: recall and specific probe. AM scores were compared with clinical and cognitive data. TLE patients showed lower performance in episodic AM than healthy controls, being significantly worst in RTLE group and after specific probe. In relation to semantic AM, LTLE retrieved higher amount of total semantic details compared to controls during recall, but not after specific probe. No significant differences were found between RTLE and LTLE, but a trend towards poorer performance in RTLE group was found. TLE patients obtained lower scores for adolescence period memories after specific probe. Our findings support the idea that the right hippocampus would play a more important role in episodic retrieval than the left, regardless of a temporal gradient.

1. Introduction

Cognitive neuroscience over the years has been trying to elucidate which are the basic mechanisms underlying autobiographical memory (AM). Despite the vast amount of studies performed in this area there is still no consensus on the role of medial temporal lobe (MTL) structures.

Medial temporal lobe epilepsy (TLE) patients provide a unique opportunity to systematically explore different aspects of AM processing considering the involvement of hippocampal structures on seizure onset and the connectivity to local and distal areas of MTL through the neural network related to epileptic spreading [1]. Epilepsy is a "pathologic model" that allows greater opportunities for research in clinical neuroscience than other neurological disorders, like stroke

or dementia, in which massive damage of anatomical structures or a degenerative process is observed. An additional advantage is that most of these patients are young adults, whose illness could have begun in childhood, adolescence, or early adult life periods, giving us the chance to compare their performance at different stages. Furthermore, retrieval in this population has not a distinguished base level performance [2] which is central in the assessment of AM.

Two prominent theories argue the role of MTL in the encoding and retrieval of remote AM after consolidation. Briefly, the standard consolidation model (SCM) [3] supports the idea that the hippocampal formation is necessary for encoding episodic and semantic memories, but after consolidation, these memories would become independent of the hippocampus and represented in the neocortex. On the other hand, multiple trace theory (MTT) [4, 5] suggests that MTL structures would be always involved in the retrieval of remote episodic memories and the hippocampus would provide spatial context that could link the details to a "fully elaborated episode memory" [4], and remote semantic memory seems to be independent of the hippocampus, although it initially contributes to its formation and assimilation [5].

Most of the research in AM was conducted in aging, mild cognitive impairment, and degenerative disorders [6–11] while there are fewer investigations in epileptic subjects [2, 12, 13]. The study of AM in TLE would contribute to understanding of the role of MTL and to assessment of daily memory complaints within an ecological approach.

AM is understood as the retrieval of situations lived across lifetime and our own personal experiences that occurred in specific time and space [12, 14, 15] and that are accompanied by the feeling of reliving [16]. The aim of our study was to investigate AM in TLE candidates for surgical treatment analyzing episodic and semantic details throughout different lifetime periods, the association with laterality of epileptic zone (EZ), and other clinical aspects like age of onset of epilepsy, gender, years of formal education, and cognitive status [17].

2. Materials and Methods

2.1. Participants. Twenty patients with pharmacoresistant TLE candidates for surgery epilepsy were consecutively examined for this study at the Epilepsy Center, Neurology Department, Ramos Mejia Hospital of Buenos Aires, Argentina. Patients aged 18–53 years (M = 31.75; SD = 9.63) had an average of 12 years of formal education and were predominantly male (12/8). Only patients with a Full Scale IQ > 70 and without history of psychiatric disorders or other neurological diseases were included. Twenty healthy control subjects were matched to the patients group by age, education, and sex (Table 1).

All subjects gave written informed consent approved by the Institutional Ethics Committee at Ramos Mejia Hospital, which follows the guidelines of the Declaration of Helsinki.

In order to determine lateralization and localization of the epileptogenic zone (EZ), video-EEG monitoring was performed in all patients over 5 days, finding 10 subjects with left EZ (LTLE) and 10 with right EZ (RTLE). An organized seizure activity with a clearly unilateral beginning was found in all patients, with a late propagation to contralateral areas only in 4 LTLE and 3 RTLE. Patients with a bilateral seizure activity from the beginning were not included. A magnetic resonance imaging (MRI) study was conducted for every patient: 19 subjects had hippocampal sclerosis, 10 right and 9 left, and one patient had a left temporal dysembryoplastic neuroepithelial tumor (Table 1).

At the time of the study, all patients were polymedicated with 2-3 AEDs. Only one patient with LTLE had generalized tonic clonic seizures, while five patients (2 left and 3 right) had sporadic secondary generalized seizures.

A neuropsychological assessment was performed according to the CE presurgical protocol [17, 18] and using a z-score

TABLE 1: Demographic and clinical features.

	TLE group		Controls
	Left EZ	Right EZ	
N	10	10	20
Age (years)*	33,2 (10,97)	30,3 (8,42)	34,07 (11,47)
Education (years)*	12,3 (3,09)	12,4 (3,09)	12,93 (2,96)
Sex M/F	7/3	5/5	12/8
Handedness	Right: 10	Left: 2/right: 8	Right: 20
MRI	HS = 9 DNT = 1	HS = 8 HS plus = 2	NA
Age at seizure onset (years)*	10,33 (7,69)	8,2 (6,23)	NA
Duration of epilepsy (years)*	23,44 (15,42)	22,1 (11,79)	NA
Seizure frequency (per month)	8,57 (10,03)	6,12 (6,93)	NA

*Mean (SD). M: male, F: female, HS: hippocampal sclerosis, DNT: dysembryoplastic neuroepithelial tumor, and NA: not applicable.

cutoff of −2. We found a normal memory performance on average of z-scores of TLE groups; four of 20 patients (1 RTLE and 3 LTLE) showed deficits in verbal memory measures as observed on the delayed recall of the Rey Auditory Verbal Learning Test. A visual memory deficit was found in 9 of 20 subjects (5 RTLE and 4 LTLE). A deficit in the Boston Naming Test was found in RTLE (6) and LTLE (5) [19] (Table 2).

2.2. Autobiographical Interview (AI). AM was assessed with the Autobiographical Interview [6] translated to Spanish language for our group. We made a pilot study to evaluate comprehension of the questions and to build a list of typical life events adjusted to Argentinean and nearby countries population (e.g., first communion, 15-year birthday (women), wedding day, etc.) keeping the same categories used by Levine et al. [6].

According to the administration instructions [6], subjects were asked to recollect memories from five different time periods (early childhood, teenage years, early adulthood, middle adulthood, and last year), for a total of five memories. Each subject had to choose at least two events for each period and assigned a single "title" per event, so that the examiner randomly chose one title per period. The interview was conducted through three different conditions as follows: (a) "free recall": subjects described the event chosen without interruption from the interviewer; (b) a "general probe" was used after the free recall when the subject did not understand the task or the event narrated was not clear or did not correspond to the lifetime assessed or to encourage the subject to add more details; (c) after all the events were narrated a "specific probe" was administered for each one of the events and in the same order they were obtained: this probe consists of a semistructured interview to collect additional details. Each one of the lifetime periods was taken into account in the analysis. If subjects were under 30 years

TABLE 2: Neuropsychological performance of subjects (TLE).

Neuropsychological test	Left EZ			Right EZ		
	Mean (SD)	Range		Mean (SD)	Range	
		Min	Max		Min	Max
WASI: *IQ scores*						
Full Scale IQ (FIQ)	94,66 (12,07)	74	116	80,44 (9,44)	70	96
Verbal IQ (VIQ)	88,37 (14,69)	70	107	78,11 (13,34)	62	95
Performance IQ (PIQ)	100,62 (15,9)	73	126	84,22 (8,46)	71	95
Verbal functioning: *z-scores*						
RAVLT (delayed recall)	−1,36 (1,25)	−2,96	0,29	−0,42 (0,67)	−1,52	0,56
BNT	−3,02 (3,17)	−7,78	1	−2,2 (1,81)	−5,02	0,76
Verbal fluency (phonemic)	−0,90 (0,62)	−2	−0,05	−0,73 (0,9)	−1,68	1,1
Visual functioning: *z-scores*						
RCFT (delayed recall)	−1,41 (1,63)	−3,52	0,56	−1,56 (1,38)	−3,32	0,66

WASI: Wechsler Abbreviated Scale of Intelligence. RAVLT = Rey Auditory Verbal Learning Test. BNT: Boston Naming Test. Phonemic verbal fluency. RCFT: Rey Complex Figure Test. z-scores <-2 were considered as deficit.

of age, they had to recollect two memories instead of one for early adulthood.

Every interview was recorded, transcribed, and segmented in detail or pieces of information. The details were classified as internal-episodic and external-semantic. These were further divided into the following categories: main event, place, time, perceptual details, and thoughts/emotions as internal-episodic information; and repetitions, other details (metacognitive, editorial statements), and factual information as external-semantic information. The information given was segmented and scored to obtain quantitative data following the scoring instructions [6]. One point was given to every detail which was tallied for each category. As was carried out in previous work [6, 12, 20, 21] we add the scores from the general probe condition to those obtained during free recall condition (henceforth found as recall condition).

Additionally, each person assigned a value between 1 and 6 related to how well they visualized the event related, the emotional change produced by the event, the importance given actually and then, and how frequently they talk or think about it. Quantitative ratings were also assigned for episodic information (time, place, perception, and thoughts/emotion) and time integration on a scale of 0 to 3 and episodic richness using a scale extended to 6 points [6]. All memories were transcribed and scored by two independent examiners achieving high interrater reliability.

AI scores were compared between all patients and control group, in RTLE/LTLE versus control, and between LTLE and RTLE. The clinical data and the cognitive status were also analyzed.

2.3. Statistical Analysis. Control and TLE group were matched for age, sex, and formal education. For each patient, the raw values of every cognitive test in the neuropsychological battery were normalized to a z-score and classified as "deficit" for values less than or equal to −2.

We compared TLE groups versus controls' performance in AI and we analyzed the composite measures considering both the total life span and each period of time. One-way ANOVA, Student's t-test, Bonferroni correction post hoc test, Pearson correlation coefficient r, Chi-squared test, and logistic regression analysis were used.

All comparisons that were significant at the $P < 0.05$ level were reported. Statistical analysis was carried out using the Statistical Package for the Social Sciences (SPSS version 20).

3. Results

3.1. Composite Measures of AM. The total number of episodic and semantic details recalled across five life periods was compared for TLE group and control subjects.

For episodic details, TLE group scores were lower during recall than control group but we did not find a statistical difference ($P = 0.286$). We found significant differences after specific probe between all patients versus control group ($P = 0.002$) and in RTLE group, retrieving fewer episodic details ($P = 0.004$) compared to controls. When we compared RTLE versus LTLE group, no significant difference was found; however, a tendency to a lower performance for RTLE was sustained (Figure 1).

In relation to semantic details, no differences were found between TLE and controls during either recall ($P = 0.80$) or specific probe ($P = 0.226$). We observed that LTLE group retrieved significantly higher amount of total semantic details ($P = 0.031$) during recall condition but the significant difference disappears after specific probe. No differences were found between RTLE and LTLE (Figure 1).

3.2. Specific Autobiographical Retrieval Categories. The number of episodic and semantic details retrieved for individual categories was compared between TLE and control group.

For episodic details, differences were found between TLE group and control only after specific probe in event details ($P = 0.020$), time details ($P = 0.022$), perceptual details ($P = 0.006$), and emotion/thoughts details ($P = 0.038$). RTLE retrieved lower details for each category compared to controls but significant differences were found only after specific

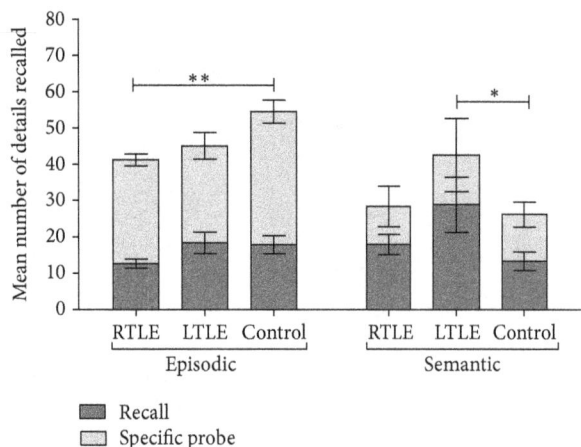

FIGURE 1: Mean number of episodic and semantic details retrieved during recall (darkest portion of the histogram) and specific probe (lighter portion of the histogram) conditions for each group: RTLE, LTLE, and control. $^*P < 0.05$, $^{**}P < 0.01$. Bars indicate the standard error of the mean (SEM).

probe for perceptual details ($P = 0.024$). No differences were found between RTLE and LTLE (Figure 2(a)).

For semantic details (Figure 2(b)), TLE scores were statistically different compared to controls only in details classified as "Oth" and during recall condition ($P = 0.035$). LTLE generated significantly higher scores during recall for semantic category factual information (LTLE versus control $P = 0.027$) and the other category metacognitive or editorial statements (LTLE versus control $P = 0.022$), but after specific probe no differences were found. It was observed that LTLE produced more semantic category details than RTLE (recall $P = 0.041$; specific probe $P = 0.037$).

3.3. Life Period Analysis of AM. Figure 3 shows the number of episodic details, semantic details, and rating composite recalled by each group at each of the five life periods. Most remarkable differences were found during the period between 10 and 18 years (adolescence). Both patient groups compared to controls performed poorly for episodic details during each life period but this difference was only statistically significant during the adolescence period and after the specific probe (RTLE $P = 0.002$; LTLE $P = 0.017$) (Figure 3(a)). Semantic details were significantly higher among LTLE compared to controls (recall $P < 0.001$; specific probe $P < 0.01$) and compared to RTLE (recall $P < 0.05$; specific probe $P < 0.05$) (Figure 3(b)) during early adulthood memories.

Ratings composites for recall condition were significantly diminished for RTLE compared to controls not only for adolescence period ($P < 0.05$), but also for early adulthood ($P < 0.05$) and last year ($P < 0.05$) memories. After the specific probe, both RTLE and LTLE obtained lower scores for adolescence period memories ($P < 0.01$) (Figure 3(c)).

3.4. Subjective Quality of Autobiographical Memories. Figure 4 indicates ratings assigned by the participants to every memory narrated. An ANOVA showed no effect of group,

laterality, or time period ($P > 0.05$) for vividness. When subjects were asked if they experienced an emotional change after the event narrated, it was observed that RTLE reported significantly lower ratings only for adulthood memories compared to controls ($P < 0.01$) and compared to LTLE ($P < 0.05$).

No differences were found when participants were asked how important the event actually is, how relevant it was at the moment of its occurrence, and how frequently they rehearse about it.

3.5. AI Scores Correlation with Other Variables. AI scores were compared to neuropsychological test results for each patient. A statistically significant correlation was only found between VIQ and episodic details during recall in RTLE (Pearson correlation coefficient $r = -0.645$). No other significant results were found.

There were no significant correlations between AI scores and age, years of education, age of onset, and disease duration. Our sample does not include cases of recent onset; the duration of the epilepsy was higher than ten years.

4. Discussion

Most of previous memory research in epileptic subjects has analyzed different aspects related to type of material, lateralization, and pre- and postsurgical performance [17, 18, 22–25] and a specific group have focused on understanding the quality of epileptic patients AM recollections in comparison to general population [2, 12, 26–28].

Different studies that have used the AI [1, 12] or other tasks to measure AM in TLE [2, 13, 26–30] showed deficits in patients recollections compared to controls. Our findings suggest a significant impaired autobiographical episodic memory only in subjects with right epileptogenic zone. Therefore, the possibility that the right hippocampus would play a more important role in episodic retrieval than the left could be considered. Studies in healthy subjects described a right temporal activation during AM retrieval [31, 32]. In epileptic population it was also found that, after right temporal lobectomy, subjects have a drop in autobiographical episodic memory measures and a poorer performance compared to healthy controls and left temporal lobectomy patients [29, 30]. RTLE episodic deficits in our study become evident only after a specific probing. One possible explanation is that for LTLE and controls the additional questions had triggered a better access to a vast amount of information. For RTLE, the use of "frontotemporal" executive retrieval compensation strategies is not effective which would imply a disruption in that pathway due to the disease. According to Markowitsch [33], the connection between right "anterolateral prefrontal and temporopolar cortices" is critical to recall of past episodic memories.

However, other authors suggest that the left hippocampus is essential to episodic retrieval [28, 34] and proposed the existence of a left-lateralized network which includes not only temporal structures, but also frontal, posterior, subcortical, and cerebellum regions [35]. Within our subjects, LTLE had

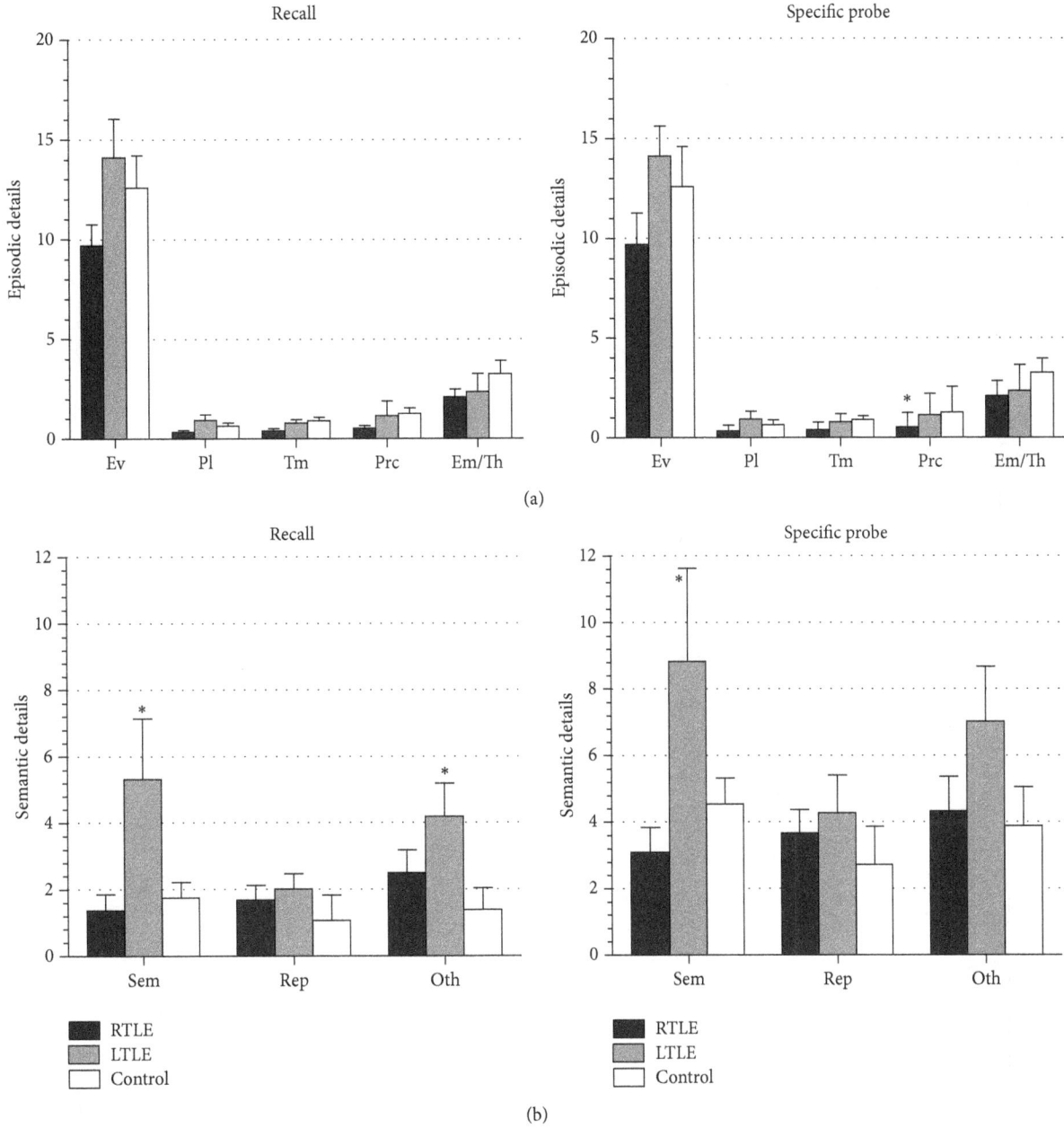

FIGURE 2: Mean number of (a) episodic and (b) semantic details retrieved for each category during recall and specific probe conditions. All significance levels were at $P < 0.05$. Bars indicate the standard error of the mean (SEM). Ev: event, Pl: place, Tm: time, Prc: perceptual details, Em/Th: emotion/thoughts, Sem: semantic, Rep: repetitions, and Oth: other details.

a lower performance compared to control group, which was not statistically significant.

In relation to episodic detail categories, RTLE presented impaired performance during retrieval after specific probe for perceptual category. No differences were found between RTLE and LTLE. St-Laurent et al. [12] suggest that the impairment in perceptual categories, but not in event categories, might support the idea that hippocampal formation would be necessary "for a rich perceptual re-experiencing" of an episode. AM entails different processes from attention and executive functions to self-reflection, emotion,

visual imagery, episodic memory, and semantic processes and according to findings in PET and fMRI studies shows activation in medial and dorsolateral prefrontal, posterior regions and MTL structures, including hippocampus and amygdala [36, 37]. Taking into account previous studies and our findings, we considered that hippocampal structures would be actively involved in episodic remote memories retrieval regardless of a temporal gradient.

Our findings showed no temporal gradient through the five life periods in episodic and semantic AM, as proposed by the consolidation theory [3]. In addition, the reminiscence

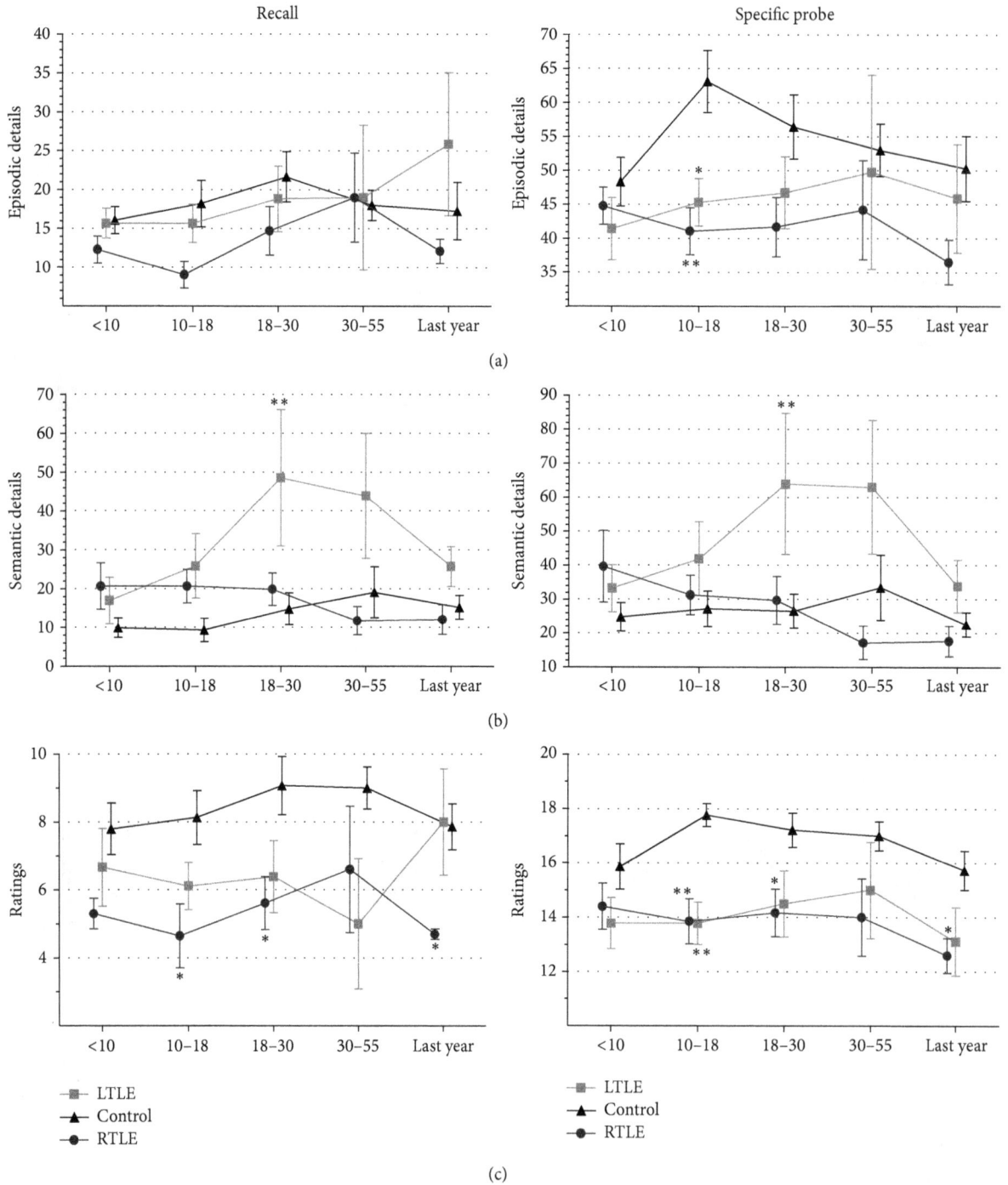

FIGURE 3: Number of details and ratings retrieved across each one of the life periods, childhood (>10 years), adolescence (10–18 years), early adulthood (18–30 years), and adulthood (30–55 years), and during the last year, for recall (left column) and after specific probe (right column). (a) shows the average number of episodic details, (b) indicates performance for semantic details, and (c) indicates the total score in different rating categories (max = 21). Bars indicate the standard error of the mean (SEM). $^*P < 0.05$, $^{**}P < 0.01$.

bump described as a period where "people produce the most memories" [38] usually between 10 and 30 years of age was observed in control group but not in TLE group. Previous studies suggest that the reminiscence bump is related to a specific period of lifetime in which identity and self are being built; therefore autobiographical memories that are

highly self-relevant would be preferably encoded [38]. In our study, both right and left TLE patients performed significantly worst for adolescence in episodic AM compared to controls. This finding could be related to important changes that occur during this stage of human development, not only in physical appearance but also in the acquirement of new

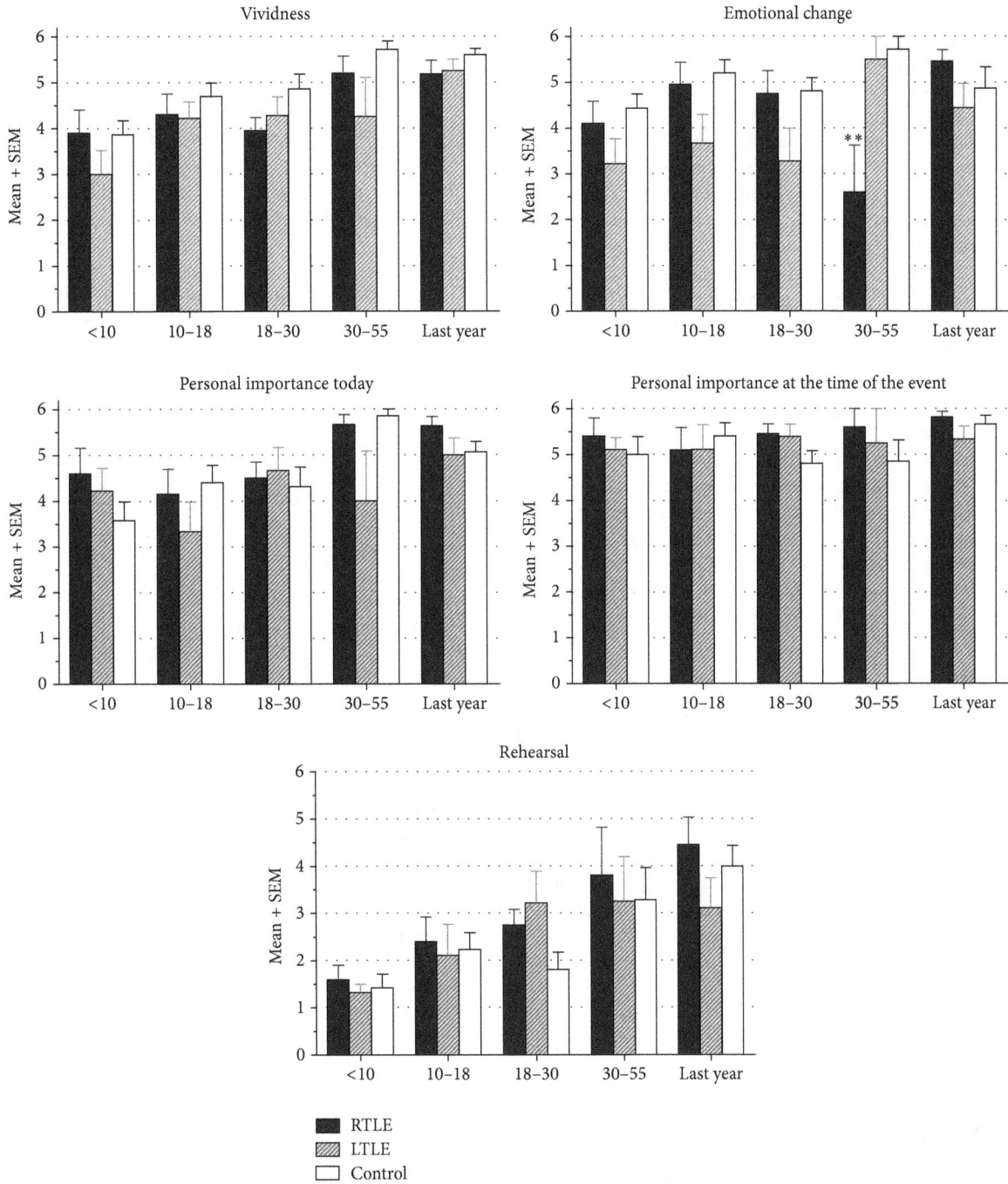

FIGURE 4: Average of subjective quality ratings for each of the five time periods regarding the vividness of the event, the emotional change experienced, how important the event was at the time of its occurrence and now and how frequently they thought or spoke about it. Bars indicate the standard error of the mean (SEM). $^*P < 0.05$, $^{**}P < 0.01$.

responsibilities, and has a crucial role in personality char acteristics [39]. These changes would be stressful in general, even more for epileptic teenagers that have to deal with discrimination, limited personal choices, and an altered quality of life [40]; thereby learning and retention of new information could be affected [41]. Authors like Berntsen and Rubin [42] suggest that the reminiscence bump would

be present only for positive memories but not for negative events.

With regard to semantic AM memory we observed higher performance of LTLE patients on recall condition that disappears after specific probe. In the same way, higher scores in semantic categories, factual information (semantic), and metacognitive statements (the other category) were found which would reflect a compensatory cognitive mechanism [6, 36].

In our work, participants showed no difference with respect to the degree of vividness, personal significance, and rehearsal of their recollections. We could assume that a lesion in MTL structures does not affect these subjects' appreciation. As far as cognitive performance is concerned, we did not observe any relation between verbal or visual memory performance and AI scores that could provide additional data to our results.

Finally, regarding the duration of epilepsy, our interest was to determine its influence in AM recollections but none of the subjects had illness duration fewer than 10 years, so this variable could not be analyzed. The impact of epilepsy across life period recollections was not analyzed either, because the age of onset for the majority of subjects was during childhood.

Our results allow us to provide additional evidence to previous work, of the hippocampal structures involvement in episodic autobiographical memories recollection, particularly the right hippocampus in TLE patients. It is important to consider that one limitation of our study is the relatively small sample size that may contribute to the lack of differences between EZ side groups. For future work, we will compare performance in TLE patients, before and after surgery.

Abbreviations

TLE: Temporal lobe epilepsy
AM: Autobiographical memory
AI: Autobiographical Interview.

Disclosure

The authors confirm that they have read the journal's position on issues involved in ethical publication and affirm that this report is consistent with those guidelines.

Conflict of Interests

The authors declare that there is no conflict of interests regarding the publication of this paper.

Acknowledgments

The authors would like to thank Dr. Brian Levine for providing the Autobiographical Interview administration and scoring manual and for allowing them to translate it to Spanish, Lucia Valeriano for helping them with the transcriptions, and all the participants for giving their time. This study was supported by a doctoral fellowship from the National Scientific and Technical Research Council (CONICET) to Claudia P. Múnera.

References

[1] D. R. Addis, M. Moscovitch, and M. P. McAndrews, "Consequences of hippocampal damage across the autobiographical memory network in left temporal lobe epilepsy," *Brain*, vol. 130, no. 9, pp. 2327–2342, 2007.

[2] I. V. Viskontas, M. P. McAndrews, and M. Moscovitch, "Remote episodic memory deficits in patients with unilateral temporal lobe epilepsy and excisions," *Journal of Neuroscience*, vol. 20, no. 15, pp. 5853–5857, 2000.

[3] L. R. Squire and P. Alvarez, "Retrograde amnesia and memory consolidation: a neurobiological perspective," *Current Opinion in Neurobiology*, vol. 5, no. 2, pp. 169–177, 1995.

[4] L. Nadel and O. Hardt, "Update on memory systems and processes," *Neuropsychopharmacology*, vol. 36, no. 1, pp. 251–273, 2011.

[5] M. Moscovitch, L. Nadel, G. Winocur, A. Gilboa, and R. S. Rosenbaum, "The cognitive neuroscience of remote episodic, semantic and spatial memory," *Current Opinion in Neurobiology*, vol. 16, no. 2, pp. 179–190, 2006.

[6] B. Levine, E. Svoboda, J. F. Hay, G. Winocur, and M. Moscovitch, "Aging and autobiographical memory: dissociating episodic from semantic retrieval," *Psychology and Aging*, vol. 17, no. 4, pp. 677–689, 2002.

[7] D. R. Addis and L. J. Tippett, "Memory of myself: autobiographical memory and identity in Alzheimer's disease," *Memory*, vol. 12, no. 1, pp. 56–74, 2004.

[8] H. E. Moss, M. D. Kopelman, M. Cappelletti, P. D. M. Davies, and E. Jaldow, "Lost for words or loss of memories? Autobiographical memory in semantic dementia," *Cognitive Neuropsychology*, vol. 20, no. 8, pp. 703–732, 2003.

[9] P. Piolino, G. Chételat, V. Matuszewski et al., "In search of autobiographical memories: a PET study in the frontal variant of frontotemporal dementia," *Neuropsychologia*, vol. 45, no. 12, pp. 2730–2743, 2007.

[10] P. L. St. Jacques, D. C. Rubin, and R. Cabeza, "Age-related effects on the neural correlates of autobiographical memory retrieval," *Neurobiology of Aging*, vol. 33, no. 7, pp. 1298–1310, 2012.

[11] E. Tramoni, O. Felician, L. Koric, M. Balzamo, S. Joubert, and M. Ceccaldi, "Alteration of autobiographical memory in amnestic mild cognitive impairment," *Cortex*, vol. 48, no. 10, pp. 1310–1319, 2012.

[12] M. St-Laurent, M. Moscovitch, B. Levine, and M. P. McAndrews, "Determinants of autobiographical memory in patients with unilateral temporal lobe epilepsy or excisions," *Neuropsychologia*, vol. 47, no. 11, pp. 2211–2221, 2009.

[13] V. Voltzenlogel, O. Despres, J. P. Vignal, P. Kehrli, and L. Manning, "One-year postoperative autobiographical memory following unilateral temporal lobectomy for control of intractable epilepsy," *Epilepsia*, vol. 48, no. 3, pp. 605–608, 2007.

[14] M. D. Kopelman, B. A. Wilson, and A. D. Baddeley, "The autobiographical memory interview: a new assessment of autobiographical and personal semantic memory in amnesic patients," *Journal of Clinical and Experimental Neuropsychology*, vol. 11, no. 5, pp. 724–744, 1989.

[15] M. C. McKinnon, S. E. Black, B. Miller, M. Moscovitch, and B. Levine, "Autobiographical memory in semantic dementia: implications for theories of limbic-neocortical interaction in remote memory," *Neuropsychologia*, vol. 44, no. 12, pp. 2421–2429, 2006.

[16] D. L. Greenberg and D. C. Rubin, "The neuropsychology of autobiographical memory," *Cortex*, vol. 39, no. 4-5, pp. 687–728, 2003.

[17] S. Oddo, P. Solís, D. Consalvo et al., "Mesial temporal lobe epilepsy and hippocampal sclerosis: cognitive function assessment in Hispanic patients," *Epilepsy and Behavior*, vol. 4, no. 6, pp. 717–722, 2003.

[18] S. Oddo, P. Solis, D. Consalvo et al., "Postoperative neuropsychological outcome in patients with mesial temporal lobe epilepsy in Argentina," *Epilepsy Research and Treatment*, vol. 2012, Article ID 370351, 5 pages, 2012.

[19] C. Lomlomdjian, P. Solis, N. Medel, and S. Kochen, "A study of word finding difficulties in Spanish speakers with temporal lobe epilepsy," *Epilepsy Research*, vol. 97, no. 1-2, pp. 37–44, 2011.

[20] R. S. Rosenbaum, M. C. McKinnon, B. Levine, and M. Moscovitch, "Visual imagery deficits, impaired strategic retrieval, or memory loss: disentangling the nature of an amnesic person's autobiographical memory deficit," *Neuropsychologia*, vol. 42, no. 12, pp. 1619–1635, 2004.

[21] S. Steinvorth, B. Levine, and S. Corkin, "Medial temporal lobe structures are needed to re-experience remote autobiographical memories: evidence from H.M. and W.R.," *Neuropsychologia*, vol. 43, no. 4, pp. 479–496, 2005.

[22] C. Helmstaedter and C. E. Elger, "Cognitive consequences of two-thirds anterior temporal lobectomy on verbal memory in 144 patients: a three-month follow-up study," *Epilepsia*, vol. 37, no. 2, pp. 171–180, 1996.

[23] C. Helmstaedter, M. Kurthen, S. Lux, M. Reuber, and C. E. Elger, "Chronic epilepsy and cognition: a longitudinal study in temporal lobe epilepsy," *Annals of Neurology*, vol. 54, no. 4, pp. 425–432, 2003.

[24] M. Jones-Gotman, R. J. Zatorre, A. Olivier et al., "Learning and retention of words and designs following excision from medial or lateral temporal lobe structures," *Neuropsychologia*, vol. 35, no. 7, pp. 963–973, 1997.

[25] T. M. C. Lee, J. T. H. Yip, and M. Jones-Gotman, "Memory deficits after resection from left or right anterior temporal lobe in humans: a meta-analytic review," *Epilepsia*, vol. 43, no. 3, pp. 283–291, 2002.

[26] K. Herfurth, B. Kasper, M. Schwarz, H. Stefan, and E. Pauli, "Autobiographical memory in temporal lobe epilepsy: role of hippocampal and temporal lateral structures," *Epilepsy and Behavior*, vol. 19, no. 3, pp. 365–371, 2010.

[27] M. Noulhiane, P. Piolino, D. Hasboun, S. Clemenceau, M. Baulac, and S. Samson, "Autobiographical memory after temporal lobe resection: neuropsychological and MRI volumetric findings," *Brain*, vol. 130, no. 12, pp. 3184–3199, 2007.

[28] V. Voltzenlogel, O. Després, J.-P. Vignal, B. J. Steinhoff, P. Kehrli, and L. Manning, "Remote memory in temporal lobe epilepsy," *Epilepsia*, vol. 47, no. 8, pp. 1329–1336, 2006.

[29] S. Lah, T. Lee, S. Grayson, and L. Miller, "Changes in retrograde memory following temporal lobectomy," *Epilepsy and Behavior*, vol. 13, no. 2, pp. 391–396, 2008.

[30] T. W. Buchanan, D. Tranel, and R. Adolphs, "Memories for emotional autobiographical events following unilateral damage to medial temporal lobe," *Brain*, vol. 129, no. 1, pp. 115–127, 2006.

[31] P. Piolino, G. Giffard-Quillon, B. Desgranges, G. Chételat, J.-C. Baron, and F. Eustache, "Re-experiencing old memories via hippocampus: a PET study of autobiographical memory," *NeuroImage*, vol. 22, no. 3, pp. 1371–1383, 2004.

[32] G. R. Fink, H. J. Markowitsch, M. Reinkemeier, T. Bruckbauer, J. Kassler, and W. D. Heiss, "Cerebral representation of one's own past: neural networks involved in autobiographical memory," *Journal of Neuroscience*, vol. 16, no. 13, pp. 4275–4282, 1996.

[33] H. J. Markowitsch, "Which brain regions are critically involved in the retrieval of old episodic memory?" *Brain Research Reviews*, vol. 21, no. 2, pp. 117–127, 1995.

[34] E. A. Maguire and C. D. Frith, "Lateral asymmetry in the hippocampal response to the remoteness of autobiographical memories," *The Journal of Neuroscience*, vol. 23, no. 12, pp. 5302–5307, 2003.

[35] E. Svoboda, M. C. McKinnon, and B. Levine, "The functional neuroanatomy of autobiographical memory: a meta-analysis," *Neuropsychologia*, vol. 44, no. 12, pp. 2189–2208, 2006.

[36] P. Martinelli, M. Sperduti, A.-D. Devauchelle et al., "Age-related changes in the functional network underlying specific and general autobiographical memory retrieval: a pivotal role for the anterior cingulate cortex," *PLoS ONE*, vol. 8, no. 12, Article ID e82385, 2013.

[37] D. L. Greenberg, H. J. Rice, J. J. Cooper, R. Cabeza, D. C. Rubin, and K. S. LaBar, "Co-activation of the amygdala, hippocampus and inferior frontal gyrus during autobiographical memory retrieval," *Neuropsychologia*, vol. 43, no. 5, pp. 659–674, 2005.

[38] C. J. Rathbone, C. J. A. Moulin, and M. A. Conway, "Self-centered memories: the reminiscence bump and the self," *Memory and Cognition*, vol. 36, no. 8, pp. 1403–1414, 2008.

[39] S. Choudhury, S.-J. Blakemore, and T. Charman, "Social cognitive development during adolescence," *Social Cognitive and Affective Neuroscience*, vol. 1, no. 3, pp. 165–174, 2006.

[40] M. J. McEwan, C. A. Espie, and J. Metcalfe, "Quality of life and psychosocial development in adolescents with epilepsy: a qualitative investigation using focus group methods," *Seizure*, vol. 13, no. 1, pp. 15–31, 2004.

[41] N. Laugesen, M. J. Dugas, and W. M. Bukowski, "Understanding adolescent worry: the application of a cognitive model," *Journal of Abnormal Child Psychology*, vol. 31, no. 1, pp. 55–64, 2003.

[42] D. Berntsen and D. C. Rubin, "Cultural life scripts structure recall from autobiographical memory," *Memory and Cognition*, vol. 32, no. 3, pp. 427–442, 2004.

17

Neurocognitive and Seizure Outcomes of Selective Amygdalohippocampectomy versus Anterior Temporal Lobectomy for Mesial Temporal Lobe Epilepsy

Alireza Mansouri,[1,2] **Aria Fallah,**[1,2,3] **Mary Pat McAndrews,**[2,4,5,6] **Melanie Cohn,**[2,4,6]
Diana Mayor,[2,6,7] **Danielle Andrade,**[2,8] **Peter Carlen,**[2,8] **Jose M. del Campo,**[2,8] **Peter Tai,**[2,8]
Richard A. Wennberg,[2,8] **and Taufik A. Valiante**[1,2,6,7]

[1] *Division of Neurosurgery, University of Toronto, Toronto, ON, Canada M5G 1X8*
[2] *Toronto Western Hospital, University Health Network, 399 Bathurst Street, Toronto, ON, Canada M5T 2S8*
[3] *Department of Clinical Epidemiology and Biostatistics, McMaster University, Hamilton, Canada L8S 4K1*
[4] *Psychology Department, University of Toronto, Toronto, ON, Canada M5T 2S8*
[5] *Institute of Medical Sciences, University of Toronto, Toronto, Canada M5T 2S8*
[6] *Krembil Neuroscience Center, University Health Network, Toronto, Canada M5T 2S8*
[7] *Division of Fundamental Neurobiology, Toronto Western Research Institute, Toronto Western Hospital, Toronto, ON, Canada M5T 2S8*
[8] *Department of Neurology, University of Toronto, Toronto, ON, Canada M5T 2S8*

Correspondence should be addressed to Taufik A. Valiante; taufik.valiante@uhn.ca

Academic Editor: Louis Lemieux

Objective. To report our institutional seizure and neuropsychological outcomes for a series of patients with mesial temporal lobe epilepsy (mTLE) undergoing anterior temporal lobectomy (ATL) or selective amygdalohippocampectomy (SelAH) between 2004 and 2011. *Methods.* A retrospective study of patients with mTLE was conducted. Seizure outcome was reported using time-to-event analysis. Cognitive outcome was reported using the change principal in component factor scores, one each, for intellectual abilities, visuospatial memory, and verbal memory. The Boston Naming Test was used for naming assessment. Language dominant and nondominant resections were compared separately. Student's *t*-test was used to assess statistical significance. *Results.* Ninety-six patients (75 ATL, 21 SelAH) were included; fifty-four had complete neuropsychological follow-up. Median follow-up was 40.5 months. There was no statistically significant difference in seizure freedom or any of the neuropsychological outcomes, although there was a trend toward greater postoperative decline in naming in the dominant hemisphere group following ATL. *Conclusion.* Seizure and neuropsychological outcomes did not differ for the two surgical approaches which is similar to most prior studies. Given the theoretical possibility of SelAH sparing language function in patients with epilepsy secondary to mesial temporal sclerosis and the limited high-quality evidence creating equipoise, a multicenter randomized clinical trial is warranted.

1. Introduction

Anterior temporal lobectomy (ATL) is a well-established and efficacious surgical procedure for the treatment of medically refractory mTLE [1–3]. However, in some patients with mTLE, the ATL procedure has been associated with worsening of cognitive functions, particularly language and memory,

when surgery involves the dominant hemisphere [4–7]. Thus, for the appropriate patient population, a more specific resection of the mesial structures through a selective amygdalohippocampectomy (SelAH) has been recommended by some groups [1, 8–10]. The rationale is that SelAH allows for sparing of the nonepileptogenic structures of the neocortex that are potentially involved in language and cognition, potentially resulting in less neuropsychological morbidity [11, 12].

A fair number of studies have been conducted to compare the efficacy of the two surgical approaches with regard to seizure outcome [1, 12–22], neuropsychological outcomes [9, 23–29], or both [10, 30–34] in adults with mTLE. As most of these are retrospective analyses of case series, conclusions are difficult to make given the heterogeneity of pathologies managed, surgical technique, follow-up frequency and duration, neuropsychological test battery, and reporting of seizure outcomes.

Two recent systematic reviews and meta-analyses have been conducted in order to determine the benefit of one procedure over the other with regard to either strictly seizure outcomes [35] or both seizure and neuropsychological outcomes, with the latter focusing on global assessment of intellectual functioning [36]. Importantly, none of the studies included were randomized controlled trials (RCTs) but rather a mix of mainly retrospective and a few prospective studies. Both reviews found that the ATL procedure conferred a higher chance of seizure freedom [35, 36]. Hu and colleagues were not able to identify a statistically significant difference with regard to IQ measurements [36].

As these reviews demonstrate, individual studies may not have sufficient power to detect statistically significant or clinically meaningful differences. However, each can provide valuable data points for meta-analyses. Herein, we seek to contribute the Toronto Western Hospital (TWH) experience, as one of the major sites for adult epilepsy care across Canada. This is a retrospective observational study at TWH, assessing seizure control and neuropsychological outcomes in patients with hippocampal sclerosis as the underlying pathology undergoing either SelAH or ATL, based on a prospectively collected database of a single surgeon (TAV). In all patients examined, cognitive outcome variables that were assessed have been previously validated as sensitive predictors of change in language and cognition [37].

2. Methods

2.1. Subjects. A retrospective review of a prospectively collected database of patients undergoing SelAH or ATL by a single surgeon (TAV) at the Toronto Western Hospital from January 2004 to December 2011 was conducted. All patients included in the study had medically refractory epilepsy attributable to hippocampal sclerosis, as confirmed on preoperative MRI and postoperative histopathological analysis. All patients included in neuropsychological analyses had complete pre- and postoperative testing. All neuropsychological and seizure evaluations were performed by a consistent team of neuropsychologists and epileptologists, respectively. Additional standard preoperative evaluation included MRI imaging (1.5T scanner, mTLE protocol) and video-EEG through admission to the Epilepsy Monitoring Unit (EMU).

2.2. Selection of Surgical Approach. The patients undergoing the SelAH approach were part of a cohort in time, July 2009–July 2010, when our center undertook the SelAH approach in consecutive patients as a trial of a variation to the prior approach of ATL. During this time, patients with MTS but with EEG evidence of neocortical epilepsy were offered ATL while the remainder underwent SelAH. Prior to and after this period, all patients were offered ATL, the standard procedure at our institution for medically refractory mTLE.

2.3. Selective Amygdalohippocampectomy. A 2 cm × 0.5 cm corticectomy through the middle temporal gyrus just ventral to the superior temporal sulcus (STS) provides the access window. A subpial approach is utilized following the STS as a plane towards the ventricle. Once the ventricle is entered, the ventricular opening is enlarged. The parahippocampal gyrus is then aspirated in a piecemeal fashion. The hippocampus is removed en bloc. Frameless stereotaxy is subsequently utilized to ensure that the extent of hippocampal resection is to a point behind the tectal plate. The amygdala is resected flush with the roof of the ventricle.

2.4. Anterior Temporal Lobectomy. In this approach, the extent of the hippocampal resection is similar to the SelAH with an additional resection of the anterior 4.5 cm or 5.5 cm of the temporal neocortex on the dominant or nondominant side, respectively. The superior temporal gyrus is spared, except the anterior 1 cm. The resection of the amygdala is similar to that of SelAH.

2.5. Neuropsychological Testing Battery. Only patients with a full neuropsychological examination prior to and at least 6 months following surgery were included in this component of the analysis. Excluded patients had partial neuropsychological testing which did not allow us to use component measures (e.g., missing verbal component is common in our patients with English as their second language, those who were not seen for postoperative assessment, or individuals who had impaired intellectual functioning assessed as verbal IQ (VIQ) or performance IQ (PIQ) < 70).

Cognitive outcomes were measured using scores from a principal component analysis (PCA), which allows one to reduce data from multiple cognitive measures into single latent components. We have previously demonstrated that these memory PCA scores provide robust estimates of material-specific memory change in mTLE patients; specifically the presurgery verbal memory component predicts postsurgery verbal memory decline, while the presurgery visuospatial memory component predicts visuospatial memory decline [37]. The IQ component score is composed of the Wechsler Abbreviated Scale of Intelligence (WASI), VIQ estimate, and PIQ estimate. The verbal memory component is based on the Rey Auditory Verbal Learning Test (RAVLT) total learning, RAVLT percent retained, and Warrington Recognition Memory Test for words. The visual memory component is composed of Rey Visual Design Learning Test (RVDLT) total learning, Warrington Recognition Memory Test (WRMT) for faces, and Spatial Conditional Associative

TABLE 1: Patient demographics and preoperative evaluation.

	SelAH ($n = 21$)	ATL ($n = 75$)	P value
Gender (%female)	57	53	0.76
Age at first seizure (Yr)	16.1	13.9	0.52
Age at surgery (Yr)	36	41.9	0.03
History of febrile seizures (%)	6 (29%)	39 (52%)	0.06
Freq. of seizures at time of surgery (per month)	8	9.7	0.40
On multiple AEDs (%)	19 (90%)	62 (83%)	0.60
Initial EEG lateralizing (%)	13 (60%)	45 (60%)	0.99
Contralateral ictal propagation in EMU (%)	3 (14%)	12 (16%)	0.85
Bilateral interictal abnormalities in EMU (%)	3 (14%)	21 (28%)	0.20
Invasive recording needed (%)	1 (5%)	18 (24%)	0.05

P values < 0.05 were considered significant.
AED: Antiepileptic drug; EMU: Epilepsy Monitoring Unit.

Learning Test (SCALT) trials to criterion. A detailed method of determining these components has been described previously [37]. In brief, it relies on calculating individual test z-scores (based on the distribution of scores in the original patient sample used for the PCA), multiplying each by the latent coefficient associated with the measure, and summing these products to arrive at a PCA score for a particular component.

Visual confrontation naming, shown to be reliably reduced in dominant side ATL, was also tested using the Boston Naming Test (BNT) [38]. The total correct score without phonemic cues was the dependent variable.

2.6. Statistical Analysis. All data were analyzed with IBM SPSS Statistics Version 20. Quantitative baseline characteristics were compared between the two groups (ATL or SelAH) using the Student's t-test and categorical characteristics were compared using the Chi-squared test.

Student's t-test was also used to assess the mean difference for the neuropsychological scores (PCA components and BNT performance) between the two surgical approaches. Analyses were done separately for the dominant and the nondominant groups. Four left-sided temporal lobe epilepsy (TLE) patients had atypical language dominance (one SelAH and three ATL) and were included in the nondominant groups. P values less than 0.05 were deemed significant.

Kaplan-Meier curves were generated to determine the relationship between seizure recurrence and the surgical approach. A time-to-event analysis was performed to compare the recurrence rates among the two surgical groups. An "event" was classified as any seizure that occurred after the first postoperative week; seizures occurring in the first postoperative week were excluded. We limited our analysis to a two-year follow-up period to enhance our sample size.

3. Results

Overall, 96 patients were included in the study (75 ATL, 21 SelAH); of these, fifty-four (37 ATL, 17 SelAH) completed a full neuropsychological examination prior to and at least 6 months following surgery (median = 11.3 months). Median

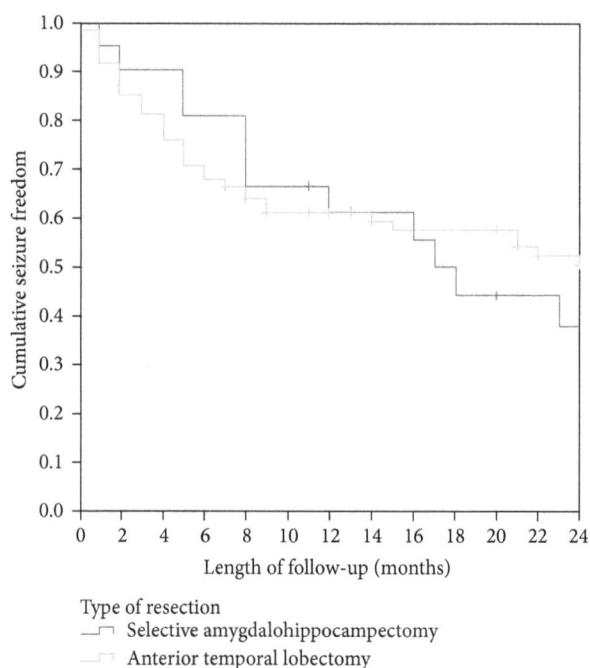

FIGURE 1: Postoperative seizure freedom in patients with mesial temporal lobe epilepsy as a function of surgical procedure. Analysis time point of two-year follow-up period.

follow-up was 41 months (range 6–104 months). Patient demographics and a summary of the preoperative evaluations are presented in Table 1. The two groups were well-matched on most variables, except that patients in the SelAH group were slightly younger at the time of surgery and a higher proportion of patients in the ATL group required invasive monitoring prior to surgery (24% versus 5%; Table 1).

A trend toward earlier seizure recurrence was observed in the ATL group. In the ATL cohort not experiencing early seizures, seizure freedom appeared to be more durable (Figure 1). However, this difference was not statistically significant (HR: 0.85; 95% CI 0.45–1.59; $P = 0.61$).

Invasive EEG (iEEG) monitoring was required in 19 patients; one patient belonging to the SelAH group and the

TABLE 2: Characteristics of patients requiring invasive EEG monitoring.

	Invasive EEG required	Invasive EEG not required
Frequency	19	77
SelAH procedure	1	20
ATL procedure	18	57
Gender (%female)	9 (47%)	45 (58%)
Age at surgery (Year)	37.2	40.9
Initial EEG lateralizing/localizing (%)	9 (47%)	47 (62%)
MRI concordance	14 (72%)	67 (87%)
Multifocal spikes in EMU*	18 (95%)	19 (25%)
Bilateral interictal abnormalities in EMU (%)*	9 (47%)	13 (17%)
Average duration of seizure freedom (months)^	18.1	13.7

*$P < 0.05$.
^$P = 0.08$.
EEG: electroencephalography; EMU: Epilepsy Monitoring Unit.

remaining 18 belonging to the ATL group. At our institution, the criteria for iEEG monitoring generally include ictal video EEG findings that are nonconcordant with imaging and neuropsychological examinations, bilateral interictal abnormalities, or multifocal ictal findings. Given that the need for iEEG monitoring is an indication of the complexity of the underlying neuronal network, these patients were more likely to undergo ATL. In patients with bitemporal spikes a standard bitemporal implantation, with hippocampal depth electrodes, in addition to subdural strip electrodes was used. Grid electrodes were used for patients with suspected neocortical involvement. Characteristic differences between the cohort of patients requiring iEEG and those identified as candidates for surgery without iEEG have been outlined in Table 2. While there were no major pre-EMU differences between these two cohorts (outpatient MRI and scalp EEG), a significantly greater proportion of the iEEG cohort was found to have multifocal ictal spikes ($P < 0.001$) and bilateral interictal abnormalities ($P < 0.001$) during video EEG monitoring. While the heterogeneity of these two cohorts suggests a greater complexity with regard to seizure onset localization, there was no statistically significant impact on duration of seizure freedom among them ($P = 0.08$).

Neuropsychological outcomes are shown in Table 3. The PCA change scores can be thought of as "standardized" scores, with a mean of 0 and standard deviation (sd) of 1, based on the distribution of scores in a large population of mTLE patients who have undergone surgery in our centre. They represent postoperative scores minus preoperative scores for each component; a score of −1.0 indicates a decline in performance that is one sd greater than the normative sample of left and right mTLE surgical cohort and therefore a moderate-to-large decline. Here, none of the PCA change scores differed significantly between the ATL and SelAH groups (all P values > 0.3), and all were within one standard deviation of the average change seen in the "normative" sample. Critically for the current hypothesis, there was no systematic advantage seen with respect to memory sparing in the selective procedures; memory was affected equivalently in both groups. Scores for the BNT represent the raw number of

items named at postsurgery minus presurgery; again negative scores reflect decline. There was no statistically significant difference amongst groups, although there was a trend for dominant ATL to show a greater decline than other groups (dominant ATL versus nondominant ATL: $t = 1.58$, one-tailed $P = 0.06$; versus nondominant SelAH: $t = 1.37$, one-tailed $P = 0.09$; versus dominant SelAH: $t = 0.96$; one-tailed $P = 0.20$).

4. Discussion

The goal of surgery for epilepsy patients is to attain seizure freedom while preventing or minimizing surgical morbidity such as impairments of cognition and memory. As recent meta-analyses suggest, ATL is likely associated with a reduced rate of seizure recurrence relative to SelAH [35, 36]. Given the greater technical challenges of the SelAH procedure [30, 39], it is important to ascertain whether it confers neurocognitive benefits. Both mesial and neocortical temporal lobe structures have roles in acquiring, consolidating, and retrieving material-specific information and the temporal neocortex in the dominant hemisphere is critically involved in naming and other semantic abilities. Given the lack of randomized controlled studies, it is important to consider both seizure and cognitive outcomes in a well-characterized surgical cohort. Furthermore, with respect to the evaluation of cognitive outcomes, validated standardized neuropsychological scores should be included to reduce variability of results.

No statistically significant differences in seizure outcomes were observed in our study. Among studies performed to date, only a few have included patients with hippocampal sclerosis as the sole underlying pathology [15, 21, 23, 25]. Three studies have reported the outcomes of a single surgeon [15, 24, 31], as our study has. Most published series have not identified a significant difference in seizure outcome between the two approaches [23, 26, 30, 31, 34]. Three studies have shown more favorable seizure outcomes in patients undergoing ATL [16, 17, 32]; no studies to date have shown favorable seizure outcomes in patients undergoing SelAH. The meta-analyses of Josephson et al. [35] and Hu et al. [36]

TABLE 3: Neuropsychological outcome comparison between dominant and nondominant SelAH and ATL surgical groups.

	Dominant SelAH (n = 8)	Dominant ATL (n = 12)	Nondominant SelAH (n = 9)	Nondominant ATL (n = 25)
Change verbal memory PC	−0.7 (1.3)	−0.5 (0.8)	0.2 (0.5)	0.4 (0.7)
Change visuospatial memory PC	0.2 (0.6)	0.3 (0.8)	0.1 (1.2)	0.3 (1.0)
Change IQ PC	−0.4 (0.9)	0.0 (0.8)	−0.2 (0.7)	0.1 (1.0)
Change BNT	−1.0 (7.0)	−4.0 (8.6)	0.1 (2.7)	−0.6 (4.7)

Note: change in BNT for the dominant ATL group is based on N = 11. PC: principal component score; BNT is postop-preop total score. Mean and standard deviation for PC and naming scores; no differences are observed between SelAH and ATL in the dominant groups or in the nondominant groups (P > 0.31).

demonstrated that ATL conferred an increased likelihood of achieving control from disabling seizures, defined as Engel class I, with an NNT of 10–13 for 1 additional patient to achieve control from seizures (RR 1.32, 95% CI 1.12–1.57) [35]. This benefit was maintained when subgroup analysis was performed on patients who had hippocampal sclerosis as the lone pathology (RR 1.26, 95% confidence interval [1.05–1.51]) [35].

Regarding the question of neuropsychological morbidity, one important aspect of our study was the use of measures that assessed not only IQ, as in several previous studies, but also verbal and visuospatial memory and naming which represent domains that are more specifically related to temporal-lobe function. While we did not observe a statistically significant difference in neuropsychological outcomes between the two procedures, we did observe a trend toward better preservation of naming in patients undergoing SelAH versus ATL on the dominant side. While there are fewer studies that can be amalgamated to evaluate cognitive outcomes and the measures are often heterogeneous, one large-scale series from the Montreal Neurological Institute (123 ATL and 133 SelAH cases) reported that SelAH patients showed better scores compared to patients with ATL in both full-scale and PIQ. Although material-specific memory deficits were apparent following surgery, there were no striking differences between the two approaches [31]. It is possible that there is no clinically meaningful difference between the two approaches with respect to memory measures that are more closely aligned with medial temporal functioning, as was shown by the Montreal Neurological Institute and our results, whereas other cortically mediated functions, such as those reflecting semantic processing, are more likely to show differences.

It is well established that ATL can result in postoperative memory deficits, particularly for verbal memory following dominant hemisphere resection [40]. The magnitude of postoperative decline is strongly influenced by the presence of mesial temporal lobe pathology and the functional integrity of the resected mesial temporal lobe as demonstrated on preoperative memory testing [41–43]. In addition, naming deficits have been documented with the standard ATL on the dominant side [38]. While this is thought to be secondary to resection of relevant functional areas at the temporal base and tip, reduced language comprehension and fluency have been observed in patients undergoing SelAH on the dominant side as well; two narrative reviews [7, 44] reported

a greater risk of decline in naming and verbal memory components after resection of the mesial structures on the dominant hemisphere, regardless of the surgical approach. This may reflect deafferentiation in cortical areas, disruption of basal temporal language area pathways, or neocortical lesions secondary to surgical intervention [45]. While there are no meta-analyses directly comparing SelAH and ATL with respect to memory and language, a large number of studies have failed to show a difference in neuropsychological outcomes [23, 24, 26, 28, 46]. However, several studies have reported favorable neuropsychological outcomes in patients undergoing SelAH [10, 12, 18, 19, 25]. Hadar et al. [33] reported an advantage of SelAH in verbal recall based on the RAVLT test, but no difference when overall Wechsler Memory Scale test was used. Goldstein and Polkey found a beneficial effect on immediate verbal recall for paragraphs and verbal paired associate learning for SelAH [4] but could not demonstrate the same results when using Rivermead Behavioral Memory Test to evaluate memory in a more global context [27]. These results open the discussion as to whether the differences on neuropsychological outcomes depend exclusively on the baseline pathology and the surgical approach or whether the specific neuropsychological tests used, and their relative reliance on operations that depend on medial versus neocortical temporal regions, are influential as well.

Whereas the SelAH procedure is restricted to the temporomesial structures [25], ATL involves resections in the dominant (3.5 to 4.0 cm) or nondominant (up to 5 cm) temporal neocortex in combination with an amygdalo-hippocampectomy [25, 32]. Even in patients with strictly hippocampal sclerosis apparent on preoperative imaging, abnormalities (metabolic, histological, and electrical) have been detected in the temporal neocortex as well [47–49]. Thus, a theoretical advantage of ATL may be attributed to the possible incorporation of epileptogenic foci in addition to the mesial region [35] or by the disconnection of an epileptogenic circuit, preventing seizure propagation and neocortical epileptogenesis. In interpreting the findings in the extant literature, it also must be borne in mind that older studies may not have been as stringent in differentiating mTLE and neocortical TLE, which would erroneously result in a seizure outcome favoring ATL. This is also an important potential confound in considering the lack of compelling differences in cognitive outcome. The expectation is that surgical resection of functionally intact regions should come at a cost. It may be that greater precision in both patient and task selection is required to appropriately estimate the cost associated with resection of the anterior temporal cortex. Even if SelAH can be found to confer an advantage with respect to some aspect of cognitive functioning, there is an argument to be made that patients receiving ATL may fare better over a longer period given the psychosocial benefits derived from improved seizure control [35, 50–52].

Similar to many previous studies, our analysis was limited by its retrospective, nonrandomized nature. In addition, the SelAH procedure was performed within a one-year period; the presence of a learning curve effect could potentially affect outcomes. Furthermore, the database included a greater number of ATL patients. Nonetheless, our findings have contributed a relatively large sample of patients subjected to robust neuropsychological analyses and assessed with stringent seizure recurrence criteria. In addition, our study has the advantage of incorporating data from the experience of a single surgeon, with a homogenous cohort limited only to patients with mTLE with evidence of hippocampal sclerosis. Furthermore, our neuropsychological assessment has implemented data reduction techniques to derive composite scores from a uniform battery of tests pre- and postoperatively. As was demonstrated by St-Laurent et al. [37], this technique has an important value for simplifying measurements while remaining sensitive enough to detect group differences and predict postoperative changes.

Recently, the interest in comparing the two surgical approaches has been rekindled [35] and multicenter randomized control trial (RCT) has been recommended. This is particularly important given that the evidence in favor of ATL for seizure control is growing while the evidence for SelAH for better neuropsychological outcomes remains equivocal. The optimal RCT would be one whereby both seizure and neuropsychological outcomes are assessed. Logistically, however, it may be difficult to obtain a large enough sample that is powered to assess for both outcomes in both dominant and nondominant resections in a single surgical centre. Given that most studies favoring SelAH for neuropsychological outcomes have found that patients with dominant side resections fare better [4, 19], we would advocate for randomization of patients undergoing dominant lobe resections only. Furthermore, it is necessary to establish a unified surgical approach for each procedure and all patients must undergo a standard battery of pre- and postoperative neuropsychological assessments that include measures known to be sensitive to anterior temporal neocortex dysfunction (e.g., naming and semantic fluency) as well as verbal memory. In addition, a standard definition of seizure recurrence and method of analysis must be established and follow-up periods must be predefined. As practice is variable across and within centres, only such Level 1 evidence is appropriate to guide surgical decision-making in weighing seizure and cognitive outcomes of epilepsy surgery.

Conflict of Interests

The authors declare that there is no conflict of interests regarding the publication of this paper.

References

[1] H. Clusmann, J. Schramm, T. Kral et al., "Prognostic factors and outcome after different types of resection for temporal lobe epilepsy," *Journal of Neurosurgery*, vol. 97, no. 5, pp. 1131–1141, 2002.

[2] J. J. Engel, P. C. van Ness, T. B. Rasmussen, and L. M. Ojemann, "Outcome with respect to epileptic seizures," in *Surgical Treatment of the Epilepsies*, J. Engel Jr., Ed., pp. 609–621, New-York Raven Press, New York, NY USA, 2nd edition, 1993.

[3] R. L. Wolf, R. J. Ivnik, K. A. Hirschorn, F. W. Sharbrough, G. D. Cascino, and W. R. Marsh, "Neurocognitive efficiency following left temporal lobectomy: standard versus limited resection," *Journal of Neurosurgery*, vol. 79, no. 1, pp. 76–83, 1993.

[4] L. H. Goldstein and C. E. Polkey, "Short-term cognitive changes after unilateral temporal lobectomy or unilateral amygdalo-hippocampectomy for the relief of temporal lobe epilepsy," *Journal of Neurology, Neurosurgery & Psychiatry*, vol. 56, no. 2, pp. 135–140, 1993.

[5] S. Baxendale, P. Thompson, W. Harkness, and J. Duncan, "Predicting memory decline following epilepsy surgery: a multivariate approach," *Epilepsia*, vol. 47, no. 11, pp. 1887–1894, 2006.

[6] M. Jones-Gotman, R. J. Zatorre, A. Olivier et al., "Learning and retention of words and designs following excision from medial or lateral temporal lobe structures," *Neuropsychologia*, vol. 35, no. 7, pp. 963–973, 1997.

[7] E. M. S. Sherman, S. Wiebe, T. B. Fay-Mcclymont et al., "Neuropsychological outcomes after epilepsy surgery: systematic review and pooled estimates," *Epilepsia*, vol. 52, no. 5, pp. 857–869, 2011.

[8] M. G. Yaşargil, H. G. Wieser, A. Valavanis, K. von Ammon, and P. Roth, "Surgery and results of selective amygdala-hippocampectomy in one hundred patients with nonlesional limbic epilepsy," *Neurosurgery Clinics of North America*, vol. 4, no. 2, pp. 243–261, 1993.

[9] C. Helmstaedter and C. E. Elger, "Cognitive consequences of two-thirds anterior temporal lobectomy on verbal memory in 144 patients: a three-month follow-up study," *Epilepsia*, vol. 37, no. 2, pp. 171–180, 1996.

[10] E. Pauli, S. Pickel, H. Schulemann, M. Buchfelder, and H. Stefan, "Neuropsychologic findings depending on the type of the resection in temporal lobe epilepsy," *Advances in Neurology*, vol. 81, pp. 371–377, 1999.

[11] P. Niemeyer, "The transventricular amygdala-hippocampectomy in temporal lobe epilepsy," in *Temporal Lobe Epilepsy*, M. Baldwin and P. Bailey, Eds., Springfield, Mass, USA, pp. 461–482, Charles Thomas, 1958.

[12] M. G. Yaşargil, P. J. Teddy, and P. Roth, "Selective amygdalohippocampectomy. Operative anatomy and surgical technique," *Advances and Technical Standards in Neurosurgery*, vol. 12, pp. 93–123, 1985.

[13] F. Arruda, F. Cendes, F. Andermann et al., "Mesial atrophy and outcome after amygdalohippocampectomy or temporal lobe removal," *Annals of Neurology*, vol. 40, no. 3, pp. 446–450, 1996.

[14] E. Paglioli, A. Palmini, J. C. Da Costa et al., "Survival analysis of the surgical outcome of temporal lobe epilepsy due to hippocampal sclerosis," *Epilepsia*, vol. 45, no. 11, pp. 1383–1391, 2004.

[15] T. Tanriverdi, A. Olivier, N. Poulin, F. Andermann, and F. Dubeau, "Long-term seizure outcome after mesial temporal

lobe epilepsy surgery: corticalamygdalohippocampectomy versus selective amygdalohippocampectomy," *Journal of Neurosurgery*, vol. 108, no. 3, pp. 517–524, 2008.

[16] H. Bate, P. Eldridge, T. Varma, and U. C. Wieshmann, "The seizure outcome after amygdalohippocampectomy and temporal lobectomy," *European Journal of Neurology*, vol. 14, no. 1, pp. 90–94, 2007.

[17] R. A. Mackenzie, J. Matheson, M. Ellis, and J. Klamus, "Selective versus non-selective temporal lobe surgery for epilepsy," *Journal of Clinical Neuroscience*, vol. 4, no. 2, pp. 152–154, 1997.

[18] E. Paglioli, A. Palmini, M. Portuguez et al., "Seizure and memory outcome following temporal lobe surgery: selective compared with nonselective approaches for hippocampal sclerosis," *Journal of Neurosurgery*, vol. 104, no. 1, pp. 70–78, 2006.

[19] S. A. Renowden, Z. Matkovic, C. B. T. Adams et al., "Selective amygdalohippocampectomy for hippocampal sclerosis: postoperative MR appearance," *The American Journal of Neuroradiology*, vol. 16, no. 9, pp. 1855–1861, 1995.

[20] O. Sagher, "Epilepsy surgery," *Journal of Neurosurgery*, vol. 118, no. 1, pp. 167–168, 2013.

[21] A.-S. Wendling, E. Hirsch, I. Wisniewski et al., "Selective amygdalohippocampectomy versus standard temporal lobectomy in patients with mesial temporal lobe epilepsy and unilateral hippocampal sclerosis," *Epilepsy Research*, vol. 104, no. 1-2, pp. 94–104, 2013.

[22] O. E. Schijns, C. G. Bien, M. Majores et al., "Presence of temporal gray-white matter abnormalities does not influence epilepsy surgery outcome in temporal lobe epilepsy with hippocampal sclerosis," *Neurosurgery*, vol. 68, no. 1, pp. 98–106, 2011.

[23] T. Tanriverdi and A. Olivier, "Cognitive changes after unilateral cortico-amygdalo-hippocampectomy or unilateral selective-amyg-dalohippocampectomy for mesial temporal lobe epilepsy," *Turkish Neurosurgery*, vol. 17, no. 2, pp. 91–99, 2007.

[24] M.-S. Shin, S. Lee, S.-H. Seol et al., "Changes in neuropsychological functioning following temporal lobectomy in patients with temporal lobe epilepsy," *Neurological Research*, vol. 31, no. 7, pp. 692–701, 2009.

[25] C. Helmstaedter, S. Richter, S. Röske, F. Oltmanns, J. Schramm, and T. N. Lehmann, "Differential effects of temporal pole resection with amygdalohippocampectomy versus selective amygdalohippocampectomy on material-specific memory in patients with mesial temporal lobe epilepsy," *Epilepsia*, vol. 49, no. 1, pp. 88–97, 2008.

[26] T. Lee, R. A. Mackenzie, A. J. Walker, J. M. Matheson, and P. Sachdev, "Effects of left temporal lobectomy and amygdalohippocampectomy on memory," *Journal of Clinical Neuroscience*, vol. 4, no. 3, pp. 314–319, 1997.

[27] L. H. Goldstein and C. E. Polkey, "Behavioural memory after temporal lobectomy or amygdalo-hippocampectomy," *The British Journal of Clinical Psychology*, vol. 31, no. 1, pp. 75–81, 1992.

[28] M. E. Lacruz, G. Alarcón, N. Akanuma et al., "Neuropsychological effects associated with temporal lobectomy and amygdalohippocampectomy depending on Wada test failure," *Journal of Neurology, Neurosurgery and Psychiatry*, vol. 75, no. 4, pp. 600–607, 2004.

[29] C. Helmstaedter, M. Reuber, and C. C. Elger, "Interaction of cognitive aging and memory deficits related to epilepsy surgery," *Annals of Neurology*, vol. 52, no. 1, pp. 89–94, 2002.

[30] M. Morino, T. Uda, K. Naito et al., "Comparison of neuropsychological outcomes after selective amygdalohippocampectomy versus anterior temporal lobectomy," *Epilepsy and Behavior*, vol. 9, no. 1, pp. 95–100, 2006.

[31] T. Tanriverdi, R. W. R. Dudley, A. Hasan et al., "Memory outcome after temporal lobe epilepsy surgery: corticoamygdalohippocampectomy versus selective amygdalohippocampectomy," *Journal of Neurosurgery*, vol. 113, no. 6, pp. 1164–1175, 2010.

[32] H. Clusmann, T. Kral, U. Gleissner et al., "Analysis of different types of resection for pediatric patients with temporal lobe epilepsy," *Neurosurgery*, vol. 54, no. 4, pp. 847–860, 2004.

[33] E. Hadar, W. Bingaman, M. Foldvary, G. J. Chelune, and Y. G. Comair, "Prospective analysis of outcome after selective amygdalohippocampectomy and anterior temporal lobectomy for refractory epilepsy," in *Congress of Neurological Surgeons*, San Diego, Calif, USA, 2001.

[34] A. Grivas, J. Schramm, T. Kral et al., "Surgical treatment for refractory temporal lobe epilepsy in the elderly: seizure outcome and neuropsychological sequels compared with a younger cohort," *Epilepsia*, vol. 47, no. 8, pp. 1364–1372, 2006.

[35] C. B. Josephson, J. Dykeman, K. M. Fiest et al., "Systematic review and meta-analysis of standard vs selective temporal lobe epilepsy surgery," *Neurology*, vol. 80, no. 18, pp. 1669–1676, 2013.

[36] W.-H. Hu, C. Zhang, K. Zhang, F.-G. Meng, N. Chen, and J.-G. Zhang, "Selective amygdalohippocampectomy versus anterior temporal lobectomy in the management of mesial temporal lobe epilepsy: a meta-analysis of comparative studies a systematic review," *Journal of Neurosurgery*, vol. 119, no. 5, pp. 1089–1097, 2013.

[37] M. St-Laurent, C. McCormick, M. Cohn, B. Mišić, I. Giannoylis, and M. P. McAndrews, "Using multivariate data reduction to predict postsurgery memory decline in patients with mesial temporal lobe epilepsy," *Epilepsy and Behavior*, vol. 31, pp. 220–227, 2014.

[38] V. L. Ives-Deliperi and J. T. Butler, "Naming outcomes of anterior temporal lobectomy in epilepsy patients: a systematic review of the literature," *Epilepsy and Behavior*, vol. 24, no. 2, pp. 194–198, 2012.

[39] B. Adada, "Selective amygdalohippocampectomy via the transsylvian approach," *Neurosurgical Focus*, vol. 25, no. 3, article E5, 2008.

[40] B. D. Bell and A. R. Giovagnoli, "Memory after temporal lobe epilepsy surgery: risk and reward," *Neurology*, vol. 71, no. 17, pp. 1302–1303, 2008.

[41] G. J. Chelune, "Hippocampal adequacy versus functional reserve: predicting memory functions following temporal lobectomy," *Archives of Clinical Neuropsychology*, vol. 10, no. 5, pp. 413–432, 1995.

[42] E. Stroup, J. Langfitt, M. Berg, M. McDermott, W. Pilcher, and P. Como, "Predicting verbal memory decline following anterior temporal lobectomy (ATL)," *Neurology*, vol. 60, no. 8, pp. 1266–1273, 2003.

[43] N. Elshorst, B. Pohlmann-Eden, S. Horstmann, R. Schulz, F. Woermann, and M. P. McAndrews, "Postoperative memory prediction in left temporal lobe epilepsy: the Wada test is of no added value to preoperative neuropsychological assessment and MRI," *Epilepsy and Behavior*, vol. 16, no. 2, pp. 335–340, 2009.

[44] J. Schramm, "Temporal lobe epilepsy surgery and the quest for optimal extent of resection: a review," *Epilepsia*, vol. 49, no. 8, pp. 1296–1307, 2008.

[45] L. Bartha, E. Trinka, M. Ortler et al., "Linguistic deficits following left selective amygdalohippocampectomy: a prospective study," *Epilepsy and Behavior*, vol. 5, no. 3, pp. 348–357, 2004.

[46] C. Helmstaedter, A. Hufnagel, and C. E. Elger, "Seizures during cognitive testing in patients with temporal lobe epilepsy: possibility of seizure induction by cognitive activation," *Epilepsia*, vol. 33, no. 5, pp. 892–897, 1992.

[47] M.-C. Cheung, A. S. Chan, J. M. K. Lam, and Y.-L. Chan, "Pre- and postoperative fMRI and clinical memory performance in temporal lobe epilepsy," *Journal of Neurology, Neurosurgery and Psychiatry*, vol. 80, no. 10, pp. 1099–1106, 2009.

[48] S. Chabardès, P. Kahane, L. Minotti et al., "The temporopolar cortex plays a pivotal role in temporal lobe seizures," *Brain*, vol. 128, no. 8, pp. 1818–1831, 2005.

[49] K. N. Fountas, I. Tsougos, E. D. Gotsis, S. Giannakodimos, J. R. Smith, and E. Z. Kapsalaki, "Temporal pole proton preoperative magnetic resonance spectroscopy in patients undergoing surgery for mesial temporal sclerosis," *Neurosurgical Focus*, vol. 32, no. 3, article E3, 2012.

[50] C. E. Elger, C. Helmstaedter, and M. Kurthen, "Chronic epilepsy and cognition," *The Lancet Neurology*, vol. 3, no. 11, pp. 663–672, 2004.

[51] A. Jacoby, G. A. Baker, N. Steen, P. Potts, and D. W. Chadwick, "The clinical course of epilepsy and its psychosocial correlates: findings from a U.K. community study," *Epilepsia*, vol. 37, no. 2, pp. 148–161, 1996.

[52] C. Helmstaedter, M. Kurthen, S. Lux, M. Reuber, and C. E. Elger, "Chronic epilepsy and cognition: a longitudinal study in temporal lobe epilepsy," *Annals of Neurology*, vol. 54, no. 4, pp. 425–432, 2003.

18

Efficacy and Safety of Levetiracetam and Carbamazepine as Monotherapy in Partial Seizures

Swaroop Hassan Suresh,[1] **Ananya Chakraborty,**[2]
Akash Virupakshaiah,[2] **and Nithin Kumar**[3]

[1]*Cipla Ltd, 117/1, Anjanadri, Pantharapalya, Bangalore 560039, India*
[2]*Department of Pharmacology, Vydehi Institute of Medical Sciences and Research Centre, No. 82 EPIP Area, Whitefield, Bangalore 560037, India*
[3]*Department of Neurology, Columbia Asia Hospital, Whitefield, Bangalore 560066, India*

Correspondence should be addressed to Swaroop Hassan Suresh; swap_hs@yahoo.co.in

Academic Editor: Roy G. Beran

Introduction. Levetiracetam (LEV) is a newer antiepileptic drug with better pharmacokinetic profile. Currently, it is frequently used for the treatment of partial seizures. The present study was undertaken to compare the efficacy and safety of LEV and Carbamazepine (CBZ) in partial epilepsy. *Methods.* This was a prospective, open labeled, randomized study. It was conducted in participants suffering from partial seizures after the approval of ethics committee and written informed consent. The first group received Tab LEV (500 to 3000 mg/day) and the second group received Tab CBZ (300 to 600 mg/day). The primary outcomes were efficacy and safety. The secondary outcome was the Quality of Life (QOL). Efficacy was assessed by comparing the seizure freedom rates at the end of 6 months. Safety profile was evaluated by comparing the adverse effects. QOL was assessed by QOLIE-10 scale. *Results.* The overall seizure freedom rate at the end of 6 months was 71.42% in CBZ group compared to 78.57% in LEV group ($p = 0.2529$). Both LEV and CBZ reported a similar incidence of adverse reactions. LEV group reported more behavioral changes like increased aggression and anxiety. Also, it showed better QOL compared to the CBZ group. *Conclusion.* LEV monotherapy and CBZ monotherapy demonstrated similar efficacy for treatment of partial epilepsy and were found to be well tolerated.

1. Introduction

Epilepsy is a chronic disorder characterized by 2 or 3 recurrent seizures of cerebral origin. It is the second most common neurological condition after headache. The estimated average prevalence of epilepsy is 6.8 per 1000 people in US, 5.5 per 1000 people in Europe, and 1.5 to 14 per 1000 people in Asia, respectively. Epilepsy is classified based on the source of seizure into partial and generalized seizures [1]. World Health Organization (WHO) and International League against Epilepsy (ILAE) have estimated that, out of 50 million people, 34 million with epilepsy live in developing countries. Out of them, nearly 80% are not on treatment [2]. In India, it is estimated that, out of over 1.23 billion population, there are around 6–10 million people with epilepsy. It accounts for nearly 1/5th of global epilepsy burden [3]. Epilepsy is classified based on the source of seizure into partial and generalized seizures. Partial seizures arise in specific, often small, loci of cortex in one hemisphere of the brain. About 2/3rd of newly diagnosed epilepsies are partial or secondarily generalized. The treatment of the epilepsy depends on appropriate classification of seizure type and the epileptic syndrome [4].

The mainstay of treatment of epilepsy is pharmacological therapy with antiepileptic drugs (AEDs). In epilepsy, optimal treatment is important as the condition is associated with increased morbidity and mortality and unexpected deaths without clear structural or pathological cause [5, 6]. AEDs are selected based on the nature of the disease, the efficacy and tolerability of the agent, and the characteristics of the patient [7]. Treatment options for epilepsy include the older AEDs (carbamazepine, ethosuximide, phenytoin, phenobarbital, primidone, and valproic acid) as well as several newer drugs (Levetiracetam, felbamate, gabapentin, lacosamide, lamotrigine, oxcarbazepine, pregabalin, rufinamide, tiagabine, topiramate, vigabatrin, and zonisamide) [8]. Carbamazepine (CBZ) is the preferred drug for the treatment of partial seizures but it has the disadvantages of requirement for frequent dosing, dose related adverse reactions, and drug interactions. Recently, Levetiracetam (LEV) has become one of the most frequently prescribed newer drugs for the treatment of partial seizures. It offers several advantages like twice daily dosing, better safety profile, less drug interactions, and no requirement of serum level monitoring. This advantageous pharmacologic profile makes LEV an attractive first-line or adjunctive therapy for epileptic seizures [9, 10].

Till date, there have been a very few studies on the efficacy and safety of LEV and CBZ in partial epilepsy. Hence, this study was undertaken to compare the efficacy and safety of LEV and CBZ as monotherapy in partial epilepsy.

2. Materials and Methods

2.1. Study Design and Setting. This was a randomized, prospective, open label, comparative monotherapy study. The study was conducted in the Department of Neurology at Vydehi Institute of Medical Sciences and Research Center, Bengaluru, India. The institute is a 1000-bed tertiary care hospital equipped with modern diagnostic and treatment facilities. Patients visiting this hospital come from different geographical regions including Southern Karnataka, Andhra Pradesh, and West Bengal, India, with a fair representation of both urban and rural populations. The patients belong to varied socioeconomic strata. The study was conducted after receiving the approval from the Institutional Ethics Review Board. The duration of the study was one year from January 2013 to December 2013.

2.2. Selection of the Participants. The participants were included in the study after obtaining written informed consent. The study inclusion criteria included subjects of age between 18 and 60 years diagnosed newly with focal or partial seizures with or without secondary generalization. The exclusion criteria were pregnant and lactating mothers, patients with nonepileptic seizures, auras or absence of seizures, and patients with acute symptomatic seizures occurring within 14 days of an acute brain injury such as stroke and patients with history of psychiatric illness.

2.3. Data Collection. The Neurology OPD was used to recruit participants with newly diagnosed partial epilepsy. The study objectives and process were explained to the patients or their relatives in their own language. Subjects who consented to participate were then interviewed and were divided into two groups by the toss of a coin. Each group recruited 30 participants. Group 1 participants were prescribed Tab LEV, 1000–3000 mg/day/oral; and group 2 participants were prescribed Tab CBZ, 400–1200 mg/day/oral. The participants were started with minimum dose, 500 mg of LEV and 200 mg of CBZ, given twice daily after food and then titrated depending

on the seizure control. LEV dose was increased by 500 mg twice daily every 2 weeks up to a maximum of 3000 mg/day if seizure control was not achieved. Similarly, CBZ dose was increased by 200 mg twice daily up to a maximum of 1200 mg/day if seizure control was not achieved. In cases where the seizure was not controlled after titration of drug dose, the participant was shifted to adjuvant therapy based on the clinical condition. The participant was also discontinued from the study.

All the participants were given a diary and were asked to note down any adverse effects (AE). They were advised to come after 4, 12, and 26 weeks after the initiation of therapy for follow-up. During follow-up visits, the participants were thoroughly examined, history of breakthrough seizures was elicited, and any AEs were noted. QOL was assessed by using the QOLIE-10 questionnaire before initiation of the treatment and after 26 weeks of therapy [11]. QOLIE-10 comprises seven components: (1) seizure worry, (2) overall QOL, (3) emotional well-being, (4) cognitive function, (5) energy/fatigue, (6) medication effects: physical effects and psychological effects, and (7) social functioning: work, driving, and social function. The English version of QOLIE-10 was used for this study. Participants who were conversant in English completed the questionnaire themselves. Since the remaining patient population was multilingual (Kannada, Hindi, Bengali, and Telugu), the questions were explained to them in their respective languages and responses were elicited. The responses were then scored to provide subscale scores which were then averaged to provide a total score.

2.4. Data Analysis. The baseline data like demography, efficacy, and AEs were subjected to descriptive statistical analysis and expressed as mean ± SD, frequencies, and percentages. The QOLIE-10 scores were expressed as mean ± SD scores. The categorical variables were compared using Chi-square (χ^2) test. Comparison of continuous variables between groups was carried out using unpaired Student's t-test. Statistical significance was set at $p < 0.05$.

3. Results

A total of 79 subjects were screened for the study. Out of them, 60 (75.6%) participants who fulfilled the eligibility criteria were randomized into the two study groups. Following is the summarization of the observed results.

3.1. Patient Characteristics and Demographic Profile. Out of 30 participants in CBZ group, 17 were male and 13 were female. Out of 30 participants in LEV group, 13 were male and 17 were female. The mean age of the male participants in CBZ group was 30.70 ± 2.66 years, and in the LEV group it was 22.62 ± 1.152 years (p value, 0.0834). The mean age of females in CBZ group was 29.31 ± 2.44 years and in LEV group it was 28.18 ± 2.553 yrs (p value, 0.7101). Thus there was no significant difference between the mean age of males and that of females in both groups. The mean BMI of CBZ group was 22.56 ± 0.41 kg/m^2 and that of LEV group was 21.49 ± 0.41 kg/m^2 (p value of 0.0690). There was no significant difference in BMI in both groups.

TABLE 1: Overall characteristics of patients on Levetiracetam and Carbamazepine monotherapy.

	CBZ group $n = 28$	LEV group $n = 28$	p value
Male mean age	30.70 ± 2.66 yrs	22.62 ± 1.152 yrs	0.0834
Female mean age	29.31 ± 2.44 yrs	28.18 ± 2.553 yrs	0.7101
Mean BMI	22.56 ± 0.41	21.49 ± 0.41	0.0690
Pretreatment mean seizure frequency	2.83 ± 0.19	4.2 ± 0.65	0.0470
Seizure freedom at 4 weeks	85.72%	85.72%	1.0000
Seizure freedom at 12 weeks	89.29%	93.34%	0.4595
Seizure freedom at 26 weeks	96.43%	100%	0.1212
Overall seizure freedom at 6 months	71.42%	78.57%	0.2529
QOL at 0 weeks	31.14 ± 1.83	29.76 ± 1.71	0.5861
QOL at 26th week	58.41 ± 1.89	64.58 ± 2.02	0.0302

3.2. Treatment Efficacy. Thirty participants were randomized to both CBZ group and LEV group. In the LEV group, 2 participants dropped from the study, one was lost to follow-up, and one subject had serious AE. Thus, a total of 28 subjects in LEV group were assessed for efficacy. Similarly, 2 subjects in CBZ group were dropped from the study due to AE. Thus, a total of 28 subjects from CBZ group were assessed for efficacy as shown in Figure 1.

All participants were followed up at 4, 12, and 26 weeks after the initiation of monotherapy. At the 4th week of follow-up, both groups had equal seizure freedom of 85.72% which is not statistically significant (p value of 1.000). At 12 weeks of follow-up, CBZ group had 89.29% of seizure freedom compared to LEV group which had 93.34% seizure freedom which is not statistically significant (p value, 0.4595). Twenty-two (78.57%) of those taking LEV and 20 (71.42%) subjects on CBZ were seizure-free for at least 6 months during the monotherapy treatment, which is not statistically significant (p value, 0.2529). The data is shown in Figures 2 and 3.

3.3. Treatment Safety. Participants who experienced at least one AE constituted 36.66% in CBZ group and 40% in the LEV group (p value, 0.7714), which is not statistically significant. One participant (3.33%) on LEV therapy discontinued the treatment due to AE of increased nausea and vomiting and 2 patients (6.66%) discontinued the treatment due to AE of dizziness and increased nausea. In LEV group, 5 participants experienced behavioral changes like increased aggressive behavior, 1 participant experienced suicidal tendency, 3 participants had increased anxiety, 3 participants suffered from increased sleep, 2 participants reported weight gain of around 3–5 kilograms in 3 months of duration, and 2 participants reported constipation. The other AEs reported were giddiness, decreased sleep, nausea, itching, and vomiting. In CBZ group, 6 participants experienced somnolence, and 4 patients reported dizziness. The other adverse events reported were constipation, itching, poor concentration, nausea, and vomiting.

3.4. QOL Assessment. In clinical practice, QOLIE-10 score ranges from 0 to 100. A total score range of less than 50

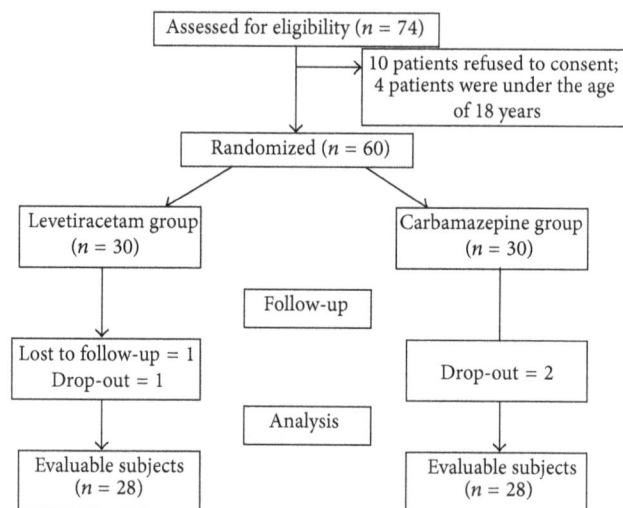

FIGURE 1: Patient disposition in the study.

indicates the poor quality of life, a score from 50 to 70 indicates the optimal QOL, and a score more than 70 implies better QOL. QOL assessment was done in the participants in both groups at 0 weeks and at the end of 24 weeks. The mean QOL score in CBZ group at 0 weeks was 31.14±1.83 and in the LEV group it was 29.76 ± 1.71 (p value, 0.5861) which is not statistically significant. The mean QOL score in CBZ group at the end of 26th week was 58.41 ± 1.89 and the mean QOL score in LEV group at the end of 26th week was 64.58±2.02 (p value of 0.0302, $p < 0.05$) which was found to be statistically significant.

Overall characteristics are shown in Table 1.

4. Discussion

The aim of AED treatment is to achieve seizure freedom with minimal or ideally no AE and with an optimal QOL. Numerous AEDs are licensed as monotherapy for focal seizure in adults. These include the older AED like CBZ. Even though CBZ has many AEs and tolerability issues, it was considered

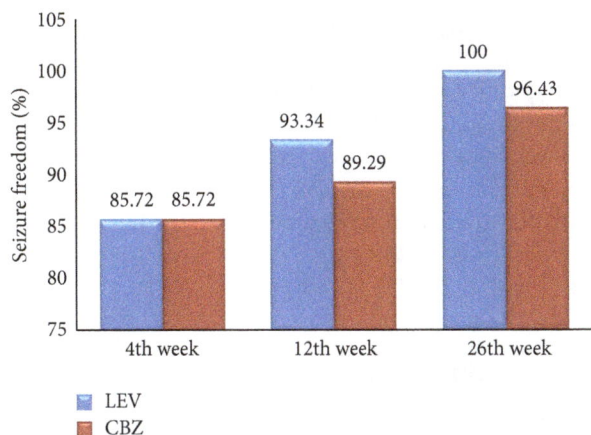

FIGURE 2: Seizure freedom at 4th, 12th, and 26th weeks.

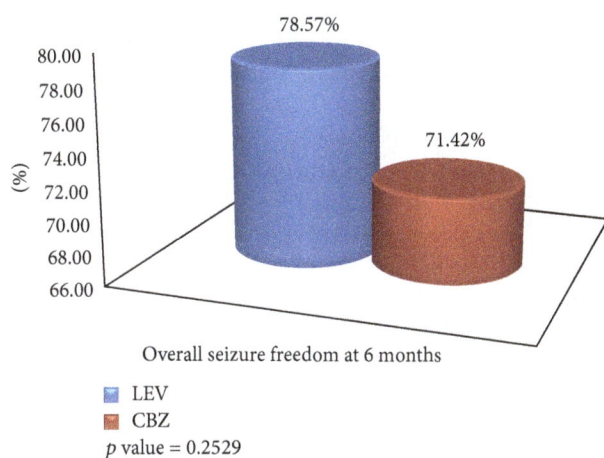

FIGURE 3: Overall seizure freedom at the end of 6 months.

as gold standard first-line drug to treat focal seizures from past many years. In 2013, ILEA has produced an updated review in epilepsy treatment, which highlighted the fact that newer AEDs like LEV and zonisamide have class 1-2 evidence to be used as monotherapy. This is based on regulatory trials showing noninferiority when compared to CBZ for 6-month remission [2, 12]. Till date, there have been very few studies to compare the efficacy and tolerability of LEV versus CBZ as monotherapy in focal seizures all over the world. Since the usage of LEV is very high in India, comparative study of efficacy and tolerability of LEV versus CBZ was expected to give more confidence for the use of the drug. Evaluation of QOL outcomes has been increasingly adopted into the standard management plan for epilepsy along with traditional measures of seizure frequency and AE.

4.1. Demographic Profile. The study sample was characterized by its relatively younger age (mean age, 27 ± 2.62 years). The mean age group of males in CBZ group was 30.70 ± 2.66 years and that of LEV group was 22.62 ± 1.152 years. The mean age group of females in CBZ group was 29.31 ± 2.44 years and that of LEV group was 28.18 ± 2.553 years. This is different from the previous studies conducted at developed countries like UK, USA, and Germany, which had relatively older age that

varied from 35 to 40 years, respectively. In this study, the CBZ group comprised 17 (56.66%) males and 13 (43.33%) females and LEV group comprised 13 (43.33%) males and 17 (56.66%) females, respectively. This is comparatively similar to the study conducted by Brodie et al., which had 58.8% males and 41.2% females in CBZ group and 51.2% males and 48.8% females in LEV group [9].

4.2. Efficacy Outcome. In this study, the efficacy was mainly assessed by seizure freedom rate. According to ILAE, a patient is considered as seizure-free following an intervention after a period without seizures has elapsed equal to three times the longest preintervention interseizure interval over the previous year [12]. In this study, we assessed seizure freedom rate at 4, 12, and 26 weeks. We also assessed the overall seizure freedom rate at the end of 6 months of the study; similarly, in LaLiMo trial, they have assessed seizure freedom rates at 6, 16, and 26 weeks [12].

Participants were asked to come for follow-up visits at 4, 12, and 26 weeks after initiation of the drug. The pretreatment mean seizure rate in LEV was 4.2 ± 0.65 per month which was comparatively higher than CBZ group with 2.83 ± 0.19 per month. At 4 weeks of follow-up, the seizure freedom rate in both CBZ and LEV groups was the same (85.72%). Since the pretreatment seizure frequency in LEV group was high, the seizure freedom at 4 weeks goes in the favor of LEV group. Similarly, in LaLiMo trial, the seizure freedom at 6 weeks in LEV group was 83.6% compared to 79.8% in Lamotrigine group ($p = 0.47$) with no statistical significance [12]. In this study, both groups showed better seizure freedom even though the results were not statistically significant. The increased seizure freedom may be due to better drug adherence.

Seizure freedom at 12 weeks of therapy in LEV group was 93.34%, while in CBZ group it was 89.29% (no statistical significance; $p = 0.4595$). Similarly, in LaLiMo trail, the seizure freedom at 16 weeks of maintenance therapy was 51.9% in LEV group and 55.7% in Lamotrigine group. Also, there was breakthrough seizures between 6 weeks and 16 weeks. Therefore, the seizure freedom rates in both groups had reduced significantly; this might be due to lack of drug adherence [12]. In this study, the seizure freedom at 12 weeks was comparatively better in LEV group than in CBZ group, even though the results were not statistically significant.

In most of the comparative studies of LEV versus CBZ, the main efficacy outcome was seizure freedom rate at 6 months and 12 months. Since this was time bound academic study, we could not follow up the cases for long term.

The final efficacy outcome was assessed on seizure freedom at the end of 6 months. In our study overall seizure freedom rate at the end of 6 months was 71.42% in CBZ group compared to 78.57% in LEV group ($p = 0.2529$), which is not statistically significant. As per Perry et al.'s study, where they have compared LEV versus CBZ as monotherapy for partial epilepsy, the efficacy outcome was seizure freedom at 6, 12, and 24 months. The seizure freedom rate at the end of 6 months was 73% in LEV group compared to 65% in CBZ group ($p = 0.58$) which showed no statistical significance like our study [10]. Similarly, in KOMET trial, the authors compared LEV with CBZ in newly diagnosed focal epilepsy; seizure freedom rate at 6 months for CBZ was 62% which was comparatively higher than LEV which had seizure freedom rate of 57.5%. The results were not statistically significant [13]. In another similar study by Brodie et al., the primary efficacy endpoint was seizure freedom rate at 6 months. At the end of 6 months, the seizure freedom rate was 73% in LEV group and 72.8% in CBZ group, which was almost similar efficacy in both groups [9].

No drug has shown superior efficacy to CBZ in randomized, head to head comparison in newly diagnosed epilepsy patients with partial or generalized tonic-clonic seizures. Though most of the studies clearly mention that newer AEDs are always comparable with older AEDs in efficacy, none of the studies till date showed a superior efficacy with newer AEDs compared to older AEDs. In our study too similar results were obtained; that is, LEV was comparable with CBZ in efficacy but it was not superior to CBZ.

4.3. Safety. The ultimate goal of treatment of epilepsy is the fact that patients should not have seizures, less AE, and an optimal QOL. In this study, both LEV and CBZ were well tolerated as initial monotherapy. Only 6.66% of patients on CBZ and 3.33% of patients on LEV withdrew from the study due to AE. There was more withdrawal of patients in the CBZ group which correlates to a previous study conducted by Brodie et al. In that study, 19.2% of patients on CBZ versus 14.4% of patients on LEV discontinued due to AE [9]. In this study, AEs were more reported from LEV (40%) compared to CBZ (36.66%) group even though the difference was not statistically significant. Similarly, in the KOMET trial, there was increased serious AE associated with LEV (13.7%) compared to CBZ group (8.2%) [13]. In contrast to these findings, in a study conducted by Perry et al., 70% of patients on CBZ experienced ADRs compared to 45% of those on LEV [10].

In this study, the participants taking CBZ mostly reported AEs like increased sleep (20%) and dizziness (13.33%) similar to the study conducted by Perry et al., where 40% of patients on CBZ reported increased sleep and 10% of patients reported dizziness. There was withdrawal of 2 subjects after 24 hours of initiation of drug, but none of the patients on CBZ reported serious AE.

In this study, subjects assigned to the LEV group most commonly (17.85%) reported behavioral changes in terms of increased aggressive behavior, increased anxiety, and suicidal tendency. Similarly, in Perry et al.'s study, LEV was associated with increased behavioral changes in terms of irritability (30.5%). Many of the case reports do suggest that LEV is associated with increased behavioral changes [14, 15]. Also, the package insert of LEV mentions the fact that LEV is contraindicated in patients with past history of psychiatric illness. A study on the safety profile of LEV mentions that 13.3% patients on LEV reported behavioral symptoms in terms of agitation, hostility, aggressiveness, anxiety, apathy, emotional liability, and depression [16]. Similarly, another study addressing the clinical experience of LEV also mentions that 33.33% of patients reported nervousness or irritability after the initiation of the drug. Also, 16.66% of patients discontinued the treatment due to the irritability [8].

In this study, 2 patients on LEV reported weight gain of 3–5 kg in 3 months. Till date, there have been reports of LEV induced weight loss. Here, weight gain can be correlated with improved QOL. Other AEs observed in this study were giddiness, increased sleep, itching, and nausea.

Long term AEs of CBZ have been reported to be leukopenia, hyponatremia, disturbances of vitamin D metabolism, agranulocytosis, and hepatitis. LEV is a comparatively new drug. The studies till date mention that the drug is well tolerated on long term use. There are reports of discontinuation of the drug due to irritability but this was related to previous history of mood disorders [17, 18]. In this regard, LEV appears to be a better option compared to CBZ for long term use. To avoid the behavioral AE, prescribers should thoroughly evaluate a patient of past psychiatric illness.

4.4. Quality of Life. The QOL evaluation is a relatively new measure to evaluate patient related outcome of treatment for epilepsy. Recently, other studies have tried to determine the effects of various demographic and clinical variables on the overall QOL among patients with epilepsy [2]. Here, we evaluated QOL with QOLIE-10 and studied the impact of both LEV and CBZ before and after the initiation of therapy. The mean score in CBZ group before the initiation of the therapy was 31.14 ± 1.83 compared to LEV group where it was 29.76 ± 1.71 ($p = 0.5861$) which is statistically not significant. The less scores correlate with the poor QOL of patients. After completing the course of therapy of 6 months, there was an increase in the mean score of both groups which was statistically significant. The mean score in CBZ group at the end of 6 months of initiation of therapy was 58.41 ± 1.89 compared to 64.58 ± 2.02 ($p = 0.0302$, $p < 0.05$), which was statistically significant. Unlike the previous KOMET trial, where QOL was assessed by QOLIE-31 scale, there were no clear differences between LEV and CBZ in the impact on health related quality of life [13]. Among both drugs, LEV has been shown to be superior to CBZ in terms of QOL, which can be due to the fact that LEV was associated with increased seizure freedom compared to CBZ. This increased seizure frequency can be correlated with decreased QOL in CBZ group. Similarly, another study conducted by Thomas et al. suggests that patients on monotherapy have a significant better QOL [2].

LEV thus demonstrated better QOL after 6 months of therapy compared to CBZ.

5. Conclusion

The efficacy of LEV was found to be comparable to CBZ as monotherapy in the treatment of partial seizures. LEV did not show superior efficacy compared to CBZ. Both drugs equally reduced the seizure frequency compared to pretreatment seizure frequency. LEV was equally tolerable to CBZ. LEV and CBZ demonstrated equal incidence of AE. LEV can be safely used as monotherapy in the treatment of partial epilepsy.

Disclosure

The work was conducted when the corresponding author was a postgraduate student at Vydehi Institute of Medical Sciences and Research Centre.

Conflict of Interests

The authors declare that there is no conflict of interests regarding the publication of this paper.

References

[1] M. Maguire, G. A. Marson, and S. Ramaratnam, "Epilepsy (generalized)," *BMJ Clinical Evidence*, vol. 2, article 1201, 2012.

[2] S. V. Thomas, S. Koshy, C. R. S. Nair, and S. P. Sarma, "Frequent seizures and polytherapy can impair quality of life in persons with epilepsy," *Neurology India*, vol. 53, no. 1, pp. 46–50, 2005.

[3] M. Gourie-Devi, P. Satishchandra, and G. Gururaj, "Epilepsy control program in India: a district model," *Epilepsia*, vol. 44, no. 1, pp. 58–62, 2003.

[4] S. Simon, *Handbook of Epilepsy Treatment*, Wiley-Blackwell, Oxford, UK, 3rd edition, 2010.

[5] R. Surges, R. D. Thijs, H. L. Tan, and J. W. Sander, "Sudden unexpected death in epilepsy: risk factors and potential pathomechanisms," *Nature Reviews Neurology*, vol. 5, no. 9, pp. 492–504, 2009.

[6] A. A. Asadi-Pooya and M. R. Sperling, "Clinical features of sudden unexpected death in epilepsy," *Journal of Clinical Neurophysiology*, vol. 26, no. 5, pp. 297–301, 2009.

[7] M. A. Stein and A. M. Kanner, "Management of newly diagnosed epilepsy: a practical guide to monotherapy," *Drugs*, vol. 69, no. 2, pp. 199–222, 2009.

[8] S. M. LaRoche, "A new look at the second-generation antiepileptic drugs: a decade of experience," *Neurologist*, vol. 13, no. 3, pp. 133–139, 2007.

[9] M. J. Brodie, E. Perucca, P. Ryvlin et al., "Comparison of levetiracetam and controlled release carbamazepine in newly diagnosed epilepsy," *Neurology*, vol. 68, pp. 402–408, 2007.

[10] S. Perry, P. Holt, and M. Benatar, "Levetiracetam versus carbamazepine monotherapy for partial epilepsy in children less than 16 years of age," *Journal of Child Neurology*, vol. 23, no. 5, pp. 515–519, 2008.

[11] J. A. Cramer, K. Perrine, O. Devinsky, and K. Meador, "A brief questionnaire to screen for quality of life in epilepsy: the QOLIE-10," *Epilepsia*, vol. 37, no. 6, pp. 577–582, 1996.

[12] F. Rosenow, C. Schade-Brittinger, N. Burchardi et al., "The LaLiMo trial: lamotrigine compared with levetiracetam in the initial 26 weeks of monotherapy for focal and generalised epilepsy—an open-label, prospective, randomised controlled multicenter study," *Journal of Neurology, Neurosurgery and Psychiatry*, vol. 83, no. 11, pp. 1093–1098, 2012.

[13] E. Trinka, A. G. Marson, W. Van Paesschen et al., "KOMET: an unblinded, randomised, two parallel-group, stratified trial comparing the effectiveness of levetiracetam with controlled-release carbamazepine and extended-release sodium valproate as monotherapy in patients with newly diagnosed epilepsy," *Journal of Neurology, Neurosurgery and Psychiatry*, vol. 84, no. 10, pp. 1138–1147, 2013.

[14] N. Kumar, H. S. Swaroop, A. Chakraborty, and S. Chandran, "Levetiracetam induced acute reversible psychosis in a patient with uncontrolled seizures," *Indian Journal of Pharmacology*, vol. 46, no. 5, pp. 560–561, 2014.

[15] A. Aggarwal, D. D. Sharma, R. C. Sharma, and R. Kumar, "Probable psychosis associated with levetiracetam: a case report," *Journal of Neuropsychiatry and Clinical Neurosciences*, vol. 23, no. 3, pp. E19–E20, 2011.

[16] C. L. Harden, "Safety profile of levetiracetam," *Epilepsia*, vol. 42, no. 4, pp. 36–49, 2001.

[17] T. Keranen and J. Sivenius, "Side effects of carbamazepine, valproate and clonazepam during long-term treatment of epilepsy," *Acta Neurologica Scandinavica*, vol. 68, supplement 97, pp. 69–80, 1983.

[18] B. S. Kang, H. J. Moon, Y.-S. Kim et al., "The long-term efficacy and safety of levetiracetam in a tertiary epilepsy centre," *Epileptic Disorders*, vol. 15, no. 3, pp. 302–310, 2013.

19

Long-Term Survival and Outcome in Children Admitted to Kilifi District Hospital with Convulsive Status Epilepticus

Agnes Prins,[1] Eddie Chengo,[1] Victor Mung'ala Odera,[1] Manish Sadarangani,[2,3] Claire Seaton,[4] Penny Holding,[5] Greg Fegan,[1,6] and Charles R. Newton[1,7,8]

[1] Centre for Geographic Medicine Research-Coast (CGMRC), Kenya Medical Research Institute (KEMRI), P.O. Box 230, Kilifi 80108, Kenya

[2] Department of Paediatrics, University of Oxford, Level 2, Children's Hospital, Oxford OX3 9DU, UK

[3] Department of Paediatrics, University of British Columbia & BC Children's Hospital, 4480 Oak Street, Vancouver, BC, Canada V6H 3V4

[4] Department of Paediatrics, John Radcliffe Hospital, Oxford University Hospitals NHS Trust, Headington, Oxford OX3 9DU, UK

[5] International Centre for Behavioral Studies, P.O. Box 34307, Mombasa 80118, Kenya

[6] Centre for Clinical Vaccinology and Tropical Medicine, Churchill Hospital, Old Road, Oxford OX3 7LJ, UK

[7] Neurosciences Unit, Institute of Child Health, University College London, 30 Guilford Street, London WC1N 1EH, UK

[8] Department of Psychiatry, University of Oxford, Oxford OX3 7JX, UK

Correspondence should be addressed to Agnes Prins; agnes_prins@yahoo.com

Academic Editor: Raffaele Manni

Objectives. The incidence of convulsive status epilepticus (CSE) is high in Africa but the long-term outcome is unknown. We examined the neurocognitive outcome and survival of children treated for CSE in a Kenyan hospital 3 to 4 years after discharge. *Methods.* The frequency and nature of neurological deficits among this group of children were determined and compared to a control group. The children were screened with the Ten Questions Questionnaire for neurodevelopmental impairment if alive and those that screened positive were invited for further assessment to determine the pattern and extent of their impairment. A verbal autopsy was performed to determine the cause of death in those that died. *Results.* In the 119 cases followed-up, 9 (8%) died after discharge, with the majority having seizures during their fatal illness. The 110 survivors (median age 5 years) had significantly more neurological impairments on the screening compared to 282 controls (34/110 (30.9%) versus 11/282 (3.9%), OR = 11.0, 95% CI 5.3–22.8). Fifteen percent of the cases had active epilepsy. *Conclusions.* This study demonstrates the considerable burden of CSE in African children. Strategies to manage children with CSE that are acceptable to the community need to be explored to improve the longer-term outcome.

1. Introduction

Convulsive status epilepticus (CSE) is the most common neurological emergency in children. It is associated with an increase in mortality and neurological sequelae, but the frequency of these outcomes varies across the world [1]. The incidence and severity of CSE are presumed to be greater in developing countries; however, data are sparse [2]. The incidence of CSE in the West is estimated at 17–23/100,000 children per year [3, 4], highest in children below the age of one year [5]. Overall, between 10% and 20% of children with epilepsy will have at least one episode of CSE during the course of the disease, most occurring in the first few years of epilepsy onset [6], but in sub-Saharan Africa CSE occurs in 25% of people with active convulsive epilepsy [7]. In the United Kingdom the short-term (within 30 days) mortality after CSE is 3–5% and 5–8% in children admitted to intensive care. The long-term mortality after a first episode of CSE is variable, ranging from 5% to 17% [8]. In Western survivors of CSE, less than 15% have focal neurological deficits, cognitive impairment, and behavioral problems; however, 13 to 74% of CSE patients develop epilepsy [8].

There are few published data on CSE in children living in Africa, despite the fact that the prevalence of epilepsy is higher than in Europe and North America [9]. In Kenya the prevalence of active epilepsy is 11/1,000 and the incidence is 187/100,000/year in children aged 6–9 years [10]. In the first reported study from Africa, the incidence of CSE in children was at least twice that of Western countries [10], with a case fatality of 15% in hospital, and 12% were discharged with neurological deficits, mostly motor impairment.

In this study we report on the long-term outcome of these children, 3 to 4 years after discharge. The frequency, nature, and extent of neurological deficits were determined and compared to that of a control group. We also assessed the long-term mortality and investigated causes of death.

2. Materials and Methods

2.1. Study Sites. The study was conducted in an area within Kilifi District on the Kenyan coast that was mapped in 2000-2001 and has a Health and Demographic Surveillance System (HDSS) with regular (usually 4 monthly) community censuses. Kilifi District Hospital (KDH) is the only hospital in the area. Details of the study area have been described previously [11].

2.2. Participants. The study cohort was identified from a group of 388 children admitted to KDH with CSE in 2002 and 2003 [11]. Ninety-five percent were 2–9 years at the time of admission. Inclusion criteria for cases were (i) confirmed CSE (according to the International League Against Epilepsy criteria at the time of this study [12]), defined as any seizure lasting for 30 minutes or longer, or intermittent seizures lasting for greater than 30 minutes during which the patient did not regain consciousness, that is, Blantyre Coma Score (BCS) < 3 [13]; (ii) probable CSE, defined by the presence of any of the following criteria: convulsing on arrival at hospital; parenteral phenobarbital or phenytoin administered to stop convulsions after the failure of two doses of the first-line medication (diazepam, paraldehyde, or both); BCS < 3 on arrival at hospital and more than one convulsion in previous 30 minutes; BCS < 3 on arrival and >10 convulsions in previous 24 hours [11]. Availability of benzodiazepines and other antiepileptic drugs in the community is very limited, so it would not be expected that the BCS would be modified due to drug administration before arrival to hospital. A list of control children was randomly selected from the HDSS database, using the most recent census round conducted prior to recruitment. They were matched for age, sex, and area of residence.

2.3. Study Procedures

2.3.1. Determination of Mortality and Screening for Impairment. Children were visited at home by a fieldworker fluent in the local language, Kigiriama. If the child had died, a verbal autopsy was conducted by a fieldworker trained in this technique to determine the cause of death [14]. In particular, evidence of epilepsy and convulsions during the agonal stages was determined. For the children that were alive the "Ten Questions Questionnaire" (TQQ) was administered to the parents or guardians to screen for neurological disability or impairment [15]. The TQQ has been validated in Kilifi for the detection of neurocognitive impairment and has a sensitivity of 71% and specificity of 98% for detecting moderate-or-severe motor impairment [15]. Children who screened positive on the TQQ were invited for further assessment at KDH to determine the pattern and extent of their sensorimotor or neurological impairments.

2.3.2. Hospital Based Assessments. During further evaluation, a full birth and medical history was obtained, in addition to sociodemographic details. A thorough neurological examination was performed by a clinician trained in neurological examinations that included assessment of the cranial nerves and motor function to detect features such as spasticity, ataxia, and fine motor dysfunction [16]. Vision was assessed using a Sonksen-Silver chart for children aged 3(1/2) years and older [17], which provided a measure of distant and near acuity using Snellen 6 meter standard specifications. Hearing was assessed with a Kamplex screening audiometer (P.C. Werth, London, UK) in children older than 5 years. Air conduction at 500 Hz, 1000 Hz, 2000 Hz, and 4000 Hz in each ear was carried out according to the recommendations of British Society of Audiology [18]. Hearing impairment was classified according to the lowest audible tone and defined as mild impairment 40–50 dB, moderate impairment 51–60 dB, severe impairment 61–70 dB, and profound impairment > 70 dB. A 20–30-minute electroencephalogram (EEG) with photic stimulation and hyperventilation was performed in those with reported seizures, to identify epileptic discharges and to help classify the seizures [19].

2.4. Data Analysis. Data were collected using standard forms and entered into an electronic database using FoxPro (version 9, Microsoft, Redmond, WA, USA) and statistical analysis was performed using SPSS (version 17.0, SPSS, Chicago, IL, USA). The cases and controls were compared with respect to neurological impairments on either the TQQ or hospital based assessments, using Pearson Chi-square analysis and Fisher's exact test if an expected cell value was <5. Differences between the groups were estimated by a calculation of the odds ratio (OR) and these are reported with 95% confidence intervals (95% CI).

2.5. Ethical Considerations. Ethical approval was obtained from the KEMRI National Ethical and Scientific committees in Nairobi (SSC-1074). Informed consent was obtained from the parents or caretakers of the participants.

3. Results

3.1. Description of Study Participants. In the period 2002-2003 a total of 388 children were admitted to hospital who fulfilled the criteria of confirmed (*n* = 155) or probable

(n = 233) CSE [11]. One hundred and nineteen children were followed up during a 5-month period in 2006 and their caretakers were identified and interviewed (Figure 1). The follow-up duration was 3-4 years. The TQQ was administered to the caretakers of 110 cases and the verbal autopsy to the caretakers of 9 cases who had died. There were no significant differences in the clinical characteristics between the 119 cases recruited and the 269 not recruited regarding age, sex, seizure type at admission, and impairment at discharge. Many children had multiple discharge diagnoses. Significantly more children that were not recruited had a discharge diagnosis of non-TB meningitis compared to the children who were recruited (Table 1). A total of 293 possible controls were randomly selected for interview, at least two controls for each case, of which we were able to interview 282 caretakers (Figure 1).

3.2. Mortality. On follow-up, 9 (7.6%) cases had died after discharge. Eight had a fever during the illness that led to death, and 8 experienced generalized seizures during their fatal illness. Seven children had experienced both fever and generalized seizures. None of the deceased children were taking AEDs at the time of their death.

3.3. Screening with the Ten Questions Questionnaire. The caretakers of 110 cases and 282 controls were interviewed with the TQQ (Figure 1). The median age was 5 years (range: 3 to 14 years), and 176 (44.9%) were male. Significantly more cases screened positive on the TQQ than controls (34/110 (30.9%) versus 11/282 (3.9%), OR = 11.0, 95% CI 5.3–22.8). In particular, significantly more cases screened positive to questions about vision, hearing, movement, cognition, and speech (Table 2). The most common neurological problem reported by the parents of cases was the child "appearing mentally backward, dull, or slow." Of the 110 cases, 12 (10.9%) had neurological deficits at time of discharge from hospital after the CSE episode. Of the 34 cases with one or more impairments reported on the TQQ, 10 had had an impairment observed at discharge, with 9 of them a motor impairment.

3.4. Assessments

3.4.1. Neurological Examination. Of the 43 children who were assessed at the clinic, there were no significant differences in the demographic characteristics or birth history of the controls compared to the cases. On neurological examination 15 cases (45.5%) and 1 control (10.0%) had neurological deficits. Using the denominators of the children screened with the TQQ, cases were significantly more likely to have deficits compared to controls (15/110 (13.6%) versus 1/282 (0.4%), $P < 0.001$). This difference was mostly due to higher prevalence of motor, speech, and visual impairment and epilepsy (Table 3).

3.4.2. Vision and Hearing. In the visual screening 20 cases and 4 controls could not be given a score, due to inability of the child to match the letters on the practice board (19/24), inability to follow the instructions of the fieldworker (4/24),

or inappropriate age for the test (1/24). These included the 3 children who were thought to have a visual problem during the neurological examination. None of the children that were assessed were found to have a visual impairment. Similarly on the hearing screening 19 cases and 4 controls were unable to do the test; most of them could not follow the instructions given to them (20/23), and 8 were too young to complete the test. Two cases and 1 control were found to have a hearing impairment, but these numbers are too small to draw firm conclusions with regard to the difference between the two groups.

3.4.3. Epilepsy. Seven of the 110 children (6.4%) alive in this cohort had a discharge diagnosis of epilepsy after their admission for CSE. Twelve cases (10.9%) were using antiepileptic drugs: either phenobarbital, carbamazepine, or phenytoin. Of the 43 children assessed at KDH, 9 did not cooperate sufficiently to undergo an EEG and data for 9 children were not collected due to technical problems. Thus EEG was performed on 19 cases and 6 controls. Epileptiform activity was observed in 7 cases (21.2%) and 1 control (10.0%) which was mostly focal temporal or focal extratemporal features. After reviewing the history 16 cases and 1 control were diagnosed with epilepsy, defined as recurrent unprovoked seizures [12].

4. Discussion

This study demonstrates that children who are discharged from hospital following CSE in a rural area of Kenya have a poorer developmental outcome compared to community controls. In total 30% of the cases had an impairment reported on the TQQ, with cognitive, motor, and speech domains being the most affected. On neurological examination significantly more cases had motor, speech, and vision impairment compared to the controls. Overall 15% of the cases had active epilepsy. Furthermore there was considerable mortality in the children discharged following CSE, with a majority (8/9) having seizures during their terminal illness.

The prevalence of neurodevelopmental impairments reported in this study is higher than that reported in the West, where it is less than 15% (excluding epilepsy) [8]. One possible explanation is that these children often present with a longer duration of seizures, since they have limited access to medical facilities in this region [2]. The longer a seizure persists, the more likely is the seizure to be unresponsive to antiepileptic drugs, the higher the mortality, and the worse the outcome in survivors [20]. In most Western studies the underlying cause of the CSE appears to be the main determinant of neurological impairment [1, 21]. However, in this study the number of children having a face-to-face assessment was low, so we were unable to examine this.

Long-term follow-up of this cohort demonstrates that the prevalence of epilepsy following an episode of CSE increases over time. At discharge 6% of children were diagnosed with epilepsy, while after three years the prevalence had doubled. This highlights that prolonged acute symptomatic seizures

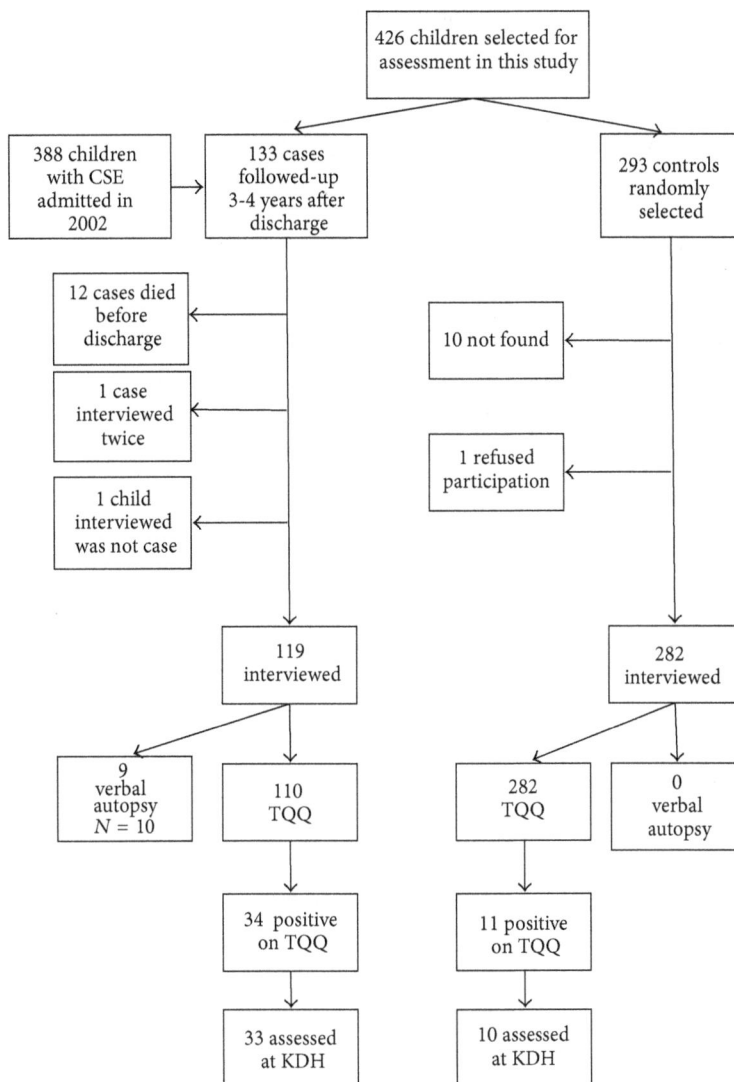

FIGURE 1

TABLE 1: Clinical characteristics of children recruited for follow-up compared to children not recruited.

Demographic and clinical characteristics at the time of admission for CSE	Found ($N = 119$)	Not found ($N = 269$)	P value
Male	52 (43.9%)	137 (50.9%)	0.189
Age in years, median (range)	2.2 (0.3–10.3)	2.1 (0.1–12.4)	—
Generalised convulsion (either initial or secondary)[§]	94 (79.7%)	189 (71.1%)	0.077
Focal onset seizure	44 (37.0%)	107 (39.8%)	0.602
Neurological impairment at discharge[§]	15 (12.7%)	31 (14.7%)	0.619
Discharge diagnosis[¥]			
Sepsis[*]	2 (1.7%)	10 (3.7%)	0.358
Malaria	79 (66.4%)	173 (64.3%)	0.693
Febrile convulsion	41 (34.5%)	68 (25.3%)	0.064
Non-TB meningitis	4 (3.4%)	36 (13.4%)	0.003
Encephalopathy of unknown cause	14 (11.8%)	39 (14.5%)	0.470
Anaemia	19 (16.0%)	56 (20.8%)	0.264

[¥]Some children had multiple diagnoses at discharge.
[*]Differences between "found" and "not found" with Fisher's exact test.
[§]Number may not be exact due to missing values.

TABLE 2: Responses to Ten Questions Questionnaire in cases and controls.

	Cases $N = 110$ Yes	Controls $N = 282$ Yes	P value
(1) Child had delay in sitting, standing, or walking	10 (9.1%)	3 (1.1%)	<0.001
(2) Child has difficulty seeing	4 (3.6%)	0 (0%)	0.006
(3) Child appears to have difficulty hearing	11 (10.0%)	7 (2.5%)	0.001
(4) Child understands what you are saying	101 (91.8%)	280 (99.6%)	<0.001
Child does not understand what you are saying	9 (8.2%)	1 (0.4%)	<0.001
(5) Child has difficulty walking or moving his/her arms or has weakness and/or stiffness in arms or legs	13 (11.8%)	1 (0.4%)	<0.001
(6a) Child sometimes has fits, becomes rigid, or loses consciousness[¥]	—	5 (1.8%)	Not done
(6b) Since admission to KDH, child has had fits, has become rigid, or has lost consciousness[§]	14 (12.7%)	—	Not done
(7) Child learns to do things like other children his/her age	102 (93.6%)	282 (100%)	<0.001
Child does not learn to do things like other children his/her age	7 (6.4%)	0 (0%)	<0.001
(8) Child speaks	99 (90.0%)	281 (99.6%)	<0.001
Child does not speak	11 (10.0%)	1 (0.4%)	<0.001
(9) Child's speech is different from normal	13 (11.8%)	1 (0.4%)	<0.001
(10) Child appears mentally backward, dull, or slow	14 (12.7%)	1 (0.4%)	<0.001
Other serious health problems	17 (15.7%)	28 (10.0%)	0.111
Child is attending school regularly, no. (%)	48 (43.6%)	143 (50.9%)	0.197

[¥]Question only for controls.
[§]Question only for cases.

TABLE 3: Neurological deficits on assessment.

Neurological deficits on assessment	Cases $N = 33$	Controls $N = 10$	P value[*]
Total screened with TQQ	$N = 110$	$N = 282$	
Any neurological deficit, no. (% of total screened with TQQ)	15 (13.6%)	1 (0.4%)	<0.001
Speech impairment	11 (10.0%)	0	<0.001
Motor impairment	11 (10.0%)	0	<0.001
Vision impairment	3 (2.7%)	0	0.022
Hearing impairment	1 (0.9%)	0	0.281
Cognitive impairment	1 (0.9%)	1 (0.4%)	0.483
Epilepsy	16 (14.5%)	1 (0.4%)	<0.001

[*]Differences between cases and controls with Fisher's exact test.

may contribute to the high incidence of epilepsy in this region [2].

4.1. TQQ and Assessments. Some of the impairments reported on the TQQ, that is, motor and speech impairment, were confirmed during the hospital based neurological assessments, but not all of them. The evaluation of sensory deficits (vision/hearing) was hampered by difficulties in engaging the children in the procedures. Although visual impairment was not found in the visual screening, most of the cases were not able to match the letters on the practice board and might not have understood the instructions due to cognitive problems. In testing the hearing, a lot of children were unable to point or use the tools or could not sit still. In other assessments a significant proportion was found to be uncooperative as well. While these findings support the high frequency of cognitive problems reported by parents, without specific measures of behaviour or cognition we are not able to validate either the sensory measures used or determine the true cause of the children's lack of cooperation.

4.2. Longer-Term Mortality. The mortality of children who survived to discharge from hospital was 8% after 3-4 years. If the children that died before discharge are added, it amounts to 23% of the children that were admitted to hospital with CSE had died within 4 years of their admission. This is higher than in the West, where the cumulative long-term mortality after a first episode of CSE ranges from 5% to 17% [8]. In most of the cases, the child appeared to die with a seizure and a febrile illness suggesting that children who have suffered status epilepticus previously are more susceptible to febrile status epilepticus.

4.3. Treatment Gap. None of the children who had died were using AEDs. The inadequate treatment of epilepsy probably plays an important role in the outcome of CSE. Nonadherence for AEDs is a risk factor for CSE in children with epilepsy. It is estimated that in the Kilifi district 70% of epilepsy patients are not receiving appropriate medication [22]. Besides the high costs of AEDs, the parent's perception of epilepsy might also explain this treatment gap, since seizures are thought to be caused by spiritual causes and thus not amenable to treatment by AEDs [23]. Traditional healers have a profound influence on the treatment of epilepsy, who are not likely to refer a child with seizures to hospital when their treatment fails. Furthermore, in this area distance to a health facility has been an important factor in treatment seeking [24]. To reduce the seizures and the associated impairments in children, intervention should focus on educating the parents in recognizing CSE as a treatable illness and forge communication between health care workers and traditional healers to improve treatment programmes for these patients.

4.4. Limitations to the Study. We were not able to compare the mortality of cases and controls since the controls were recruited from the most recent census round data, which did not include the children that had died. We could not ensure that the controls had not had any seizures, and caretakers of 5 controls reported their child had fits sometimes. We were not able to administer neuropsychological tests to estimate the degree of cognitive impairments in the children. Although the TQQ detects developmental delay, this needs to be verified with comprehensive assessments. The high number of "probable" CSE in the baseline study makes it difficult to compare the outcome to Western studies, where different criteria for CSE are used. These definitions were used, since in this context the history of seizure duration is very unreliable.

5. Conclusions

In this rural African population, a single episode of CSE requiring hospital admission is associated with significant developmental sequelae and high mortality. Nearly a quarter of children in our hospital based sample died following CSE, either as inpatients or after discharge from hospital. An additional one-third was identified as having developmental deficits after three to four years, with epilepsy developing in a considerable proportion. This data is likely to underestimate the total burden of CSE, since not all children with the condition will present to hospital. The results of this study emphasise the need for education of parents and carers, as well as community healthcare workers, to enable early, aggressive treatment of seizures that should improve longer-term outcome. In addition policy makers and health care

planners should be aware of the need to ensure an adequate supply of AEDs as well as increased access to facilities where children can receive adequate supportive care.

Conflict of Interests

The authors declare that there is no conflict of interests regarding the publication of this paper.

Acknowledgments

The authors are grateful to the clinical and nursing staff of Kilifi District Hospital and the assessment staff. They specifically thank Francis Yaah, Kenneth Rimba, Rachael Mapenzi, Grace Mtanje, Nancy Mwangemi, and Milton Karisa for participating in the fieldwork. Godfrey Otieno, for conducting the neurological examination and interpreting the EEGs, Clarice Mapenzi and Judy Tumaini, who conducted the assessments of vision and hearing, and Rachael Odhiambo for data management. The Wellcome Trust sponsored this study, through funding Charles Newton as a Wellcome Trust Senior Fellowship in Clinical Tropical Medicine (083744). Unfortunately Victor Munga'la Odera died before this paper was published.

References

[1] C. L. Novorol, R. F. M. Chin, and R. C. Scott, "Outcome of convulsive status epilepticus: a review," *Archives of Disease in Childhood*, vol. 92, no. 11, pp. 948–951, 2007.

[2] C. R. Newton, "Status epilepticus in resource-poor countries," *Epilepsia*, vol. 50, supplement 12, pp. 54–55, 2009.

[3] B. G. R. Neville, R. F. M. Chin, and R. C. Scott, "Childhood convulsive status epilepticus: epidemiology, management and outcome," *Acta Neurologica Scandinavica*, vol. 115, no. 186, pp. 21–24, 2007.

[4] R. F. Chin, B. G. Neville, C. Peckham, H. Bedford, A. Wade, and R. C. Scott, "Incidence, cause, and short-term outcome of convulsive status epilepticus in childhood: prospective population-based study," *The Lancet*, vol. 368, no. 9531, pp. 222–229, 2006.

[5] R. F. M. Chin, B. G. R. Neville, and R. C. Scott, "A systematic review of the epidemiology of status epilepticus," *European Journal of Neurology*, vol. 11, no. 12, pp. 800–810, 2004.

[6] M. Raspall-Chaure, R. F. M. Chin, B. G. Neville, H. Bedford, and R. C. Scott, "The epidemiology of convulsive status epilepticus in children: a critical review," *Epilepsia*, vol. 48, no. 9, pp. 1652–1663, 2007.

[7] S. M. Kariuki, W. Matuja, A. Akpalu et al., "Clinical features, proximate causes, and consequences of active convulsive epilepsy in Africa," *Epilepsia*, 2013.

[8] M. Raspall-Chaure, R. F. Chin, B. G. Neville, and R. C. Scott, "Outcome of paediatric convulsive status epilepticus: a systematic review," *The Lancet Neurology*, vol. 5, no. 9, pp. 769–779, 2006.

[9] A. G. Diop, D. C. Hesdorffer, G. Logroscino, and W. A. Hauser, "Epilepsy and mortality in Africa: a review of the literature," *Epilepsia*, vol. 46, no. 11, pp. 33–35, 2005.

[10] V. Munga'la-Odera, S. White, R. Meehan et al., "Prevalence, incidence and risk factors of epilepsy in older children in rural Kenya," *Seizure*, vol. 17, no. 5, pp. 396–404, 2008.

[11] M. Sadarangani, C. Seaton, J. A. G. Scott et al., "Incidence and outcome of convulsive status epilepticus in Kenyan children: a cohort study," *The Lancet Neurology*, vol. 7, no. 2, pp. 145–150, 2008.

[12] "Guidelines for epidemiologic studies on epilepsy. Commission on Epidemiology and Prognosis, International League Against Epilepsy," *Epilepsia*, vol. 34, no. 4, pp. 592–596, 1993.

[13] M. E. Molyneux, T. E. Taylor, J. J. Wirima, and A. Borgstein, "Clinical features and prognostic indicators in paediatric cerebral malaria: a study of 131 comatose Malawian children," *Quarterly Journal of Medicine*, vol. 71, no. 265, pp. 441–459, 1989.

[14] R. W. Snow, I. B. De Azevedo, D. Forster et al., "Maternal recall of symptoms associated with childhood deaths in rural East Africa," *International Journal of Epidemiology*, vol. 22, no. 4, pp. 677–683, 1993.

[15] V. Mung'ala-Odera, R. Meehan, P. Njuguna et al., "Validity and reliability of the "Ten Questions" questionnaire for detecting moderate to severe neurological impairment in children aged 6–9 years in rural Kenya," *Neuroepidemiology*, vol. 23, no. 1-2, pp. 67–72, 2004.

[16] R. Palisano, P. Rosenbaum, S. Walter, D. Russell, E. Wood, and B. Galuppi, "Development and reliability of a system to classify gross motor function in children with cerebral palsy," *Developmental Medicine and Child Neurology*, vol. 39, no. 4, pp. 214–223, 1997.

[17] A. T. Salt, P. M. Sonksen, A. Wade, and R. Jayatunga, "The maturation of linear acuity and compliance with the Sonksen-Silver Acuity System in young children," *Developmental Medicine and Child Neurology*, vol. 37, no. 6, pp. 505–514, 1995.

[18] "British Society of Audiology. Short papers meeting on experimental studies of hearing and deafness. Cambridge, 22nd and 23rd September 1988. Abstracts," *British Journal of Audiology*, vol. 23, no. 2, pp. 143–174, 1989.

[19] H. H. Jasper, "Electroencephalography," *Pediatrics*, vol. 9, no. 6, pp. 786–787, 1952.

[20] A. Neligan and S. D. Shorvon, "Prognostic factors, morbidity and mortality in tonic-clonic status epilepticus: a review," *Epilepsy Research*, vol. 93, no. 1, pp. 1–10, 2011.

[21] K. Ostrowsky and A. Arzimanoglou, "Outcome and prognosis of status epilepticus in children," *Seminars in Pediatric Neurology*, vol. 17, no. 3, pp. 195–200, 2010.

[22] T. Edwards, A. G. Scott, G. Munyoki et al., "Active convulsive epilepsy in a rural district of Kenya: a study of prevalence and possible risk factors," *The Lancet Neurology*, vol. 7, no. 1, pp. 50–56, 2008.

[23] G. E. Sharkawy, C. Newton, and S. Hartley, "Attitudes and practices of families and health care personnel toward children with epilepsy in Kilifi, Kenya," *Epilepsy and Behavior*, vol. 8, no. 1, pp. 201–212, 2006.

[24] N. H. Kendall-Taylor, C. Kathomi, K. Rimba, and C. R. Newton, "Comparing characteristics of epilepsy treatment providers on the Kenyan coast: implications for treatment-seeking and intervention," *Rural and Remote Health*, vol. 9, no. 4, p. 1253, 2009.

20

The Modified Atkins Diet in Refractory Epilepsy

Suvasini Sharma and Puneet Jain

Division of Pediatric Neurology, Department of Pediatrics, Lady Hardinge Medical College and Associated Kalawati Saran Children's Hospital, New Delhi 110001, India

Correspondence should be addressed to Suvasini Sharma; sharma.suvasini@gmail.com

Academic Editor: József Janszky

The modified Atkins diet is a less restrictive variation of the ketogenic diet. This diet is started on an outpatient basis without a fast, allows unlimited protein and fat, and does not restrict calories or fluids. Recent studies have shown good efficacy and tolerability of this diet in refractory epilepsy. In this review, we discuss the use of the modified Atkins diet in refractory epilepsy.

1. Introduction

Seizures are a frequent cause of morbidity in the pediatric age group [1]. Several severe catastrophic epilepsies present in childhood, including severe infantile myoclonic epilepsy, West syndrome, Lennox-Gastaut syndrome, and myoclonic-astatic epilepsy (Doose syndrome) [2]. Seizures in these epilepsy syndromes are difficult to control, with the added problems of multiple and toxic levels of antiepileptic medications [3]. Epilepsy surgery may not work in these patients and also the costs are prohibitively high. Uncontrolled seizures pose a variety of risks to children, including higher rates of mortality, developmental delay and/or regression, and cognitive impairment [4]. The shortcomings of antiepileptic drug therapy and epilepsy surgery have made the need for alternative treatments.

The ketogenic diet is one of the oldest available treatments for epilepsy. It is a medically supervised high fat, low carbohydrate, and restricted protein diet that maintains a chronic state of ketosis. The ketogenic diet compares favourably with the newer antiepileptic drugs (AEDs) which have been developed for the treatment epilepsy in children [5, 6]. With the ketogenic diet, 33% of patients with intractable epilepsy have more than 50% reduction in seizures and 15–20% become seizure free [7–11]. Also, many of the children who are maintained on the diet are able to have their antiepileptic drugs decreased or withdrawn. This leads to improvement in alertness, behavior, and cognition.

The traditional ketogenic diet, with 4 : 1 ratio of fat: carbohydrate + protein, has its drawbacks. It restricts calories and fluids and requires strict weighing of foods. Protein is generally restricted, with the majority of the remaining calories in the form of fat. This may lead to hypoproteinemia and growth problems. Hospitalization is generally advocated for diet initiation. Side effects of the diet include kidney stones, constipation, acidosis, diminished growth, weight loss, and hyperlipidemia [7–11].

The modified Atkins diet is a less restrictive alternative to the traditional ketogenic diet [12, 13]. This diet is started on an outpatient basis without a fast, allows unlimited protein and fat, and does not restrict calories or fluids [12–14]. In this review we discuss the use of the modified Atkins diet in refractory epilepsy.

2. The Atkins Diet

The Atkins diet was developed in the United States in 1970 by Robert C. Atkins for the purpose of weight loss. This diet allowed the intake of fat and the restriction of carbohydrates. The modified Atkins diet is "*modified*" from the Atkins diet as the "induction phase" of the diet limiting carbohydrates is maintained indefinitely, fat is encouraged (not just allowed), and seizure control is the goal rather than weight loss [15]. In contrast to the ketogenic diet, it does not restrict protein intake or daily calories. The Atkins diet allows meals containing 60% fat, 30% protein, and 10% carbohydrates [16].

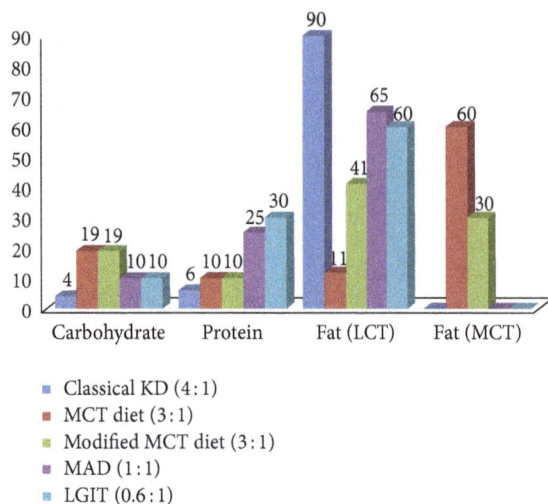

FIGURE 1: Composition of the ketogenic diets and their variants.

Figure 1 shows the composition of MAD as compared to other diets. Because of strong carbohydrate restriction, patients following the Atkins diet also produce ketones [17].

3. Use of the Modified Atkins Diet in Refractory Epilepsy

With its comparatively fewer dietary restrictions, the Atkins diet may be less restrictive than the ketogenic diet. Kossoff et al. hypothesized that the Atkins diet can induce metabolic ketosis and might reduce seizures in patients with epilepsy, similar to the ketogenic diet [12]. In 2003, they published a pilot study of six patients, aged 7 to 52 years, who were started on the Atkins diet for the treatment of intractable focal and multifocal epilepsy [12]. Five patients maintained moderate to large ketosis for periods of 6 weeks to 24 months; three patients had seizure reduction and were able to reduce antiepileptic medications. This study provided preliminary evidence that the Atkins diet may have a role as therapy for patients with medically resistant epilepsy.

The same group published their experience with the modified Atkins diet in 20 children with intractable epilepsy in 2006 [13]. Eighty percent of the patients stayed on the diet for six months. In all children, at least moderate urinary ketosis developed within 4 days of starting the modified Atkins diet. At 6 months on the diet, 65% had a >50% response, and 35% had a >90% response. This was strikingly similar to prospective studies on the traditional ketogenic diet [8].

Kang et al. evaluated the efficacy, safety, and tolerability of the modified Atkins diet in fourteen Korean children with refractory epilepsy [14]. Six months after diet initiation, seven (50%) remained on the diet, five (36%) had >50% seizure reduction, and three (21%) were seizure free. The diet was well tolerated by 12 (86%) patients, despite the fact that this was a predominantly rice eating population.

The ideal starting carbohydrate limit in the modified Atkins diet is not yet established. Preliminary studies used 10 grams of carbohydrates/day. However, in one of these studies,

10 (50%) of 20 children had increased carbohydrates to 15 g per day after the first month, and one child increased to 20 g per day after the fourth month, as assessed by the dietary chart reviews [13]. Only one of these children reported a reduction in efficacy as a result, and none described decreased levels of urinary ketosis. Based on these results, Kossoff et al. performed a study to determine the initiating carbohydrate limits in the modified Atkins diet [18]. Twenty children with intractable epilepsy were randomized to either 10 or 20 g of carbohydrates per day for the initial 3 months of the modified Atkins diet and then crossed over to the opposite amount. A significantly higher likelihood of >50% seizure reduction was noted for children started on 10 g of carbohydrate per day at 3 months: 60% versus 10% ($P = 0.03$). Most parents reported no change in seizure frequency or ketosis between groups but improved tolerability with 20 g per day. The authors concluded that a starting carbohydrate limit of 10 g per day for children starting the modified Atkins diet may be ideal, with a planned increase to a more tolerable 20 g per day after 3 months. Table 1 summarizes the pediatric studies of MAD.

In a recent randomized controlled trial [28], 102 children aged 2 to 14 years who had daily seizures despite the appropriate use of at least 3 antiepileptic drugs were randomized to receive either the modified Atkins diet ($n = 50$) or no dietary intervention ($n = 52$) for a period of three months. The ongoing antiepileptic medications were continued unchanged in both groups. Four patients discontinued the diet before the study endpoint, and three patients in the control group were lost to follow up. The median seizure frequency at 3 months, expressed as a percentage of the baseline, was significantly less in the diet group (37.3% versus 100%, $P = 0.003$). The proportion of children with >90% seizure reduction (30% versus 7.7%, $P = 0.005$) and >50% seizure reduction was significantly higher in the diet group (52% versus 11.5%, $P < 0.001$). Constipation was the commonest adverse effect (46%) among children on the diet.

Most of the studies have reported short term seizure outcome following diet initiation. Recently, Chen and Kossoff [34] reported long term follow-up of 87 MAD-treated children. Fifty-four children continued diet beyond 6 months. After a mean of 19.9 months on diet, 30/54 (55%) children with diet durations of >6 months achieved >50% improvement and 19 (35%) were seizure-free. The adverse effects were predominantly elevations in lipid profile and gastrointestinal upset.

This diet has the advantages of nonfasting initiation. Also, it can be used in resource constraint settings with limited dietician support, as it does not require tedious calculations [35]. The counseling time is reduced to 30–60 minutes. In the West, this diet has predominantly been advocated for adolescents and adults. However, in India, this diet has been found useful in young children as well. In a study of 15 children, aged 6 months to 3 years, with infantile spasms refractory to hormonal therapy and/or vigabatrin, the modified Atkins diet was found to render 6 children (40%) spasm free with EEG resolution of hypsarrhythmia at 3 months [26]. The diet was well tolerated in these young children.

Further, the efficacy of the ketogenic diet can be maintained when switching to MAD [12]. The information

TABLE 1: Summary of studies involving children treated with MAD.

Authors	Study type	Sample size	Age range	Epilepsy	At 3 months		Adverse effects
					>50%	>90%	
Kossoff et al. 2003 [12]	Open trial	6	7–52 yrs	Mixed	3	—	Not reported
Kossoff et al. 2006 [13]	Prospective	20	3–18 yrs	≥3 Sz/week on at least 2 AEDs	50%	11%	Constipation
Kossoff et al. 2007 [18]	Randomized cross-over (10 g versus 20 g)	20	3–18 yrs	At least daily countable seizures	10 g—60% 20 g—10%	10 g—30% 20 g—0%	Improved tolerability with 20 g
Kang et al. 2007 [14]	Prospective	14	Mean 7.4 yrs	≥4 Sz/month; ≥3 AEDs	50%	29%	Gastrointestinal disturbances
Porta et al. 2009 [19]	Retrospective	27	4–182 months	≥2 Sz/week, ≥3 AEDs	KD—64% MAD—20%	—	Mild digestive disorders
Weber et al. 2009 [20]	Prospective	15	2–17 yrs	≥1 Sz/week, ≥2 AEDs	40%	13%	Not significant
Tonekaboni et al. 2010 [21]	Prospective	27	1–16 yrs	≥3 AEDs tried	67%	25%	Minor
Miranda et al. 2010 [22]	Prospective	33	1–16 yrs	Medically intractable epilepsy	52%	42%	Subtle
Kossoff et al. 2011 [23]	Prospective (MAD + 1 month Ketocal)	30	3–18 yrs	At least daily countable seizures; ≥2 AEDs	At 1 month, 80% At 2 months, 70%	37% 43%	Constipation
Groomes, et al. 2011 [24]	Retrospective + prospective	21 (8-ketogenic diet, 13-MAD)	Median age at diet onset—6 yrs	Intractable childhood and juvenile absence epilepsy	82%	38%	Not mentioned
Kumada et al. 2012 [25]	Prospective	10	1.5–17 yrs	≥3 Sz/week, ≥3 AEDs	At 3 weeks, 3	2	
Sharma et al. 2012 [26]	Prospective	15	6 m–3 yrs	Daily infantile spasms		40% spasm free	Constipation
Kim et al. 2012 [27]	Retrospective	20	21 m–17 yrs	Mixed	55%*	35%*	Constipation, hypercalciuria, hyperuricemia, transient lipase elevation
Sharma et al. 2013 [28]	Randomized controlled trial	Total 102, 50 randomized to diet group	2–14 yrs	Daily seizures, or at least 7/week	52% in diet group versus 11.5% in control group	30% in diet group versus 7.7% in control group	Constipation, anorexia, vomiting, lethargy

*Efficacy during the recent or final 3 months of the diet therapy.
AEDs: antiepileptic drugs; Sz: seizures; MAD: modified Atkins diet; KD: ketogenic diet.

regarding additional seizure control when switching from MAD to ketogenic diet is limited. In one retrospective review, 37% of patients (10/27) had ≥10% additional seizure reduction with the KD over the MAD with most favorable response seen in children with myoclonic astatic epilepsy [36].

4. MAD in Adults

Three open-label studies have reported use of the MAD exclusively in adults [30, 31, 33]. Three studies have reported

on adolescents in mixed cohorts of children and adolescents [14, 20, 32]. One case series has included one adolescent and three adults [12]. Data from six studies show that, on average, 18 of 66 (27%) adolescents and adults achieved ≥50% seizure reduction; of these 66 individuals, 1 (6%) became seizure-free. Treatment may be slightly more effective in those with higher initial seizure frequencies and in younger adults.

One study found that, after an average of 3 days, all adults had positive results for urinary ketones, both in the morning and evening [31]. In another study, all 28 adults

TABLE 2: A summary of studies that include data specifically on individuals aged >12 years on MAD [29].

Study	Study design	Sample size (adolescents/adults)	Age (yrs)	Seizure types	Endpoint (mths)	Number of adolescent (12–18 yrs) responders (%) (>50% reduction)	Number of adult (>18 yrs) responders at endpoint (%) (>50% reduction)	Adverse effects
Kang et al. 2007 [14]	Prospective	1 (1/0)	14.4	DS with ATS	7	0 (0%)	NA	Vomiting
Kossoff et al. 2008 [30]	Prospective	30 (0/30)	18–53	CPS, MST, AS	6	NA	9 (30%)	Lethargy, weight loss, elevated total cholesterol, leg swelling
Carrette et al. 2008 [31]	Prospective	8 (0/8)	31–55	CPS, CPS with occasional SG, LGS	6	NA	1 (13%)	Vomiting, headache, nausea, diarrhoea, constipation, weakness, weight loss, elevated total and LDL cholesterol
Weber et al. 2009 [20]	Prospective	7 (7/0)	12–17	SFE, LGS, MAE, JME	3	3 (43%)	NA	Unknown
Kossoff et al. 2010 [32]	Prospective	2 (2/0)	13–18	SWS with CPS	6	1 (50%)	NA	Weight loss, high peak total cholesterol
Smith et al. 2011 [33]	Prospective	18 (0/18)	18–55	PS with SG, MS, CPS, SPS	12	NA	3 (17%)	Weight loss

AS: absence seizures; ATS: atonic seizures; CPS: complex partial seizures; DS: Doose syndrome; JME: juvenile myoclonic epilepsy; LGS: Lennox-Gastaut syndrome; MAE: myoclonic astatic epilepsy; MS: myoclonic seizures; MST: multiple seizure types; NA: not available; PS: partial seizures; SFE: symptomatic focal epilepsy; SG: secondary generalization; SPS: simple partial seizures; SWS: Sturge-Weber syndrome.

who remained on the diet for at least 1 week became ketotic, but only 2 of 15 (13%) had moderate-large urinary ketosis after 6 months [30]. Ketone levels do not always correlate with improved efficacy in adults [30, 33] or in mixed cohorts of children and adolescents [13, 23, 32]. Table 2 summarizes the studies of MAD in adults.

5. Other Uses of MAD

The MAD has rarely been used for other indications. Its successful use has been reported in Sturge-Weber syndrome [32] and GLUT1 deficiency syndrome [37]. Kumada et al. [38] reported resolution of nonconvulsive status epilepticus following administration of MAD to two children, one with frontal lobe epilepsy and the other with subcortical band heterotopias. Kossoff et al. reported use of MAD in adolescents with chronic daily headache. Only 3 patients out of 8 completed the three-month study. Two of them reported improvement in their headache severity [39].

6. Tolerability and Side Effects

The modified Atkins diet has generally been well tolerated. In the study by Kossoff et al., significant constipation was reported in four children [13]. Six children lost weight, median of 2.7 kg, three of whom were the heaviest in the cohort. Cholesterol values increased from a mean of 192 mg/dL to 221 mg/dL at the end of 6 months, but this increase was half of the reported increase with the ketogenic diet [40]. In the study on 30 adults who were administered the modified Atkins diet for refractory epilepsy, total cholesterol increased from 187 mg/dL to 201 mg/dL, but the LDL, HDL, and triglycerides remained in average risk ranges [30].

Gastrointestinal side effects such as constipation and vomiting have been the commonest side effects reported [12–14, 18, 30, 31]. These are most marked at the initiation of the diet, with time they improve [31]. Weight loss is prominent in obese patients [30]. One child developed aspiration pneumonia in the study by Kang et al. [14]. Kidney stones, seen in 5% of patients on the ketogenic diet, have not been reported with the modified Atkins diet to date.

7. Conclusion

MAD is an efficacious therapy for patients with refractory epilepsy. It is less restrictive and more palatable than the classical ketogenic diet. There is limited data regarding the efficacy of MAD with respect to the classical ketogenic diet. However, MAD is a prudent therapeutic option especially for older children and adolescents as it is a more "liberalized" diet as compared to classical ketogenic diet. It is also a good option for resource-constraint settings with paucity of trained dieticians.

Conflict of Interests

The authors declare that there is no conflict of interests regarding the publication of this paper.

References

[1] W. A. Hauser, "The prevalence and incidence of convulsive disorders in children," *Epilepsia*, vol. 35, supplement 2, pp. S1–S6, 1994.

[2] J. M. Pellock, "Seizures and epilepsy in infancy and childhood," *Neurologic Clinics*, vol. 11, no. 4, pp. 755–775, 1993.

[3] P. N. Patsalos and J. S. Duncan, "Antiepileptic drugs. A review of clinically significant drug interactions," *Drug Safety*, vol. 9, no. 3, pp. 156–184, 1993.

[4] S. Shorvon, F. Dreifuss, and D. Fish, *The Treatment of Epilepsy*, Blackwell Science, 1996.

[5] F. J. Ritter, I. E. Leppik, F. E. Dreifuss et al., "Efficacy of felbamate in childhood epileptic encephalopathy (Lennox-Gastaut syndrome)," *The New England Journal of Medicine*, vol. 328, no. 1, pp. 29–33, 1993.

[6] R. George, M. Salinsky, R. Kuznicky et al., "Vagus nerve stimulation for treatment of partial seizures: 3. Long-term follow-up on first 67 patients exiting a controlled study," *Epilepsia*, vol. 35, no. 3, pp. 637–643, 1994.

[7] E. P. G. Vining, J. M. Freeman, K. Ballaban-Gil et al., "A multicenter study of the efficacy of the ketogenic diet," *Archives of Neurology*, vol. 55, no. 11, pp. 1433–1437, 1998.

[8] J. M. Freeman, E. P. G. Vining, D. J. Pillas, P. L. Pyzik, J. C. Casey, and M. T. Kelly, "The efficacy of the ketogenic diet—1998: a prospective evaluation of intervention in 150 children," *Pediatrics*, vol. 102, no. 6, pp. 1358–1363, 1998.

[9] A. M. Hassan, D. L. Keene, S. E. Whiting, P. J. Jacob, J. R. Champagne, and P. Humphreys, "Ketogenic diet in the treatment of refractory epilepsy in childhood," *Pediatric Neurology*, vol. 21, no. 2, pp. 548–552, 1999.

[10] N. G. Katyal, A. N. Koehler, B. McGhee, C. M. Foley, and P. K. Crumrine, "The ketogenic diet in refractory epilepsy: the experience of Children's Hospital of Pittsburgh," *Clinical Pediatrics*, vol. 39, no. 3, pp. 153–159, 2000.

[11] P. Kankirawatana, P. Jirapinyo, S. Kankirawatana, R. Wongarn, and N. Thamanasiri, "Ketogenic diet : an alternative treatment for refractory epilepsy in children," *Journal of the Medical Association of Thailand*, vol. 84, no. 7, pp. 1027–1032, 2001.

[12] E. H. Kossoff, G. L. Krauss, J. R. McGrogan, and J. M. Freeman, "Efficacy of the Atkins diet as therapy for intractable epilepsy," *Neurology*, vol. 61, no. 12, pp. 1789–1791, 2003.

[13] E. H. Kossoff, J. R. McGrogan, R. M. Bluml, D. J. Pillas, J. E. Rubenstein, and E. P. Vining, "A modified Atkins diet is effective for the treatment of intractable pediatric epilepsy," *Epilepsia*, vol. 47, no. 2, pp. 421–424, 2006.

[14] H.-C. Kang, H. S. Lee, S. J. You, D. C. Kang, T.-S. Ko, and H. D. Kim, "Use of a modified Atkins diet in intractable childhood epilepsy," *Epilepsia*, vol. 48, no. 1, pp. 182–186, 2007.

[15] E. H. Kossoff and J. L. Dorward, "The modified Atkins diet," *Epilepsia*, vol. 49, supplement 8, pp. 37–41, 2008.

[16] E. H. Kossoff, "More fat and fewer seizures: dietary therapies for epilepsy," *The Lancet Neurology*, vol. 3, no. 7, pp. 415–420, 2004.

[17] R. Atkins, *Dr. Atkins' New Diet Revolution*, Harper-Collins Publishers, 2004.

[18] E. H. Kossoff, Z. Turner, R. M. Bluml, P. L. Pyzik, and E. P. G. Vining, "A randomized, crossover comparison of daily carbohydrate limits using the modified Atkins diet," *Epilepsy and Behavior*, vol. 10, no. 3, pp. 432–436, 2007.

[19] N. Porta, L. Vallée, E. Boutry et al., "Comparison of seizure reduction and serum fatty acid levels after receiving the ketogenic and modified Atkins diet," *Seizure*, vol. 18, no. 5, pp. 359–364, 2009.

[20] S. Weber, C. Mølgaard, K. KarenTaudorf, and P. Uldall, "Modified Atkins diet to children and adolescents with medical intractable epilepsy," *Seizure*, vol. 18, no. 4, pp. 237–240, 2009.

[21] S. H. Tonekaboni, P. Mostaghimi, P. Mirmiran et al., "Efficacy of the atkins diet as therapy for intractable epilepsy in children," *Archives of Iranian Medicine*, vol. 13, no. 6, pp. 492–497, 2010.

[22] M. J. Miranda, M. Mortensen, J. H. Povlsen, H. Nielsen, and S. Beniczky, "Danish study of a modified Atkins diet for medically intractable epilepsy in children: can we achieve the same results as with the classical ketogenic diet?" *Seizure*, vol. 20, no. 2, pp. 151–155, 2011.

[23] E. H. Kossoff, J. L. Dorward, Z. Turner, and P. L. Pyzik, "Prospective study of the modified atkins diet in combination with a ketogenic liquid supplement during the initial month," *Journal of Child Neurology*, vol. 26, no. 2, pp. 147–151, 2011.

[24] L. B. Groomes, P. L. Pyzik, Z. Turner, J. L. Dorward, V. H. Goode, and E. H. Kossoff, "Do patients with absence epilepsy respond to ketogenic diets?" *Journal of Child Neurology*, vol. 26, no. 2, pp. 160–165, 2011.

[25] T. Kumada, T. Miyajima, N. Oda, H. Shimomura, K. Saito, and T. Fujii, "Efficacy and tolerability of modified Atkins diet in Japanese children with medication-resistant epilepsy," *Brain & Development*, vol. 34, no. 1, pp. 32–38, 2012.

[26] S. Sharma, N. Sankhyan, S. Gulati, and A. Agarwala, "Use of the modified Atkins diet in infantile spasms refractory to first-line treatment," *Seizure*, vol. 21, no. 1, pp. 45–48, 2012.

[27] Y. M. Kim, V. V. Vaidya, T. Khusainov et al., "Various indications for a modified Atkins diet in intractable childhood epilepsy," *Brain & Development*, vol. 34, pp. 570–575, 2012.

[28] S. Sharma, N. Sankhyan, S. Gulati, and A. Agarwala, "Use of the modified Atkins diet for treatment of refractory childhood epilepsy: a randomized controlled trial," *Epilepsia*, vol. 54, pp. 481–486, 2013.

[29] N. E. Payne, J. H. Cross, J. W. Sander, and S. M. Sisodiya, "The ketogenic and related diets in adolescents and adults—a review," *Epilepsia*, vol. 52, no. 11, pp. 1941–1948, 2011.

[30] E. H. Kossoff, H. Rowley, S. R. Sinha, and E. P. G. Vining, "A prospective study of the modified Atkins diet for intractable epilepsy in adults," *Epilepsia*, vol. 49, no. 2, pp. 316–319, 2008.

[31] E. Carrette, K. Vonck, V. de Herdt et al., "A pilot trial with modified Atkins' diet in adult patients with refractory epilepsy," *Clinical Neurology and Neurosurgery*, vol. 110, no. 8, pp. 797–803, 2008.

[32] E. H. Kossoff, J. L. Borsage, and A. M. Comi, "A pilot study of the modified Atkins diet for Sturge-Weber syndrome," *Epilepsy Research*, vol. 92, no. 2-3, pp. 240–243, 2010.

[33] M. Smith, N. Politzer, D. MacGarvie, M.-P. McAndrews, and M. Del Campo, "Efficacy and tolerability of the modified Atkins diet in adults with pharmacoresistant epilepsy: a prospective observational study," *Epilepsia*, vol. 52, no. 4, pp. 775–780, 2011.

[34] W. Chen and E. H. Kossoff, "Long-term follow-up of children treated with the modified Atkins diet," *Journal of Child Neurology*, vol. 27, pp. 754–758, 2012.

[35] E. H. Kossoff, J. L. Dorward, M. R. Molinero, and K. R. Holden, "The modified Atkins diet: a potential treatment for developing countries," *Epilepsia*, vol. 49, no. 9, pp. 1646–1647, 2008.

[36] E. H. Kossoff, J. L. Bosarge, M. J. Miranda, A. Wiemer-Kruel, H. C. Kang, and H. D. Kim, "Will seizure control improve by switching from the modified Atkins diet to the traditional ketogenic diet?" *Epilepsia*, vol. 51, no. 12, pp. 2496–2499, 2010.

[37] Y. Ito, H. Oguni, S. Ito, M. Oguni, and M. Osawa, "A modified Atkins diet is promising as a treatment for glucose transporter type 1 deficiency syndrome," *Developmental Medicine and Child Neurology*, vol. 53, no. 7, pp. 658–663, 2011.

[38] T. Kumada, T. Miyajima, N. Kimura et al., "Modified atkins diet for the treatment of nonconvulsive status epilepticus in children," *Journal of Child Neurology*, vol. 25, no. 4, pp. 485–489, 2010.

[39] E. H. Kossoff, J. Huffman, Z. Turner, and J. Gladstein, "Use of the modified Atkins diet for adolescents with chronic daily headache," *Cephalalgia*, vol. 30, no. 8, pp. 1014–1016, 2010.

[40] P. O. Kwiterovich Jr., E. P. G. Vining, P. Pyzik, R. Skolasky Jr., and J. M. Freeman, "Effect of a high-fat ketogenic diet on plasma levels of lipids, lipoproteins, and apolipoproteins in children," *Journal of the American Medical Association*, vol. 290, no. 7, pp. 912–920, 2003.

21

Why Are Seizures Rare in Rapid Eye Movement Sleep? Review of the Frequency of Seizures in Different Sleep Stages

Marcus Ng[1] and Milena Pavlova[2]

[1] Department of Neurology, Epilepsy Service, Massachusetts General Hospital, 55 Fruit Street, Boston, MA 02114, USA
[2] Department of Neurology, Division of Epilepsy, EEG, and Sleep Neurology, Brigham and Women's-Faulkner Hospital, 1153 Centre Street, Boston, MA 02130, USA

Correspondence should be addressed to Milena Pavlova; mpavloval@partners.org

Academic Editor: M. Maestri

Since the formal characterization of sleep stages, there have been reports that seizures may preferentially occur in certain phases of sleep. Through ascending cholinergic connections from the brainstem, rapid eye movement (REM) sleep is physiologically characterized by low voltage fast activity on the electroencephalogram, REMs, and muscle atonia. Multiple independent studies confirm that, in REM sleep, there is a strikingly low proportion of seizures (~1% or less). We review a total of 42 distinct conventional and intracranial studies in the literature which comprised a net of 1458 patients. Indexed to duration, we found that REM sleep was the most protective stage of sleep against focal seizures, generalized seizures, focal interictal discharges, and two particular epilepsy syndromes. REM sleep had an additional protective effect compared to wakefulness with an average 7.83 times fewer focal seizures, 3.25 times fewer generalized seizures, and 1.11 times fewer focal interictal discharges. In further studies REM sleep has also demonstrated utility in localizing epileptogenic foci with potential translation into postsurgical seizure freedom. Based on emerging connectivity data in sleep, we hypothesize that the influence of REM sleep on seizures is due to a desynchronized EEG pattern which reflects important connectivity differences unique to this sleep stage.

1. Introduction

A bidirectional relationship between epilepsy and sleep has been observed since the time of Hippocrates [1]. It was not until the first formal characterization of sleep stages that this relationship became successively attuned to each specific sleep stage. It became apparent that seizures may preferentially occur during certain phases of sleep with the least likelihood of occurrence in rapid eye movement (REM) sleep. The purpose of this review is to focus on the impact of REM sleep on seizures. We discuss REM sleep physiology, a review of the available literature regarding seizures during REM sleep, and a consideration of the potential mechanisms which may underlie this intriguing but often overlooked phenomenon.

2. REM Sleep Physiology

Based on a wealth of animal and human data accumulated since the discovery of REM sleep in 1953 [2], an exciting and coherent model of REM sleep physiology has emerged. In the pontomesencephalic junction of the brainstem, there are two populations of cholinergic neurons in the laterodorsal tegmentum (LDT) and pedunculopontine tegmentum (PPT) [3]. Within these populations, there is a subset of cells that are most active in REM sleep, as well as another subset, which is active in both REM sleep and wakefulness [4–7].

Of the neurons whose spontaneous firing rate is highest in REM sleep, some exhibit a spontaneous bursting depolarization pattern due to a "low threshold spike" inward calcium current [8]. Through muscarinic greater than nicotinic acetylcholine receptors [9], connections from the LDT and PPT excite populations of neurons in the pontine reticular formation (PRF) and mesencephalic reticular formation (MRF) which serve as "effector cells" responsible for the following dissociable characteristics of REM sleep:

(1) low voltage fast electroencephalographic (EEG) activity,

(2) rapid eye movements (REMs),

(3) muscle atonia.

Low voltage fast activity on the EEG is due largely to depolarization of the thalamus by cholinergic MRF neurons [8]. Thalamic activation allows transmission of information to the cortex and subsequent EEG desynchronization which contrasts with the generally synchronized high-voltage activity of slow-wave sleep [10]. There is also evidence that another cholinergic subpopulation ventral to the dorsolateral PRF depolarizes the thalamus; however, the resultant EEG resembles more the waking state than REM sleep [11]. Furthermore, the LDT and PPT may directly activate cholinergic centers in the basal forebrain which has further excitatory connections to hippocampus and cortex [12–15]. In addition, there may be an element of cortical disinhibition as the basal forebrain also contains gamma-aminobutyric acid (GABA) ergic neurons which may be stimulated to deactivate inhibitory interneurons with further projections to hippocampus and cortex [16, 17].

Rapid eye movements are heralded by discharges, known as pontogeniculooccipital (PGO) waves, from a dorsorostral subpopulation of cholinergic PRF neurons which project to the occipital lobe via the lateral geniculate nucleus (LGN). The presence of PGO waves precedes REMs by 3–5 waves and low voltage fast activity by 30–60 seconds [18].

Muscle atonia is partly the result of neurons in the dorsolateral PRF [8]. Through glutamatergic and/or GABAergic connections [19], these neurons project to the bulbar reticular formation (BRF) which inhibits lower motor neurons via GABA and glycine [20]. Muscle atonia is also the result of loss of serotonergic and noradrenergic tone as these neurotransmitter systems are silent in REM sleep [21–24].

Collectively the LDT, PPT, PRF, and MRF are known as the "REM-on" neurons. In contrast, there are populations of "REM-off" neurons mainly in the serotonergic midline raphe nuclei and noradrenergic locus coeruleus (LC) [25–28]. Of the raphe nuclei, the chief nucleus is the dorsal raphe (DRN) [29] but others (such as the linearis centralis [30], centralis superior [31], raphe magnus [32, 33], and raphe pallidus [34]) have been implicated. Furthermore, there are also aminergic populations in the anterior pontine tegmentum near the pontomesencephalic junction as well as other "stray" neurons throughout the brainstem with REM-off characteristics [8]. While firing rates of REM-on neurons are the highest in REM sleep, firing of the REM-off neurons is maximal in wakefulness [35].

The REM-on and REM-off neurons mutually antagonize each other. The model first proposed by McCarley and Hobson in 1975 [36] was characterized as a reciprocal interaction model based on Lotka-Volterra equations originally used to describe interactions between prey (i.e., REM-on) and predator (i.e., REM-off) populations. In this model, REM-on neurons initially grow exponentially by positively feeding back onto each other. At the same time, they activate REM-off neurons as a form of negative feedback. After being activated, REM-off neurons inhibit REM-on neurons and simultaneously exert negative feedback pressure on themselves.

With respect to anatomical and functional correlation of REM-on neurons in the model, there exists a positive feedback connection between LDT/PPT and PRF/MRF neurons [3]. Furthermore, a negative feedback connection has been found between LDT/PPT and LC neurons [37]. Regarding REM-off neurons, serotonin and noradrenaline (presumably from the DRN and LC, resp.) have been found to inhibit bursting LDT neurons [38]. There also exist negative feedback inhibitory recurrent collateral pathways for both the DRN and LC [8].

The reciprocal interaction model provides one method of explaining the 90-minute alternations between 30-minute REM sleep periods and NREM sleep periods over the course of a usual night. In order to account for the first shorter REM episode, which typically occurs 70–120 (on average 90) minutes after sleep onset, subsequent versions of the model have included a "limit cycle" modification [39].

Furthermore, the hormone orexin (also known as hypocretin), which is secreted by neurons in the lateral hypothalamus, additionally fine-tunes transitions into and out of REM sleep by diurnally gating REM sleep over the course of the entire sleep-wake cycle [53]. One potential mechanism is through strategic and selective excitation of REM-off neurons [8, 54–57]. Also manufactured in the lateral hypothalamus by neurons intermixed with orexin neurons [58–60], melanin-concentrating hormone is another recently discovered agent which may play a similar diurnal role through an inhibitory, rather than excitatory, mechanism [58, 61, 62].

3. Clinical Observations of Seizures in REM Sleep

Initial studies on the frequency of interictal and ictal events during REM sleep were largely anecdotal and consisted primarily of case reports. Studies were heterogeneous in terms of seizure/epilepsy classification (e.g., waking epilepsy, definitely symptomatic epilepsy), patient population (e.g., severity of epilepsy, use of antiepileptic drugs), use of the EEG (e.g., 10–20 system, montages, method of detecting abnormalities, inclusion of benign variants as abnormal features), use of the polysomnogram (PSG) (e.g., use of electromyography, definition of wakefulness and sleep stages), and outcome measures of both interictal and ictal events. Gradually, however, the methodology for recording and scoring became more standardized and this permitted comparison.

In this review, the total number of events in wakefulness and each sleep stage was extracted for each study examined. Rates of interictal and ictal events in wakefulness and each sleep stage were also extracted. If rates were not explicitly provided, then they were calculated by dividing the number

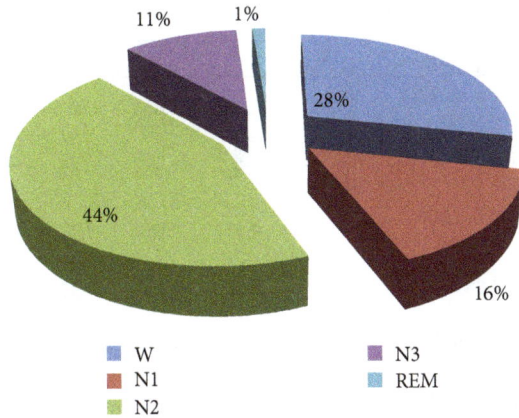

FIGURE 1: Raw sum of focal seizures.

TABLE 1: Relative focal seizure rates[*].

Paper/sleep stage	W	N1	N2	N3	REM
Minecan et al. 2002 [40]	0.00	6.00	7.00	5.00	1.00
Crespel et al. 1998 [41]—FLE	133.42	14.59	14.59	14.59	1.00
Crespel et al. 1998 [41]—TLE	55.08	1.67	1.67	1.67	1.00
Terzano et al. 1991 [42]	0.00	5.52	2.16	3.77	1.00
Weighted mean	7.83	87.25	67.84	50.78	1.00

[*]Herman et al. 2001 [43] was included in weighted mean but could not be displayed as a relative rate because no seizures occurred in REM sleep.

TABLE 2: Relative generalized discharge rates.

Paper/sleep stage	W	N1	N2	N3	REM
Halász et al. 2002 [44]	8.14	14.53	10.47	3.49	1.00
Parrino et al. 2001 [45]		3.50	3.50	3.50	1.00
Horita et al. 1991 [46]	1.43	3.54	0.75	0.00	1.00
Autret et al. 1987 [47] /1997 [48]	1.37	1.50	1.50	2.25	1.00
Autret et al. 1987 [47] /1997 [48]—Pediatrics	2.30	3.66	3.66	4.91	1.00
Touchon 1982 [49]	5.05	3.26	0.10		1.00
Kellaway et al. 1980 [50]	1.68	5.63	5.63	5.63	1.00
Sato et al. 1973 [51]		3.32	16.04	43.45	1.00
Ross et al. 1966 [52]	4.94	3.12	3.94	11.06	1.00
Weighted mean	3.25	3.10	3.13	6.59	1.00

of events by the duration of wakefulness and/or each sleep stage when available. To facilitate comparison, each rate was then divided by the rate for REM sleep in order to determine an "indexed" rate. In averaging these indexed rates, each study was not treated equally. Rather, a "weighted mean" was produced by weighting each study based on the number of patients contained with each.

If individual sleep stages were not separated, then the same rate was used for each constituent stage (e.g., a combined N1/N2 rate was used individually as a rate for N1 and a rate for N2). With respect to numbers of events, this was divided equally among the constituent stages (e.g., a total of 33 seizures for N1/N2/N3 were counted as 11 for each stage). Formerly stage III and stage IV sleep were combined into stage N3 for analysis. Depending on the study, the definition of wakefulness may have included wake periods after sleep onset (WASO), nocturnal awakenings, morning awakenings, and/or samples of fully alert daytime wakefulness. As studies were divergent, statistical significance could not be calculated.

3.1. Focal Seizures. A total of 542 patients with a collective 1990 seizures over 9 studies [40–43, 75–79] from 1987 to 2006 were included. Two studies [78, 79] were conducted using intracranial depth electrodes on patients classified with temporal or extratemporal epilepsy. The distribution of the 1990 seizures in wakefulness and specific sleep stages is shown in Figure 1.

The percentage of focal seizures during REM sleep over total recording time was extremely low (1%) over all these studies. However, because these studies did not provide specific durations, the length of recording may have led to artificial overinflation or underinflation of data. To address this issue, Table 1 provides a rate of focal seizure activity from four of these studies [40–43] where duration was provided.

Relative to REM sleep, the focal seizure rate was 7.83 times higher in wakefulness, 87 times higher in stage N1 sleep, 68 times higher in stage N2 sleep, and 51 times higher in stage N3 sleep. These data imply that focal seizures were most frequent in NREM sleep, intermediate in wakefulness, and lowest in REM sleep. However, the increased rate in wakefulness was

highly variable with the weighted mean being powered by a single study [41]. In comparison, the study with the largest number of patients conducted by Herman et al. [43] yielded no seizures in either REM sleep or wakefulness.

3.2. Primary Generalized Seizures. A total of 256 patients with idiopathic generalized epilepsy were included among 7–9 studies [44–52] who ranged in age from 4 to 46. Specific subsets of idiopathic generalized epilepsy included juvenile myoclonic epilepsy, childhood absence epilepsy, and more generally "petit mal" and "grand mal" seizures in older studies.

Table 2 demonstrates that, relative to REM sleep, the generalized discharge rate was 3.25 times higher in wakefulness, 3.1 times higher in stage N1 sleep, 3.13 times higher in stage N2 sleep, and 6.59 times higher in stage N3 sleep. In contrast to focal epilepsy, where data was available as shown in Table 3, no patients demonstrated maximal generalized discharges in REM sleep.

3.3. Specific Epilepsy Syndromes. Benign epilepsy of childhood with rolandic spikes (BECRS) is the best studied focal syndrome in terms of discharge frequency in REM sleep. A total of 110 patients aged 3–16 were examined by

TABLE 3: % patients with maximal generalized discharges per state.

Paper/sleep stage	W (%)	N1 (%)	N2 (%)	N3 (%)	REM (%)
Horita et al. 1991 [46]	0.0	100.0	0.0	0.0	0.0
Sato et al. 1973 [51]		0.0	8.3	91.7	0.0
Ross et al. 1966 [52]	23.1	7.7	7.7	61.5	0.0
Weighted mean	22.8	14.8	5.9	56.4	0.0

TABLE 4: Relative rolandic discharge rates.

Paper/sleep stage	W	N1	N2	N3	REM
Billiard et al. 1990 [63]	0.54	1.19	1.19	1.19	1.00
Dalla Bernardina et al. 1982 [64]	0.22	0.97	1.08	1.28	1.00
Weighted mean	0.27	1.00	1.10	1.27	1.00

Billiard et al. [63] and Dalla Bernardina et al. [64] in 2 separate studies.

Table 4 demonstrates that, relative to REM sleep, discharges were about 4 times lower in wakefulness, about the same in stage N1 sleep, 1.1 times higher in stage N2 sleep, and 1.27 times higher in stage N3 sleep. In another study by Dalla Bernardina et al. in 1975 [80], comment was made that children with rolandic spikes but without seizures have a marked deactivation of discharges in REM sleep while those with seizures do not.

In addition to focal syndromes, a few case reports have also explored the impact of REM sleep on the epileptic encephalopathies. In 1981, Billiard et al. [70] presented 2 patients with Landau-Kleffner Syndrome aged 3 and 6 years who had higher interictal discharge rates in stage N1/2 (113% of REM) and N3 (127% of REM) sleep. However, Genton et al. [81] later published a case report of a 3.5-year-old girl with lateralized activation of right temporal spike-wave complexes in REM sleep.

In 1982, Tassinari [82] described 19 cases of electrical status epilepticus in slow wave sleep (ESES). He noted that, in REM sleep, all electrical status disappeared with only 3 instances of electrographic seizures resuming at the end of the REM sleep period. Similarly in 1981, Hrachovy et al. [83] described 32 patients aged 1–43 months with infantile spasms. He also noted that all patients demonstrated less or no hypsarrhythmia on the EEG during REM sleep.

3.4. Focal Interictal Discharges. A total of 214 patients were included among 7–10 different studies [47, 48, 65–73] who ranged in age from 2 to 61 years. Three studies [71–73] were conducted using intracranial depth electrodes on patients classified with temporal, frontal, occipital, parietal, or limbic seizures.

Table 5 demonstrates that, relative to REM sleep, the focal interictal discharge rate was 1.11 times higher in wakefulness, 1.75 times higher in stage N1 sleep, 1.69 times higher in stage

TABLE 5: Relative focal interictal discharge rates.

Paper/sleep stage	W	N1	N2	N3	REM
Clemens et al. 2005 [65]	1.52	2.50	1.85	2.67	1.00
Clemens et al. 2003 [66]	0.41	1.56	1.48	2.46	1.00
Ferillo et al. 2000 [67]		0.91	1.09	1.81	1.00
Malow et al. 1998 [68]		2.45	3.79	7.39	1.00
Malow et al. 1997 [69]		2.38	4.50	7.13	1.00
Billiard et al. 1981 [70]—Symptomatic	0.84	1.68	1.68	1.68	1.00
Billiard et al. 1981 [70]—Definite	0.70	1.43	1.43	1.43	1.00
Autret et al. 1987 [47]/1997 [48]	0.44	1.18	1.18	1.15	1.00
Rossi et al. 1984 [71, 72]*	1.17	1.33	1.33	1.18	1.00
Montplaisir et al. 1982 [73]*	1.21		2.43		1.00
Weighted mean	1.11	1.75	1.69	2.46	1.00

* Intracranial depth electrode study.

TABLE 6: % patients with maximal focal discharges per state.

Paper/sleep stage	W (%)	N1 (%)	N2 (%)	N3 (%)	REM (%)
Clemens et al. 2005 [65]	11.1	11.1	0.0	66.7	11.1
Ferrillo et al. 2000 [67]		19.4	11.1	61.1	8.3
Sammaritano et al. 1991 [74]	2.5	3.8	3.8	77.5	12.5
Weighted mean	5.9	8.7	5.1	69.5	10.9

N2 sleep, and 2.46 times higher in stage N3 sleep. These data imply that discharge rates are highest in NREM sleep (particularly stage N3) and comparable between wakefulness and REM sleep with the latter having a slightly lower firing rate.

Although REM sleep had the lowest rate of focal interictal discharges overall, this did not mean that each individual patient necessarily had lower rates of discharges in REM sleep. As Table 6 shows, where data was available, a weighted mean 10.9% of patients had maximal interictal discharge rates in REM sleep. This was second only to stage N3 sleep. In the context of the findings in Table 1, this implies that while these patients had maximal discharge rates in REM sleep compared to wakefulness or other sleep stages, the absolute rate remained low.

In intracranial depth recordings, Rossi et al. [71, 72] showed that, in REM sleep, there was a selective increase in the rate of interictal discharges over the epileptogenic zone (defined as the region which after resection resulted in seizure freedom) when compared to other sampled parts of the brain. While Wieser [84] commented on previous similar findings of increased REM sleep interictal discharge rates over the amygdala and supplementary motor area, he noted that these studies often considered benign variants as epileptiform [85, 86].

3.5. Selective Localization of Epilepsy in REM Sleep. Like seizure frequency in REM sleep, the impact of REM sleep on the distribution of interictal and ictal phenomena is controversial. The most powerful argument for clinically useful localization of an epileptogenic focus in REM sleep comes from a subset of tuberous sclerosis patients and a single temporal lobe epilepsy patient in studies by Ochi et al. [87] and Malow and Aldrich [88], respectively. In 6 of Ochi's patients, the semiology, neuroimaging, and other EEG were discordant in localizing the epileptogenic focus. Focal resection was undertaken in the hemisphere to which discharges were selectively lateralized in REM sleep. Four of six patients did well after surgery (Engel class I or II). In Malow's case report, 1 patient with bitemporal discharges selectively lateralized in REM sleep. After amygdalohippocampectomy in this hemisphere, the patient was rendered seizure-free for at least 3 years. For these patients, lateralization based on REM sleep alone was able to localize the epileptogenic zone in the midst of discordant data and predict seizure freedom.

Other studies have explored the localizing ability of REM sleep in relation to a "final" localization based on general concordance of all available data. 100% of unilateral temporal lobe patients with REM-lateralized interictal discharges or seizures were lateralized to the same hemisphere as the "final" localization. For NREM sleep, the concordance rate of interictal discharges and seizures was 100% and 94%, respectively. For wakefulness, it was a respective 88% and 94%. In patients where discharges were bitemporal, REM localization agreed with the final localization 100% of the time (compared to 81% in NREM and 100% in wakefulness). In an intracranial study by Lieb et al. [89], eight of 10 patients with REM-lateralized interictal discharges demonstrated statistically significant concordance with the final localization. Statistical significance for lower rates of concordance could not be established for wakefulness, "light sleep", or "deep sleep".

However, there remains controversy regarding the localizing value of interictal discharges. For example, in Lieb's study [89], two of 10 patients with REM-lateralized discharges were discordant with the final localization. Furthermore, Genton et al. [81] have described a case of Landau-Kleffner Syndrome in which spike rate dramatically increased and spread contralaterally during REM sleep. In an intracranial depth electrode study of 15 temporal lobe epilepsy patients, Montplaisir et al. [73] noted that spikes were often seen in areas outside the epileptogenic zone in the ipsilateral hemisphere as well as in homologous regions to the epileptogenic zone over the contralateral hemisphere.

4. How REM Sleep Could Affect Seizures

As previously discussed, the observed desynchronized EEG of REM sleep is the result of cholinergic MRF neurons depolarizing the thalamus which allows transmission of information to the cortex. Like REM sleep, the EEG of wakefulness is also desynchronized because cholinergic activity is likewise present.

In contrast, cholinergic neurons are less active in NREM sleep with the least activity occurring in deep slow-wave sleep (i.e., stage N3) [10]. Without afferent mesencephalic cholinergic stimulation, the thalamus is not depolarized. An inactive thalamus does not allow transmission of information to the cortex. Without the inhomogeneous stimulation afforded by afferently transmitted information through the thalamus, cortical neurons are then able to intrinsically fire in a synchronized fashion. This is reflected by the maximally synchronized EEG of stage N3 sleep.

To summarize, REM sleep and wakefulness represent states of maximal cortical synchrony, stages N1 and N2 sleep are states of intermediate synchrony, and stage N3 sleep represents a state of maximal cortical desynchrony.

4.1. Focal Interictal Discharges. When neurons exhibit asynchronous discharging behaviour at baseline, there is a reduced opportunity for spatial and temporal summation of any additional spontaneous depolarization [90, 91]. Such spontaneous depolarizations by populations of abnormally excitable neurons, in other words the "paroxysmal depolarizing shift", have been hypothesized to be the mechanism behind focal epilepsy and interictal epileptiform discharges [92].

The reduced opportunity for spatial and temporal summation of such abnormal depolarizations may account for the results contained within Table 5. These data demonstrate that the highest rate of focal interictal discharges is in stage N3 sleep. This is in contrast to the lowest discharge rate which occurs comparably across REM sleep and wakefulness.

Another possible mechanism by which cortical desynchrony may account for this disparity in focal discharge rates is through the emergence of regional antiepileptic "microrhythms". In contrast to the uniform global cortical synchrony of stage N3 sleep, there usually are distinct regional rhythms in more desynchronized states. For example, a posterior dominant alpha rhythm often exists in wakefulness. Even during the intermediately synchronized EEG of stage N2 sleep, there are regional sleep spindles located in the frontocentral regions bilaterally which, by definition, disappear with the onset of slow-wave sleep. Furthermore, a recent study has commented on "islands of hyperconnectivity" in REM sleep [93].

While the regional rhythms mentioned above are not known to be antiepileptic, another rhythm has been described, the hippocampal theta rhythm, which is also present in the desynchronized states of REM sleep and wakefulness [94]. In animal models, this rhythm has been shown to exert an antiepileptic effect [95].

However, the opposite may also be true and there could exist proepileptic regional rhythms in certain individuals. This may account for the interindividual variability in Table 6 which examined in which state of consciousness did a particular individual have the greatest rate of focal interictal discharging. Despite comparable overall rates of focal interictal discharges in REM sleep and wakefulness among patients from all studies included for analysis, a respective 5.9% and 10.9% of individuals achieved maximal discharge firing rates in wakefulness and REM sleep.

4.2. Focal Seizures and Generalized Epilepsy. Similar to focal interictal discharges, focal seizures are also hypothesized to arise from the "paroxysmal depolarizing shift" [96]. However, subsequent organization is required to sufficiently activate and recruit surrounding neurons in order to transform a focal interictal epileptiform discharge into an ictal event [96]. Recruitment of surrounding neurons leads to loss of surround inhibition, and seizure activity then spreads contiguously via local "short" cortical-cortical connections [96]. Secondary generalization may occur if there is spread to more distant areas via "long" association pathways such as the corpus callosum [96].

Like secondarily generalized seizures, primary generalized epilepsy also involves spread via long pathways but through a mechanism distinct from the paroxysmal depolarizing shift. Both primary generalized ictal and interictal phenomena have been hypothesized to be the result of abnormally synchronized and reverberating thalamocortical networks [97]. The distinction between ictal from interictal events rests mainly on discharge duration (i.e., greater than 10 seconds) and presence of clinical correlate [98].

Tables 1 and 2 demonstrate that rates of focal seizures and generalized discharges occur most often in NREM sleep when compared to either REM sleep or wakefulness. The same mechanisms proposed to account for a relatively higher rate of focal interictal discharges in NREM sleep would also apply to focal seizures and primary generalized epilepsy.

Namely, the lower likelihood for spatial and temporal summation of aberrant spontaneous depolarizations in the cortically desynchronized states of REM sleep and wakefulness reduces the chance of spread along "short" pathways to surrounding neurons in focal epilepsy and "long" thalamocortical and association pathways in generalized epilepsy. Furthermore, should a desynchronized cortical milieu permit the emergence of regional antiepileptic microrhythms, this would present a further impediment to the spread of any aberrant depolarization.

However, unlike focal interictal discharges, the potential presence of proepileptic regional rhythms in certain individuals would not be expected to impact a primary generalized phenomenon. This is consistent with the results of Table 3 which demonstrate that among all patients in studies included for analysis, no individuals (0%) demonstrated a maximal discharge firing rate in REM sleep.

Returning to Tables 1 and 2, not only is it shown that rates of focal seizures and generalized discharges are lower in REM sleep and wakefulness, but rates are additionally lower in REM sleep compared to wakefulness. While both states of consciousness share a desynchronized EEG due to cholinergic activity, they differ greatly in terms of other neurotransmitter activity and in terms of connectivity.

Serotonergic neurons primarily located in the raphe nuclei, noradrenergic neurons in the locus coeruleus, and histaminergic neurons from the tuberomammillary nucleus demonstrate maximal firing rates in wakefulness and lowest firing rates during REM sleep [10]. These neurotransmitters are generally considered to produce arousal through widespread and usually excitatory effects on target neurons [10]. Such effects, present in wakefulness and absent in REM sleep, may account for recently discovered significant differences in connectivity between REM sleep and wakefulness.

An fMRI study [99] of the default network demonstrated substantially reduced connectivity in REM sleep when compared to wakefulness. The greatest difference appeared to be disconnection of the dorsomedial prefrontal cortex. This was validated by another study [100] examining functional connectivity by multichannel EEG which disclosed disconnection of anterior from posterior cortical areas in REM sleep. Loss of the organizing influence from the frontal lobes may be reflected by the often illogical and nonsensical content of dreams in REM sleep [101].

Because a loss of connectivity precludes the presence of synchrony, strategic losses of brain connectivity in REM sleep compared to wakefulness might explain any extra antiepileptic effect of REM sleep. As previously discussed, the greater the degree of desynchronization, the less likely the spatial and temporal summation of any aberrant spontaneous depolarization which would allow "spread" along "short" or "long" pathways in the brain.

4.3. Specific Epilepsy Syndromes. From the aforementioned case reports on the epileptic encephalopathies, REM sleep has been noted to usually have an antiepileptic effect. As an encephalopathy is, by definition, a spread-out and diffuse process, the reduced potential for such spread in the desynchronized environment of REM sleep may explain this observed antiepileptic effect.

In contrast, Table 4 demonstrates that the rate of rolandic interictal discharges in BECRS is higher in REM sleep than wakefulness. Like Table 2 which demonstrates a higher maximal rate of focal interictal discharges in REM sleep for certain individuals, the finding in Table 4 can also be explained by the presence of a proepileptic regional rhythm which may promote interictal discharging in the rolandic region.

4.4. Selective Localization. From the reviewed studies involving multifocal (i.e., tuberous sclerosis [87]) and focal [89] (i.e., temporal lobe [74, 88]) epilepsy, interictal discharges during REM sleep usually have a greater predictive value in selectively localizing an epileptogenic focus. Like the postulated mechanisms behind a lower rate of focal seizures and generalized discharges in REM sleep, selective localization may also be explained by the reduced chance of an aberrant spontaneous depolarization spreading—be it from a lower probability of spatial and temporal summation in a desynchronized cortical environment or the emergence of regional antiepileptic microrhythms.

However, there are also clearly described instances of false localization in the literature [73, 81, 89]. Like the postulated mechanism behind a higher rate of interictal discharges in certain individuals and in certain syndromes such as BECRS, the presence of a proepileptic regional rhythm may skew the propagation patterns of focal interictal discharges so as to point to a false localization of the epileptogenic focus.

5. Conclusion

Sixty years after the discovery of REM sleep, a wealth of literature has commented on the effect of REM sleep on seizures. In our review, we have demonstrated that, compared to NREM sleep, REM sleep has a strong antiepileptic effect against focal interictal discharges, focal seizures, and generalized seizures. We also found that REM sleep has an additional antiepileptic effect compared to wakefulness against focal and generalized seizures.

While cases of false localization have been described, REM sleep has been demonstrated to have promise in helping localize epileptogenic foci with possible translation into postsurgical seizure freedom. The potential selective localizing value of REM sleep may argue for the use of dedicated sleep recordings in the presurgical evaluation of epilepsy.

Finally, we hypothesize that the impact of REM sleep on epilepsy is due to a maximally desynchronized EEG pattern which reduces the likelihood of spatial and temporal summation of aberrant depolarizations. Although at first glance similar to wakefulness, recent connectivity studies demonstrate a further strategic loss of connectivity in REM sleep which we hypothesize accounts for its unique antiepileptic influence on seizures.

Acknowledgment

Dr. Pavlova has received research support from the Harvard Catalyst (Grant no. UL1 RR 02758) in 2010-2011.

References

[1] P. Passouant, "Historical views on sleep and epilepsy," in *Sleep and Epilepsy*, M. B. Sterman, Ed., pp. 1–6, Academic Press, New York, NY, USA, 1982.

[2] E. Aserinsky and N. Kleitman, "Regularly occurring periods of eye motility, and concomitant phenomena, during sleep," *Science*, vol. 118, no. 3062, pp. 273–274, 1953.

[3] A. Mitani, K. Ito, A. E. Hallanger, B. H. Wainer, K. Kataoka, and R. W. McCarley, "Cholinergic projections from the laterodorsal and pedunculopontine tegmental nuclei to the pontine gigantocellular tegmental field in the cat," *Brain Research*, vol. 451, no. 1-2, pp. 397–402, 1988.

[4] R. W. McCarley, R. W. Greene, D. Rainnie, and C. M. Portas, "Brainstem neuromodulation and REM sleep," *Seminars in the Neurosciences*, vol. 7, no. 5, pp. 341–354, 1995.

[5] C. S. Leonard and R. Llinás, "Serotonergic and cholinergic inhibition of mesopontine cholinergic neurons controlling rem sleep: an in vitro electrophysiological study," *Neuroscience*, vol. 59, no. 2, pp. 309–330, 1994.

[6] J. I. Luebke, R. W. Greene, K. Semba, A. Kamondi, R. W. McCarley, and P. B. Reiner, "Serotonin hyperpolarizes cholinergic low-threshold burst neurons in the rat laterodorsal tegmental nucleus in vitro," *Proceedings of the National Academy of Sciences of the United States of America*, vol. 89, no. 2, pp. 743–747, 1992.

[7] M. M. Thakkar, R. E. Strecker, and R. W. McCarley, "Behavioral state control through differential serotonergic inhibition in the mesopontine cholinergic nuclei: a simultaneous unit recording and microdialysis study," *Journal of Neuroscience*, vol. 18, no. 14, pp. 5490–5497, 1998.

[8] S. Chokroverty, "Neurobiology of rapid eye movement and non-rapid eye movement sleep," in *Sleep Disorders Medicine: Basic Science, Technical Considerations, and Clinical Aspects*, S. Chokroverty, Ed., pp. 29–58, Saunders Elsevier, Philadelphia, Pa, USA, 3rd edition, 2009.

[9] M. Steriade and R. W. McCarley, *Brain Control of Sleep and Wakefulness*, Kluwer Academic Publishers, New York, NY, USA, 2005.

[10] R. A. España and T. E. Scammell, "Sleep neurobiology from a clinical perspective," *Sleep*, vol. 34, no. 7, pp. 845–858, 2011.

[11] R. Boissard, D. Gervasoni, M. H. Schmidt, B. Barbagli, P. Fort, and P. H. Luppi, "The rat ponto-medullary network responsible for paradoxical sleep onset and maintenance: a combined microinjection and functional neuroanatomical study," *European Journal of Neuroscience*, vol. 16, no. 10, pp. 1959–1973, 2002.

[12] S. Boucetta and B. E. Jones, "Activity profiles of cholinergic and intermingled gabaergic and putative glutamatergic neurons in the pontomesencephalic tegmentum of urethane-anesthetized rats," *Journal of Neuroscience*, vol. 29, no. 14, pp. 4664–4674, 2009.

[13] M. El Mansari, K. Sakai, and M. Jouvet, "Unitary characteristics of presumptive cholinergic tegmental neurons during the sleep-waking cycle in freely moving cats," *Experimental Brain Research*, vol. 76, no. 3, pp. 519–529, 1989.

[14] M. G. Lee, I. D. Manns, A. Alonso, and B. E. Jones, "Sleep-wake related discharge properties of basal forebrain neurons recorded with micropipettes in head-fixed rats," *Journal of Neurophysiology*, vol. 92, no. 2, pp. 1182–1198, 2004.

[15] M. Steriade, S. Datta, D. Paré, G. Oakson, and R. Curró Dossi, "Neuronal activities in brain-stem cholinergic nuclei related to tonic activation processes in thalamocortical systems," *Journal of Neuroscience*, vol. 10, no. 8, pp. 2541–2559, 1990.

[16] P. Henny and B. E. Jones, "Projections from basal forebrain to prefrontal cortex comprise cholinergic, GABAergic and glutamatergic inputs to pyramidal cells or interneurons," *European Journal of Neuroscience*, vol. 27, no. 3, pp. 654–670, 2008.

[17] I. Gritti, L. Mainville, M. Mancia, and B. E. Jones, "GABAergic and other non-cholinergic basal forebrain neurons, together with cholinergic neurons, project to the mesocortex and isocortex in the rat," *Journal of Comparative Neurology*, vol. 383, pp. 163–177, 1997.

[18] K. Ito, M. Yanagihara, H. Imon, L. Dauphin, and R. W. McCarley, "Intracellular recordings of pontine medial gigantocellular tegmental field neurons in the naturally sleeping cat: behavioral state-related activity and soma size difference in order of recruitment," *Neuroscience*, vol. 114, no. 1, pp. 23–37, 2002.

[19] K. Sakai, J. P. Sastre, D. Salvert, M. Touret, M. Tohyama, and M. Jouvet, "Tegmentoreticular projections with special reference to the muscular atonia during paradoxical sleep in the cat: an HRP study," *Brain Research*, vol. 176, no. 2, pp. 233–254, 1979.

[20] D. R. Curtis, L. Hösli, G. A. R. Johnston, and I. H. Johnston, "The hyperpolarization of spinal motoneurones by glycine and related amino acids," *Experimental Brain Research*, vol. 5, no. 3, pp. 235–258, 1968.

[21] Y. Y. Lai, T. Kodama, and J. M. Siegel, "Changes in monoamine release in the ventral horn and hypoglossal nucleus linked to pontine inhibition of muscle tone: an in vivo microdialysis study," *Journal of Neuroscience*, vol. 21, no. 18, pp. 7384–7391, 2001.

[22] A. Jelev, S. Sood, H. Liu, P. Nolan, and R. L. Horner, "Microdialysis perfusion of 5-HT into hypoglossal motor nucleus differentially modulates genioglossus activity across natural sleep-wake states in rats," *Journal of Physiology*, vol. 532, no. 2, pp. 467–481, 2001.

[23] J. F. Perrier and R. Delgado-Lezama, "Synaptic release of serotonin induced by stimulation of the raphe nucleus promotes plateau potentials in spinal motoneurons of the adult turtle," *Journal of Neuroscience*, vol. 25, no. 35, pp. 7993–7999, 2005.

[24] B. Fedirchuk and Y. Dai, "Monoamines increase the excitability of spinal neurones in the neonatal rat by hyperpolarizing the threshold for action potential production," *Journal of Physiology*, vol. 557, no. 2, pp. 355–361, 2004.

[25] S. L. Foote, G. Aston-Jones, and F. E. Bloom, "Impulse activity of locus coeruleus neurons in awake rats and monkeys is a function of sensory stimulation and arousal," *Proceedings of the National Academy of Sciences of the United States of America*, vol. 77, no. 5, pp. 3033–3037, 1980.

[26] G. Aston-Jones and F. E. Bloom, "Activity of norepinephrine-containing locus coeruleus neurons in behaving rats anticipates fluctuations in the sleep-waking cycle," *Journal of Neuroscience*, vol. 1, no. 8, pp. 876–886, 1981.

[27] G. Aston-Jones and F. E. Bloom, "Norepinephrine-containing locus coeruleus neurons in behaving rats exhibit pronounced responses to non-noxious environmental stimuli," *Journal of Neuroscience*, vol. 1, no. 8, pp. 887–900, 1981.

[28] J. A. Hobson, R. W. Mccarley, and P. W. Wyzinski, "Sleep cycle oscillation: reciprocal discharge by two brainstem neuronal groups," *Science*, vol. 189, no. 4196, pp. 55–58, 1975.

[29] D. J. McGinty and R. M. Harper, "Dorsal raphe neurons: depression of firing during sleep in cats," *Brain Research*, vol. 101, no. 3, pp. 569–575, 1976.

[30] J. A. Hobson, R. W. McCarley, and J. P. Nelson, "Location and spike-train characteristics of cells in anterodorsal pons having selective decreases in firing rate during desynchronized sleep," *Journal of Neurophysiology*, vol. 50, no. 4, pp. 770–783, 1983.

[31] K. Rasmussen, J. Heym, and B. L. Jacobs, "Activity of serotonin-containing neurons in nucleus centralis superior of freely moving cats," *Experimental Neurology*, vol. 83, no. 2, pp. 302–317, 1984.

[32] C. Fornal, S. Auerbach, and B. L. Jacobs, "Activity of serotonin-containing neurons in nucleus raphe magnus in freely moving cats," *Experimental Neurology*, vol. 88, no. 3, pp. 590–608, 1985.

[33] R. Cespuglio, H. Faradji, M. E. Gomez, and M. Jouvet, "Single unit recordings in the nuclei raphe dorsalis and magnus during the sleep-waking cycle of semi-chronic prepared cats," *Neuroscience Letters*, vol. 24, no. 2, pp. 133–138, 1981.

[34] K. Sakai, G. Vanni Mercier, and M. Jouvet, "Evidence for the presence of PS-OFF neurons in the ventromedial medulla oblongata of freely moving cats," *Experimental Brain Research*, vol. 49, no. 2, pp. 311–314, 1983.

[35] Y. Kayama, M. Ohta, and E. Jodo, "Firing of "possibly" cholinergic neurons in the rat laterodorsal tegmental nucleus during sleep and wakefulness," *Brain Research*, vol. 569, no. 2, pp. 210–220, 1992.

[36] R. W. Mccarley and J. A. Hobson, "Neuronal excitability modulation over the sleep cycle: a structural and mathematical model," *Science*, vol. 189, no. 4196, pp. 58–60, 1975.

[37] B. E. Jones, "The organization of central cholinergic systems and their functional importance in sleep-waking states," *Progress in Brain Research*, vol. 98, pp. 61–71, 1993.

[38] R. Lydic, R. W. McCarley, and J. A. Hobson, "Serotonin neurons and sleep. I. Long term recordings of dorsal raphe discharge frequency and PGO waves," *Archives Italiennes de Biologie*, vol. 125, no. 4, pp. 317–343, 1987.

[39] R. W. McCarley and S. G. Massaquoi, "A limit cycle mathematical model of the REM sleep oscillator system," *American Journal of Physiology*, vol. 251, no. 6, pp. 1011–1029, 1986.

[40] D. Minecan, A. Natarajan, M. Marzec, and B. Malow, "Relationship of epileptic seizures to sleep stage and sleep depth," *Sleep*, vol. 25, no. 8, pp. 899–904, 2002.

[41] A. Crespel, M. Baldy-Moulinier, and P. Coubes, "The relationship between sleep and epilepsy in frontal and temporal lobe epilepsies: practical and physiopathologic considerations," *Epilepsia*, vol. 39, no. 2, pp. 150–157, 1998.

[42] M. G. Terzano, L. Parrino, P. G. Garofalo, C. Durisotti, and C. Filati-Roso, "Activation of partial seizures with motor signs during cyclic alternating pattern in human sleep," *Epilepsy Research*, vol. 10, no. 2-3, pp. 166–173, 1991.

[43] S. T. Herman, T. S. Walczak, and C. W. Bazil, "Distribution of partial seizures during the sleep-wake cycle: differences by seizure onset site," *Neurology*, vol. 56, no. 11, pp. 1453–1459, 2001.

[44] P. Halász, J. Filakovszky, A. Vargha, and G. Bagdy, "Effect of sleep deprivation on spike-wave discharges in idiopathic generalised epilepsy: a 4 × 24 h continuous long term EEG monitoring study," *Epilepsy Research*, vol. 51, no. 1-2, pp. 123–132, 2002.

[45] L. Parrino, A. Smerieri, and M. G. Terzano, "Combined influence of cyclic arousability and EEG synchrony on generalized interictal discharges within the sleep cycle," *Epilepsy Research*, vol. 44, no. 1, pp. 7–18, 2001.

[46] H. Horita, E. Uchida, and K. Maekawa, "Circadian rhythm of regular spike-wave discharges in childhood absence epilepsy," *Brain and Development*, vol. 13, no. 3, pp. 200–202, 1991.

[47] A. Autret, B. Lucas, and F. Laffont, "Two distinct classifications of adult epilepsies: by time of seizures and by sensitivity of the interictal paroxysmal activities to sleep and waking," *Electroencephalography and Clinical Neurophysiology*, vol. 66, no. 3, pp. 211–218, 1987.

[48] A. Autret, B. Lucas, C. Hommet, P. Corcia, and B. de Toffol, "Sleep and the epilepsies," *Journal of Neurology*, vol. 244, pp. S10–S17, 1997.

[49] J. Touchon, "Effect of awakening on epileptic activity in primary generalized myoclonic epilepsy," in *Sleep and Epilepsy*, M. B. Sterman, Ed., pp. 239–248, Academic Press, New York, NY, USA, 1982.

[50] P. Kellaway, J. D. Frost, and J. W. Crawley, "Time modulation of spike-and-wave activity in generalized epilepsy," *Annals of Neurology*, vol. 8, no. 5, pp. 491–500, 1980.

[51] S. Sato, F. E. Dreifuss, and J. K. Penry, "The effect of sleep on spike wave discharges in absence seizures," *Neurology*, vol. 23, no. 12, pp. 1335–1345, 1973.

[52] J. J. Ross, L. C. Johnson, and R. D. Walter, "Spike and wave discharges during stages of sleep," *Archives of Neurology*, vol. 14, no. 4, pp. 399–407, 1966.

[53] J. M. Zeitzer, C. L. Buckmaster, K. J. Parker, C. M. Hauck, D. M. Lyons, and E. Mignot, "Circadian and homeostatic regulation of hypocretin in a primate model: implications for the consolidation of wakefulness," *Journal of Neuroscience*, vol. 23, no. 8, pp. 3555–3560, 2003.

[54] P. Bourgin, S. Huitron-Resendiz, A. D. Spier et al., "Hypocretin-1 modulates rapid eye movement sleep through activation of locus coeruleus neurons," *Journal of Neuroscience*, vol. 20, no. 20, pp. 7760–7765, 2000.

[55] R. E. Brown, O. Sergeeva, K. S. Eriksson, and H. L. Haas, "Orexin A excites serotonergic neurons in the dorsal raphe nucleus of the rat," *Neuropharmacology*, vol. 40, no. 3, pp. 457–459, 2001.

[56] E. Eggermann, M. Serafin, L. Bayer et al., "Orexins/hypocretins excite basal forebrain cholinergic neurones," *Neuroscience*, vol. 108, no. 2, pp. 177–181, 2001.

[57] J. N. Marcus, C. J. Aschkenasi, C. E. Lee et al., "Differential expression of Orexin receptors 1 and 2 in the rat brain," *Journal of Comparative Neurology*, vol. 435, no. 1, pp. 6–25, 2001.

[58] L. Verret, R. Goutagny, P. Fort et al., "A role of melanin-concentrating hormone producing neurons in the central regulation of paradoxical sleep," *BMC Neuroscience*, vol. 4, article 19, 2003.

[59] M. N. Alam, H. Gong, T. Alam, R. Jaganath, D. McGinty, and R. Szymusiak, "Sleep-waking discharge patterns of neurons recorded in the rat perifornical lateral hypothalamic area," *Journal of Physiology*, vol. 538, no. 2, pp. 619–631, 2002.

[60] Y. Koyama, K. Takahashi, T. Kodama, and Y. Kayama, "State-dependent activity of neurons in the perifornical hypothalamic area during sleep and waking," *Neuroscience*, vol. 119, no. 4, pp. 1209–1219, 2003.

[61] A. Ahnaou, W. H. I. M. Drinkenburg, J. A. Bouwknecht, J. Alcazar, T. Steckler, and F. M. Dautzenberg, "Blocking melanin-concentrating hormone MCH1 receptor affects rat sleep-wake architecture," *European Journal of Pharmacology*, vol. 579, no. 1–3, pp. 177–188, 2008.

[62] J. T. Willie, C. M. Sinton, E. Maratos-Flier, and M. Yanagisawa, "Abnormal response of melanin-concentrating hormone deficient mice to fasting: hyperactivity and rapid eye movement sleep suppression," *Neuroscience*, vol. 156, no. 4, pp. 819–829, 2008.

[63] C. Billard, A. Autret, S. Markabi et al., "The influence of vigilance states on paroxysmal EEG activities and clinical seizures in children," *Electroencephalography and Clinical Neurophysiology*, vol. 75, no. 3, pp. 127–135, 1990.

[64] B. Dalla Bernardina, S. Bondavalli, and V. Colamaria, "Benign epilepsy of childhood with rolandic spikes (BERS) during sleep," in *Sleep and Epilepsy*, M. B. Sterman, Ed., pp. 239–248, Academic Press, New York, NY, USA, 1982.

[65] Z. Clemens, J. Janszky, B. Clemens, A. Szucs, and P. Halász, "Factors affecting spiking related to sleep and wake states in temporal lobe epilepsy (TLE)," *Seizure*, vol. 14, no. 1, pp. 52–57, 2005.

[66] Z. Clemens, J. Janszky, A. Szucs, M. Békésy, B. Clemens, and P. Halász, "Interictal epileptic spiking during sleep and wakefulness in mesial temporal lobe epilepsy: a comparative study of scalp and foramen ovale electrodes," *Epilepsia*, vol. 44, no. 2, pp. 186–192, 2003.

[67] F. Ferrillo, M. Beelke, F. De Carli et al., "Sleep-EEG modulation of interictal epileptiform discharges in adult partial epilepsy: a spectral analysis study," *Clinical Neurophysiology*, vol. 111, no. 5, pp. 916–923, 2000.

[68] B. A. Malow, X. Lin, R. Kushwaha, and M. S. Aldrich, "Interictal spiking increases with sleep depth in temporal lobe epilepsy," *Epilepsia*, vol. 39, no. 12, pp. 1309–1316, 1998.

[69] B. A. Malow, R. Kushwaha, X. Lin, K. J. Morton, and M. S. Aldrich, "Relationship of interictal epileptiform discharges to sleep depth in partial epilepsy," *Electroencephalography and Clinical Neurophysiology*, vol. 102, no. 1, pp. 20–26, 1997.

[70] C. Billiard, A. Autret, F. Laffont et al., "Aphasie acquise de l'enfant avec épilepsie à propos de 4 observations avec état de mal électrique infraclinique du sommeil," *Revue d'Electroencéphalographie et de Neurophysiologie Clinique*, vol. 11, pp. 457–467, 1981.

[71] G. F. Rossi, G. Colicchio, P. Pola, and R. Roselli, "Sleep and epileptic activity," in *Epilepsy, Sleep and Sleep Deprivation*, R. Degen, Ed., pp. 35–46, Elsevier Science Publishers B.V., Amsterdam, The Netherlands, 1984.

[72] G. F. Rossi, G. Colicchio, and P. Pola, "Interictal epileptic activity during sleep: a stereo-EEG study in patients with partial epilepsy," *Electroencephalography and Clinical Neurophysiology*, vol. 58, no. 2, pp. 97–106, 1984.

[73] J. Montplaisir, M. Laverdière, and J. M. Saint-Hilaire, "Sleep and focal epilepsy: contribution of depth recording," in *Sleep and Epilepsy*, M. B. Sterman, Ed., pp. 301–314, Academic Press, New York, NY, USA, 1982.

[74] M. Sammaritano, G. L. Gigli, and J. Gotman, "Interictal spiking during wakefulness and sleep and the localization of foci in temporal lobe epilepsy," *Neurology*, vol. 41, no. 2, pp. 290–297, 1991.

[75] C. W. Bazil and T. S. Walczak, "Effects of sleep and sleep stage on epileptic and nonepileptic seizures," *Epilepsia*, vol. 38, no. 1, pp. 56–62, 1997.

[76] S. Sinha, M. Brady, C. A. Scott, and M. C. Walker, "Do seizures in patients with refractory epilepsy vary between wakefulness and sleep?" *Journal of Neurology, Neurosurgery and Psychiatry*, vol. 77, no. 9, pp. 1076–1078, 2006.

[77] M. Billiard, A. Besset, Z. Zachariev, J. Touchon, M. Baldy-Moulinier, and J. Cadilhac, "Relation of seizures and seizure discharges to sleep stages," in *Advances in Epileptology*, P. Wolf, Ed., pp. 665–670, Raven Press, New York, NY, USA, 1987.

[78] B. A. Malow, R. J. Bowes, and D. Ross, "Relationship of temporal lobe seizures to sleep and arousal: a combined scalp-intracranial electrode study," *Sleep*, vol. 23, no. 2, pp. 231–234, 2000.

[79] J. Montplaisir, M. Laverdière, J. M. Saint-Hilaire, and I. Rouleau, "Nocturnal sleep recording in partial epilepsy: a study with depth electrodes," *Journal of Clinical Neurophysiology*, vol. 4, no. 4, pp. 383–388, 1987.

[80] B. Dalla Bernardina, F. Pajno-Ferrara, and G. Beghini, "Proceedings: rolandic spike activation during sleep in children with and without epilepsy," *Electroencephalography and Clinical Neurophysiology*, vol. 39, no. 5, p. 537, 1975.

[81] P. Genton, B. Maton, M. Ogihara et al., "Continuous focal spikes during REM sleep in a case of acquired aphasia (Landau-Kleffner syndrome)," *Sleep*, vol. 15, no. 5, pp. 454–460, 1992.

[82] C. A. Tassinari, "Electrical status epilepticus during sleep in children (ESES)," in *Sleep and Epilepsy*, M. B. Sterman, Ed., pp. 465–479, Academic Press, New York, NY, USA, 1982.

[83] R. A. Hrachovy, J. D. Frost, and P. Kellaway, "Sleep characteristics in infantile spasms," *Neurology*, vol. 31, no. 6, pp. 688–694, 1981.

[84] H. G. Wieser, "Temporal lobe epilepsy, sleep and arousal: stereo-EEG findings," in *Epilepsy, Sleep and Sleep Deprivation*,

R. Degen, Ed., pp. 137–167, Elsevier Science Publishers B.V., Amsterdam, The Netherlands, 1984.

[85] D. W. Klass, "Electroencephalographic manifestations of complex partial seizures," *Advances in Neurology*, vol. 11, pp. 113–140, 1975.

[86] J. R. Hughes and S. F. Olson, "An investigation of eight different types of temporal lobe discharges," *Epilepsia*, vol. 22, no. 4, pp. 421–435, 1981.

[87] A. Ochi, R. Hung, S. Weiss et al., "Lateralized interictal epileptiform discharges during rapid eye movement sleep correlate with epileptogenic hemisphere in children with intractable epilepsy secondary to tuberous sclerosis complex," *Epilepsia*, vol. 52, pp. 1986–1994, 2011.

[88] B. A. Malow and M. S. Aldrich, "Localizing value of rapid eye movement sleep in temporal lobe epilepsy," *Sleep Medicine*, vol. 1, no. 1, pp. 57–60, 2000.

[89] J. P. Lieb, J. P. Joseph, J. Engel, J. Walker, and P. H. Crandall, "Sleep state and seizure foci related to depth spike activity in patients with temporal lobe epilepsy," *Electroencephalography and Clinical Neurophysiology*, vol. 49, no. 5-6, pp. 538–557, 1980.

[90] M. N. Shouse, J. M. Siegel, M. F. Wu, R. Szymusiak, and A. R. Morrison, "Mechanisms of seizure suppression during rapid-eye-movement (REM) sleep in cats," *Brain Research*, vol. 505, no. 2, pp. 271–282, 1989.

[91] M. N. Shouse, P. R. Farber, and R. J. Staba, "Physiological basis: how NREM sleep components can promote and REM sleep components can suppress seizure discharge propagation," *Clinical Neurophysiology*, vol. 111, no. 2, pp. S9–S18, 2000.

[92] R. A. B. Badawy, A. S. Harvey, and R. A. L. Macdonell, "Cortical hyperexcitability and epileptogenesis: understanding the mechanisms of epilepsy—part 1," *Journal of Clinical Neuroscience*, vol. 16, no. 3, pp. 355–365, 2009.

[93] C. W. Wu, P. Y. Liu, Y. C. Wu et al., "Variations in connectivity in the sensorimotor and default-mode networks during the first nocturnal sleep cycle," *Brain Connectivity*, vol. 2, pp. 177–190, 2012.

[94] L. V. Colom, "Septal networks: relevance to theta rhythm, epilepsy and Alzheimer's disease," *Journal of Neurochemistry*, vol. 96, no. 3, pp. 609–623, 2006.

[95] J. W. Miller, G. M. Turner, and B. C. Gray, "Anticonvulsant effects of the experimental induction of hippocampal theta activity," *Epilepsy Research*, vol. 18, no. 3, pp. 195–204, 1994.

[96] E. B. Bromfield, J. E. Cavazos, and J. I. Sirven, "Basic mechanisms underlying seizures and epilepsy," in *An Introduction to Epilepsy*, pp. 1–30, American Epilepsy Society, West Hartford, Conn, USA, 2006.

[97] R. A. B. Badawy, A. S. Harvey, and R. A. L. Macdonell, "Cortical hyperexcitability and epileptogenesis: understanding the mechanisms of epilepsy—Part 2," *Journal of Clinical Neuroscience*, vol. 16, no. 4, pp. 485–500, 2009.

[98] D. J. Chong and L. J. Hirsch, "Which EEG patterns warrant treatment in the critically ill? Reviewing the evidence for treatment of periodic epileptiform discharges and related patterns," *Journal of Clinical Neurophysiology*, vol. 22, no. 2, pp. 79–91, 2005.

[99] T. Koike, S. Kan, M. Misaki, and S. Miyauchi, "Connectivity pattern changes in default-mode network with deep non-REM and REM sleep," *Neuroscience Research*, vol. 69, no. 4, pp. 322–330, 2011.

[100] S. I. Dimitriadis, N. A. Laskaris, Y. Del Rio-Portilla, and G. C. Koudounis, "Characterizing dynamic functional connectivity across sleep stages from EEG," *Brain Topography*, vol. 22, no. 2, pp. 119–133, 2009.

[101] M. Massimini, F. Ferrarelli, M. J. Murphy et al., "Cortical reactivity and effective connectivity during REM sleep in humans," *Cognitive Neuroscience*, vol. 1, no. 3, pp. 176–183, 2010.

22

Both Maternal and Pup Genotype Influence Ultrasonic Vocalizations and Early Developmental Milestones in $Tsc2^{+/-}$ Mice

Emily A. Greene-Colozzi, Abbey R. Sadowski, Elyza Chadwick, Peter T. Tsai, and Mustafa Sahin

The F.M. Kirby Neurobiology Center, Translational Neuroscience Center, Department of Neurology, Children's Hospital Boston, Harvard Medical School, 300 Longwood Avenue CLSB 14073, Boston, MA 02115, USA

Correspondence should be addressed to Mustafa Sahin; mustafa.sahin@childrens.harvard.edu

Academic Editor: Heidrun Potschka

Tuberous sclerosis complex (TSC) is an autosomal dominant disorder characterized by tumor growth and neuropsychological symptoms such as autistic behavior, developmental delay, and epilepsy. While research has shed light on the biochemical and genetic etiology of TSC, the pathogenesis of the neurologic and behavioral manifestations remains poorly understood. TSC patients have a greatly increased risk of developmental delay and autism spectrum disorder, rendering the relationship between the two sets of symptoms an extremely pertinent issue for clinicians. We have expanded on previous observations of aberrant vocalizations in $Tsc2^{+/-}$ mice by testing vocalization output and developmental milestones systematically during the early postnatal period. In this study, we have demonstrated that $Tsc2$ haploinsufficiency in either dams or their pups results in a pattern of developmental delay in sensorimotor milestones and ultrasonic vocalizations.

1. Introduction

Tuberous sclerosis complex (TSC) is an autosomal dominant disease presenting with hamartomatous tumor development and neurological symptoms, including autism spectrum disorder, epilepsy, and developmental delays [1]. TSC results from mutation in either the *TSC1* or *TSC2* genes, which encode for hamartin and tuberin, respectively. These two proteins inhibit the pathway of the mammalian target of rapamycin (mTOR) through negative regulation of the GTPase Rheb [2]. The mTOR pathway plays essential roles in protein synthesis and translation that are necessary for cell proliferation [3, 4].

Approximately 25–50% of TSC patients are diagnosed with autism spectrum disorder (ASD), a developmental disorder presenting with stereotyped behavioral patterns, social impairments, and communication deficits [5]. This represents a significantly increased risk for ASD among TSC patients as compared to individuals without TSC. The neuropathology and etiology of autism remain undefined although the relationship between TSC and associated autistic symptoms continues to be explored [6]. Several studies have suggested that the neurological disruption evoked by infantile spasms as well as the presence of cortical tubers or cerebellar abnormalities increases the risk for development of ASD [7–10]. Emerging evidence from neuroimaging studies also indicates that hypomyelination, a common phenotype in the TSC brain, may be correlated with neurocognitive disabilities in patients (reviewed in [3]).

TSC patients also show an increased incidence of intellectual disability, with up to 80% of patients experiencing developmental delay [11]. In addition, epileptic symptoms associated with TSC promote risk for moderate to severe psychomotor developmental delay among patients

[12]. Importantly, there is a proposed association between the type of *TSC* mutation (e.g., *TSC1* or *TSC2*) and the risk of developmental delay, with a greater proportion of patients with *TSC2* mutations suffering from moderate to severe delay as compared to patients with *TSC1* mutations [13–15].

While most animal studies have attempted to elucidate the relationship between *TSC* and ASD, no model has completely reproduced the social impairment, communicative deficits, and stereotyped behaviors seen in autism. One particular model, the $Tsc2^{+/-}$ model, involves a nonlethal deletion of a single allele of the *Tsc2* gene [16]. These mice display a mild disease phenotype as well as neurocognitive impairments in spatial learning, both of which are reversible with rapamycin treatment [17]. Previous work on the $Tsc2^{+/-}$ model has focused on identification of an adult behavioral phenotype, but a recent study reported increased ultrasonic vocalizations (USVs) in both heterozygous and wildtype (WT) mouse pups born to *Tsc2* heterozygous dams, indicating that maternal genotype is critical for pup vocalization output [18]. However, somewhat surprisingly, this study also noted that compared to WT mothers, $Tsc2^{+/-}$ mothers displayed more vigilant maternal behavior, which might be expected to reduce the call rate of pups. Additionally, a study on USVs in the BTBR T+tf/J mouse model of autism demonstrated increased USVs in BTBR T+tf/J mice as compared to C57BL/6J WT mice, as well as abnormal development of sensorimotor milestones [19]. We therefore asked whether the previously reported association between maternal haploinsufficiency and atypical pup vocalizations is related to a more global delay in sensorimotor development. Based on previously described tests, we systematically investigated $Tsc2^{+/-}$ and WT pups from heterozygous and WT mothers for both sensory and motor development, concentrating on early development and ultrasonic vocalizations. We found increased ultrasonic vocalizations among WT pups compared to heterozygous counterparts from both WT and heterozygous mothers, indicating that pup and maternal genotype affect changes to pup vocalizations. This is also the first study to report delays in early development in the $Tsc2^{+/-}$ model that are dependent on both mother and pup genotype.

2. Methods

2.1. Animals. Tsc2 animals from a C57BL/6J background, backcrossed for five generations (see [16]), were mated in crosses containing one heterozygous animal and one WT animal. In approximately half of the crosses, the female was heterozygous. For all tests, more than nine pups were used. Pups in each group were derived from a variety of mothers within each respective genotype group. Mice were identified using toe clippling, and date of birth was considered postnatal day (pnd) 0 for all pups. All experimental procedures were reviewed and approved by the Animal Research at Children's Hospital Boston Committee.

2.2. Ultrasonic Vocalizations. Beginning at pnd 4, WT and heterozygous pups from *Tsc2* WT and heterozygous dams were separated from their mother for 5 minutes and placed in a sound proof Noldus controlled acoustics chamber equipped with three microphones tuned to 50, 75, and 90 Hz. USVs were recorded using Ultravox software and were analyzed for number of calls. Testing was performed at the same time each day until pnd 10.

2.3. Developmental Milestones. Testing commenced on pnd 4 and continued every other day until pnd 14 for all animals. The regimen of developmental milestones included righting reflex, negative geotaxis, level screen test, cliff aversion, forelimb grasping reflex, bar holding test, and auditory startle, described in detail below [19]. Pups were weighed prior to each testing period and were reunited with their mother immediately after testing. All experiments were conducted on a heating pad (approximately 170 degrees Fahrenheit) and total daily testing lasted approximately 5 minutes per animal. Testing environment, time period, and investigator were consistent across all trials. Pup genotyping was completed after all testing had been finished in order to conduct each experiment in blinded fashion.

Righting Reflex. Pups were placed on their backs on a heated pad and latency to turn over (place all four paws on the surface) was recorded.

Negative Geotaxis. Pups were placed facing down on a piece of wire mesh ($1/16''$; $8'' \times 10''$) positioned at a 45-degree angle. Latency to rotate 180 degrees and reposition facing towards the top of the screen was recorded.

Level Screen Test. Pups were placed on a piece of wire mesh positioned horizontally on flat surface and were gently dragged down the length of the screen by the tail. Strength of grip (measured by resistance to pulling) was recorded and scored 0 (worst) to 3 (best).

Cliff Aversion. Pups were positioned on wire mesh held horizontally 6 inches above the heating pad so that both front paws were hanging over the edge of the screen. Pups were scored on how rapidly they retreated from the edge of the screen (0–3).

Bar Holding Test. Pups were allowed to rest on a heating pad while a thin segment of wire was placed beneath the front paws. Strength of the grasping reflex was recorded and scored 0–3.

Bar Hanging Test. A thin segment of wire was held 6 inches above a heating pad and pups were positioned so both front paws could grasp the wire while hanging vertically. Hanging ability was scored 0–3 and was based on duration of the hang.

Auditory Startle. Pups were allowed to rest on the heating pad while the experimenter snapped directly behind pup's head. Startle response was recorded and scored 0–3.

2.4. Statistical Analysis. For all data, statistical analysis was performed using Student's *t*-test (two-way, unpaired) and Analysis of Variance (ANOVA; rep. measures). Bonferroni

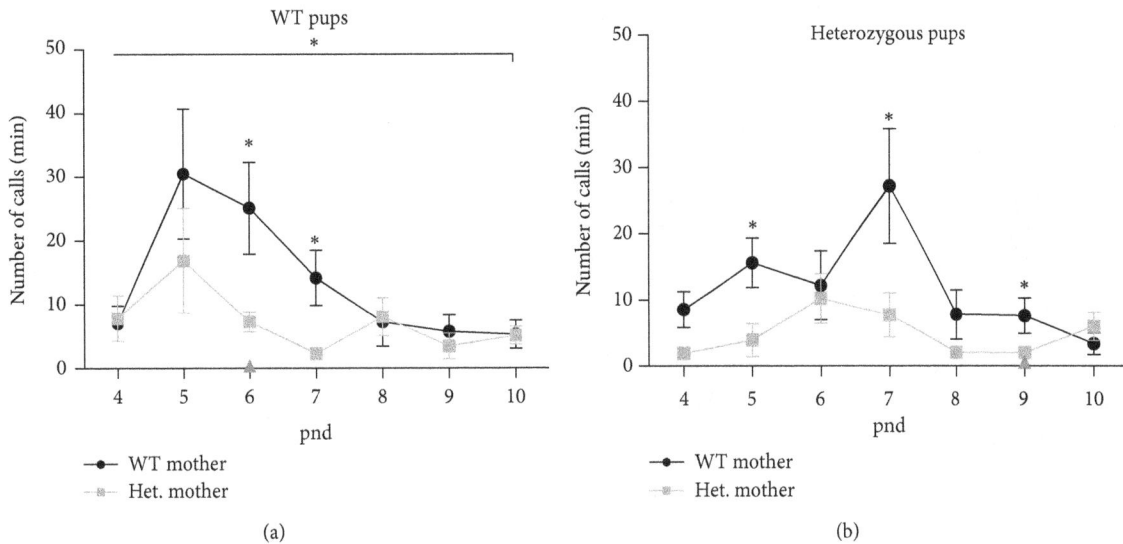

FIGURE 1: Pups born to WT or *Tsc2* heterozygous mothers emit differing numbers of calls dependent on maternal genotype. (a) WT pups from heterozygous mothers have fewer calls per minute than WT pups from WT mothers overall and at time points pnds 6 and 7. (b) *Tsc2* heterozygous pups from heterozygous mothers emit fewer calls than heterozygous pups from WT mothers at pnds 5, 7, and 9. $^*P < 0.05$.

post-hoc tests were performed on vocalization data to identify specific points of difference. $P < 0.05$ was considered significant.

3. Results

3.1. Maternal Tsc2 Haploinsufficiency Affects Pup Vocalizations. To evaluate early communication between mother and pups, we analyzed pup vocalizations recorded at 50–90 Hz, concentrating on rate of calls per minute. The number of calls per minute emitted by WT pups born to either *Tsc2* heterozygous or WT mothers varied by maternal genotype $[F(1) = 12.29; P < 0.05]$ (Figure 1(a)). Bonferroni post-hoc tests identified pnd 6 as a strong point of variation ($t = 4, 1$; $P < 0.001$), which was also supported with two-way t-tests of correlation at each time point. At pnds 6 and 7, WT pups born to *Tsc2* heterozygous dams released fewer calls than age-matched animals born to WT dams (t-test; $P < 0.05$; Figure 1(a)). The difference did not persist into a later age, however, and by pnd 8 WT pups from heterozygous mothers had similar call numbers to WT pups from WT mothers. All WT pups emitted a peak number of vocalizations at pnd 5, although there was a trend of pups from heterozygous mothers emitting fewer calls than counterparts from WT mothers.

Heterozygous pups from WT mothers displayed distinct USV patterns from heterozygous pups born to *Tsc2* heterozygous mothers. While the overall differences did not achieve statistical significance ($F(1, 84) = 3.26; P = 0.09$), number of calls per minute on certain postnatal days differed according to maternal genotype. Heterozygous pups from WT mothers vocalized more than age-matched heterozygous pups from *Tsc2* heterozygous mothers at pnds 5, 7, and 9 (t-test; $P < 0.05$; Figure 1(b)). Heterozygous pups born to a WT mother reached their peak number of calls on pnd 7

while heterozygous pups born to heterozygous mothers had a smaller but earlier peak number of calls at pnd 6. Their mean number of calls was lower than that of matched heterozygous pups from WT mothers.

3.2. Maternal Haploinsufficiency Affects the Acquisition and Performance of Developmental Milestones. Since maternal genotype affected pup vocalizations, we asked whether maternal *Tsc2* genotype might also affect early sensorimotor milestone acquisition. Analysis of developmental milestones, which compared pup results based on the genotype of the dam, yielded multiple points of significant difference when WT pups from heterozygous mothers were compared to WT pups from WT mothers. WT pups from heterozygous mothers displayed delayed geotaxis at pnd 9 (t-test; $P < 0.05$; Figure 2(c)) and impaired reflexive grasp during the level screen test on pnds 7, 9, and 12 (t-test; $P < 0.05$; Figure 2(d)). On the forelimb grasp test, WT pups from heterozygous mothers displayed a decline in ability when counterparts from WT mothers were plateauing at pnd 11 (t-test; $P < 0.05$; Figure 2(e)) and had a similar and longer-lasting impairment in bar hang, differing significantly from controls at pnds 6, 7, 9, and 11 (t-test; $P < 0.05$; Figure 2(g)). In addition, they displayed an increased startle response to auditory stimulation at pnds 12 and 14 (t-test; $P < 0.05$; Figure 2(h)). No difference in the righting reflex or cliff aversion was detected (Figures 2(b) and 2(f)). With the exception of the auditory startle test, all observed delays were not permanent and did not persist into the final day of testing (pnd 14). WT pups from heterozygous mothers weighed less than their WT counterparts from WT mothers, starting at pnd 4, continuing to be underweight until pnd 8 (t-test; $P < 0.05$; Figure 2(a)). We analyzed the other milestones from pnds 4–8 to determine if the underweight animals displayed similarly timed delays in development, which might indicate an effect

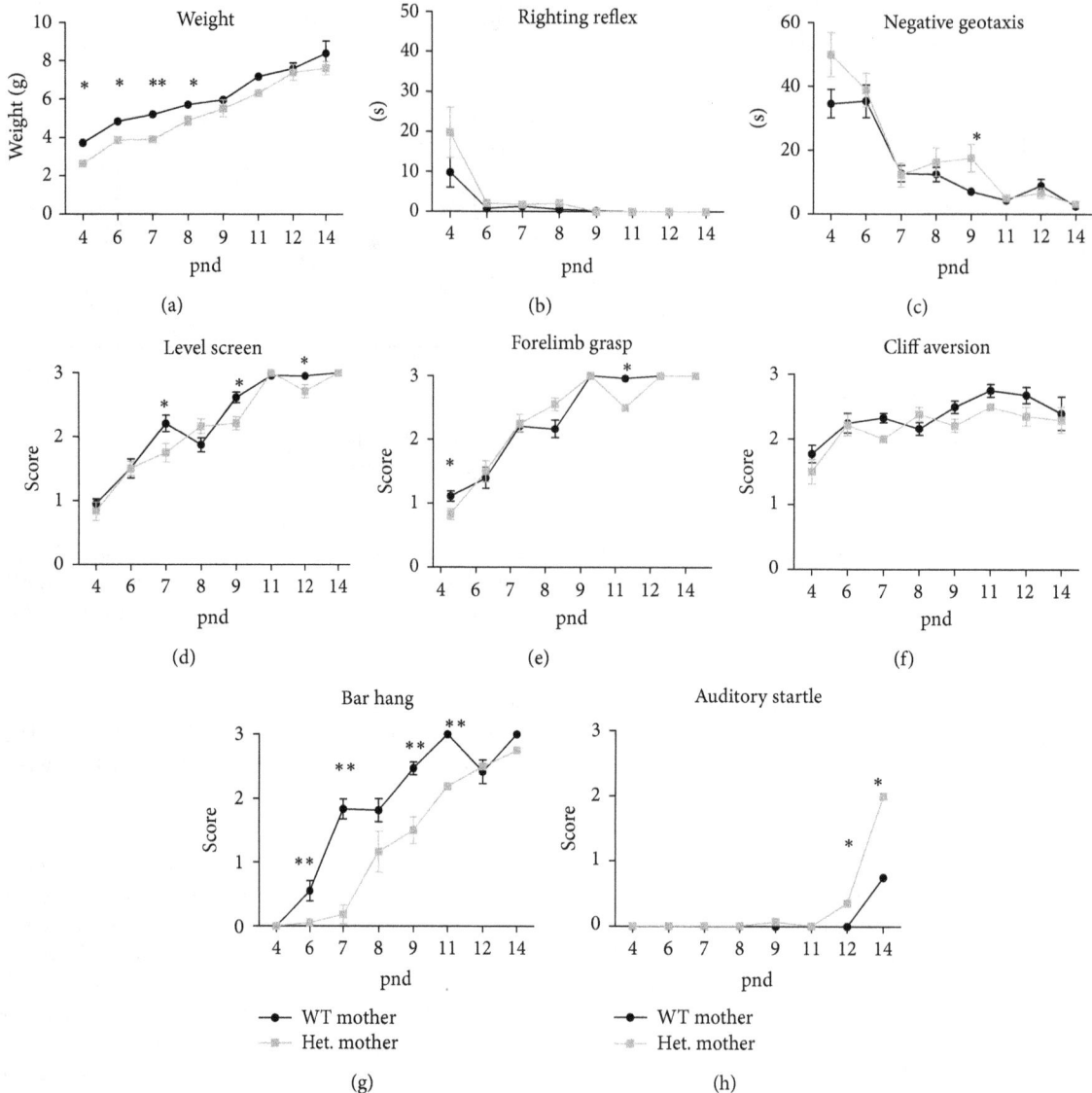

FIGURE 2: WT pups born to WT or *Tsc2* heterozygous mothers display developmental delay dependent on maternal genotype. (a) WT pups from heterozygous mothers weigh less than WT pups from WT mothers at pnds 4–8. (b) WT pups from WT and heterozygous mothers show no differences in righting reflex. (c). WT pups from heterozygous mothers delayed on negative geotaxis at pnd 9. (d) WT pups from heterozygous mothers impaired on level screen test at pnds 7, 11, and 12. (e) WT pups from heterozygous mothers show impaired forelimb grasp on pnds 4 and 11. (f) WT pups born to WT or *Tsc2* heterozygous mothers display no differences on cliff aversion. (g) WT pups from heterozygous mothers show significant impairment on bar hang at pnds 6, 7, 9, and 11. (h) WT pups from heterozygous mothers have decreased auditory startle response at pnds 12 and 14. $^{*}P < 0.05$; $^{**}P < 0.005$.

of weight rather than genotype, and observed that weight differences did not correlate with any significant delays.

The effect of maternal genotype on developmental milestones in heterozygous pups was also examined. However, when statistical comparisons were made between all heterozygous pups born to WT and heterozygous mothers, no significant differences were observed based on maternal genotype (Figures 3(a)–3(h)).

3.3. Pup Tsc2 Haploinsufficiency Affects Vocalizations. Although our and previous results show that maternal genotype is critical in determining pup vocalizations, we also wanted

to investigate the impact of pup genotype on vocalizations and development. While previous studies did not observe an effect of pup genotype on USVs, we analyzed our data for an effect of pup genotype and discovered significant differences parallel to those observed for maternal genotype. WT pups (from WT dams) displayed a peak number of <30 calls per minute on pnd 5. The number of calls subsequently declined until pnd 9, when they reached a plateau of >10 calls per minute (Figure 4(a)). *Tsc2* heterozygous pups from WT mothers emitted fewer calls than WT littermates at pnds 5 and 6 and reached their peak number of calls per minute at pnd 7 at a time when WT littermates displayed a marked decrease

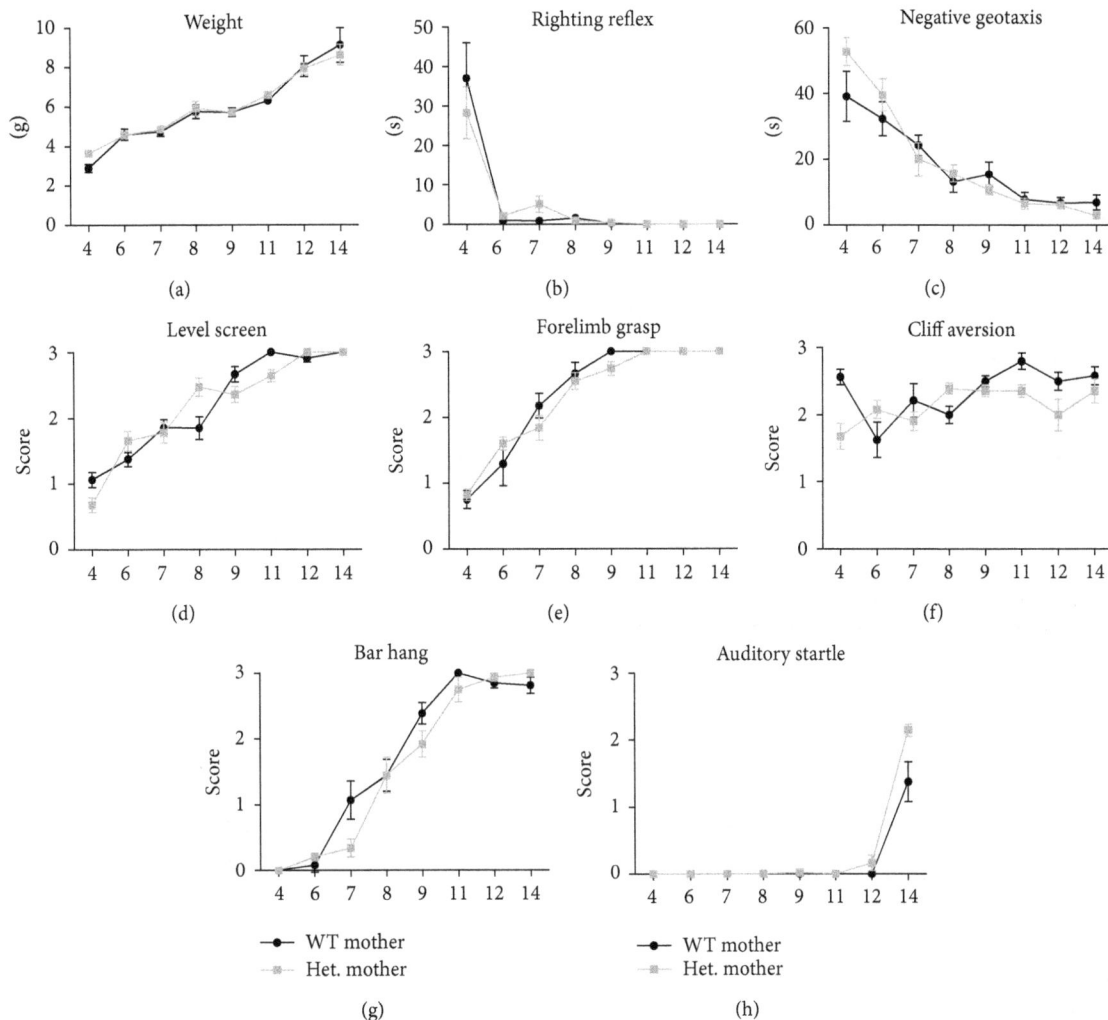

FIGURE 3: *Tsc2* heterozygous pups from WT or heterozygous mothers display no significant difference in developmental milestones.

in calling (Figure 4(a)). The differences observed between WT and heterozygous pups from WT mothers failed to reach statistical significance at specific time points; however, a repeated measures analysis of variance showed significant difference in number of calls with an overall effect of genotype over the entire multiday testing period [$F(13) = 4.06$; $P < 0.001$].

Pups from heterozygous mothers also displayed distinct vocalization patterns based on their genotype (Figure 4(b)). As with WT mothers, heterozygous pups showed a trend towards a later and smaller peak number of vocalizations than WT littermates, reaching their maximum number of calls at pnd 7, as opposed to WT pups, which reached maximum calls at pnd 5. These differences however did not reach statistical significance, likely related to baseline low levels of calls in all pups born to heterozygous mothers.

3.4. Pup Tsc2 Haploinsufficiency Affects the Acquisition and Performance of Developmental Milestones.

Since pup genotype affected vocalizations in pups born to WT mothers, we then analyzed the milestone data for an effect of pup genotype

and found that heterozygous and WT pups from WT mothers (Figure 5) displayed greater differences in their performance of developmental tests than did heterozygous and WT pups from a heterozygous mother (Figure 6). WT and heterozygous pups with consistent WT maternal genotype showed statistically significant differences in righting reflex, negative geotaxis, forelimb grasp, cliff aversion, and bar hang (Figures 5(a)–5(d) and 5(f)-5(g)). Most differences manifested only between pnds 4 and 9, suggesting that the developmental delay is early and temporary. At pnd 4, heterozygous pups from a WT mother showed delayed righting reflex (*t*-test; $P < 0.05$; Figure 5(b)) and impaired forelimb grasping reflex and cliff aversion (*t*-test; $P < 0.05$; Figures 5(e) and 5(f)) as compared to WT littermates. Cliff aversion was also impaired at pnd 6 (*t*-test; $P < 0.05$; Figure 5(f)), but that difference did not persist past this time point. At pnd 7, heterozygous pups demonstrated a delay in latency to complete negative geotaxis (*t*-test; $P < 0.05$; Figure 5(c)) and impairment in bar hanging (*t*-test; $P < 0.05$; Figure 5(g)) when compared to WT littermates. Heterozygous pups displayed continued bar hang impairment at pnd 8 (*t*-test; $P < 0.05$; Figure 5(g))

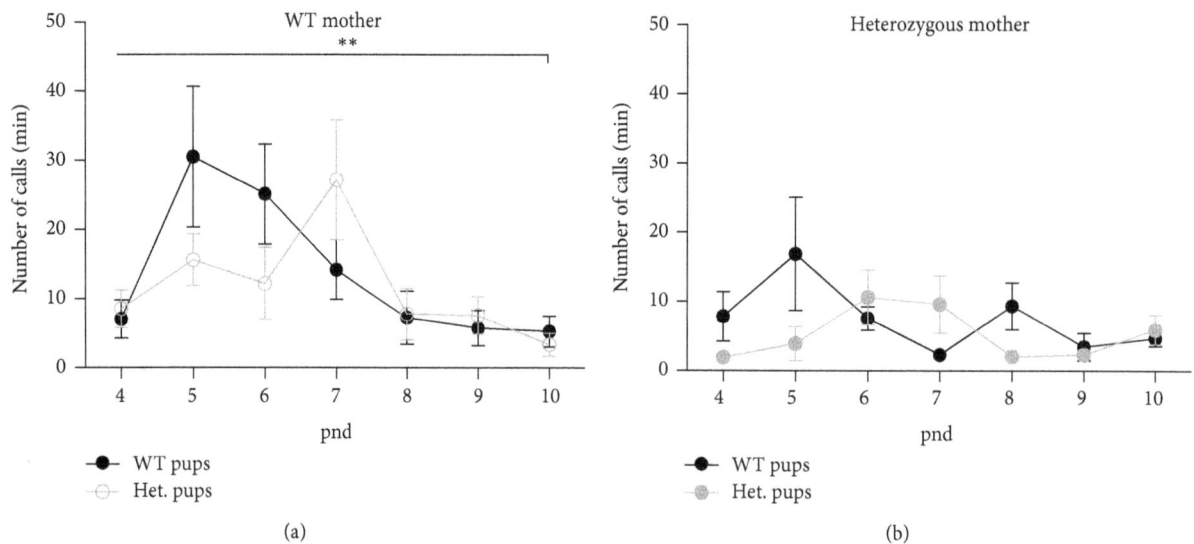

FIGURE 4: WT and *Tsc2* heterozygous pups born to WT or *Tsc2* heterozygous mothers display differences in overall number of calls dependent on pup genotype. (a) Heterozygous pups from WT mothers have delayed peak number of vocalizations. (b) WT and heterozygous pups from *Tsc2* heterozygous mothers show no significant differences in number of calls; although not statistically relevant, heterozygous pups have delayed peak number of calls. $^{**}P < 0.005$.

and showed a delay in latency to negative geotaxis during that time point (t-test; $P < 0.05$; Figure 5(b)). After pnd 9, heterozygous and WT pups had comparable results for all tests excluding negative geotaxis, which remained delayed in heterozygous pups until pnd 11 (t-test; $P < 0.05$; Figure 5(b)).

Heterozygous and WT pups born to heterozygous mothers were closely matched in performance and acquisition of all milestones, likely due to a strong effect of maternal haploinsufficiency. No significant differences were noted in developmental milestone tests based on pup genotype (Figures 6(a)–6(h)).

4. Discussion

USVs, which range from 50 to 90 Hz, are reliable indicators of the mother-pup relationship and of early pup development. They begin 3-4 days after birth and reach a peak between 6 and 8 days [20]. Socially, they enable the juvenile pups to communicate with their mother during and after separation by eliciting searching behavior during separation and retrieval during reunion. Although the possible role of pup vocalizations in communication is still being investigated, it has been shown that vocalizations by juvenile pups do elicit searching behavior in the mother during periods of separation [21]. Vocalizations also appear to be dependent on mouse strain, suggesting that they are sensitive to genetic differences [22]. A previous study showed increases in $Tsc2^{+/-}$ pup vocalizations based on maternal genotype and reported greater maternal attention from heterozygous mothers [18]. Our results are congruent with previous reports of increased maternal attention from heterozygous mothers: pups born to heterozygous mothers emit fewer distress calls than those born to WT mothers, suggesting that heterozygous mothers display more vigilant search and retrieval behavior. Fewer

pup calls generally indicate increased maternal vigilance with resulting reductions in pup calls. Our reports of decreased numbers of vocalizations based on pup and maternal heterozygosity differ from the observations published by Young and colleagues in 2010, which presented evidence that WT pups from heterozygous dams vocalized more; that is, they were potentiated after isolation. One possible explanation for this discrepancy is the difference in experimental design: our methods closely followed those detailed in Scattoni's multiday study of the BTBR mice [19] while Young and colleagues focused on pups at pnd 10. Nonetheless, our results are consistent with their reports of increased maternal attention in heterozygote mothers.

We show a novel effect of both maternal and pup haploinsufficiency on vocalizations and also report a trend of developmental delay dependent on haploinsufficiency. TSC is associated with high instance of developmental delay and autistic phenotype; previous studies looking at early development and vocalizations in $Tsc2^{+/-}$ mice found that maternal heterozygosity at the *Tsc2* locus is linked to changes in duration and number of calls per minute of pup USVs [18]. However, our results shed new light on the relationship between *Tsc2* haploinsufficiency and risk for early developmental delay both in sensorimotor development and in communication. In all genotypic scenarios (*Tsc2* haploinsufficiency in either dam or pup), heterozygosity had a consistently suppressive effect on either production of USVs or performance of sensorimotor milestones. All pups with heterozygous mothers, regardless of individual genotype, produced reduced numbers of USVs than age-matched counterparts from WT mothers or showed a delay in peak number of calls. Additionally, all heterozygous pups from either WT or heterozygous mothers displayed a delay in peak number of calls when compared to WT pups.

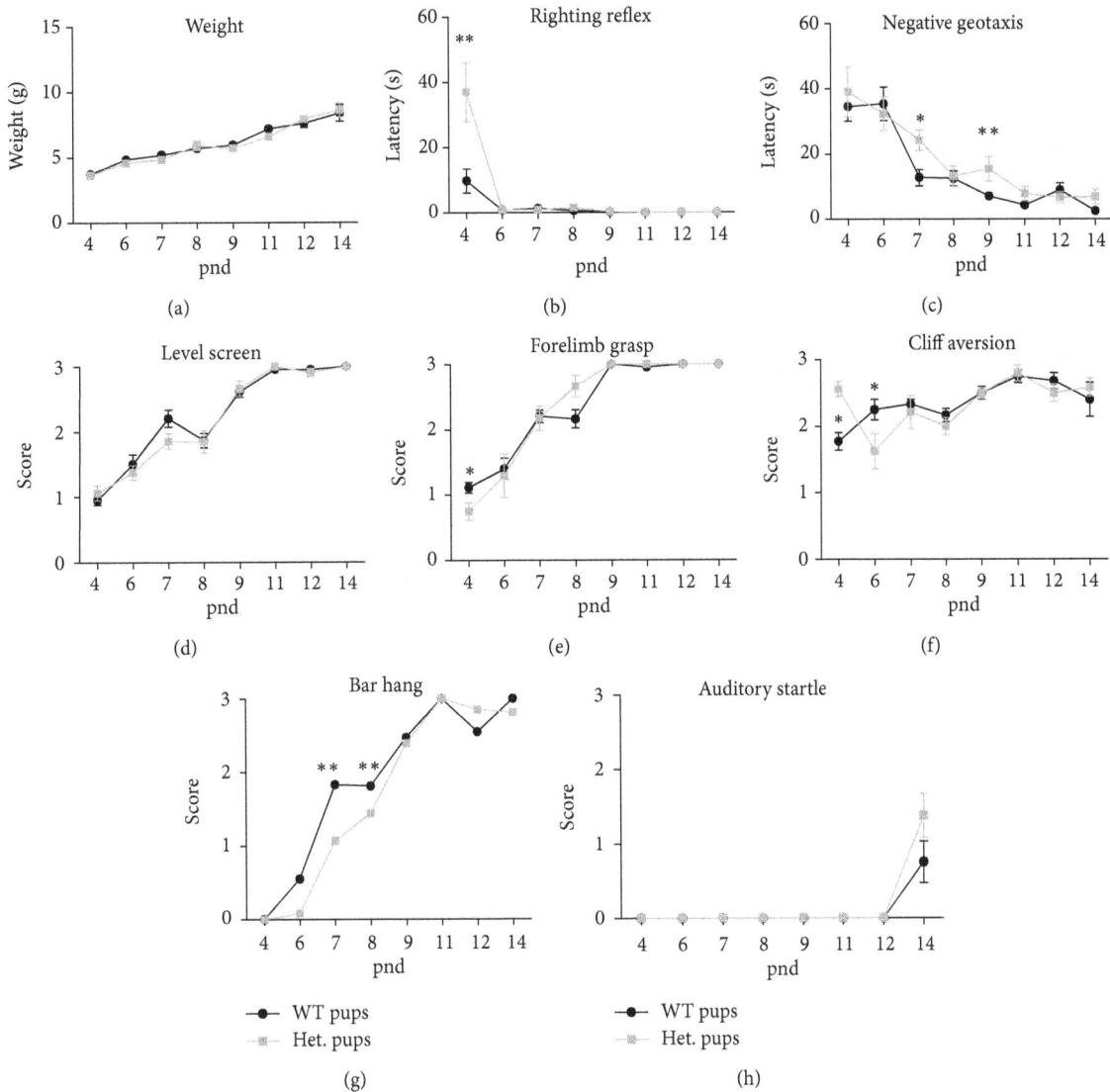

FIGURE 5: WT and *Tsc2* heterozygous pups born to WT mothers display delayed development for certain milestones. (a) WT and heterozygous pups have no differences in weight. (b) *Tsc2* heterozygous pups from WT mothers display delayed righting reflex compared to WT pups at pnd 4. (c) Heterozygous pups have delayed geotaxis at pnds 7 and 9 as compared to WT pups. (d) WT and heterozygous pups show no significant differences in forelimb grasp. (e) WT and heterozygous pups show no significant differences in level screen test. (f) WT and heterozygous pups show no significant differences in cliff aversion. (g) Heterozygous pups have impaired bar hang as compared to WT pups at pnds 7 and 8. (h) WT and heterozygous pups have no significant differences in auditory startle response. $^{*}P < 0.05$; $^{**}P < 0.005$.

The greatest overall differences in calls per minute arise among WT pups from WT dams and counterparts with any heterozygosity: maternal, pup, or both. This suggests further evidence that haploinsufficiency, whether contributing to a behavioral phenotype in the mother or causing intrinsic delays in pup sensorimotor development, may exert a suppressive force on pup development strong enough to prevent significant differences among heterozygous pups and pups from heterozygous mothers.

While USVs analysis provides convincing evidence for socially evoked vocalization abnormalities being due to maternal genotype, both developmental milestones and vocalizations, when analyzed for an effect of pup genotype, provide evidence for additional developmental delay that is dependent on pup, rather than dam, genotype. Heterozygous pups born to WT mothers showed delayed righting reflex and geotaxis as well as impaired bar holding and grasping skills when compared to WT littermates, and WT pups from heterozygous dams displayed similarly consistent delays across tests. Taken together, these observations indicate that the delay observed during the sensorimotor and vocalization testing is not only a consequence of differential maternal behavior, as previously suggested [18], but also an autonomous genetically determined phenotype. However, the behavioral phenotype of the pups likely arises from a combination of genetic predisposition and the mother-pup relationship rather than occurring as a sole consequence of environment or genes only.

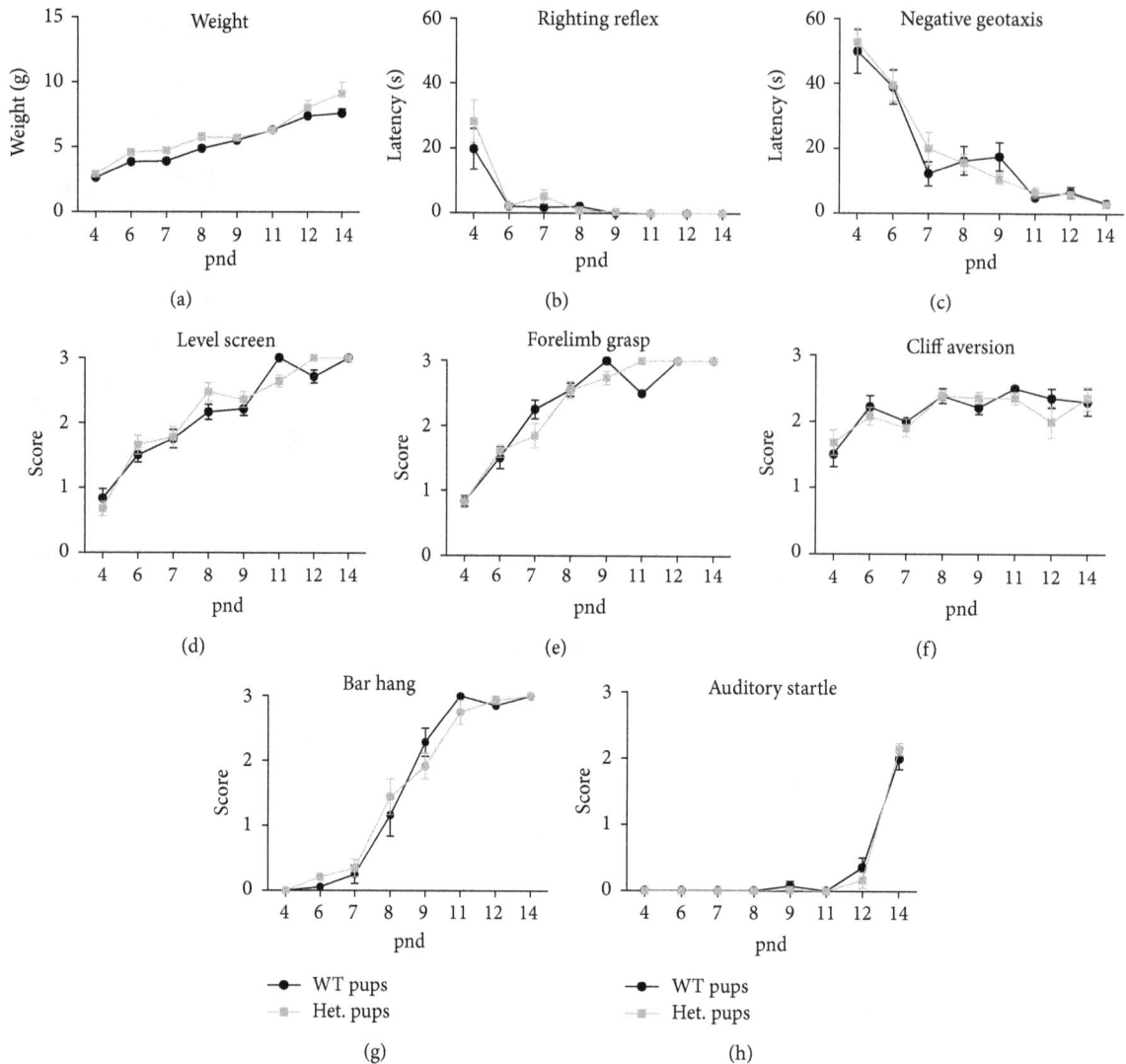

FIGURE 6: WT and *Tsc2* heterozygous pups born to *Tsc2* heterozygous mothers display no significant differences in developmental milestones.

We find that maternal genotype plays a determining role in the number of pup vocalizations while pup genotype affects the timing of the peak number of calls per minute, delaying it in the case of pup heterozygosity. Maternal heterozygosity also has an effect on pup sensorimotor development, causing delays especially in WT offspring. Additionally, pup heterozygosity delays acquisition of certain developmental skills among pups born to WT dams. These findings indicate a strong genetic relationship between *Tsc2* heterozygosity and developmental delay, providing further evidence that the *Tsc2* mutation is associated with impaired development, as has been previously suggested clinically [23]. Loss of both alleles of *Tsc1* or *Tsc2* in mice impairs neuronal migration [24, 25], while haploinsufficiency leads to disrupted connectivity between retinal neurons and their thalamic targets [26]. *Tsc1* or *Tsc2* mutant animals also have reduced CNS myelination [25, 27]. Thus far, the $Tsc2^{+/-}$ mouse has demonstrated deficits in hippocampal-dependent learning and social communication without the presence of the epileptic seizures that

are proposed to trigger these neuropsychological symptoms [17, 18]. The deficits, as evidenced by the developmental milestone tests, show that the atypical pup USVs in this animal model are strongly linked to an intrinsic condition and environmental factors. Of note, it is widely thought that epilepsy itself may significantly contribute to psychomotor delay in humans. There are other mouse models of TSC that display spontaneous seizures and can be used to investigate the relationship between epilepsy and psychomotor delay. Future investigation into and characterization of these delayed skills will be essential in elucidating the complete behavioral phenotype of the $Tsc2^{+/-}$ mice and other TSC animal models. While the mechanistic association between the disrupted neuronal pathways and the manifestation of neurologic symptoms is still under investigation, the high instance of such symptoms among TSC patients necessitates further research, and this study provides a method to investigate the pathogenesis of early developmental delay and the ASD phenotype.

Conflict of Interests

The authors declare that there is no conflict of interests regarding the publication of this paper.

Authors' Contribution

Emily A. Greene-Colozzi and Abbey R. Sadowski contributed equally to this paper.

Acknowledgments

The authors thank Michela Fagiolini for assistance with ultrasonic vocalizations. They are grateful to members of the Sahin Laboratory for critical reading of the paper. Peter T. Tsai received support from the Developmental Neurology Training Grant (T32 NS007473) and NIH K08 NS083733, American Academy of Neurology, and the Nancy Lurie Marks Family Foundation. This work and Mustafa Sahin are supported in part by the Children's Hospital Boston Translational Research Program, Autism Speaks, Nancy Lurie Marks Family Foundation, and the Children's Hospital Boston Intellectual and Developmental Disabilities Research Center (P30 HD18655).

References

[1] P. B. Crino, K. L. Nathanson, and E. P. Henske, "The tuberous sclerosis complex," *The New England Journal of Medicine*, vol. 355, no. 13, pp. 1345–1356, 2006.

[2] P. Tsai and M. Sahin, "Mechanisms of neurocognitive dysfunction and therapeutic considerations in tuberous sclerosis complex," *Current Opinion in Neurology*, vol. 24, no. 2, pp. 106–113, 2011.

[3] J. M. Han and M. Sahin, "TSC1/TSC2 signaling in the CNS," *FEBS Letters*, vol. 585, no. 7, pp. 973–980, 2011.

[4] S. Wullschleger, R. Loewith, and M. N. Hall, "TOR signaling in growth and metabolism," *Cell*, vol. 124, no. 3, pp. 471–484, 2006.

[5] S. Jeste, M. Sahin, P. Bolton, G. Ploubidis, and A. Humphrey, "Characterization of autism in young children with tuberous sclerosis complex," *Journal of Child Neurology*, vol. 23, no. 5, pp. 520–525, 2008.

[6] D. Ehninger, P. J. de Vries, and A. J. Silva, "From mTOR to cognition: Molecular and cellular mechanisms of cognitive impairments in tuberous sclerosis," *Journal of Intellectual Disability Research*, vol. 53, no. 10, pp. 838–851, 2009.

[7] P. F. Bolton and P. D. Griffiths, "Association of tuberous sclerosis of temporal lobes with autism and atypical autism," *The Lancet*, vol. 349, no. 9049, pp. 392–395, 1997.

[8] G. Ertan, S. Arulrajah, A. Tekes, L. Jordan, and T. A. G. M. Huisman, "Cerebellar abnormality in children and young adults with tuberous sclerosis complex: MR and diffusion weighted imaging findings," *Journal of Neuroradiology*, vol. 37, no. 4, pp. 231–238, 2010.

[9] G. C. Gutierrez, S. L. Smalley, and P. E. Tanguay, "Autism in tuberous sclerosis complex," *Journal of Autism and Developmental Disorders*, vol. 28, no. 2, pp. 97–103, 1998.

[10] S. Seri, A. Cerquiglini, F. Pisani, and P. Curatolo, "Autism in tuberous sclerosis: evoked potential evidence for a deficit in auditory sensory processing," *Clinical Neurophysiology*, vol. 110, no. 10, pp. 1825–1830, 1999.

[11] A. Hunt and C. Shepherd, "A prevalence study of autism in tuberous sclerosis," *Journal of Autism and Developmental Disorders*, vol. 23, no. 2, pp. 323–340, 1993.

[12] S. Jozwiak, M. Goodman, and S. H. Lamm, "Poor mental development in patients with tuberous sclerosis complex: clinical risk factors," *Archives of Neurology*, vol. 55, no. 3, pp. 379–384, 1998.

[13] S. L. Dabora, S. Jozwiak, D. N. Franz et al., "Mutational analysis in a cohort of 224 tuberous sclerosis patients indicates increased severity of TSC2, compared with TSC1, disease in multiple organs," *The American Journal of Human Genetics*, vol. 68, no. 1, pp. 64–80, 2001.

[14] A. C. Jones, C. E. Daniells, R. G. Snell et al., "Molecular genetic and phenotypic analysis reveals differences between TSC1 and TSC2 associated familial and sporadic tuberous sclerosis," *Human Molecular Genetics*, vol. 6, no. 12, pp. 2155–2161, 1997.

[15] A. C. Jones, M. M. Shyamsundar, M. W. Thomas et al., "Comprehensive mutation analysis of *TSC1* and *TSC2*—and phenotypic correlations in 150 families with tuberous sclerosis," *American Journal of Human Genetics*, vol. 64, no. 5, pp. 1305–1315, 1999.

[16] H. Onda, A. Lueck, P. W. Marks, H. B. Warren, and D. J. Kwiatkowski, "$Tsc2^{+/-}$ mice develop tumors in multiple sites that express gelsolin and are influenced by genetic background," *Journal of Clinical Investigation*, vol. 104, no. 6, pp. 687–695, 1999.

[17] D. Ehninger, S. Han, C. Shilyansky et al., "Reversal of learning deficits in a $Tsc2^{+/-}$ mouse model of tuberous sclerosis," *Nature Medicine*, vol. 14, no. 8, pp. 843–848, 2008.

[18] D. M. Young, A. K. Schenk, S. Yang, Y. N. Jan, and L. Y. Jan, "Altered ultrasonic vocalizations in a tuberous sclerosis mouse model of autism," *Proceedings of the National Academy of Sciences of the United States of America*, vol. 107, no. 24, pp. 11074–11079, 2010.

[19] M. L. Scattoni, S. U. Gandhy, L. Ricceri, and J. N. Crawley, "Unusual repertoire of vocalizations in the BTBR T+tf/J mouse model of autism," *PLoS ONE*, vol. 3, no. 8, Article ID e3067, 2008.

[20] H. N. Shair, "Acquisition and expression of a socially mediated separation response," *Behavioural Brain Research*, vol. 182, no. 2, pp. 180–192, 2007.

[21] G. Ehret, "Infant rodent ultrasounds—a gate to the understanding of sound communication," *Behavior Genetics*, vol. 35, no. 1, pp. 19–29, 2005.

[22] W. Nitschke, R. W. Bell, and T. Zachman, "Distress vocalizations of young in three inbred strains of mice," *Developmental Psychobiology*, vol. 5, no. 4, pp. 363–370, 1972.

[23] F. E. Jansen, O. Braams, K. L. Vincken et al., "Overlapping neurologic and cognitive phenotypes in patients with TSC1 or TSC2 mutations," *Neurology*, vol. 70, no. 12, pp. 908–915, 2008.

[24] Y. Choi, A. Di Nardo, I. Kramvis et al., "Tuberous sclerosis complex proteins control axon formation," *Genes and Development*, vol. 22, no. 18, pp. 2485–2495, 2008.

[25] L. Meikle, D. M. Talos, H. Onda et al., "A mouse model of tuberous sclerosis: neuronal loss of Tsc1 causes dysplastic and ectopic neurons, reduced myelination, seizure activity, and limited survival," *Journal of Neuroscience*, vol. 27, no. 21, pp. 5546–5558, 2007.

[26] D. Nie, A. Di Nardo, J. M. Han et al., "Tsc2-Rheb signaling regulates EphA-mediated axon guidance," *Nature Neuroscience*, vol. 13, no. 2, pp. 163–172, 2010.

[27] S. W. Way, J. Mckenna III, U. Mietzsch, R. M. Reith, H. C. Wu, and M. J. Gambello, "Loss of Tsc2 in radial glia models the brain pathology of tuberous sclerosis complex in the mouse," *Human Molecular Genetics*, vol. 18, no. 7, pp. 1252–1265, 2009.

23

Transcranial Magnetic Stimulation for Status Epilepticus

F. A. Zeiler,[1] M. Matuszczak,[2] J. Teitelbaum,[3] L. M. Gillman,[4,5] and C. J. Kazina[1]

[1]Section of Neurosurgery, Department of Surgery, University of Manitoba, Winnipeg, MB, Canada R3A 1R9
[2]Undergraduate Medicine, University of Manitoba, Winnipeg, MB, Canada R3A 1R9
[3]Section of Neurology, Montreal Neurological Institute, McGill, Montreal, QC, Canada H3A 2B4
[4]Section of Critical Care Medicine, Department of Medicine, University of Manitoba, Winnipeg, MB, Canada R3A 1R9
[5]Section of General Surgery, Department of Surgery, University of Manitoba, Winnipeg, MB, Canada R3A 1R9

Correspondence should be addressed to F. A. Zeiler; umzeiler@cc.umanitoba.ca

Academic Editor: József Janszky

Background. Our goal was to perform a systematic review on the use of repetitive transcranial magnetic stimulation (rTMS) in the treatment of status epilepticus (SE) and refractory status epilepticus (RSE). *Methods.* MEDLINE, BIOSIS, EMBASE, Global Health, Healthstar, Scopus, Cochrane Library, the International Clinical Trials Registry Platform, clinicaltrials.gov (inception to August 2015), and gray literature were searched. The strength of evidence was adjudicated using Oxford and GRADE methodology. *Results.* We identified 11 original articles. Twenty-one patients were described, with 13 adult and 8 pediatric. All studies were retrospective. Seizure reduction/control with rTMS occurred in 15 of the 21 patients (71.4%), with 5 (23.8%) and 10 (47.6%) displaying partial and complete responses, respectively. Seizures recurred after rTMS in 73.3% of the patients who had initially responded. All studies were an Oxford level 4, GRADE D level of evidence. *Conclusions.* Oxford level 4, GRADE D evidence exists to suggest a potential impact on seizure control with the use of rTMS for FSE and FRSE, though durability of the therapy is short-lived. Routine use of rTMS in this context cannot be recommended at this time. Further prospective study of this intervention is warranted.

1. Introduction

Repetitive transcranial magnetic stimulation (rTMS) has recently been employed as a treatment option for psychiatric conditions [1], chronic pain [2], movement disorders [3], and epilepsy [4, 5]. The use of rTMS for the control of medically refractory epilepsy has increased in the last 15 years, with over 30 publications since 1990 [5].

The exact mechanism of action of rTMS in seizure control is unknown. It is proposed that the long term effects in terms of seizure reduction are related to a reduction in cortical excitability secondary to long term depression or potentiation [5], with long term depression/potentiation referring to a use-dependent modulation of synaptic strength.

Animal kindling models in epilepsy have displayed the antiepileptic effect of rTMS [6, 7], with a potential frequency dependent impact on seizure control [7, 8]. In humans, a recent systematic review of rTMS for refractory epilepsy has displayed the safety and tolerability with improvement in seizure frequency in the majority of studies [5]. Furthermore,

recent arguments have surfaced supporting the cost effectiveness of rTMS for refractory epilepsy over standard failed antiepileptic drug (AED) based therapies [9]. Overall, recent evidence based guidelines support level C evidence for rTMS in the treatment of epilepsy [10].

Status epilepticus (SE) and refractory status epilepticus (RSE) pose difficult therapeutic challenges. Novel therapies such as rTMS have been sought out to treat RSE cases [10, 11], with a small number of cases reported in the literature to date [12–23]. The efficacy of rTMS in the setting of SE and RSE is currently unclear.

Our goal was to perform a systematic review of the literature on the use of rTMS for the treatment of SE and RSE.

2. Materials and Methods

A systematic review using the methodology outlined in the Cochrane Handbook for Systematic Reviewers [24] was conducted. The data was reported following the Preferred

Reporting Items for Systematic Reviews and Meta-Analyses (PRISMA) [25]. The review questions and search strategy were decided upon by the primary author (F. A. Zeiler) and supervisor (C. J. Kazina).

2.1. Search Question, Population, and Inclusion and Exclusion Criteria. The question posed for systematic review was the following: What is the effectiveness of rTMS in the treatment of SE/RSE? We utilized the Neurocritical Care Society guidelines on the management of SE based definition of SE and RSE [26]. The term generalized refractory status epilepticus (GRSE) was used to refer to generalized RSE. The term focal refractory status epilepticus (FRSE) was used to refer focal RSE. The term multifocal refractory status epilepticus (MFRSE) was used to refer to RSE that had a multifocal nature. The term nonconvulsive refractory status epilepticus (NCRSE) was used for nonconvulsive seizures that fulfilled the criteria for RSE.

All studies, prospective and retrospective of any size based on human subjects, were included. The reason for an all-inclusive search was based on the small number of studies of any type identified by the primary author during a preliminary search of MEDLINE and EMBASE.

The primary outcome measure was electrographic seizure control, defined as complete resolution, partial seizure reduction, and failure. Secondary outcome measures were patient outcome (if reported), and adverse effects to rTMS.

Inclusion criteria were as follows: all studies including human subjects whether prospective or retrospective, all study sizes, any age category, and the documented use of rTMS treatment for the purpose of seizure control in the setting of SE/RSE. Exclusion criteria were as follows: animal and non-English studies.

2.2. Search Strategy. MEDLINE, BIOSIS, EMBASE, Global Health, Healthstar, SCOPUS, and Cochrane Library from inception to August 2015 were searched using individualized search strategies for each database. The search strategy for MEDLINE can be seen in Appendix A of the Supplementary Material available online at http://dx.doi.org/10.1155/2015/ 678074, with a similar search strategy utilized for the other databases. In addition, the World Health Organizations International Clinical Trials Registry Platform and ClinicalTrials.gov were searched looking for studies planned or underway, with none identified.

Additionally, meeting proceedings for the last 10 years looking for ongoing and unpublished work based on TMS for SE/RSE were examined. The meeting proceedings of the following professional societies were searched: Canadian Neurological Sciences Federation (CNSF), American Association of Neurological Surgeons (AANS), Congress of Neurological Surgeons (CNS), European Neurosurgical Society (ENSS), World Federation of Neurological Surgeons (WFNS), American Neurology Association (ANA), American Academy of Neurology (AAN), European Federation of Neurological Science (EFNS), World Congress of Neurology (WCN), Society of Critical Care Medicine (SCCM), Neurocritical Care Society (NCS), World Federation of Societies of

Intensive and Critical Care Medicine (WFSICCM), American Society for Anesthesiologists (ASA), World Federation of Societies of Anesthesiologist (WFSA), Australian Society of Anesthesiologists, International Anesthesia Research Society (IARS), Society of Neurosurgical Anesthesiology and Critical Care (SNACC), Society for Neuroscience in Anesthesiology and Critical Care, and the Japanese Society of Neuroanesthesia and Critical Care (JSNCC).

Finally, reference lists of any review articles or systematic reviews on seizure management were reviewed for relevant studies on the use of rTMS for the treatment of SE/RSE that were missed during the database and meeting proceeding search.

2.3. Study Selection. Utilizing two reviewers (F. A. Zeiler and M. Matuszczak), a two-step review of all articles returned by our search strategies was performed. First, the reviewers independently screened all titles and abstracts of the returned articles to decide if they met the inclusion criteria. Second, full text of the chosen articles was then assessed to confirm if they met the inclusion criteria and that the primary outcome of seizure control was reported in the study. Any discrepancies between the two reviewers were resolved by a third party (C. J. Kazina).

2.4. Data Collection. Data was extracted from the selected articles and stored in an electronic database. Data fields included patient demographics, type of study (prospective or retrospective), number of patients, rTMS coil used, timing to rTMS treatment, rTMS treatment parameters, time to effect of rTMS, how many other AEDs were utilized prior to implementation of rTMS, degree of seizure control (as described previously), adverse effects to rTMS, and patient outcome (if recorded).

2.5. Quality of Evidence Assessment. Assessment of the level of evidence for each included study was conducted by a panel of two independent reviewers, utilizing the Oxford criteria [27] and the Grading of Recommendation Assessment Development and Education (GRADE) criteria [28–33] for level of evidence. We elected to utilize two different systems to grade level of evidence given that these two systems are amongst the most commonly used. We believe this would allow a larger audience to follow our systematic approach in the setting of unfamiliarity with a particular grading system.

The Oxford criteria consists of a 5-level grading system for literature. Level 1 is split into subcategories 1a, 1b, and 1c which represent a systematic review of randomized control trials (RCT) with homogeneity, individual RCT with narrow confidence interval, and all or none studies, respectively. Oxford level 2 is split into 2a, 2b, and 2c representing systematic review of cohort studies with homogeneity of data, individual cohort study or low quality RCT, and outcomes of research, respectively. Oxford level 3 is split into 3a and 3b representing systematic review of case-control studies with homogeneity of data and individual case-control study, respectively. Oxford level 4 represents case series and poor cohort studies. Finally, Oxford level 5 represents expert opinion.

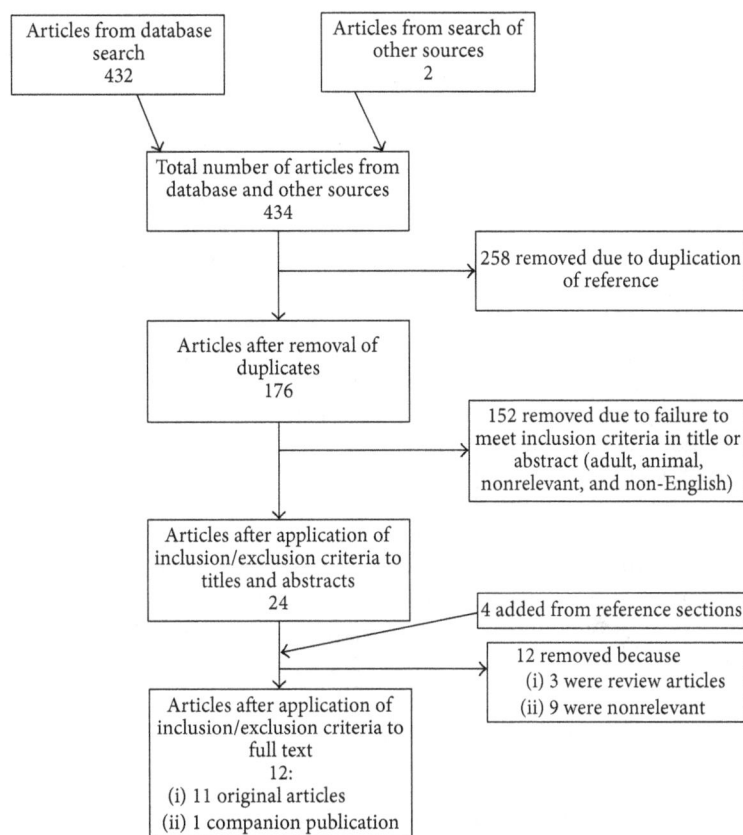

FIGURE 1: Flow diagram of search results.

The GRADE level of evidence is split into 4 levels: A, B, C, and D. GRADE level A represents high evidence with multiple high quality studies having consistent results. GRADE level B represents moderate evidence with one high quality study, or multiple low quality studies. GRADE level C evidence represents low evidence with one or more studies with severe limitations. Finally, GRADE level D represents very low evidence based on either expert opinion or few studies with severe limitations.

Any discrepancies between the grading of the two reviewers (F. A. Zeiler and M. Matuszczak) were resolved via a third party (C. J. Kazina).

2.6. Statistical Analysis. A meta-analysis was not performed in this study due to the heterogeneity of data within the articles and the presence of a small number of low quality retrospective studies.

3. Results

The results of the search strategy across all databases and other sources are summarized in Figure 1. Overall a total of 434 articles were identified, with 432 from the database search and 2 from the search of published meeting proceedings. After removing duplicates, there were 176 articles. By applying the inclusion/exclusion criteria to the title and abstract, we identified 24 articles that fit these criteria with 22 from the

database search and 2 from published meeting proceedings. Applying the inclusion/exclusion criteria to the full text documents, only 8 articles were eligible for inclusion, with 6 from database and 2 from meeting proceedings. The other articles were excluded because they either did not report details around the use of rTMS for seizure control, or because they were review articles. Reference sections from review articles were searched for any other articles missed in the database search, with 4 being identified. These were subsequently added to make a total of 12 articles for the final review.

Of the 12 articles included in the review [12–23], 11 were original studies [12–22] and 1 was a companion publication [23] with duplicate patient data. Rotenberg et al. [23] was a case report of Rasmussen's encephalitis treated with rTMS, which was subsequently also reported in the case series of rTMS for FSE, Rotenberg et al. [18]. In order to avoid duplication of patient data, Rotenberg et al. [23] was not included in the final data summary.

All 11 original studies were retrospective studies [12–22], with 5 retrospective case series [12, 14, 16, 18, 20] and 6 retrospective case reports [13, 15, 17, 19, 21, 22]. All were single center reports. Six studies described the use of rTMS for SE/RSE in adult patients only [14, 15, 17, 19, 21, 22]. Four studies described the use of rTMS in pediatric patients only [12, 13, 16, 20]. One study described the use of rTMS in both adult and pediatric patients [18].

Across all studies, a total of 21 patients were documented as having being treated with rTMS for SE/RSE (mean: 1.9 patients/study; range: 1–7 patients/study). Eight pediatric patients were treated, with a mean age of 8.3 years (age range: 2.66 years to 16 years). Thirteen patients were adult with a mean age of 42.3 years (age range: 18 to 79 years).

Seizures were classified as FSE in 10 patients [15, 18, 20], GRSE in 2 patients [14, 17], FRSE in 8 patients [12, 14, 16, 19, 21, 22], and nondefined SE/RSE in 1 patients [13].

The etiology of SE/RSE varied significantly and was as follows: primary epilepsy in 5 patients [12, 14, 21], stroke in 2 patients [16, 18], hypoglycemia in 2 patients [18], Rasmussen's encephalitis in 2 patients [18, 22], Dravet syndrome in 1 patient [13], focal cortical dysplasia in 1 patient [15], lipofuscinosis in 1 patient [16], postanoxic brain injury in 1 patient [17], post vascular malformation resection in 1 patient [18], herpes simplex encephalitis in 1 patient [19], Alpert's disease in 1 patient [20], nondefined "cortical malformation" in 1 patient [20], and unknown in 2 patients [18].

Study demographics and patient characteristics for all studies can be seen in Table 1, while treatment characteristics and seizure outcome are reported in Table 2.

3.1. rTMS Treatment Characteristics.

Nine of the 11 original articles provided [12, 14–21] details around the treatment parameters for rTMS. The 2 remaining articles referred to the use of rTMS in the management of SE/RSE, without providing any further information [13, 22].

Fourteen patients were treated with a figure 8 coil configuration [12, 14–16, 18, 19]. Two patients were treated with a "round" coil [16, 17]. Finally, 5 patients were treated with a nonspecified coil type [13, 20–22]. The stimulation parameters were highly heterogeneous between the patients described. The number of trains applied varied from 1 to 15. The frequency of stimulation varied from 0.5 Hz to 20 Hz. The train duration varied from 2 to 1800 seconds. The intertrain delay was poorly documented. Many patients received different treatment regimens on separate days [18].

The duration of rTMS treatment for these studies also varied dramatically. Some studies described a single treatment [14, 18], while others described 2 or more (range: 2 consecutive days up to 2 weeks) treatment sessions with the most aggressive schedule describing an 8-day course with varying once or twice per day stimulation settings [19].

Duration of treatment prior to the use of rTMS was documented in 3 articles [14, 17, 19], ranging from 7 to 44 days (mean = 22.0 days). The remaining 8 articles failed to mention the duration of therapy prior to rTMS. The number of AEDs administered prior to TMS was variable and was documented in 8 studies [12, 14–17, 19, 21, 22], with the total number ranging from 1 to 15 (mean = 7.5, median = 7.5).

Treatment characteristics for the adult studies can be seen in Table 2.

3.2. Seizure Response.

Seizure response to rTMS in the setting of SE/RSE occurred in 15 of the 21 patients (71.4%) included in the review, with 5 patients [14, 15, 20] (23.8%) displaying partial EEG based response and 10 patients [12, 13, 17–19,

21] (47.6%) displaying complete resolution of seizures. Six patients (28.6%) had no response to rTMS [12, 16, 18, 22]. The time to seizure response with rTMS was documented in only 2 studies [12, 18] with response occurring either during treatment [18] or following therapy up to 24 hours [12].

Looking at seizure subtype: 8 of the 10 (80.0%) FSE patients responded, 4 of the 8 (50.0%) FRSE patients responded, the 2 GRSE patients responded (100%), and the 1 "unknown" SE/RSE patient (100%) responded to TMS.

Seizure recurrence occurred in 11 of the 15 patients (73.3%) who initially responded. The time frame to seizure recurrence was quite variable, ranging from 72 hours up to 4 months. The duration of response was not documented in 5 patients in whom a response to rTMS was noted [13, 16, 20, 21].

3.3. Adverse Effects of rTMS.

Nine studies documented the presence or absence of adverse events related to rTMS [12, 14–21]. Two studies failed to mention any assessment for adverse events [13, 22]. Only 1 patient was described as having an adverse event secondary to rTMS. This patient developed transient leg sensory problems which completely resolved [16].

3.4. Outcome.

Outcome data was poorly recorded in the majority of the studies included within the review. Data on patient outcome longer than 6 months was unavailable in all studies included in the review. The majority of rTMS responders had recurrence of seizures at variable time frames after treatment, as described above. This led to either repeated treatment with rTMS, or other interventions such as operative disconnection procedures or vagal nerve stimulators. Outcomes are summarized in Table 2.

No identifiable trend in outcomes could be seen based on seizure subtype or etiology of seizure.

3.5. Level of Evidence for rTMS.

Based on the 11 original articles included in the final review, all fulfill Oxford level 4, GRADE D evidence to suggest some potential impact of rTMS on seizure control for FSE and FRSE. The role of rTMS for GRSE is unclear given the limited data.

Summary of the level of evidence can be seen in Table 3.

4. Discussion

We decided to perform an extensive systemic review of the literature in order to determine the effect of rTMS in the setting of SE/RSE. During the review we identified 11 original articles [12–22]. Twenty-one patients were described within these articles, with 13 being adult and 8 being pediatric. For the 8 pediatric patients who were treated, the mean age was 8.3 years (age range: 2.66 years to 16 years). For the 13 adult patients the mean age was 42.3 years (age range: 18 to 79 years). All studies were retrospective in nature. Seizure reduction/control with rTMS occurred in 15 of the 21 patients (71.4%), with 5 (23.8%) and 10 (47.6%) displaying partial and complete responses, respectively. Seizures recurred after rTMS in 73.3% of the patients who had initially responded.

TABLE 1: Adult study characteristics and patient demographics.

Reference	Number of patients treated with rTMS	Study type/design	Article location	Mean age (years)	Etiology of seizures and type of SE/RSE	Mean # AED prior to rTMS	Mean time until rTMS administration (days)
Graff-Guerrero et al. [12]	2	Retrospective case series	Journal manuscript	9 (11 and 7 yrs)	*Etiology*: primary epilepsy (2) *Type*: FRSE	4	N/A
Hyllienmark and Åmark [13]	1	Retrospective case report	Journal manuscript	5	*Etiology*: Dravet syndrome *Type*: cryptogenic SE	N/A	N/A
Liu et al. [14]	2	Retrospective case series	Journal manuscript	49 (46 and 51 yrs)	*Etiology*: primary epilepsy (2) *Type*: 1 → GRSE 2 → FRSE	8	15
Misawa et al. [15]	1	Retrospective case report	Journal manuscript	31	*Etiology*: FCD *Type*: FSE	1	N/A
Morales et al. [16]	2	Retrospective case series	Journal manuscript	12 (8 and 16 yrs)	*Etiology*: lipofuscinosis (1) and congenital infarct (1) *Type*: FRSE	4	N/A
Naro et al. [17]	1	Retrospective case report	Journal manuscript	35	*Etiology*: Postanoxic brain injury *Type*: GRSE	3	7
Rotenberg et al. [18]	7	Retrospective case series	Journal manuscript	41 (range: 11 to 79 yrs)	*Etiology*: hypoglycemia (2); postvascular malformation resection (1); stroke (1); Rasmussen's encephalitis (1); unknown (2) *Type*: FSE	N/A	N/A
Thordstein and Constantinescu [19]	1	Retrospective case report	Journal manuscript	68	*Etiology*: HSV encephalitis *Type*: FRSE	8	44
Thordstein et al. [20]	2	Retrospective case series	Meeting abstract	4.5 (2 yrs, 8 mons and 6 yrs, 3 mons)	*Etiology*: Alpert's (1) and cortical malformations (1) *Type*: 1 → FSE 2 → FSE	N/A	N/A
Van Haerents et al. [21]	1	Retrospective case report	Meeting abstract	24	*Etiology*: primary epilepsy *Type*: FRSE	7	N/A
Wusthoff et al. [22]	1	Retrospective case report	Journal manuscript	29	*Etiology*: Rasmussen's encephalitis *Type*: FRSE	15	N/A
Rotenberg et al. [23]	1	Retrospective case report	Journal manuscript	14	*Etiology*: Rasmussen's encephalitis *Type*: FRSE	8	N/A

rTMS: repetitive transcranial magnetic stimulation; AED: antiepileptic drug; N/A: not available; SE: status epilepticus; FSE: focal status epilepticus; FRSE: focal refractory status epilepticus; GRSE: generalized refractory status epilepticus; yrs: years; mons: months; FCD: focal cortical dysplasia; HSV: herpes simplex virus. Rotenberg et al. [18] contains a series of patients including the case description from Rotenberg et al. [23]. Thus, the data from Rotenberg et al. [23] was not included in the final summary and analysis of data in order to avoid duplication of patient data.

TABLE 2: rTMS treatment characteristics, seizure response, and outcome.

Reference	Number of patients treated with rTMS	rTMS coil type	rTMS treatment regimen (trains/freq./train duration)	Other AEDs on board	Electrographic seizure response	Duration of response	Adverse effects to rTMS	Patient outcome
Graff-Guerrero et al. [12]	2	Figure of 8	15/20 Hz/2 s train with intertrain of 58 s	1 → Valproic acid Phenytoin Primidone Topiramate 2 → Phenytoin Clobazam Valproic acid Oxcarbazepine	1 → seizure cessation after 24 h 2 → slight frequency decrease in epileptic spikes	1 → 2 weeks 2 → N/A	None	1 → required hemispherectomy: biopsy showed Rasmussen's encephalitis 2 → minimal improvement
Hyllienmark and Åmark [13]	1	N/A	N/A	Lidocaine Midazolam Thiopental	Burst suppression	N/A	N/A	Good, seizures ceased
Liu et al. [14]	2	Figure of 8	1 → 1/1 Hz/1200 s 2 → 1/1 Hz/1800 s	1 → Phenobarbital Pregabalin Lamotrigine Fosphenytoin Lacosamide Levetiracetam Pentobarbital 2 → Lamotrigine Levetiracetam Felbatol Lorazepam Lacosamide	1 → seizure frequency and spike detections decreased 2 → seizure frequency decreased	1 → until discharge (4 weeks) 2 → 72 hours	None	1 → discharged and sent to rehab on day 47 2 → required further vagus nerve stimulation; returned to baseline and discharged on 11 days after TMS
Misawa et al. [15]	1	Figure of 8	100 pulses at 0.5 Hz	Clonazepam Phenytoin	FSE suppression in hand but FSE in foot persisted	3 months	None	Patient underwent second TMS treatment which resulted in FSE suppression for 2 months
Morales et al. [16]	2	1 → round coil (5 cm diameter) 2 → figure of 8	1 → 2 sessions: 4/1 Hz/600 s and 10/6 Hz/5 s trains with 25-second intertrain interval followed by 1/1 Hz/600 s 2 → 2 sessions: 1/1 Hz/900 s and 10/6 Hz/5 s with 25 s intertrain interval followed by 1/1 Hz/900 s	1 → Zonisamide Phenobarbital Coenzyme Q Levetiracetam Carnitine 2 → Lamotrigine Clobazam	1 → no response 2 → no response	N/A	1 none 2 increased leg pain and mild headache. Both resolved	1 → brain biopsy showed neuronal ceroid lipofuscinosis Patient died 3 months later 2 → patient opted for surgery but no cortical resection could be done

TABLE 2: Continued.

Reference	Number of patients treated with rTMS	rTMS coil type	rTMS treatment regimen (trains/freq./train duration)	Other AEDs on board	Electrographic seizure response	Duration of response	Adverse effects to rTMS	Patient outcome
Naro et al. [17]	1	Round	4 trains with 300 pulses/1 Hz with 30-second intertrain interval	Levetiracetam Valproate Lorazepam	Complete remission	6 days	None	Myoclonic jerks reappeared though less frequent and intense
Rotenberg et al. [18]	7	Figure of 8	1 → 3/1 Hz/1800 s; 2 → 1/1 Hz/1600 s and 40/20 Hz/2 s followed by 1/1 Hz/1600 s; 3 → 40/20 Hz/1660 s; 4 → 2/1 Hz/1600 s; 5 → 1/1 Hz/200 s; 6 → 15/100 Hz/0.05–1.25 s & 10/1 Hz/1600–1800 s; 7 → 1/1 Hz/1800 s; 20/20 Hz/4 s	N/A	No effect = 2; Seizure ceased during TMS = 3; Seizure cessation after TMS = 2	Seizures ceased during TMS lasting 30 minutes; 1 patient = 2 days; 1 patient = >4 months	None	2/7 had no EEG response to TMS; 3/7 had a short-lived response lasting 20-30 min after TMS train before relapse of clinical seizures; 2/7 had lasting anticonvulsive effect throughout follow-up (2 days for 1 patient and >4 months for another)
Thordstein and Constantinescu [19]	1	Figure of 8	1/0.5 Hz/3600 s 2 days of 1/day and 6 days of 2/day	Fosphenytoin Levetiracetam Topiramate	Continuous seizures stopped, localized epileptiform activity recorded	2.5 months	None	Patient clinically improved slowly and has no epileptiform potentials 2.5 months later
Thordstein et al. [20]	2	N/A	1/0.5 Hz/3600 s daily for 2 weeks	N/A	Seizure severity decreased	N/A	None	Seizure frequency and severity both decreased
Van Haerents et al. [21]	1	N/A	3/1 Hz/600 s 11 sessions	Zonisamide Lamotrigine Phenobarbital Phenytoin	Seizure frequency progressively declined and then ceased	N/A	None	Complete seizure control and stabilization of epilepsy allowed patient to return to normal life
Wusthoff et al. [22]	1	N/A	N/A	N/A	No effect	N/A	N/A	Patient responded to ketogenic diet
Rotenberg et al. [23]	1	Figure of 8	1/1 Hz/1800 s (9 consecutive days)	Fosphenytoin Oxcarbazepine Levetiracetam Valproate Diazepam Lorazepam	Seizure suppression during treatment	Effect only during treatment	None	Patient returned to baseline seizures

rTMS: repetitive transcranial magnetic stimulation; AED: anti-epileptic drug; TMS: transcranial magnetic stimulation; AED: antiepileptic drug; N/A: not available; SE: status epilepticus; FSE: focal status epilepticus; FRSE: focal refractory status epilepticus; GRSE: generalized refractory status epilepticus; yrs: years; mons: months; h: hours; s: seconds. Rotenberg et al. [18] contains a series of patients including the case description from Rotenberg et al. [23]. Thus, the data from Rotenberg et al. [23] was not included in the final summary and analysis of data in order to avoid duplication of patient data.

TABLE 3: Oxford and GRADE level of evidence.

Reference	Study type	Oxford [29] level of evidence	GRADE [28, 30–33] level of evidence
Graff-Guerrero et al. [12]	Retrospective case series	4	D
Hyllienmark and Åmark [13]	Retrospective case report	4	D
Liu et al. [14]	Retrospective case series	4	D
Misawa et al. [15]	Retrospective case report	4	D
Morales et al. [16]	Retrospective case series	4	D
Naro et al. [17]	Retrospective case report	4	D
Rotenberg et al. [18]	Retrospective case series	4	D
Thordstein and Constantinescu [19]	Retrospective case report	4	D
Thordstein et al. [20]	Retrospective case series	4	D
Van Haerents et al. [21]	Retrospective case report	4	D
Wusthoff et al. [22]	Retrospective case report	4	D
Rotenberg et al. [23]	Retrospective case report	4	D

Rotenberg et al. [18] contains a series of patients including the case description from Rotenberg et al. [23]. Thus, the data from Rotenberg et al. [23] was not included in the final summary and analysis of data in order to avoid duplication of patient data.

One patient had a transient adverse event after rTMS which completely resolved. Patient outcome data was too sparingly documented for any strong conclusion, with no identifiable trend in outcomes for the responders versus the nonresponders, or based on seizure subtype or etiology. All studies were an Oxford level 4, GRADE D level of evidence. Thus, based on this review, we can currently provide Oxford level 4, GRADE D recommendations that rTMS may provide some impact on seizure control in the setting of FSE and FRSE.

A few important points can be seen within our review. First, rTMS seems quite effective for FSE with an 80% overall response rate. Second, rTMS for FRSE has a moderate efficacy of 50% compared to the results in FSE. This highlights the ongoing resistance to therapies seen with progressive and uncontrolled seizures. Furthermore, it suggests that the role for rTMS in FSE/FRSE is earlier rather than later in the treatment algorithm. Further prospective analysis of rTMS for this indication needs to occur. Third, we are unfortunately unable to comment on the efficacy of rTMS for GSE/GRSE given the limited cases described to date. Fourth, the treatment durability of rTMS is limited, with recurrence of seizures occurring within 72 hours up to 4 months in 73.3% of initial responders. This highlights that rTMS for FSE/FRSE is a technique for potentially rapid and acute control, thus acting as a transition therapy to an altered oral AED regimen or future regular rTMS treatment protocol. Fifth, the optimal rTMS stimulation parameters that lead to seizure control/reduction in SE/RSE are not well defined and, based on this review, remain currently unclear. Finally, there were a small number of complications described within the literature included in the review. This appears to mirror the data available for other pathologies treated with rTMS [1–5].

Despite the interesting results, our systematic review has significant limitations. First, the small number of studies identified, all with small patient populations, makes it difficult to generalize to all SE/RSE patients. Furthermore, our comments on the impact of rTMS for SE/RSE are currently limited to FSE/FRSE given the limited data for other subsets refractory seizures. Second, we were unable to perform a meta-analysis given the retrospective heterogeneous nature of the data. Third, as acknowledged previously, the optimal rTMS stimulation parameters which lead to seizure response in SE/RSE are unclear. The heterogenous treatment plans for the patients identified in the review produce a confusing picture on optimal stimulation strategy. Further prospective studies will need to be conducted in order to determine efficacy and treatment regimens. Fourth, the seizure response to rTMS may not be related entirely to the stimulation alone, and may represent a reflection of the combination of multiple AEDs. Fifth, and probably most importantly, there is a potential for publication bias in the articles reviewed. We suspect that publication bias is quite high in the literature identified. It is likely that there are many more failed cases of rTMS for SE/RSE that have not been published. Finally, comments related to patient outcomes are limited, and the impact of rTMS on long term patient outcome cannot be made at this time.

Routine use of rTMS for SE/RSE cannot be recommended at this time. The results of this review point to a potential impact rTMS may have on seizure control in FSE/FRSE. Further prospective study is clearly warranted in order to better define the role of rTMS in the context of SE/RSE. International databases for SE/RSE patients with prospectively maintained data could potentially bolster the data set for rTMS, and other salvage therapies for refractory seizures.

5. Conclusions

Oxford level 4, GRADE D evidence exists to suggest a potential impact on seizure control with the use of rTMS for FSE and FRSE, though durability of the therapy is short-lived. Routine use of rTMS in this context cannot be recommended at this time. Further prospective study of this intervention is warranted in order to determine its true efficacy in FSE/FRSE, amongst other subtypes of SE and RSE.

Conflict of Interests

The authors declare that there is no conflict of interests regarding the publication of this paper.

References

[1] E. Cretaz, A. R. Brunoni, and B. Lafer, "Magnetic seizure therapy for unipolar and bipolar depression: a systematic review," *Neural Plasticity*, vol. 2015, Article ID 521398, 9 pages, 2015.

[2] R. Galhardoni, G. S. Correia, H. Araujo et al., "Repetitive transcranial magnetic stimulation in chronic pain: a review of the literature," *Archives of Physical Medicine and Rehabilitation*, vol. 96, no. 4, supplement, pp. S156–S172, 2015.

[3] Y. H. Chou, P. T. Hickey, M. Sundman, A. W. Song, and N. K. Chen, "Effects of repetitive transcranial magnetic stimulation on motor symptoms in Parkinson disease: a systematic review and meta-analysis," *JAMA Neurology*, vol. 72, no. 4, pp. 432–440, 2015.

[4] M. A. Nitsche and W. Paulus, "Noninvasive brain stimulation protocols in the treatment of epilepsy: current state and perspectives," *Neurotherapeutics*, vol. 6, no. 2, pp. 244–250, 2009.

[5] E. H. Bae, L. M. Schrader, K. Machii et al., "Safety and tolerability of repetitive transcranial magnetic stimulation in patients with epilepsy: a review of the literature," *Epilepsy and Behavior*, vol. 10, no. 4, pp. 521–528, 2007.

[6] H. Moradi Chameh, M. Janahmadi, S. Semnanian, A. Shojaei, and J. Mirnajafi-Zadeh, "Effect of low frequency repetitive transcranial magnetic stimulation on kindling-induced changes in electrophysiological properties of rat CA1 pyramidal neurons," *Brain Research*, vol. 1606, pp. 34–43, 2015.

[7] A. Yadollahpour, S. M. Firouzabadi, M. Shahpari, and J. Mirnajafi-Zadeh, "Repetitive transcranial magnetic stimulation decreases the kindling induced synaptic potentiation: effects of frequency and coil shape," *Epilepsy Research*, vol. 108, no. 2, pp. 190–201, 2014.

[8] C.-Y. Lin, K. Li, L. Franic et al., "Frequency-dependent effects of contralateral repetitive transcranial magnetic stimulation on penicillin-induced seizures," *Brain Research*, vol. 1581, pp. 103–116, 2014.

[9] S. Van Haerents, S. T. Herman, T. Pang, A. Pascual-Leone, and M. M. Shafi, "Repetitive transcranial magnetic stimulation; a cost-effective and beneficial treatment option for refractory focal seizures," *Clinical Neurophysiology*, vol. 126, no. 9, pp. 1840–1842, 2015.

[10] J.-P. Lefaucheur, N. André-Obadia, A. Antal et al., "Evidence-based guidelines on the therapeutic use of repetitive transcranial magnetic stimulation (rTMS)," *Clinical Neurophysiology*, vol. 125, no. 11, pp. 2150–2206, 2014.

[11] S. Shorvon and M. Ferlisi, "The outcome of therapies in refractory and super-refractory convulsive status epilepticus and recommendations for therapy," *Brain*, vol. 135, no. 8, pp. 2314–2328, 2012.

[12] A. Graff-Guerrero, J. Olvera, M. Ruiz-García, U. Avila-Ordoñez, V. Vaugier, and J. C. García-Reyna, "rTMS reduces focal brain hyperperfusion in two patients with EPC," *Acta Neurologica Scandinavica*, vol. 109, no. 4, pp. 290–296, 2004.

[13] L. Hyllienmark and P. Åmark, "Continuous EEG monitoring in a paediatric intensive care unit," *European Journal of Paediatric Neurology*, vol. 11, no. 2, pp. 70–75, 2007.

[14] A. Liu, T. Pang, S. Herman, A. Pascual-Leone, and A. Rotenberg, "Transcranial magnetic stimulation for refractory focal status epilepticus in the intensive care unit," *Seizure*, vol. 22, no. 10, pp. 893–896, 2013.

[15] S. Misawa, S. Kuwabara, K. Shibuya, K. Mamada, and T. Hattori, "Low-frequency transcranial magnetic stimulation for epilepsia partialis continua due to cortical dysplasia," *Journal of the Neurological Sciences*, vol. 234, no. 1-2, pp. 37–39, 2005.

[16] O. G. Morales, M. E. Henry, M. S. Nobler, E. M. Wassermann, and S. H. Lisanby, "Electroconvulsive therapy and repetitive transcranial magnetic stimulation in children and adolescents: a review and report of two cases of epilepsia partialis continua," *Child and Adolescent Psychiatric Clinics of North America*, vol. 14, no. 1, pp. 193–210, 2005.

[17] A. Naro, L. R. Pisani, A. Leo, F. Molonia, P. Bramanti, and R. S. Calabrò, "Treatment of refractory generalized status epilepticus in a patient with unresponsive wakefulness syndrome: is neuro-modulation the future?" *Epilepsy & Behavior*, vol. 50, pp. 96–97, 2015.

[18] A. Rotenberg, E. H. Bae, M. Takeoka, J. M. Tormos, S. C. Schachter, and A. Pascual-Leone, "Repetitive transcranial magnetic stimulation in the treatment of epilepsia partialis continua," *Epilepsy and Behavior*, vol. 14, no. 1, pp. 253–257, 2009.

[19] M. Thordstein and R. Constantinescu, "Possibly lifesaving, noninvasive, EEG-guided neuromodulation in anesthesia-refractory partial status epilepticus," *Epilepsy and Behavior*, vol. 25, no. 3, pp. 468–472, 2012.

[20] M. Thordstein, G. Pegenius, A. Andreasson, and T. Hallböök, "P41—1877 Low-frequency repetitive transcranial magnetic stimulation (r-TMS) treatment in children with refractory focal epilepsy: two case reports," *European Journal of Paediatric Neurology*, vol. 17, supplement 1, p. S65, 2013.

[21] S. Van Haerents, S. Herman, T. Pang, A. Pascual-Leone, and M. Shafi, "Repetitive transcranial magnetic stimulation for refractory focal status epilepticus," *Epilepsy Currents*, vol. 15, no. 5, pp. 92–93, 2015.

[22] C. J. Wusthoff, S. M. Kranick, J. F. Morley, and A. G. C. Bergqvist, "The ketogenic diet in treatment of two adults with prolonged nonconvulsive status epilepticus," *Epilepsia*, vol. 51, no. 6, pp. 1083–1085, 2010.

[23] A. Rotenberg, D. Depositario-Cabacar, E. H. Bae, C. Harini, A. Pascual-Leone, and M. Takeoka, "Transient suppression of seizures by repetitive transcranial magnetic stimulation in a case of Rasmussen's encephalitis," *Epilepsy and Behavior*, vol. 13, no. 1, pp. 260–262, 2008.

[24] J. P. T. Higgins and S. Green, Eds., *Cochrane Handbook for Systematic Reviews of Interventions Version 5.1.0*, 2015, http://handbook.cochrane.org/.

[25] D. Moher, A. Liberati, J. Tetzlaff, and D. G. Altman, "Preferred reporting items for systematic reviews and meta-analysis: the PRISMA statement," *Annals of Internal Medicine*, vol. 151, no. 4, pp. 264–269, 2009.

[26] G. M. Brophy, R. Bell, J. Claassen et al., "Guidelines for the evaluation and management of status epilepticus," *Neurocritical Care*, vol. 17, no. 1, pp. 3–23, 2012.

[27] B. Phillips, C. Ball, D. Sackett, S. Straus, B. Haynes, and M. Dawes, "Oxford Centre for Evidence-Based Medicine Levels

of Evidence. Version 2009," June 2015, http://www.cebm.net/?o=1025.

[28] G. H. Guyatt, A. D. Oxman, G. E. Vist et al., "GRADE: an emerging consensus on rating quality of evidence and strength of recommendations," *British Medical Journal*, vol. 336, no. 7650, pp. 924–926, 2008.

[29] G. H. Guyatt, A. D. Oxman, R. Kunz, G. E. Vist, Y. Falck-Ytter, and H. J. Schünemann, "Rating quality of evidence and strength of recommendations: what is 'quality of evidence' and why is it important to clinicians?" *British Medical Journal*, vol. 336, no. 7651, pp. 995–998, 2008.

[30] H. J. Schünemann, A. D. Oxman, J. Brozek et al., "Grading quality of evidence and strength of recommendations for diagnostic tests and strategies," *British Medical Journal*, vol. 336, no. 7653, pp. 1106–1110, 2008.

[31] G. H. Guyatt, A. D. Oxman, R. Kunz et al., "Rating quality of evidence and strength of recommendations: incorporating considerations of resources use into grading recommendations," *British Medical Journal*, vol. 336, no. 7654, pp. 1170–1173, 2008.

[32] G. H. Guyatt, A. D. Oxman, R. Kunz et al., "Rating quality of evidence and strength of recommendations: going from evidence to recommendations," *British Medical Journal*, vol. 336, no. 7652, pp. 1049–1051, 2008.

[33] R. Jaeschke, G. H. Guyatt, P. Dellinger et al., "Use of GRADE grid to reach decisions on clinical practice guidelines when consensus is elusive," *British Medical Journal*, vol. 337, article a744, 2008.

24

Bridging the Gap between Evidence and Practice for Adults with Medically Refractory Temporal Lobe Epilepsy: Is a Change in Funding Policy Needed to Stimulate a Shift in Practice?

Alireza Mansouri,[1,2,3] **Abdulrahman Aldakkan,**[1,2,4] **Magda J. Kosicka,**[2]
Jean-Eric Tarride,[3] **and Taufik A. Valiante**[1,2,5,6,7]

[1]*Division of Neurosurgery, University of Toronto, Toronto, ON, Canada*
[2]*Toronto Western Hospital, University Health Network, Toronto, ON, Canada M5T 2S8*
[3]*Department of Clinical Epidemiology and Biostatistics, McMaster University, Hamilton, ON, Canada L8P 1H1*
[4]*Division of Neurosurgery, King Saud University, Riyadh, Saudi Arabia*
[5]*Institute of Medical Sciences, University of Toronto, Toronto, ON, Canada*
[6]*Division of Fundamental Neurobiology, Toronto Western Research Institute, Toronto Western Hospital, Toronto, ON, Canada M5T 2S8*
[7]*Krembil Neuroscience Center, Toronto, Canada*

Correspondence should be addressed to Alireza Mansouri; alireza.mansouri@utoronto.ca

Academic Editor: József Janszky

Objective. Surgery for medically refractory epilepsy (MRE) in adults has been shown to be effective but underutilized. Comprehensive health economic evaluations of surgery compared with continued medical management are limited. Policy changes may be necessary to influence practice shift. *Methods.* A critical review of the literature on health economic analyses for adults with MRE was conducted. The MEDLINE, EMBASE, CENTRAL, CRD, and EconLit databases were searched using relevant subject headings and keywords pertaining to adults, epilepsy, and health economic evaluations. The screening was conducted independently and in duplicate. *Results.* Four studies were identified (1 Canadian, 2 American, and 1 French). Two were cost-utility analyses and 2 were cost-effectiveness evaluations. Only one was conducted after the effectiveness of surgery was established through a randomized trial. All suggested surgery to be favorable in the medium to long term (7-8 years and beyond). The reduction of medication use was the major cost-saving parameter in favor of surgery. *Conclusions.* Although updated evaluations that are more generalizable across settings are necessary, surgery appears to be a favorable option from a health economic perspective. Given the limited success of knowledge translation endeavours, funder-level policy changes such as quality-based purchasing may be necessary to induce a shift in practice.

1. Introduction

At an approximate global prevalence of 1%, epilepsy is among the most common serious neurological disorders worldwide [1]. Despite evidence in favor of the effectiveness of surgery for medically refractory epilepsy (MRE) [2–6], referral rates for evaluation of surgical candidacy are low [7–10]. Thus, many patients are maintained on ineffective and potentially harmful antiepileptic drugs (AEDs).

The economic impact of epilepsy should not be underestimated. The direct costs account for 25% of the societal economic burden [1, 11, 12]. In addition, there are indirect [12–14] and intangible costs [15]. Although seizure frequency has been shown to have a direct correlation with resource consumption [16], with seizure-free patients consuming 1/9th the resource, these figures should be balanced against the costs associated with presurgical evaluation, surgery, and its complications, along with accounting for possibility of ineffective surgery [17]. In implementing policy changes aimed at addressing possible societal welfare losses, funding organizations must balance effectiveness and costs associated with alternative interventions. Given the increasing demand for health care, rising costs, and the scarcity of resources, comprehensive health economic evaluations are necessary ingredients for guiding the decision-making process. Such economic evaluation, particularly since the landmark randomized trial suggesting the efficacy of surgery over best medical therapy [5], is however limited.

In this study, a systematic review of the literature was conducted to critically assess health economic evaluations specifically comparing surgery against continued AEDs in adults with medically refractory TLE. The overall findings have been evaluated in terms of their generalizability to other regions/health care systems. Furthermore, current obstacles to achieving efficient and equitable outcomes for MRE patients are considered. The merits of quality-based purchasing as a potential funder-level policy modification to overcome these obstacles are discussed.

2. Methods

2.1. Electronic Search. The MEDLINE, EMBASE, and Cochrane Library electronic databases were searched on February 14th, 2015. The Centre for Reviews and Dissemination (CRD) database (containing the Database of Abstracts of Reviews of Effects, Health Technology Assessment, and the NHS Economic Evaluation Database) along with the EconLit database was also searched. No limitations were placed on date of publication or language.

2.2. Search Strategy. The MEDLINE and EMBASE databases were searched separately, based on appropriate MeSH and EMTREE terms, respectively. Further details regarding the search strategy for these and other databases can be found in Appendix I in Supplementary Material available online at http://dx.doi.org/10.1155/2015/675071. Hand searching of the references for the selected articles was used to identify further relevant studies.

2.3. Title and Abstract Review. Titles and abstracts were reviewed independently and in duplicate (AM, AA); interobserver agreement was assessed using Cohen's Kappa score. Reviews, preliminary reports, protocols, and evaluations of alternative interventions for MRE (e.g., vagal nerve stimulators) were excluded.

2.4. Full-Text Review. The selected abstracts were reviewed independently and in duplicate (AM, AA) and full-texts were included if they pertained to adults with MRE in which a health economic evaluation comparing surgery and best medical therapy at the time was conducted; simple cost-analysis studies were excluded.

2.5. Data Extraction. Characteristics of the study with regard to design, population, and approach to health economic evaluation were extracted into a data extraction form that had been piloted and approved by the authors.

3. Results

Four studies were included (Figure 1); interobserver agreement at abstract (Kappa: 0.82) and full-text (Kappa: 0.89) was almost perfect. A summary of the characteristics of the included studies, along with the reason for exclusion of additional articles following full-text review, has been provided in Table 1. The specifics of the health economic evaluation in the included studies have been provided in Table 2.

3.1. Wiebe et al. (1995) [18]. In this Canadian study, a CEA from the provider perspective was undertaken. The primary effectiveness outcome was seizure-freedom status. Costs (1993 Canadian dollars) are comprised of AEDs, perioperative care, presurgical evaluation, and physician fees. These were obtained through surveying a small sample of the regional epilepsy population, assessment of the local patient cohort, hospital cost database, and physician reimbursement fees. A decision tree was constructed with transition probabilities obtained from the literature and verified by a panel of experts who also provided estimates of probabilities when not available. The model was applied to a hypothetical cohort of 100 patients in each arm and spanned a lifetime horizon (projected 35 years) discounted at 5%. A myriad of sensitivity analyses were performed; AEDs would be more cost-effective only if seizure-free rates in surgical cohort were <41% and >30% in AED cohort. Indirect costs were not addressed.

The cost per seizure-free patients was $895,119 and $142,419 in the medical and surgical cohorts, respectively. The upfront costs of surgery were recouped by the 9th year, after which costs continued to decline compared to medical cohort. The authors concluded that AEDs account for a large fraction of costs averted by surgery and although surgical costs are high, they are outweighed by those of medical management for TLE. Furthermore, the earlier the surgery is performed, the greater the savings are.

3.2. King et al. (1997) [19]. In this American study, a CUA from the societal perspective was conducted to compare presurgical evaluation and surgery against continued AEDs for MRE patients. The outcome was QALYs, derived from the literature. AED costs were assessed through a sample of 30 patients. Indirect costs were "explored" based on future earnings. Transition probabilities within the Markov model were obtained from direct data collection, published clinical trials, expert consensus, and clinical judgment. A lifetime horizon was considered, discounted at 5%.

Surgery was assumed to confer no survival benefit, but a mortality of 0.25% was assumed. From the simulations, average accumulated and discounted lifetime costs of AEDs were $8,000 USD for the surgically treated patients and $13,000 for medically treated patients. The marginal cost

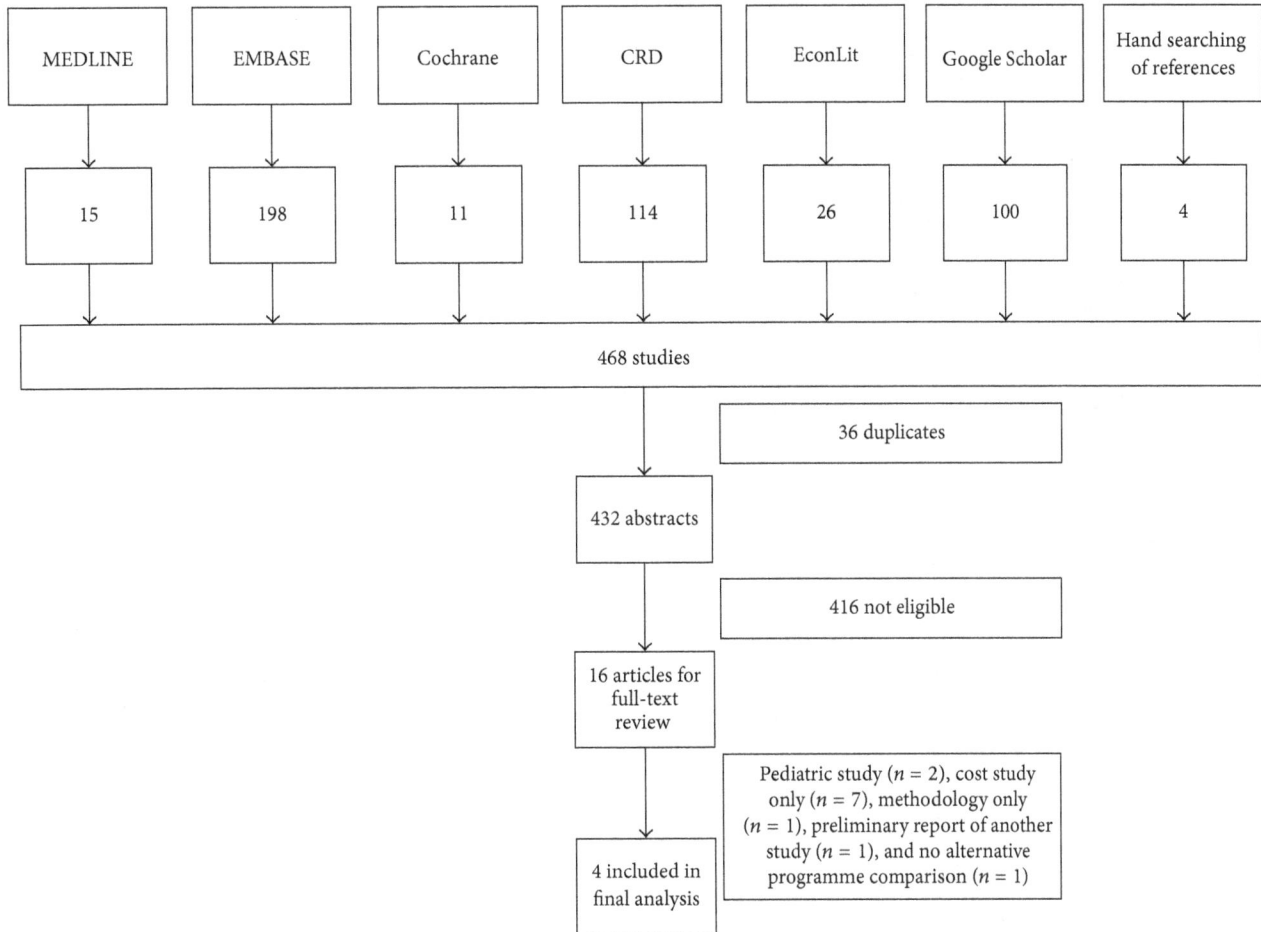

FIGURE 1: Flow diagram summarizing the results of the search strategy, followed by abstract and title screening.

for evaluating and treating those with TLE was $29,800 USD (1994). The cost per QALY was $27,200, placing it well within the $50,000 threshold of what the authors considered reasonable for acceptable interventions.

3.3. Langfitt (1997) [20]. This American study was a CUA based on QALY difference in adults with medically refractory TLE. The provider perspective was considered and only direct medical costs were included; these were estimated from the local institution charges. Presurgical evaluation costs were obtained from 25 consecutive patients at the institution (1995 USD), whereas estimates of the complication costs were obtained from two patients who sustained intracranial hematomas. Follow-up costs were estimated from the literature and were a function of the extent of seizure control [21]. The authors argued against the validity of including indirect costs. All costs were discounted at 5%. A decision tree analysis was used, incorporating probabilities obtained from published values.

Base case analysis found an ICUR of $15,581 USD/QALY for surgery, below the upper ICUR threshold of $19,000 USD/QALY at the time (1995) [22]. In addition to various issues of generalizability with both the current analysis and

that of King et al., the latter was based on an intent-to-treat analysis whereby all patients evaluated for surgical candidacy were assumed to belong to the surgical cohort; patients who are not candidates but continue on AEDs can erroneously increase costs in this cohort. Furthermore, Langfitt assumed that patients with Engel class I seizure status would not require any further follow-up, which would lower the AED and follow-up costs in the (likely more effective) surgical cohort. Sensitivity analyses suggested that efficiency of patient selection, the chance of being seizure-free after surgery, evaluation and follow-up costs, and exact estimate of QOL adjustments as a function of seizure frequency all affected the acceptability of the ICUR.

3.4. Picot et al. (2008) [23]. In this multicenter study based in France, a CEA was applied to a cohort of 280 patients with MRE (119: surgery, 161: AED). The primary effectiveness outcome was 1-year seizure-freedom rate. A Monte Carlo simulation of 1,000 patients based on the Markov transition model was used to expand the analysis to a lifetime horizon. The probability of seizure-freedom was based on study patients. Transition probabilities for the first four cycles were based on trial data while the rest were obtained from the literature. Mortality rates were assumed to be

TABLE 1: Characteristics of included and excluded studies, following full-text review.

(a) Studies that were included in final analysis

First author/year	Home nation	Study population	Source of costs	Source of outcomes	Funding	Recommendations
Wiebe/1995 [18]	Canada	MRE adults with presumed TLE (hypothetical cohort of 100 patients in each alternative option)	*Preliminary resource consumption* Survey of 33 representative local patients *Confirmation of resource use* Expert panel *Perioperative costs* Cohort of 30 consecutive local patients (1993 Cdn) *Physician costs* Provincial fee schedule (1992 Cdn)	*Clinical outcome probability estimates,* Literature search, local experience, and expert panel	N/A	Surgery is cost-effective $895,119/seizure-free patient with BMT versus $142,419/seizure-free patient with surgery Surgery dominates BMT at around 8-9 years
King/1997 [19]	USA	51 MRE adults with TLE	*Hospital costs* Cost/charge ratios from local finance department (1994 USD) *Outpatient investigations/physician costs* Medicare fee schedule (1994 USD) *AED cost* Local bulk acquisition cost (1994 USD)	*One-year seizure status,* Cohort of 51 local patients *Postoperative mortality,* Review of the literature and local data *Nonsurgical mortality,* Review of the literature *QALYs,* Review of the literature	N/A	ATL is preferred for MRE (ICUR** of surgery = $27,200/QALY)
Langfitt/1997 [20]	USA	Hypothetical cohort of MRE adults with TLE	*Medical services* Local hospital and providers plus review of the literature (1995 USD) *Surgical evaluation* Based on select cohort of 25 local patients (1991–1993 USD) *Surgical complication costs* Based on postoperative hematoma costs of 2 patients in larger operative cohort of 150 patients (1991–1993 USD) *Follow-up costs* Lifetime estimate, using local unit costs (year not clear) *AED costs* Hospital pharmacy costs based on average AED dosage (year not clear)	*Clinical event probabilities,* Review of the literature *QALY,* Review of the literature	N/A	ATL is preferred for MRE (MCUR** of surgery = $15,581/QALY)

(a) Continued

First author/year	Home nation	Study population	Source of costs	Source of outcomes	Funding	Recommendations
Picot/2008 [23]	France	280 adults with MRE thought to be surgical candidates (not necessarily TLE)	*Hospital costs* Published fees (2004 Euros) *Outpatient costs* Published professional fees (2004 Euros) *Direct, nonmedical costs* Estimated from mode of transportation, distances, and transport fees (2003 Euros), elicited from patients *Indirect costs* Working days lost, elicited from patients	*Seizure freedom rates,* Review of outcomes for 280 patients in study *Transition probabilities,* Review of the literature *Mortality rates,* General population data *Quality of life,* Questionnaires administered to patients in study	National PHRC (1998) and Pfizer	Surgery is cost-effective in medium-term projections (productivity not considered) ICER of surgery at 5 years: ~1,900 Euros/seizure-free year Surgery is cost-effective at around 7-8 years postoperatively (ICER becomes 0, direct costs only)

(b) Studies that were NOT included in final analysis

First author/year	Home nation	Title	Journal	Reason for exclusion	Main conclusions
Rao/2000 [24]	India	Is Epilepsy Surgery Possible in Countries with Limited Resources?	Epilepsia	Isolated cost analysis	(i) Surgery for MRE is feasible in developing nations (ii) Surgery is cost-effective
Platt/2002 [25]	USA	A Comparison of Surgical and Medical Costs for Refractory Epilepsy	Epilepsia	This was a cost analysis to assess the impact of incorporating direct and indirect costs	(i) Surgery is cost-effective (ii) Reduction of direct costs occurs in the long term (>10 years) (iii) Income gains more significant to society than payers; therefore, societal perspective is necessary
Picot/2004 [26]	France	Cost-Effectiveness of Epilepsy Surgery in a Cohort of Patients with Medically Intractable Partial Epilepsy—Preliminary Results	Revue Neurologique	Preliminary report of longer-term study already included in this review	Surgery was cost-effective at around 7-8 years after intervention
Chen/2014 [27]	China	Surgery: A Cost-Effective Option for Drug-Resistant Epilepsy in China	World Neurosurgery	Review of cost studies pertaining to surgery for MRE in China	Surgery is a cost-effective option for patients not responding to medications

MRE, medically refractory epilepsy; TLE, temporal lobe epilepsy, QALY, quality-adjusted life year, and AED, antiepileptic drug; BMT, best medical therapy; ICER, incremental cost-effectiveness ratio, MCER, marginal cost-effectiveness ratio, and ICUR, incremental cost-utility ratio; ATL, anterior temporal lobectomy.
** Authors reported ICER in original publication.

TABLE 2: Specific components of health economic evaluation conducted in selected studies.

First author	Type of economic evaluation	Outcome measure	Perspective	Modeling	Time horizon (years)	Discounting (rates in %)
Wiebe [18]	Intent-to-treat, CEA	Seizure freedom rate overall	Provider	Decision analysis modeling	Lifetime (35 years)	5
King [19]	Intent-to-treat, CUA*	QALY	Societal	Markov state transition model	Lifetime	5
Langfitt [20]	CUA*	QALY	Provider	Decision analysis modeling	Lifetime	5
Picot [23]	CEA alongside clinical study (280 patients total)	Seizure-freedom rate at 1 year	Societal	Monte Carlo simulation based on Markov transition model	Lifetime	3

*Although referred to as a CEA, this was technically a CUA.

the age-equivalent population rates in France. Costs included inpatient/outpatient costs (2004 Euros), direct nonmedical costs (primarily transportation related, elicited from patients, 2003 Euros), and indirect costs (health capital approach, elicited from patients). The costs associated with patients undergoing intracranial EEG monitoring (27.7%) were also included. Costs were discounted at 3%.

Seizure-freedom rates at 1 year were 81.2% and 10.1% in the surgical and AED cohorts, respectively. These differences were stable beyond year 1. TLE was the diagnosis in ~85% of the surgical patients but only 58% of the medical cohort. Differences in costs were significantly in favor of the surgical cohort beyond 2 years, primarily attributed to reduction of AEDs. At the 5th postoperative year, the ICER for 1 seizure-free year for the surgical option was 1,900 Euros (direct costs only, 2004) and surgery became dominant at 7-8 years postoperatively. This benefit was delayed by ~1 year if a discount rate of 5% or if seizure-freedom rates from the literature were used. Significant variations were also noted when considering the extremes of surgical cost. Employment status was not significantly different. The authors concluded that if only direct costs are considered and effectiveness is defined as being seizure-free for 1 year, then the surgical option is cost-effective at ~7-8 years postoperatively. ICER thresholds were not used to determine cost-effectiveness.

4. Discussion

The effectiveness of surgery for medically refractory TLE has been established through various studies [5, 6, 28, 29]. In the current study, four health economic evaluations of surgery for MRE were identified through a systematic review, only one of which had been conducted following the RCT by Wiebe et al. [5]. All concluded surgery to be a favorable alternative to continued AEDs. However, the methodological details of these studies must be considered cautiously prior to applying their findings across various settings.

4.1. Critical Evaluation. In the Wiebe study, a hypothetical cohort (with limited description of patient characteristics

such as MRE definition) was used and neither the quantity nor unit cost of many diagnostic investigations was provided. Modern day technology, costs, and practice protocol have changed since 1993. The definition of MRE used by King is no longer valid [30] and, similar to Wiebe, the cost data are likely outdated. In addition, the QALYs were based on health-related quality of life scales which had not been adjusted to reflect individual health state preferences for epilepsy patients. Furthermore, the QALYs at 1 year were summated and discounted to obtain lifetime values, assuming a constant relationship with time until death, which is not necessarily valid. Langfitt also used QALYs that had not been validated for individual health states. Furthermore, these were assumed to be dependent solely on seizure frequency. Similar to the above, cost values are likely outdated. The study by Picot was the only European study. Here an imbalance of baseline characteristics, with regard to proportion of TLE patients, was evident in the two treatment arms. Furthermore, costs were presented in aggregate format only. Together, these factors impact comparability across studies and generalizability to other settings.

Although the specific methodologies/assumptions of these studies may vary, the general conclusion is uniform. Cost analyses in other developing countries [24, 27, 31] have also demonstrated surgery to be cost-saving in the long term. Furthermore, two recent analyses conducted in Canada pertaining to children with MRE [9, 32] have also suggested the cost-effectiveness of surgery.

4.2. The Disconnect between Evidence and Practice. Despite the established effectiveness of surgery, referral rates for surgical evaluation continue to be low. In 2010, <750 individuals in Ontario (3.75% of the potential 20,000 surgical candidates) were assessed for candidacy [33]. The estimated wait-time from first seizure to surgery can be as long as 22 years [34–37]. Ontario is not unique for this "treatment gap," which is reflective of the state of epilepsy care in Canada, North America, and much of the rest of the world [7]. The medical community's skepticism toward surgery [38, 39] and variable definitions of MRE [39, 40] have contributed to these statistics. However, despite class I evidence in favor of early referral for surgical assessment, a change in practice has not been observed [41].

A delay in the comprehensive management of patients with epilepsy has various negative biopsychosocial and ethical repercussions [42–46]. The Ontario health technology assessment committee states that patients with MRE should be considered as surgical candidates unless proven otherwise [42]. The American Academy of Neurology has recommended that patients are reassessed for surgical candidacy every 3 years as part of quality-care indicators [47]. Given such positions and the limited success of knowledge translation endeavours, consideration of funder-level policy changes to promote a shift in practice may be warranted. The limitation of resources such as specially trained health care professionals and appropriate diagnostic tools is certainly a contributing factor. However, this scarcity expands across the entire economic landscape of medicine and simply increasing available resources will not be a sustainable solution. As an alternative funder-level policy adaptation, quality-based purchasing (QBP) is an option for ensuring delivery of high quality care [48]. In the following section, the strengths and limitations of various strategies toward achieving QBP are discussed.

4.3. Quality-Based Purchasing. In the principal-agent framework that describes the relationship between the funder (principal) and providers (agents) [49], the principal strives to provide necessary information and incentives to align the agent toward a unified goal: quality care. The information can be guidelines/performance targets while incentives can be financial/nonfinancial. Physician personality traits (e.g., personal motivation for improvement and altruism) are strong nonfinancial factors and should be explored [50, 51]. Related to physician personality, some suggest that providing financial incentives based on patient satisfaction surveys rather than productivity goals may be better received [52]. While reasonable, these measures are potentially subjective and therefore difficult to quantify. Consideration of options for financial incentives based on quality care criteria is discussed below.

4.4. Parameters to Consider. Any incentive scheme is likely associated with positives and negatives; careful consideration of several factors is necessary. Baseline characteristics of physicians and structure of practice are influential as habits and established practice patterns are harder to modify [53]. The perception of the target group on the attainability of the quality index matters; physicians may be more open to measures based on the structure/process of care delivery (e.g., appropriate timely referrals) compared to outcome measures (e.g., number of seizure-free patients) [54]. The decision to impose penalties or incentives is paramount; while it is conceivable that the former is more likely to be influential, the repercussions must also be considered.

4.5. Penalty-Based Schemes. The imposition of penalty-based reforms in Germany (1993) [55] and British Columbia

(early 1990s) [56] targeting the rising expenditures on medications resulted in a swift change in practice and reduction of costs. However, dissatisfaction was an issue in both cases. Imposition of funding penalties to the restricted setting of physicians/clinics caring for epilepsy patients based on well-defined referral criteria may increase referral rates with minimal adverse effects on other interventions. Considering the myriad of evidence in favor of the effectiveness (from health and economics perspective) and the established quality-based standards, this approach may be justified. However, this represents a rather antagonistic approach that decreases overall satisfaction and hampers the collaborative approach to patient care. Furthermore, physicians may choose against enrolling epilepsy patients based on concerns of being penalized for inappropriate care.

4.6. Pay-for-Performance (PFP). Incentives for performance promote a more positive approach and ideally improve quality care [57]. However, success has been limited. In Ontario (2002), a PFP strategy was initiated to optimize several preventative care services. Incentives (as high as 10% of the physicians' gross annual income) pertained to both the initiations of contact with eligible patients and of achieving cumulative preventative care targets [58]. Only modest increases were noted, likely attributable to the inability to affect patient demand, the amount of the incentive being too small, and the range of services affected by these incentives being too broad and confusing [58]. The UK NHS implemented a similar strategy though incentives were higher and yet improvement in quality of care was not observed for all intended programs; some areas not covered by the incentives declined further [59]. Elements from these and other failed initiatives provide useful insight [60, 61]. It is clear that the type of bonus matters and the amount must make the endeavour worthwhile [62, 63]. The guidelines should be simple to understand and implement [63]. The potential for "cream skimming" is a concern [60]. Furthermore, strategies are necessary to ensure care in other areas is not compromised [63]. The selection of appropriate performance targets and their appropriate measurement would be a challenge.

In Ontario, a provincial strategy for improving epilepsy care was proposed in 2011 to expand on infrastructure and to promote regionalization of care [64]. District epilepsy centers serve as nodes of contact between community physicians and regional epilepsy centers of excellence (ECEs). These districts provide initial diagnostic evaluation, connect patients with advocacy groups, provide recommendations, and coordinate with ECEs regarding further assessment and care. Such a network provides the ideal setting for the implementation of a comprehensive yet simple PFP strategy. A similar framework (e.g., accountable care organizations) can be implemented in other healthcare funding models as well [65]. The possibility for establishing and strengthening existing collaborations with patient advocacy groups within the network to increase patient awareness regarding available resources is one key benefit. Further, districts provide the ideal hub for the dissemination of evidence, guidelines, and expectations to community physicians. Reimbursing community physicians and ECE epileptologists/neurosurgeons set amounts for the *collective* management of the region's epilepsy patients recognizes all stakeholders, increasing buy-in and thus collaboration. Incentives directed at community physicians (for accepting new patients and referring MRE patients according to guidelines) and ECE physicians (for timely assessment and provision of care) can improve patient flow. To avoid "cream skimming" for patients who are good surgical candidates, a capitation approach, funding based on number and variety of epilepsy patients enrolled, would be necessary. To ensure continuity, guidelines for discharging seizure-free patients should be provided. Although the ideal size of the bonus would be challenging to determine, it must outweigh the opportunity cost for physicians. Frequent evaluation of the results and long-term financial implications of this policy change are necessary as well.

4.7. Future Directions. There is a need for updated health economic evaluations incorporating modern day costs. Ideally these would be conducted through RCTs and would be multinational to increase generalizability, particularly given the large variations in global costs of AEDs and surgery [20, 25, 31]. Although indirect costs are controversial and difficult to quantify, a systematic approach toward assessing them in epilepsy patients would be worthwhile. Furthermore, all of the studies reviewed pertained to established epilepsy centers; none considered the capital costs of establishing epilepsy centers/expanding the existing infrastructure. This is relevant considering the potential need for expansion of ECEs in anticipation of the potentially increased streamlining of referrals.

4.8. Conclusions. The expanding body of evidence and the uniform conclusions of the analyses reviewed suggest that, for MRE patients, surgery is likely to be in fact cost-saving over the long term [18, 23]. Despite published guidelines, referral rates of MRE patients for surgical evaluation continue to be low on a global level. Therefore, funding reforms may need to be considered to stimulate change. Ultimately reforms in funding alone are not sufficient until large-scale shifts in the medical culture are implemented, this may be a worthwhile alternative [66].

Conflict of Interests

None of the authors has any conflict of interests to disclose.

References

[1] E. H. Reynolds, "The ILAE/IBE/WHO epilepsy global campaign history," *Epilepsia*, vol. 43, supplement 6, pp. 9–11, 2002.

[2] J. F. Tellez-Zenteno, M. Pondal-Sordo, S. Matijevic, and S. Wiebe, "National and regional prevalence of self-reported epilepsy in Canada," *Epilepsia*, vol. 45, no. 12, pp. 1623–1629, 2004.

[3] S. S. Spencer, "When should temporal-lobe epilepsy be treated surgically?" *Lancet Neurology*, vol. 1, no. 6, pp. 375–382, 2002.

[4] S. S. Spencer, "Long-term outcome after epilepsy surgery," *Epilepsia*, vol. 37, no. 9, pp. 807–813, 1996.

[5] S. Wiebe, W. T. Blume, J. P. Girvin, and M. Eliasziw, "A randomized, controlled trial of surgery for temporal-lobe epilepsy," *The New England Journal of Medicine*, vol. 345, no. 5, pp. 311–318, 2001.

[6] J. Engel Jr., M. P. McDermott, S. Wiebe et al., "Early surgical therapy for drug-resistant temporal lobe epilepsy: a randomized trial," *The Journal of the American Medical Association*, vol. 307, no. 9, pp. 922–930, 2012.

[7] P. de Flon, E. Kumlien, C. Reuterwall, and P. Mattsson, "Empirical evidence of underutilization of referrals for epilepsy surgery evaluation," *European Journal of Neurology*, vol. 17, no. 4, pp. 619–625, 2010.

[8] G. Erba, L. Moja, E. Beghi, P. Messina, and E. Pupillo, "Barriers toward epilepsy surgery. A survey among practicing neurologists," *Epilepsia*, vol. 53, no. 1, pp. 35–43, 2012.

[9] J. M. Bowen, O. C. Snead, K. Chandra, G. Blackhouse, and R. Goeree, "Epilepsy care in Ontario: an economic analysis of increasing access to epilepsy surgery," *Ontario Health Technology Assessment Series*, vol. 12, no. 18, pp. 1–41, 2012.

[10] M. E. Lim, J. M. Bowen, O. C. Snead et al., "Access to surgery for paediatric patients with medically refractory epilepsy: a systems analysis," *Epilepsy Research*, vol. 107, no. 3, pp. 286–296, 2013.

[11] O. C. Cockerell, Y. M. Hart, J. W. A. S. Sander, and S. D. Shorvon, "The cost of epilepsy in the United Kingdom: an estimation based on the results of two population-based studies," *Epilepsy Research*, vol. 18, no. 3, pp. 249–260, 1994.

[12] C. E. Begley, M. Famulari, J. F. Annegers et al., "The cost of epilepsy in the United States: an estimate from population-based clinical and survey data," *Epilepsia*, vol. 41, no. 3, pp. 342–351, 2000.

[13] C. W. Bazil, "Comprehensive care of the epilepsy patient—control, comorbidity, and cost," *Epilepsia*, vol. 45, supplement 6, pp. 3–12, 2004.

[14] D. Heaney, "Epilepsy at work: evaluating the cost of epilepsy in the workplace," *Epilepsia*, vol. 40, supplement 8, pp. 44–47, 1999.

[15] G. A. Baker, C. Camfield, P. Camfield et al., "Commission on outcome measurement in epilepsy, 1994–1997: final report," *Epilepsia*, vol. 39, no. 2, pp. 213–231, 1998.

[16] C. E. Begley, D. R. Lairson, T. F. Reynolds, and S. Coan, "Early treatment cost in epilepsy and how it varies with seizure type and frequency," *Epilepsy Research*, vol. 47, no. 3, pp. 205–215, 2001.

[17] "National institutes of health consensus conference. Surgery for epilepsy," *The Journal of the American Medical Association*, vol. 264, no. 6, pp. 729–733, 1990.

[18] S. G. Wiebe, A. Gafni, W. T. Blume, and J. P. Girvin, "An economic evaluation of surgery for temporal lobe epilepsy," *Journal of Epilepsy*, vol. 8, no. 3, pp. 227–235, 1995.

[19] J. T. King Jr., M. R. Sperling, A. C. Justice, and M. J. O'Connor, "A cost-effectiveness analysis of anterior temporal lobectomy for intractable temporal lobe epilepsy," *Journal of Neurosurgery*, vol. 87, no. 1, pp. 20–28, 1997.

[20] J. T. Langfitt, "Cost-effectiveness of anterotemporal lobectomy in medically intractable complex partial epilepsy," *Epilepsia*, vol. 38, no. 2, pp. 154–163, 1997.

[21] C. E. Begley, J. F. Annegers, D. R. Lairson, T. F. Reynolds, and W. A. Hauser, "Cost of epilepsy in the United States: a model based on incidence and prognosis," *Epilepsia*, vol. 35, no. 6, pp. 1230–1243, 1994.

[22] A. Laupacis, D. Feeny, A. S. Detsky, and P. X. Tugwell, "How attractive does a new technology have to be to warrant adoption

and utilization? Tentative guidelines for using clinical and economic evaluations," *Canadian Medical Association Journal*, vol. 146, no. 4, pp. 473–481, 1992.

[23] M.-C. Picot, A. Jaussent, P. Kahane et al., "Medicoeconomic assessment of epilepsy surgery in adults with medically intractable partial epilepsy. Three-year outcomes from a multicenter French cohort," *Neurochirurgie*, vol. 54, no. 3, pp. 484–495, 2008.

[24] M. B. Rao and K. Radhakrishnan, "Is epilepsy surgery possible in countries with limited resources?" *Epilepsia*, vol. 41, supplement 4, pp. S31–S34, 2000.

[25] M. Platt and M. R. Sperling, "A comparison of surgical and medical costs for refractory epilepsy," *Epilepsia*, vol. 43, supplement 4, pp. 25–31, 2002.

[26] M.-C. Picot, D. Neveu, P. Kahane et al., "Cost-effectiveness of epilepsy surgery in a cohort of patients with medically intractable partial epilepsy—preliminary results," *Revue Neurologique*, vol. 160, no. 5, pp. S354–S367, 2004.

[27] J. Chen and D. Lei, "Surgery: a cost-effective option for drug-resistant epilepsy in China," *World Neurosurgery*, vol. 82, no. 1-2, pp. E375–E376, 2014.

[28] W.-H. Hu, C. Zhang, K. Zhang, F.-G. Meng, N. Chen, and J.-G. Zhang, "Selective amygdalohippocampectomy versus anterior temporal lobectomy in the management of mesial temporal lobe epilepsy: a meta-analysis of comparative studies," *Journal of Neurosurgery*, vol. 119, no. 5, pp. 1089–1097, 2013.

[29] C. B. Josephson, J. Dykeman, K. M. Fiest et al., "Systematic review and meta-analysis of standard vs selective temporal lobe epilepsy surgery," *Neurology*, vol. 80, no. 18, pp. 1669–1676, 2013.

[30] P. Kwan, A. Arzimanoglou, A. T. Berg et al., "Definition of drug resistant epilepsy: consensus proposal by the ad hoc task force of the ILAE commission on therapeutic strategies," *Epilepsia*, vol. 51, no. 6, pp. 1069–1077, 2010.

[31] I. E. Tureczek, J. Fandiño-Franky, and H.-G. Wieser, "Comparison of the epilepsy surgery programs in Cartagena, Colombia, and Zurich, Switzerland," *Epilepsia*, vol. 41, supplement 4, pp. S35–S40, 2000.

[32] E. Widjaja, B. Li, C. D. Schinkel et al., "Cost-effectiveness of pediatric epilepsy surgery compared to medical treatment in children with intractable epilepsy," *Epilepsy Research*, vol. 94, no. 1-2, pp. 61–68, 2011.

[33] Health Quality Ontario (HQO), *Making Evidence Relevant*, Ontario Health Technology Assessment Service, 2011, http://www.ontla.on.ca/library/repository/ser/255421/2011//2011no16dec.pdf.

[34] G. D. Cascino, M. R. Trenerry, E. L. So et al., "Routine EEG and temporal lobe epilepsy: relation to long-term EEG monitoring, quantitative MRI, and operative outcome," *Epilepsia*, vol. 37, no. 7, pp. 651–656, 1996.

[35] V. Salanova, O. Markand, and R. Worth, "Temporal lobe epilepsy surgery: outcome, complications, and late mortality rate in 215 patients," *Epilepsia*, vol. 43, no. 2, pp. 170–174, 2002.

[36] H. Choi, R. Carlino, G. Heiman, W. A. Hauser, and F. G. Gilliam, "Evaluation of duration of epilepsy prior to temporal lobe epilepsy surgery during the past two decades," *Epilepsy Research*, vol. 86, no. 2-3, pp. 224–227, 2009.

[37] A. T. Berg, J. Langfitt, S. Shinnar et al., "How long does it take for partial epilepsy to become intractable?" *Neurology*, vol. 60, no. 2, pp. 186–190, 2003.

[38] C. Garcia Gracia, R. Yardi, M. W. Kattan et al., "Seizure freedom score: a new simple method to predict success of epilepsy surgery," *Epilepsia* , vol. 56, no. 3, pp. 359–365, 2015.

[39] A. S. Hakimi, M. V. Spanaki, L. A. Schuh, B. J. Smith, and L. Schultz, "A survey of neurologists' views on epilepsy surgery and medically refractory epilepsy," *Epilepsy and Behavior*, vol. 13, no. 1, pp. 96–101, 2008.

[40] E. Kumlien and P. Mattsson, "Attitudes towards epilepsy surgery: a nationwide survey among Swedish neurologists," *Seizure*, vol. 19, no. 4, pp. 253–255, 2010.

[41] Z. Haneef, J. Stern, S. Dewar, and J. Engel, "Referral pattern for epilepsy surgery after evidence-based recommendations: a retrospective study," *Neurology*, vol. 75, no. 8, pp. 699–704, 2010.

[42] Epilepsy Implementation Task Force, *Provincial Guidelines for the Management of Epilepsy in Adults and Children*, Epilepsy Implementation Task Force, 2015, http://www.braininstitute.ca/sites/default/files/provincial_guidelines_for_the_management_of_epilepsy_is_adults_and_children_janurary_2015.pdf.

[43] M. W. Kellett, D. F. Smith, G. A. Baker, and D. W. Chadwick, "Quality of life after epilepsy surgery," *Journal of Neurology Neurosurgery and Psychiatry*, vol. 63, no. 1, pp. 52–58, 1997.

[44] M. R. Sperling, "The consequences of uncontrolled epilepsy," *CNS Spectrums*, vol. 9, no. 2, pp. 98–109, 2004.

[45] J. T. Langfitt and S. Wiebe, "Early surgical treatment for epilepsy," *Current Opinion in Neurology*, vol. 21, no. 2, pp. 179–183, 2008.

[46] O. Madore, "The Canada Health Act: overview and options," 2005, http://www.parl.gc.ca/content/lop/researchpublications/944-e.htm.

[47] N. B. Fountain, P. C. Van Ness, R. Swain-Eng, S. Tonn, and C. T. Bever Jr., "Quality improvement in neurology: AAN epilepsy quality measures: report of the quality measurement and reporting subcommittee of the American Academy of Neurology," *Neurology*, vol. 76, no. 1, pp. 94–99, 2011.

[48] R. A. Dudley and H. S. Luft, "Managed care in transition," *The New England Journal of Medicine*, vol. 344, no. 14, pp. 1087–1092, 2001.

[49] J. E. Hurley, *Health Economics*, Edited by J. Sturrup, McGraw-Hill Ryerson, 2010.

[50] B. S. Frey, "On the relationship between intrinsic and extrinsic work motivation," *International Journal of Industrial Organization*, vol. 15, no. 4, pp. 427–439, 1997.

[51] M. Kuhn, *Quality in Primary Care: Economic Approaches to Analysing Quality-Related Physician Behavior*, Office of Health Economics, London, UK, 2003.

[52] K. Grumbach, D. Osmond, K. Vranizan, D. Jaffe, and A. B. Bindman, "Primary care physicians' experience of financial incentives in managed-care systems," *The New England Journal of Medicine*, vol. 339, no. 21, pp. 1516–1521, 1998.

[53] R. M. Andersen, "Revisiting the behavioral model and access to medical care: does it matter?" *Journal of Health and Social Behavior*, vol. 36, no. 1, pp. 1–10, 1995.

[54] G. Amundson, L. I. Solberg, M. Reed, E. M. Martini, and R. Carlson, "Paying for quality improvement: compliance with tobacco cessation guidelines," *Joint Commission Journal on Quality and Safety*, vol. 29, no. 2, pp. 59–65, 2003.

[55] M. Hoopmann, F. W. Schwartz, and J. Weber, "Effects of the German 1993 health reform law upon primary care practitioners' individual performance: results from an empirical study in sentinel practices," *Journal of Epidemiology and Community Health*, vol. 49, supplement 1, pp. 33–36, 1995.

[56] P. Grootendorst, L. Goldsmith, J. Hurley, B. O'Brien, and L. Dolovich, "Financial incentives to dispense low-cost drugs: a case study of British Columbia pharmacare," Working Paper

96-8, McMaster University Centre for Health Economics and Policy Analysis, 1996.

[57] R. A. Berenson and E. C. Rich, "US approaches to physician payment: the deconstruction of primary care," *Journal of General Internal Medicine*, vol. 25, no. 6, pp. 613–618, 2010.

[58] J. Li, J. Hurley, P. Decicca, and G. Buckley, "PHYSICIAN response to pay-for-performance: evidence from a natural experiment," *Health Economics*, vol. 23, no. 8, pp. 962–978, 2014.

[59] S. M. Campbell, D. Reeves, E. Kontopantelis, B. Sibbald, and M. Roland, "Effects of pay for performance on the quality of primary care in England," *The New England Journal of Medicine*, vol. 361, no. 4, pp. 368–378, 2009.

[60] M. W. Friedberg, D. G. Safran, K. Coltin, M. Dresser, and E. C. Schneider, "Paying for performance in primary care: potential impact on practices and disparities," *Health Affairs*, vol. 29, no. 5, pp. 926–932, 2010.

[61] A. M. Epstein, "Pay for performance at the tipping point," *The New England Journal of Medicine*, vol. 356, no. 5, pp. 515–517, 2007.

[62] R. A. Dudley, A. Frolich, D. L. Robinowitz, J. A. Talavera, P. Broadhead, and H. S. Luft, *Strategies To Support Quality-Based Purchasing: A Review of the Evidence*, Agency for Healthcare Research and Quality, Rockville, Md, USA, 2004.

[63] T. F. Gavagan, H. Du, B. G. Saver et al., "Effect of financial incentives on improvement in medical quality indicators for primary care," *Journal of the American Board of Family Medicine*, vol. 23, no. 5, pp. 622–631, 2010.

[64] Health Quality Ontario, "Epilepsy surgery: an evidence summary," *Ontario Health Technology Assessment Series*, vol. 12, no. 1, pp. 1–28, 2012.

[65] R. Mayes and J. Walradt, "Pay-for-performance reimbursement in health care: chasing cost control and increased quality through 'new and improved' payment incentives," *Health Law Review*, vol. 19, no. 2, pp. 39–43, 2011.

[66] R. E. Mechanic and S. H. Altman, "Payment reform options: episode payment is a good place to start," *Health Affairs*, vol. 28, no. 2, pp. w262–w271, 2009.

25

The Perception of Family Function by Adolescents with Epilepsy in a Rural Nigerian Community

Edwin E. Eseigbe,[1] **Folorunsho T. Nuhu,**[2] **Taiwo L. Sheikh,**[2] **Sam J. Adama,**[3] **Patricia Eseigbe,**[4] **and Okechukwu J. Oguizu**[2]

[1] *Department of Paediatrics, Ahmadu Bello University Teaching Hospital, Zaria 810001, Nigeria*
[2] *Federal Neuropsychiatric Hospital (FNPH), Kaduna, Nigeria*
[3] *Department of Paediatrics, 44 Nigerian Army Reference Hospital, Kaduna, Nigeria*
[4] *Department of Family Medicine, Ahmadu Bello University Teaching Hospital, Zaria 810001, Nigeria*

Correspondence should be addressed to Edwin E. Eseigbe; eeeseigbe@yahoo.com

Academic Editor: Giangennaro Coppola

The family plays a significant role in epilepsy management in sub-Saharan Africa and how this role is perceived by persons with epilepsy could influence epilepsy outcomes. The objective of the study was to assess perception of family function by adolescents with epilepsy (AWE). The sociodemographic and epilepsy characteristics of AWE in a rural Nigerian community were assessed and the Family APGAR tool was used in assessing their perception of satisfaction with family functioning. Adolescents ($n = 1708$) constituted 26% of the community's population and 18 (10.5/1000) had epilepsy. The AWE age range was 11–19 years (mean 16.7 ± 2.6 years) with a male preponderance (15, 83.3%). The family was the only source of care. Family dysfunction (Family APGAR Score <7) was indicated by 15 (83.3%) of the AWE. The strongest perception of family function was in adaptability while the weakest was with growth. The indication of family dysfunction was significant ($P < 0.05$) in the older (age 14–19 years) AWE when compared with the younger AWE (11–13 years) in the study. Most of the AWE indicated living in a dysfunctional family setting. The study highlights the need to address the role of the family in the provision of comprehensive epilepsy care.

1. Introduction

Epilepsy affects 70 million persons worldwide and a high age specific incidence is associated with the adolescent population [1, 2]. The worldwide mean prevalence of epilepsy is 8.9/1000 [3]. Epilepsy prevalence rates of 4.3–26.1/1000 have been reported from several child and adolescent populations globally [4]. A significant proportion of those with the disease live in low and middle income countries (LMICs) where there is limited access to effective treatment [1, 2]. Poor outcomes of epilepsy such as stigma, depression, poor quality of life, and even death have been associated with epilepsy in the adolescent [5–11]. Ignorance, poor sociocultural epilepsy perspectives, weak health systems, epilepsy treatment gap, weak social support system, and family dysfunction are some factors that are contributory to these poor epilepsy outcomes [1–3, 5–12].

Studies have shown that adolescent perspectives on epilepsy have significant impact on the outcomes of the disease [7–10, 13, 14]. Most of these studies have been on awareness and knowledge of epilepsy and attitudes towards and the Health Related Quality of Life (HRQOL) in adolescents with epilepsy (AWE). Reports from these studies have indicated poor academic achievement, a comparatively lower HRQOL than that of the general population, lowered self-esteem, depression, poor attitudes, and a limited knowledge of epilepsy among AWE [7–10, 13, 14]. The identification of these perspectives facilitates the development and institution of interventions that could ensure adequate access to needed therapy.

In most of the LMICs statutory care or support for adolescents is lacking in health and social systems resulting in an almost total dependence on family settings for care [15].

In the African region weaknesses in health systems, stigma, and communal isolation associated with epilepsy entrust care of persons with epilepsy primarily to families and in family settings [2]. Consequently the effective functioning of the family in the region would have implications on the outcome of chronic diseases such as epilepsy.

Family functioning has been defined as the way in which family members communicate, relate, and maintain relationships among each other, as well as the way they make decisions to solve problems [16]. Satisfactory family functioning has been associated with positive outcomes in epilepsy [12, 17]. Also factors that disrupt family functioning such as low socioeconomic status, poor epilepsy awareness, stress, and parental psychopathologies have been associated with poorer epilepsy outcomes [1–3, 8, 17]. Thus outcomes in AWE in LMICs could be significantly influenced by the quality of family functioning.

Overall, the adolescent period provides opportunities and vulnerabilities with its wellbeing hinging on the development of help seeking behavior of the adolescent [15]. Perception of others and helping institutions, as helpful and trustworthy, has been identified as one of the factors that influence the help seeking behavior of adolescents [15]. Therefore in settings such as ours, where family support is the main source of care for adolescents with epilepsy, understanding adolescents' perception of this support and other family functions could have significant impact on epilepsy outcomes. Reports on AWE perception of family functioning from Nigeria are scarce. Adewuya et al. [7] reported perception of high family functioning among a majority of AWE in an urban Nigerian setting. To provide more insight on the perception of family functioning by AWE, and its impact on epilepsy outcomes, more studies are required.

The objective of the study was to assess perception of family function by AWE in a rural Nigerian community.

2. Materials and Methods

The study was conducted in Katari community of Kachia Local Government Area (LGA) in Kaduna State, northwest Nigeria. The community was randomly selected from the 22 communities that make up the LGA. The estimated population of the community is 6,572 [18]. Most of the inhabitants are small scale farmers and traders. Health care in the community is provided mainly by traditional healers, patent medicine shops, and a primary healthcare centre in the community. The nearest General Hospital to the community is 30 Km away and serves as a referral centre to Katari's PHC.

Adolescents in the community were defined as regular inhabitants of the community whose age ranged from 10 to 19 years [19]. Age was determined by evidence of birth records or corroborated oral evidence. AWE were identified via a house-to-house epilepsy survey in the community. For epidemiological surveys, and in this study, epilepsy was defined as recurrent unprovoked epileptic seizures occurring at least 24 hours apart [20, 21].

After a house-to-house survey is conducted by the authors a total of 18 adolescents were identified as having epilepsy out of a total adolescent population of 1,708 [22].

TABLE 1: Age and sex distribution of the AWE.

Age group (years)	Sex		Number of AWE (%)
	M (%)	F (%)	
11–13	4 (26.7)	0	4 (22.2)
14–16	2 (13.3)	0	2 (11.1)
17–19	9 (60)	3 (100)	12 (66.7)
Total	15 (100)	3 (100)	18 (100)

AWE: adolescents with epilepsy.

Parameters of AWE assessed included age, sex, social class, educational status, clinical features of epilepsy, current and past treatment options utilized, history of central nervous system infections, perinatal history, and assessment of intelligence using Raven's Progressive Matrix. Social class distribution was determined using the Ogunlesi et al. classification [23]. The Family APGAR tool was used in assessing perceived family function by the AWE. The tool has been validated and found to be reliable in assessing family function [24]. The Family APGAR Score uses the family's member perception of satisfaction to assess 5 dimensions of family functioning, namely, Adaptability, Partnership, Growth, Affection, and Resolve [24]. Each parameter is assessed on a 3-point scale ranging from 0 (hardly ever) to 2 (almost always). The final grading is based on the cumulative score and is graded as 0–3 (highly dysfunctional family), 4–6 (moderately dysfunctional family), and 7–10 (highly functional family) [24].

Ethical approval for the study was obtained from the Research Ethics Committee of the FNPH Kaduna. Informed consent was obtained from the community and household heads in Katari community and the AWE who were 18 years old or older while assent was obtained from those younger. A month's dose of the AED phenobarbitone was provided to all the AWE who needed to be on AED therapy but were not and they were referred to the Child and Adolescent Mental Health (CAMH) Unit of the Federal Neuropsychiatric Hospital (FNPH), Kaduna, for further management. The CAMH Unit has adequate facilities for the management of epilepsy. Furthermore, the AWE and their families were introduced to a nongovernmental organization that supports the management of persons with epilepsy and their families.

Data was analyzed using Epi Info 3.5.3 statistical package. Chi-square test, with Yates' correction where applicable, was used in determining the relationship between the characteristics of the AWE and their perception of family function. A P value less than 0.05 was regarded as significant.

3. Results

Adolescents ($n = 1708$) constituted 26% of the community's population out of which 18 (10.5/1000) had epilepsy. The age range of the subjects was 11–19 years (mean 16.7 ± 2.6 years) with a male preponderance (15, 83.3%) (Table 1). All 3 females were married but 2 were currently separated from their husbands as a result of inability of their spouses to cope with their epilepsy. All (18, 100%) were in the lower (classes IV and V) social classes. Also all had had a primary education, 4

(22%) had completed a secondary education, and 4 (22%) had experienced school rejection as a result of having epilepsy.

All the AWE had active epilepsy with generalized seizures occurring at least once weekly and monthly in 10 and 8 AWE, respectively. The seizures were tonic-clonic (12, 66.7%), tonic (5, 27.8%), and absence (1, 0.5%), respectively. All were currently on traditional herbal medication. None was currently on orthodox medical treatment even though 3 (16.7%) had accessed orthodox medical treatment, at the community's Primary Healthcare Centre (PHC), in the past. Those who visited the PHC were further referred to the nearest General Hospital for further management. After initial visits to the General Hospital, where they were seen and commenced on oral phenobarbitone, all three stopped subsequent follow-up visits and AED treatment due to financial constraints. The family was the only source of care and support for the AWE.

There was a family history of epilepsy in 8 (44.4%) of the AWE. Two (11.1%) of them were siblings, and in the remaining 6 (88.9%) AWE there was history of epilepsy in adult relatives.

There was no history of trauma to the head or that suggestive of a central nervous system infection in the AWE.

Most (14, 77.8%) of the AWE were delivered at home by traditional birth attendants while the others (4, 22.2%) were delivered in the community's PHC. The deliveries and the neonatal period of all the AWE were described as normal.

Assessment of intelligence using Raven's Progressive Matrix indicated normal intelligence in all the AWE.

Moderate family dysfunction (Family APGAR Score <7 and >3) was indicated by 15 (83.3%) of the AWE while the others (3, 16.7%) acknowledged living in a highly functional (Family APGAR > 7) setting. None indicated being in a highly dysfunctional setting. The AWE that are siblings, and all the female AWE, indicated moderate family dysfunction. The strongest perception of family function was in Adaptability while the weakest was with Growth (Table 2). The indication of family dysfunction was significant ($P < 0.05$) in the older (age 14–19 years) AWE when compared with the younger AWE (11–13 years) in the study (Table 3).

4. Discussion

The perception of family function by the AWE was predominantly dysfunctional particularly with regard to satisfaction in the Growth, Affection, and Partnership parameters of the Family APGAR. The satisfaction with the Adaptability parameter, one that assesses the family as an institution that could easily adapt and be referred to at the time of a need, was the strongest attribute of family function indicated. The study also identified the family as the only source of care and support for the AWE.

Studies have indicated that families of children with epilepsy have generally fared worse than controls [12]. Thornton et al. [12] reported poorer scores with regard to role performance among families of children with epilepsy. Additionally, these families have been found out to have lower levels of communication, family social support, and financial wellbeing [25]. Coping with frequently occurring epileptic seizures, widened epilepsy treatment gap, and lack of institutional support, which were all observed in this

study, could be quite challenging to families and impair their functioning [26]. Conversely in a study by Adewuya et al. [7] AWE rated their families as highly functional. However the study was conducted in an urban setting where most of the AWE were in more affluent mid and upper social classes and had access to AEDs as well as quality epilepsy care [7].

Studies from Nigeria indicate that AWE have perceptions of shame, depression, lowered self-esteem, and stigmatization [7–9]. Other reports also indicate poor knowledge of epilepsy, impaired HRQoL, and negative attitudes among AWE [10, 17]. To the best of our knowledge this is the first study, from northern Nigeria, that focuses specifically on the perception of AWE on family function. However the perceptions of AWE on social relationships could be gleaned from studies concerning their HRQoL. In one of such studies from southwest Nigeria, findings reported by Lagunju et al. [8] included family disruption in 50% of the families with a child who had epilepsy and marital disharmony leading to divorce in 7.6% of them. Other findings in that study included the expression of family neglect by siblings of affected children and caregivers' loss of income and financial benefits. Also the feelings of stigma, being fed up with life, inadequacy and lowered self-esteem were expressed by the children with epilepsy [8]. Also reports by Eseigbe et al. [26] and Nuhu et al. [27], from northern Nigeria, indicate stigma and socioeconomic challenges as well as significant caregiver burden in families providing care for epilepsy in childhood. The family settings in these studies are similar, and some even fairer, when compared to those in our study. The epilepsy related family burden and challenges highlighted in these studies could have influenced the poor perception of family functioning, particularly in the Family APGAR parameters of partnership (satisfaction with the way my family shares my problem with me) and Growth (satisfaction with my family's acceptance and support in my taking upon new activities), by the AWE in our study. Poor knowledge and misconceptions about epilepsy which are also common in the African region often result in fear, stigma, and discrimination among caregivers and other family members towards persons with epilepsy [2, 8, 28]. These resultant negative attitudes by family members could have contributed to the dissatisfaction associated with the Growth and Affection (satisfaction with family's expression of affection and regards towards my feelings) parameters, which were indicated by most of the AWE. The more positive responses indicated with regard to Adaptability (satisfaction with turning to my family whenever troubled) and Resolve (satisfaction with the way family and I share time together) underscores the dominant role of families in the provision of care for the AWE [26]. This role, as well as limited health and social support services for persons with epilepsy, has been reported severally from low and middle income countries (LMICs) where the burden of epilepsy is high [2].

Age was the only characteristic of the AWE that was significantly associated with perceived family dysfunction in this study. The likelihood of being more critical of relationships and having lofty expectations which increases with age could explain the significant dysfunctional appraisal by the older adolescents in the study. This could further explain the poor scores associated with the Adaptability, Growth,

TABLE 2: Distribution of optimal score (2, almost always) in the Family APGAR [11] Scores of the AWE.

Family APGAR parameter [24]	Family APGAR interpretation [24]	Number of AWE indicating optimal score (%)
Adaptability	I can turn to my family for help when something is troubling me	13 (72.2)
Partnership	I am satisfied with the way my family shares my problem with me	4 (22.2)
Growth	I am satisfied that my family accepts and supports my wishes to take on new activities	2 (11.1)
Affection	I am satisfied with the way my family expresses affection and regard to my emotions, anger, sorrow, and love	3 (16.7)
Resolve	I am satisfied with the way my family and I share time together	10 (55.6)

[24].

TABLE 3: Relationship between some variables of the AWE and their perception of family function (Family APGAR).

AWE variables	Number of AWE $n = 18$ (%)	Family APGAR		P value
		Functional $n = 3$ (%)	Dysfunctional $n = 15$ (%)	
Age (years)				
>14	14 (77.8)	0	14 (93.3)	0.01*
<14	4 (22.2)	3 (100)	1 (6.7)	
Sex				
Male	15 (83.3)	3 (100)	12 (80)	0.40*
Female	3 (16.7)	0	3 (20)	
Seizure frequency				
Weekly	10 (55.6)	3 (100)	7 (46.7)	0.29*
Monthly	8 (44.4)	0	8 (53.3)	
School rejection				
Yes	4 (22.2)	2 (66.7)	2 (13.3)	0.21*
No	14 (77.8)	1 (33.3)	13 (86.7)	
2nd school completion				
Yes	4 (22.2)	0	4 (26.7)	0.80*
No	14 (77.8)	3 (100)	11 (73.3)	
Family history (epilepsy)				
Positive	8 (44.4)	2 (66.7)	6 (40)	0.83*
Negative	10 (55.6)	1 (33.3)	9 (60)	

AWE: adolescents with epilepsy; *: with Yates' correction.

and Affection parameters of the Family APGAR. The other sociodemographic variables of the AWE did not significantly influence the perception of family function. The small sample size of the AWE and the relative homogeneity of their existing circumstances could have been accountable. Also the characteristics of epilepsy did not significantly influence the perceptions of the AWE. Epilepsy variables, particularly its severity, have been observed to correlate with greater perceived impact on the family unit [29]. The possibility of severe forms of epilepsy fostering more family attention in those affected could have had a positive influence on the perceptions of the AWE. This could have countered the negative perceptions of family function that could have arisen from the severity of the disease. Thornton et al. [12] also reported the nonsignificance of epilepsy variables on family

function even though they acknowledged that the number of those with intractable epilepsy in their study was very small.

Generally the perspectives of adolescents on issues are vital to their coping skills and health or help seeking behavior [15]. These perspectives could also influence development of abnormal behavior, psychopathology, substance abuse, and an increased risk of mortality [15]. Family function has been demonstrated to be very important in predicting adaptive, cognitive, and behavioral function in childhood epilepsy [12]. Poor academic achievement, impaired HRQoL, behavioral abnormalities, and an increased burden of disease are adverse epilepsy outcomes that have been associated with family dysfunction [8, 12, 30]. Consequently the perception and reality of family dysfunction among AWE could have grave implications for epilepsy outcomes particularly in regions where these outcomes are already grim. Dissemination of appropriate epilepsy information to the community and persons with epilepsy, improved access to treatment, provision of social support for affected families, and protection of the rights of persons with epilepsy could all strengthen family functioning and help improve its perception by AWE with desirable outcomes.

5. Limitations

The perceptions in this study were those of AWE in a rural community and of a predominantly low socioeconomic status; the perceptions of AWE in urban settings and in upper socioeconomic settings which have increased access to epilepsy care and information could be different. Also the role of family variables such as family size and presence of other chronic illnesses was not included in our study. However, majority of persons with epilepsy in LMICs live in similar settings as the AWE in this study.

6. Conclusion

The perception of living in a dysfunctional family setting was indicated by most of the AWE in a rural Nigerian community. Weak perception of satisfaction with family function was mainly with Growth (satisfaction with family's acceptance and support towards my taking on new activities) and Affection (satisfaction with family's expression of affection and regards towards my feelings) parameters of the Family APGAR assessment tool while the strongest was with Adaptability (satisfaction with turning to my family whenever troubled). The study highlights the need to address the role of the family in the provision of comprehensive epilepsy care particularly in regions with poor epilepsy outcomes.

Conflict of Interests

The authors declare that there is no conflict of interests regarding the publication of this paper.

References

[1] J. Katchanov and G. L. Birbeck, "Epilepsy care guidelines for low- and middle- income countries: from WHO mental health GAP to national programs," *BMC Medicine*, vol. 10, article 107, 2012.

[2] "Epilepsy in the World Health Organization African Region: Bridging the Gap," http://www.who.int/mental_health/management/epilepsy_in_African-region.pdf.

[3] J. H. Chin, "Epilepsy treatment in sub-Saharan Africa: closing the gap," *African Health Sciences*, vol. 12, no. 2, pp. 186–192, 2012.

[4] M. Topbaş, Ş. Özgün, M. F. Sönmez et al., "Epilepsy prevalence in the 0–17 age group in Trabzon, Turkey," *Iranian Journal of Pediatrics*, vol. 22, no. 3, pp. 344–350, 2012.

[5] R. Baskind and G. L. Birbeck, "Epilepsy-associated stigma in sub-Saharan Africa: the social landscape of a disease," *Epilepsy & Behavior*, vol. 7, no. 1, pp. 68–73, 2005.

[6] L. C. Ong, "Anxiety and depression in children with epilepsy," *Neurology Asia*, vol. 18, no. 1, pp. 39–41, 2013.

[7] A. O. Adewuya, S. B. A. Oseni, and J. A. O. Okeniyi, "School performance of Nigerian adolescents with epilepsy," *Epilepsia*, vol. 47, no. 2, pp. 415–420, 2006.

[8] I. A. Lagunju, O. Akinyinka, A. Orimadegun et al., "Health-related quality of life of Nigerian children with epilepsy," *African Journal of Neurological Sciences*, vol. 28, no. 1, 2009.

[9] C. A. Gbiri and A. D. Akingbohungbe, "Determinants of quality of life in Nigerian children and adolescents with epilepsy: a hospital-based study," *Asia Pacific Disability Rehabilitation Journal*, vol. 22, no. 3, pp. 89–96, 2011.

[10] D. Stevanovic, I. Tadic, and T. Novakovic, "Health-related quality of life in children and adolescents with epilepsy: a systematic review," in *Epilepsy in Children—Clinical and Social Aspects*, Z. P. Gadze, Ed., pp. 162–182, InTech, Rijeka, Croatia, 2011.

[11] S. D. Lhatoo and J. W. A. S. Sander, "Cause-specific mortality in epilepsy," *Epilepsia*, vol. 46, no. 11, pp. 36–39, 2005.

[12] N. Thornton, L. Hamiwka, E. Sherman, E. Tse, M. Blackman, and E. Wirrell, "Family function in cognitively normal children with epilepsy: impact on competence and problem behaviors," *Epilepsy and Behavior*, vol. 12, no. 1, pp. 90–95, 2008.

[13] G. A. Baker, S. Spector, Y. McGrath, and H. Soteriou, "Impact of epilepsy in adolescence: a UK controlled study," *Epilepsy & Behavior*, vol. 6, no. 4, pp. 556–562, 2005.

[14] C. K. Frizzell, A. M. Connolly, E. Beavis, J. A. Lawson, and A. M. Bye, "Personalised epilepsy education intervention for adolescents and impact on knowledge acquisition and psychosocial function," *Journal of Paediatrics and Child Health*, vol. 47, no. 5, pp. 271–275, 2011.

[15] G. Barker, *Adolescents, Social Support and Help-Seeking Behaviour: An International Literature Review and Programme Consultation with Recommendations for Action*, World Health Organization, Geneva, Switzerland, 2007, http://whqlibdoc.who.int/publications/2007/9789241595711_eng.pdf.

[16] A. Pujadas Botey and J. C. Kulig, "Family functioning following wildfires: recovering from the 2011 slave lake fires," *Journal of Child and Family Studies*, vol. 23, no. 8, pp. 1471–1483, 2014.

[17] M. A. Ferro, C. S. Camfield, S. D. Levin et al., "Trajectories of health-related quality of life in children with epilepsy: a cohort study," *Epilepsia*, vol. 54, no. 11, pp. 1889–1897, 2013.

[18] National Population Commission, Kaduna, Kaduna, Nigeria, 2012.

[19] State of World Population, "The Promise of Equality: Gender Equity, Reproductive Health and the Millennium Development Goals," United Nations Population Fund (UNFPA), New York, NY, USA, 2005, http://www.unfpa.org/swp/2005/pdf/en_swp05.pdf.

[20] Commission on Epidemiology and Prognosis of the International League Against Epilepsy, "Guidelines for epidemiologic studies on epilepsy," *Epilepsia*, vol. 34, no. 4, pp. 592–596, 1993.

[21] R. S. Fisher, C. Acevedo, A. Arzimanoglou et al., "ILAE official report: a practical clinical definition of epilepsy," *Epilepsia*, vol. 55, no. 4, pp. 475–482, 2014.

[22] E. E. Eseigbe, T. L. Sheikh, A. Aderinoye et al., "Factors associated with treatment gap in children and adolescents with epilepsy in a rural Nigerian community," *Nigerian Journal of Paediatrics*, vol. 41, no. 1, pp. 22–27, 2014.

[23] T. A. Ogunlesi, I. O. F. Dedeke, and O. T. Kuponiyi, "Socioeconomic classification of children attending specialist paediatric centres in Ogun State, Nigeria," *The Nigerian Medical Practitioner*, vol. 54, no. 1, pp. 21–25, 2008.

[24] G. Smilkstein, "The family APGAR: a proposal for a family function test and its use by physicians," *The Journal of Family Practice*, vol. 6, no. 6, pp. 1231–1239, 1978.

[25] J. K. Austin, "Childhood epilepsy: child adaptation and family resources," *Journal of Child and Adolescent Psychiatric and Mental Health Nursing*, vol. 1, no. 1, pp. 18–24, 1988.

[26] E. E. Eseigbe, T. L. Sheikh, and F. T. Nuhu, "Childhood epilepsy in a tropical child psychiatric unit: challenges of providing care in a resource-constrained environment," *Annals of African Medicine*, vol. 12, no. 4, pp. 236–242, 2013.

[27] F. T. Nuhu, A. J. Yusuf, A. Akinbiyi et al., "The burden experienced by family caregivers of patients with epilepsy attending the government psychiatric hospital, Kaduna, Nigeria," *The Pan African Medical Journal*, vol. 5, article 16, 2010.

[28] F. T. Nuhu, J. O. Fawole, O. J. Babalola, O. O. Ayilara, and Z. T. Sulaiman, "Social consequences of epilepsy: a study of 231 Nigerian patients," *Annals of African Medicine*, vol. 9, no. 3, pp. 170–175, 2010.

[29] C. Camfield, L. Breau, and P. Camfield, "Impact of pediatric epilepsy on the family: a new scale for clinical and research use," *Epilepsia*, vol. 42, no. 1, pp. 104–112, 2001.

[30] D. W. Dunn, "Neuropsychiatric aspects of epilepsy in children," *Epilepsy & Behavior*, vol. 4, no. 2, pp. 101–106, 2003.

26

Caregiver Burden in Epilepsy: Determinants and Impact

Ioannis Karakis,[1] Andrew J. Cole,[2] Georgia D. Montouris,[3] Marta San Luciano,[4] Kimford J. Meador,[1,5] and Charitomeni Piperidou[6]

[1] *Department of Neurology, Emory University School of Medicine, Atlanta, GA, USA*
[2] *MGH Epilepsy Service, Massachusetts General Hospital, Harvard Medical School, Boston, MA, USA*
[3] *Department of Neurology, Boston Medical Center, Boston University School of Medicine, Boston, MA, USA*
[4] *Department of Neurology, University California San Francisco, San Francisco, CA, USA*
[5] *Department of Neurology, Stanford School of Medicine, Stanford, CA, USA*
[6] *Department of Neurology, Democritus University of Thrace, Alexandroupolis, Greece*

Correspondence should be addressed to Ioannis Karakis; ioannis.karakis@emory.edu

Academic Editor: Raffaele Manni

Aim. Caregiver burden (CB) in epilepsy constitutes an understudied area. Here we attempt to identify the magnitude of this burden, the factors associated with it, and its impact to caregiver quality of life (QOL). *Methods.* 48 persons with epilepsy (PWE) underwent video-EEG monitoring and their caregivers completed questionnaires providing demographic, disease-related, psychiatric, cognitive, sleep, QOL, and burden information. *Results.* On regression analysis, higher number of antiepileptic drugs, poorer patient neuropsychological performance, lower patient QOL score, and lower caregiver education level were associated with higher CB. Time allocated to patient care approximated but did not attain statistical significance. A moderate inverse correlation between CB and caregiver QOL physical component summary score and a stronger inverse correlation between CB and caregiver QOL mental component summary score were seen. *Conclusion.* In a selected cohort of PWE undergoing video-EEG monitoring, we identified modest degree of CB, comparable to that reported in the literature for other chronic neurological conditions. It is associated with specific patient and caregiver characteristics and has a negative effect on caregiver QOL.

1. Introduction

Epilepsy is an unpredictable, often chronic and debilitating disorder that impacts not only those bearing with it but also those who care for them. Epilepsy is thought to affect more than 100 million individuals and their families worldwide at some point of their lives, thus constituting a major, universal, public health issue [1].

It is well established that epilepsy impacts the quality of life (QOL) of patients. Loss of control and independence, low self-esteem, fear, depression, stigmatization, lifestyle, social and employment restrictions, and financial strains are ways in which this impact occurs [2]. The same factors also indirectly affect care providers for those patients.

In contrast to other chronic medical conditions such as congestive heart failure [3], chronic obstructive pulmonary disease [4], chronic renal failure [5], cancer [6], and chronic neurological disorders such as stroke [7], Alzheimer's disease [8], Parkinson's disease [9], multiple sclerosis [10], amyotrophic lateral sclerosis [11], traumatic brain [12], or spinal cord injury [13], the impact of epilepsy on the family constitutes an understudied area. As illustrated in Figure 1, despite being the fourth most common neurological condition, caregiver burden in epilepsy has attracted disproportionally less attention than in less prevalent neurological conditions such as Alzheimer's disease, multiple sclerosis, Parkinson's disease, and amyotrophic lateral sclerosis. When caregiver burden and QOL-related issues have been explored, most studies have focused on the pediatric population [2, 14–28]. The data on caregivers of adult patients remains sparse [29–35] and most studies have been performed outside the United States.

Given the scarcity in the literature in this area, we sought to quantify caregiver burden in epilepsy, determine

Caregiver Burden publications per disease prevalence

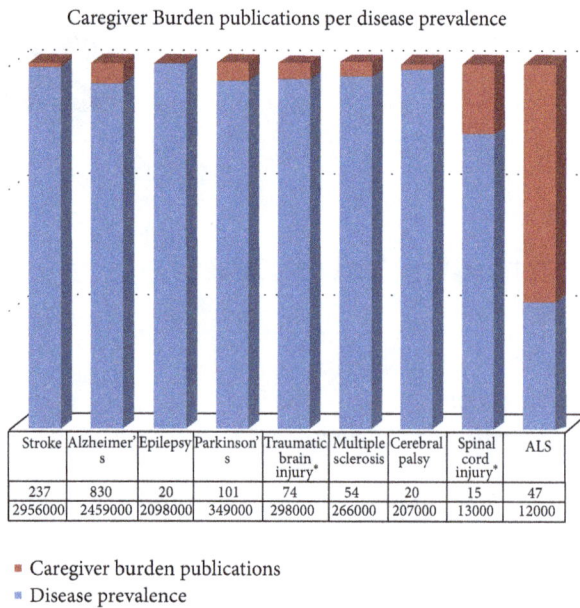

	Stroke	Alzheimer's	Epilepsy	Parkinson's	Traumatic brain injury*	Multiple sclerosis	Cerebral palsy	Spinal cord injury*	ALS
	237	830	20	101	74	54	20	15	47
	2956000	2459000	2098000	349000	298000	266000	207000	13000	12000

- Caregiver burden publications
- Disease prevalence

FIGURE 1: Publications on caregiver burden (pubmed search, accessed April 2013) for various neurologic disorders in proportion to disease prevalence (incidence for disease with *) [48].

the relative contributions of patient- and caregiver-related factors, and ascertain the impact that this burden has to the caregiver health-related QOL. We also identify implications of our findings and future directions in the field of caregiver burden and QOL in epilepsy both from clinical and research standpoints.

2. Methods

2.1. Participants. This is a cross-sectional study conducted between September 2009 and June 2011 at Massachusetts General Hospital (MGH). Adult patients admitted electively to the Epilepsy Monitoring Unit (EMU) for continuous video-EEG monitoring were asked to participate by completing a series of questionnaires and undergoing bed-side cognitive evaluation. Patients who were non-English speakers or unable to read and write due to cognitive impairment were excluded. Caregivers who accompanied them were also asked to complete questionnaires. Caregiver was defined as the family member who was primarily responsible for providing every-day care for the patient. After the monitoring was completed, only the patients with documented epileptic seizures whose caregivers completed their questionnaires were included in the analysis, while patients without a caregiver participant or patients with nonepileptic seizures, mixed disorder, or unclear diagnosis were excluded along with their caregivers. Out of 190 admissions during this study period, 14 were invasive recordings where the anesthesia/postoperative state of the patients may have interfered with their ability to reliably answer all surveys administered and another 12 admissions were repeated admissions. The total number of admitted available patients was therefore 164, out of which 126 were elected to participate leading

to responder's rate of approximately 77%. From those, 80 were proven to have epilepsy. The remaining 46 patients were diagnosed with psychogenic or other non epileptic events, mixed epileptic and nonepileptic events or had no events recorded during their stay. 48 of the 80 persons with epilepsy (PWE) had a caregiver escorting them to the EMU and those 48 patient-caregiver pairs comprised the final study population. Consent for participation was obtained from all eligible available caregivers. More male patients had an available caregiver present. Otherwise, PWE with an available caregiver did not differ significantly compared to those without one. That recruitment process yielded 48 PWE-caregiver pairs which was the focus of the study. The study was approved by the institutional review board.

2.2. Questionnaires and Procedures. Participating patients completed questionnaires providing demographic (age, gender, race, religion, employment, education, living situation, and marital status) and epilepsy-related (age of epilepsy onset, epilepsy duration in years, average number of seizures per month in the past year, number of AED, and self-reported compliance) information. The information collected was cross-validated with medical records review.

Anxiety and depression levels were measured using the Beck anxiety [36] and Beck depression [37] inventories, respectively. Those are 21-item inventories that assess the presence and degree of affective, cognitive, motivational, and psychomotor components. Each item is scored from 0 to 3 and the aggregate score is 0–63. Higher scores depict higher levels of psychopathology (depression: 1–10: normal, 11–16: mild depression, 17–20: borderline depression, 21–30: moderate depression, 31–40: severe depression, and >41: extreme depression; anxiety: 0–21: very low anxiety, 22–35: moderate anxiety, and >36: high anxiety). Both have been extensively used previously in epilepsy research [38]. Sleep quality was assessed by completing the Epworth sleepiness scale [39] and the sleep apnea section of the sleep disorder questionnaire (SDQ-SA) [40]. The Epworth sleepiness scale is a brief questionnaire rating the chances that they would doze off or fall asleep when in eight different situations commonly encountered in daily life. A score of 0–3 is given to each situation and the aggregate score is 0–24. Higher scores are suggestive of higher sleepiness level (a cutoff of >10 is generally interpreted as daytime sleepiness) [39]. While not specific to patients with epilepsy, it has been widely used to assess sleepiness in a host of diseases including epilepsy [41]. The SDQ-SA has also been commonly applied to the epilepsy population [42]. A score equal to or more than 36 for men and 32 for women is considered to have approximately 80% sensitivity and specificity for polysomnographically proven sleep apnea [40]. QOL was evaluated by completing the QOLIE-31 instrument. QOLIE-31 is one of the most commonly applied QOL instruments in epilepsy with good reliability and validity [43]. The 31-item self-administered questionnaire has seven subscales: seizure worry, overall QOL, emotional well-being, energy/fatigue, cognitive function, medication effects, and social functioning. A score ranging from 1 to 100 is obtained from each subscale with higher scores indicating better QOL. Cognitive evaluation was performed by a neurologist via administration of the Montreal Cognitive Assessment (MoCA) test [44]. This is a brief screening tool that has been shown to be superior to the commonly used minimental status examination for the detection of mild cognitive impairment in the epilepsy population [45]. By assessing multiple cognitive functions (visuospatial/executive, naming, memory, attention, language, abstraction, delayed recall, and orientation) an aggregate score of 0–30 is created. Higher scores are associated with better cognitive state (a cutoff of <26 is considered abnormal). All these evaluations took place on the day of the admission under electrographic guidance to ensure the absence of subclinical electrographic seizure activity affecting some of the responses. At the time of the testing, the patients were maintained on their home AED(s) and had not been yet sleep deprived with the intent that their answers would be representative of their baseline state in the ambulatory setting.

Caregivers accompanying the patients also completed questionnaires providing demographic information (age, gender, race, religion, employment, education, marital status, cohabitation, and time spent for patient care in hours per week). The latter was loosely defined as the time devoted to everyday activities where caregiver participation was indispensable including AED provision, outpatient and emergency department visits, and driving for any patient-related activity. Given the lack of a disease-specific questionnaire to assess their burden, the Zarit caregiver burden inventory was used. This is a 22-item inventory derived from the original 29-item inventory [46]. It is the most widely used standardized, validated scale to assess caregiver burden, administered previously in various neurological disorders, including epilepsy [14, 34]. The 22 items evaluate the effect of disease on the caregiver's QOL, psychological suffering, financial difficulty, shame, guilt, and difficulty in social and family relationships. Scores range from 0 to 88 with higher scores indicating higher burden (<20: little or no burden, 21–40: mild-to-moderate burden, 41–60: moderate-to severe burden, 61–88: severe burden). Their health-related QOL was assessed by administering the second version of the SF-36 generic questionnaire (SF36v2) [47]. This is a generic QOL instrument that assesses eight health concepts (physical functioning, role limitation caused by physical problems, bodily pain, general health perception, vitality, social functioning, role limitation caused by emotional problems, and mental health). Scores standardized to norms and weighted averages are used to create a physical component summary (PCS) and a mental component summary (MCS) composed by the first and last four of the aforementioned health concepts, respectively. All health dimension scores are standardized to normal by employing a linear transformation of data originally scored on a 0–100 scale Norm-based scores have a mean of 50 and a standard deviation of 10 in the general US population. Therefore, any score <50 for any health dimension and component scale falls below the general population mean and each point represents 1/10 of a standard deviation. This allows direct comparison among different populations [47] and has established precedence in epilepsy caregiver research.

Various paraclinical (e.g., laboratory, electroencephalographic and radiological) data were collected as part of standard of care. Routine AED levels were drawn on admission prior to initiation of gradual withdrawal. For patients on more than one AED, they were deemed to be above, within, or below the antiepileptic drug reference range of their regimen depending on the serum level of the majority of drugs in their regimen. EEG data pertained to the initial recording during the completion of the questionnaires (normal, slow, epileptiform) including the maximal posterior dominant rhythm at the time of completion and the final epilepsy monitoring unit report for classification of their seizure type (partial with or without secondary generalization and primarily generalized), epilepsy type (unitemporal right or left, bitemporal, extratemporal right or left, multilobar or idiopathic generalized epilepsy), and etiology (symptomatic, cryptogenic, or idiopathic). Radiological data included findings of the last patient's brain magnetic resonance imaging (normal, mesial temporal sclerosis, diffuse atrophy, vascular, developmental, or other abnormality) obtained before, during, or right after this monitoring.

2.3. Analysis. Summary scores were created for all the aforementioned variables and descriptive statistics were used. Univariate associations between the Zarit burden score as the outcome of interest and the various patient and caregiver related predictors were explored by using t-test or one-way ANOVA and Pearson correlation or nonparametric equivalents when appropriate. Statistical significance was set at 0.05. Those variables identified as statistically significant in the univariate analysis were subsequently fitted in a multivariate linear regression model in order to conduct an adjusted evaluation of associated factors of caregiver burden. Finally, Pearson correlation coefficient was used to investigate the association between the caregiver burden score and each of the caregiver QOL scale score. Statistical analysis was performed in SAS 9.3 (North Carolina) and STATA 11 (College Station, TX).

3. Results

Demographics are detailed in Table 1. The mean age of the patients was 36 years. The majority of the patients were men, Caucasian, and had obtained higher education. Nearly half were married and two-thirds were employed. Patients had epilepsy for approximately 16 years, averaging 4 seizures per month, mainly partial with secondary generalization and taking on average 2 AED. The majority had symptomatic temporal lobe epilepsy. Their AED levels on admission were mostly in the reference range and their average score on the MoCA assessment of cognitive function was 25. Their average depression score was nearly 11, and anxiety score was 13. Mean Epworth sleepiness scale score was 8 and mean SDQ-SA score was approximately 25. The overall QOLIE-31 score was nearly 56.

The mean age of the caregivers was 46. Most were Caucasian women, married, employed, of higher education, and cohabitated with the patients they cared for. Their average

TABLE 1: Subject characteristics.

(a) Patient characteristics

	Epilepsy patients $N = 48$
Demographic characteristics	
Age (mean ± SD)	36.52 ± 12.47
Gender (n, % female)	28 (58.33%)
Race (n, % caucasian)	45 (93.75%)
Religion (n, % Christian)	38 (80.85%)
Employment (n, % employed)	32 (66.67%)
Education (n, % some college and beyond)	38 (79.17%)
Living situation (n, % living with family or others)	44 (91.67%)
Marital status (n, % married)	23 (47.92%)
Epilepsy characteristics	
Age of onset of epilepsy (mean ± SD)	19.75 ± 14.71
Duration of epilepsy in years (mean ± SD)	16.05 ± 13.58
Number of seizures per month (median, IQR)	4 (6)
Number of AED (median, IQR)	2 (2)
Compliance (n, % compliant)	39 (84.78%)
Type of seizures	
Partial without generalization	12 (25%)
Primarily generalized	4 (8.3%)
Partial with secondary generalization	32 (66.67%)
Etiology	
Symptomatic	31 (64.58%)
Cryptogenic	13 (27.08%)
Idiopathic	4 (8.33%)
Paraclinical characteristics	
AEDs level	
Within reference range	27 (75%)
Below reference range	5 (13.89%)
Above reference range	4 (11.11%)
EEG posterior dominant rhythm	9.43 ± 1.15
EEG findings	
Slowing	6 (12.77%)
Interictal spikes	23 (48.94%)
Normal	18 (38.30%)
EMU diagnosis	
Left TLE	14 (29.17%)
Right TLE	13 (27.08%)
Bitemporal	2 (4.17%)
Left extra-TLE	8 (16.67%)
Right extra-TLE	2 (4.17%)
Multilobar	5 (10.42%)
IGE	4 (8.33%)
MRI Findings (n, % abnormal)	33 (68.75%)

(a) Continued.

	Epilepsy patients $N = 48$
Neuropsychological and sleep characteristics	
Montreal Cognitive Assessment Score (MoCA)	25 ± 4.22
Beck Depression Inventory	10.93 ± 8.65
Beck Anxiety Inventory	13.02 ± 11.08
Epworth Sleepiness Scale	8.19 ± 4.19
Sleep disordered questionnaire for sleep apnea (SDQ-SA)	24.70 ± 8.91
Quality of life characteristics (QOLIE-31)	
Seizure worry	48.53 ± 30.23
Overall quality of life	61.68 ± 22.27
Emotional Wellbeing	64.57 ± 20.94
Energy/Fatigue	46.46 ± 22.42
Cognitive Functioning	55.35 ± 25.76
Medication Effects	49.09 ± 25.86
Social Functioning	51.60 ± 29.69
Overall Score	55.98 ± 18.44

SD: standard deviation, IQR: inter-quartile range, AEDs: antiepileptic drugs, EMU: epilepsy monitoring unit, EEG: electroencephalogram, TLE: temporal lobe epilepsy, IGE: idiopathic generalized epilepsy, MRI: magnetic resonance imaging, QOLIE-31: Quality of Life 31 questionnaire.

(b) Caregiver characteristics

	Caregivers $N = 48$
Demographic characteristics	
Age (mean ± SD)	46.18 ± 13.20
Gender (n, % female)	33 (68.75%)
Race (n, % caucasian)	45 (93.75%)
Religion (n, % Christian)	36 (75%)
Relationship to patient (n, %)	
Spouse/partner	28 (58.34%)
Parent/sibling	18 (37.50%)
Other	2 (4.17%)
Employment (n, % employed)	34 (70.83%)
Education (n, % some college and beyond)	39 (81.25%)
Marital status (n, % married)	38 (79.17%)
Cohabitation with patient (n, %)	43 (89.58%)
Time spent for patient care (hours) per week	11.43 ± 21.22
Quality of life characteristics (SF36v2)	
Physical Component Summary (PCS)	53.91 ± 8.86
Mental Component Summary (MCS)	45.51 ± 11.31
Burden characteristics	
Zarit Burden Inventory	20.02 ± 14.47

SD: standard deviation, SF36v2: short form 36 health survey version 2.

TABLE 2: Caregiver burden in epilepsy compared to other chronic neurological conditions.

Author/year	Disease	Caregivers number	Zarit burden interview mean score
Carod-Artal et al., 2009 [7]	Stroke	200	27.2
Schölzel-Dorenbos et al., 2009 [8]	Alzheimer's disease	97	12.8
Martínez-Martín et al., 2007 [9]	Parkinson's disease	79	26.5
Rivera-Navarro et al., 2009 [10]	Multiple sclerosis	278	22
Pagnini et al., 2011 [11]	Amyotrophic lateral sclerosis	37	19.5
Bayen et al., 2013 [12]	Traumatic brain injury	66	25.1
Current study	Epilepsy	48	20

Zarit burden score was 20, that is, on the cusp of mild-to-moderate range, overall comparable with other chronic neurological conditions where the same burden questionnaire was applied (Table 2). The physical component scale of their QOL score averaged 54 points, while the mental component scale averaged 45 points.

In the univariate analysis, higher AED number, lower patient's neuropsychological scores, lower scores in many of the subscales of patient's QOL scale (i.e., seizure worry, emotional well-being, cognitive functioning, and social functioning) including the overall score as well as lower caregiver education level, and increase in the time spent with the patient were shown to be associated with higher disease burden to the caregiver (Table 3). In the multivariate analysis, the same factors of caregiver burden were confirmed but time allocated to patient care approximated but did not retain statistical significance (Table 4).

There were a statistically significant moderate inverse correlation between caregiver burden and caregiver QOL physical component summary score ($r = -0.35$, $P = 0.01$) and a stronger inverse correlation between caregiver burden and caregiver QOL mental component summary score ($r = -0.57$, $P \leq 0.0001$) (Figure 2).

4. Discussion

In this selected cohort of PWE undergoing video-telemetry and their caregivers, we identified the following: (a) epilepsy is associated with modest degree of burden to the caregiver, which is overall comparable to burden from other chronic neurologic conditions reported in the literature; (b) the number of AED, the patient's neuropsychological state, the patient's quality of life, and caregiver education are associated with caregiver burden; and (c) caregiver burden has a negative impact on caregiver health-related quality of life.

As illustrated in Table 2, regardless of differences in the pathophysiology of other neurological disorders and methodological variability in their research, the identified magnitude of caregiver burden in epilepsy in our study is overall comparable to other neurological conditions where similar instruments were administered, including stroke [7], Alzheimer's disease [8], Parkinson's disease [9], multiple sclerosis [10], amyotrophic lateral sclerosis [11], and traumatic brain [12] or spinal cord injury [13]. In addition to the chronicity seen in those neurological conditions, epilepsy

can often start much earlier in life; it is characterized by a paroxysmal course that introduces the unique strain of unpredictability and it is related to high grade of stigmatization. Also, caregiver QOL scores in other neurological conditions do not deviate significantly from what is reported here for epilepsy, when similar scales were used. This further underscores the aforementioned disparity between caregiver research in the 4th most common neurological condition (past migraine, stroke, and Alzheimer) [48] compared to less prevalent diseases.

Our prior knowledge of the caregiver burden in epilepsy and its associated effect on caregiver QOL is deficient. Most extant studies have focused on the pediatric population. In the adult population, most studies have been performed in the outpatient setting and outside the United States. In particular, outpatient studies performed in the Netherlands identified a trend of decreased mental component of QOL in caregivers of refractory patients [33]. No specific patient or disease characteristic appeared to drive caregiver QOL [33]. On the contrary, caregiver self-perceived burden of care [33] and coping style [32] were deemed to be more reliable indicators. Using a control group for comparison, a study of 257 caregivers escorting patients to outpatient clinics in Sudan revealed lower QOL scores for caregivers who were children of the patients, female, and had lower education attainment [35]. Another study of 231 caregivers of patients attending an outpatient clinic in Nigeria identified a median Zarit burden score of 25 [30]. Higher burden was associated with younger patient's age, patient's unemployment, longer disease duration, shorter periods of seizure freedom, family history of epilepsy, and rural residence, possibly accounting for poorer access to health care [30]. In Brazil, Westphal-Guitti et al. compared 50 adolescent and adult patients with juvenile myoclonic epilepsy (JME) and another 50 with temporal lobe epilepsy (TLE) along with their caregivers [34]. Mild-moderate caregiver burden, averaging 22 for JME and 30 for TLE in the Zarit scale, was identified. For JME patients that burden correlated with poorer emotional, social, and physical domains of the caregivers' QOL measured with SF-36, while for TLE patients the emotional component was primarily affected [34]. Another study of 65 patient-caregiver pairs from Hong Kong identified below average scores on the QOL measure applied and severe levels of depression and anxiety in 14% and 22% of caregivers, respectively [29]. The authors indicated that seizure severity and age at onset are negatively correlated with psychosocial adjustment of

TABLE 3: Factors associated with caregiver burden: univariate analysis.

(a) Patient characteristics associated with caregiver burden

Variable	P value
Demographic characteristics	
Patient age	0.79
Patient gender	0.77
Patient race	0.62
Patient religion	0.85
Patient employment	0.48
Patient education	0.83
Living situation	0.07
Marital status	0.76
Epilepsy characteristics	
Age of onset epilepsy	0.36
Duration of epilepsy	0.16
Number of seizures per month	0.89
Number of AEDs	**0.0009 (r = 0.46)**
Compliance	0.40
Type of seizures	0.78
Etiology	0.52
Paraclinical characteristics	
AEDs level	0.70
EEG posterior dominant rhythm	0.58
EEG findings	0.95
EMU diagnosis	0.51
MRI findings	0.10
Neuropsychological and sleep characteristics	
Patient MoCA	**0.003 (r = −0.41)**
Patient Beck Depression	0.18
Patient Beck Anxiety	0.10
Patient Epworth	0.11
Patient SDQ-SA	0.84
Quality of life characteristics (QOLIE-31)	
Seizure worry	**0.005 (r = −0.39)**
Overall quality of life	0.07
Emotional well-being	**0.04 (r = −0.30)**
Energy/Fatigue	0.4413
Cognitive functioning	**0.006 (r = −0.39)**
Medication effects	0.32
Social Functioning	**0.05**
Overall score	**0.004 (r = −0.40)**

(b) Caregiver characteristics associated with caregiver burden

Variable	P-value
Age	0.15
Gender	0.50
Race	0.62
Religion	0.44
Relationship to patient	0.16
Employment	0.94

(b) Continued.

Variable	P-value
Education	**0.05 (r = −0.27)**
Marital status	0.60
Cohabitation	0.44
Time spent for patient care	**0.01 (r = 0.37)**

caregivers; on the other hand, perceived support level had a positive impact in their well-being and QOL [29]. Earlier exploratory investigation of 44 families living with epilepsy in the United Kingdom suggested increased levels of anxiety and depression in caregivers of patients with severe drop attacks and history of status epilepticus [31]. Social dissatisfaction and low levels of support were again voiced as major concerns by the caregivers [31].

Our findings partially concur with the preexisting literature. Similar to Westphal-Guitti et al. [34] and Tajudeen Nuhu et al. [30], we were also able to identify burden related to the care of patients with epilepsy, yet relatively milder than previously reported. In agreement with the Brazilian [34] and the Dutch studies [33], we also recognized heavier impact in the mental component of caregiver QOL. The variability of burden magnitude and predictors reported in the literature including our study probably accounts for the broad difference in study populations, the multifaceted nature of epilepsy, and the variable research methodology applied.

There are certain advantages to our study. The focus was on adult patients, where most of the literature is sparse, who could complete the surveys independently. That prevented potential bias inevitably incurred by proxy-reports in the pediatric caregiver literature [49]. The patients recruited had well-defined epilepsy proven with inpatient video-EEG monitoring. That excluded potential misclassification that may inadvertently occur when such methods are applied in the outpatient setting. We monitored and minimized factors that may have interfered with patient's testing such as seizures or commonly applied procedures in the EMU (e.g., antiepileptic medication withdrawal or sleep deprivation). Cross-reference with medical records provided an additional checkpoint for accuracy. The data collected were thorough and covered most of the parameters reported to be associated with health-related QOL in epilepsy, including paraclinical data such as AED levels, an understudied field previously. Thus, multiple patient- and caregiver-related factors were taken into account when assessing caregiver burden.

On the other hand, there are limitations to acknowledge. First, self-reporting nature of the study bears a risk of recall bias. Yet, self-report scales are widely used, cost-effective methods for both diagnostic assessment and for outcome evaluation. Admittedly though they are not as exhaustive and objective as standardized cognitive and psychiatric interviews or physiologic sleep recording procedures. Second, the modest sample size of caregiver participants may have underpowered our study for the detection of additional associations. Third, despite the extensive evaluation of patient-associated factors, caregiver-related aspects that may have

TABLE 4: Factors associated with caregiver burden: multivariate analysis.

Variable	Beta coefficient	Standard error	P value
Number of AEDs	5.14	2.03	**0.01**
Patient MoCA	−0.78	0.38	**0.05**
QOLIE-31 overall score	−0.22	0.09	**0.02**
Caregiver education	−11.76	3.98	**0.005**
Time spent for patient care	0.15	0.08	0.06

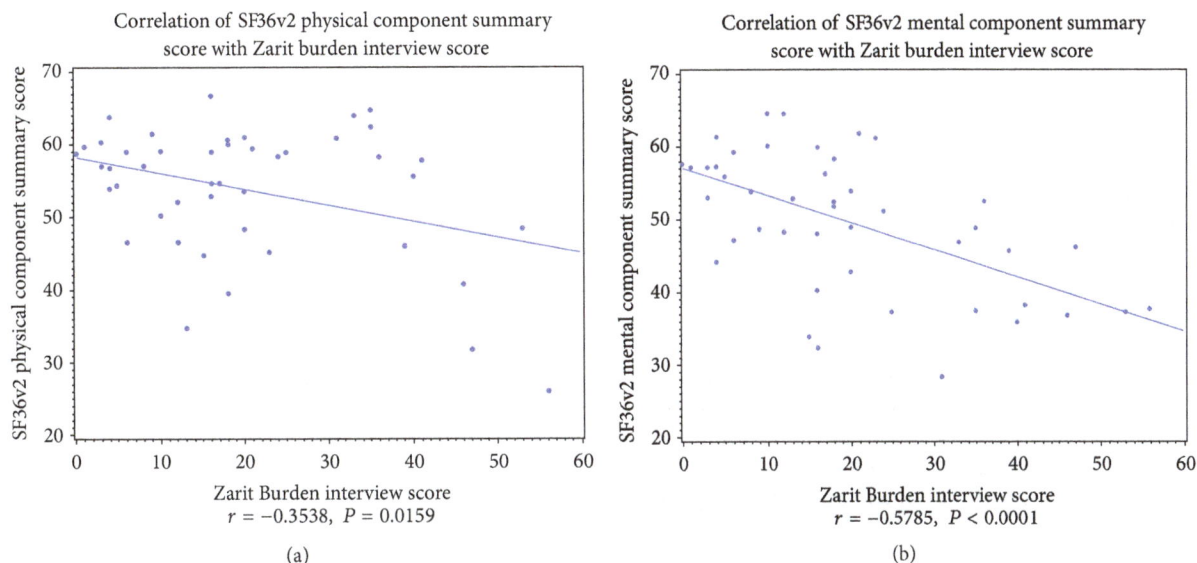

(a)

(b)

FIGURE 2: Correlation between caregiver burden and each of the components of caregiver quality of life (i.e., physical component scale (PCS) and mental component scale (MCS)).

been associated with their burden, such as social support, financial information, comorbidities, and depression and anxiety scales, were not directly addressed. They constitute, however, components of the Zarit burden inventory used. Fourth, the cross-sectional nature of the study prevented further insight into the evolution of these associations longitudinally as well as inference of causation. Fifth, we restricted our analysis to PWE who were accompanied by caregivers who completed their questionnaires. Although the patients who were not escorted by caregivers did not differ substantially from those who did, our study sample may still not be fully representative of the caregiver population for PWE. Similarly, the study population was mostly in families of higher socioeconomic and educational status. They were recruited in the EMU of a tertiary referral center of a US hospital. While this recruitment strategy allowed rigorous characterization of their epilepsy, QOL, and burden associations, it may have significantly limited generalizability of our findings to the community and to other countries where different socioeconomic barriers exist. The hospitalization itself for further epilepsy evaluation and treatment may have inadvertently affected some of the burden and QOL scores that both PWE and their caregivers provided. Finally, the absence of a nonepilepsy patient-caregiver control group

limited our ability to directly compare our findings with other chronic neurologic or medical disorders in which caregivers also play a significant role.

The findings of this study have potential implications both for clinical practice and research paradigms. In clinical practice, physicians should consider incorporating the caregiver into their assessment and treatment plan in an effort to eventually improve the patient's quality of life. Caregiver counseling and education, evaluation and treatment of evolving caregiver psychopathology, and individualized and/or group multidisciplinary interventions to provide physical, emotional, social, and financial support to the caregiver may ameliorate caregiver burden. This may in turn provide significant reciprocal benefit to the QOL of the patient which appears to be inextricably interwoven as shown in our study. Previous studies on caregivers of patients with dementia have corroborated that potential [50]. Further, advocacy groups should include caregiver feelings and needs into their agenda and expert opinion panel reviews as well as national clinical guidelines should further emphasize caregiver QOL as one of the core quality measures in the evaluation and management of epilepsy [51]. In the research field, the focus of investigation should expand to incorporate the family well-being. Our findings suggest associations that warrant further examination in future studies and especially in broader socioeconomic settings in order to elucidate further both the predictors as well as the influence of caregiver burden to their QOL and ultimately to the patient's QOL. Epilepsy specific QOL measures need to be created and validated for the caregivers of PWE and incorporated into future medication and intervention related clinical trials in epilepsy. As also underscored by the recently published Institute of Medicine report on epilepsy, there is need for rigorous research in this understudied field [52], and funding agencies should consider this important issue.

5. Conclusion

In a selected cohort of persons with epilepsy undergoing video-EEG monitoring, we identified modest caregiver burden. This burden is comparable to that reported in the literature for other less prevalent, chronic neurological conditions, although it has been under investigated, particularly for the adult epilepsy population. It appears to be associated with three patient-related factors (i.e., AED number, cognitive performance, and quality of life) and one caregiver-related factor (i.e., education attainment). This burden places a toll to the stakeholders of epilepsy care both for their physical and even more for their psychological well-being. These findings call for further investigation of caregiver burden and quality of life in epilepsy in broader socioeconomic settings and for their inclusion in the physicians' treatment plan and epilepsy care quality measures.

Disclosure

None of the authors has any conflict of interests to disclose related to this unfunded project. This work was presented in part at the 9th European Congress of Epileptology in Rhodes, 2010.

Conflict of Interests

The authors declare that there is no conflict of interests regarding the publication of this paper.

References

[1] E. H. Reynolds, "The ILAE/IBE/WHO Global Campaign against Epilepsy: bringing epilepsy 'out of the shadows'," *Epilepsy and Behavior*, vol. 1, no. 4, pp. S3–S8, 2000.

[2] C. O'Dell, J. W. Wheless, and J. Cloyd, "The personal and financial impact of repetitive or prolonged seizures on the patient and family," *Journal of Child Neurology*, vol. 22, no. 5, supplement, pp. 61S–70S, 2007.

[3] R. B. Trivedi, J. Piette, S. D. Fihn, and D. Edelman, "Examining the interrelatedness of patient and spousal stress in heart failure: conceptual model and pilot data," *Journal of Cardiovascular Nursing*, vol. 27, no. 1, pp. 24–32, 2012.

[4] R. A. Pinto, M. A. Holanda, M. M. C. Medeiros, R. M. S. Mota, and E. D. B. Pereira, "Assessment of the burden of caregiving for patients with chronic obstructive pulmonary disease," *Respiratory Medicine*, vol. 101, no. 11, pp. 2402–2408, 2007.

[5] F. Alvarez-Ude, C. Valdés, C. Estébanez, and P. Rebollo, "Health-related quality of life of family caregivers of dialysis patients," *Journal of Nephrology*, vol. 17, no. 6, pp. 841–850, 2004.

[6] E. Grunfeld, D. Coyle, T. Whelan et al., "Family caregiver burden: results of a longitudinal study of breast cancer patients and their principal caregivers," *Canadian Medical Association Journal*, vol. 170, no. 12, pp. 1795–1801, 2004.

[7] F. J. Carod-Artal, L. Ferreira Coral, D. S. Trizotto, and C. Menezes Moreira, "Burden and perceived health status among caregivers of stroke patients," *Cerebrovascular Diseases*, vol. 28, no. 5, pp. 472–480, 2009.

[8] C. J. M. Schölzel-Dorenbos, I. Draskovic, M. J. Vernooij-Dassen, and M. G. M. Olde Rikkert, "Quality of life and burden of spouses of Alzheimer disease patients," *Alzheimer Disease and Associated Disorders*, vol. 23, no. 2, pp. 171–177, 2009.

[9] P. Martínez-Martín, M. J. Forjaz, B. Frades-Payo et al., "Caregiver burden in Parkinson's disease," *Movement Disorders*, vol. 22, no. 7, pp. 924–931, 2007.

[10] J. Rivera-Navarro, J. Benito-León, C. Oreja-Guevara et al., "Burden and health-related quality of life of Spanish caregivers of persons with multiple sclerosis," *Multiple Sclerosis*, vol. 15, no. 11, pp. 1347–1355, 2009.

[11] F. Pagnini, C. Lunetta, G. Rossi et al., "Existential well-being and spirituality of individuals with amyotrophic lateral sclerosis is related to psychological well-being of their caregivers," *Amyotrophic Lateral Sclerosis*, vol. 12, no. 2, pp. 105–108, 2011.

[12] E. Bayen, P. Pradat-Diehl, C. Jourdan et al., "Predictors of informal care burden 1 year after a severe traumatic brain injury: results from the PariS-TBI study," *The Journal of Head Trauma Rehabilitation*, vol. 28, no. 6, pp. 408–418, 2013.

[13] L. Blanes, M. I. S. Carmagnani, and L. M. Ferreira, "Health-related quality of life of primary caregivers of persons with paraplegia," *Spinal Cord*, vol. 45, no. 6, pp. 399–403, 2007.

[14] K. R. Kim, E. Lee, K. Namkoong, Y. M. Lee, J. S. Lee, and H. D. Kim, "Caregiver's burden and quality of life in mitochondrial disease," *Pediatric Neurology*, vol. 42, no. 4, pp. 271–276, 2010.

[15] K. Gallop, D. Wild, A. Nixon, L. Verdian, and J. A. Cramer, "Impact of Lennox-Gastaut Syndrome (LGS) on health-related quality of life (HRQL) of patients and caregivers: literature review," *Seizure*, vol. 18, no. 8, pp. 554–558, 2009.

[16] G. Ramaglia, A. Romeo, M. Viri, M. Lodi, S. Sacchi, and G. Cioffi, "Impact of idiopathic epilepsy on mothers and fathers: strain, burden of care, worries and perception of vulnerability," *Epilepsia*, vol. 48, no. 9, pp. 1810–1813, 2007.

[17] M. A. Ferro and K. N. Speechley, "Examining clinically relevant levels of depressive symptoms in mothers following a diagnosis of epilepsy in their children: a prospective analysis," *Social Psychiatry and Psychiatric Epidemiology*, vol. 47, no. 9, pp. 1419–1428, 2012.

[18] M. R. Asato, R. Manjunath, R. D. Sheth et al., "Adolescent and caregiver experiences with epilepsy," *Journal of Child Neurology*, vol. 24, no. 5, pp. 562–571, 2009.

[19] B. Desnous, E. Bourel-Ponchel, E. Raffo et al., "Assessment of education needs of adolescents and parents of children with epilepsy," *Revue Neurologique*, vol. 169, no. 1, pp. 67–75, 2013.

[20] J. Taylor, A. Jacoby, G. A. Baker, and A. G. Marson, "Self-reported and parent-reported quality of life of children and adolescents with new-onset epilepsy," *Epilepsia*, vol. 52, no. 8, pp. 1489–1498, 2011.

[21] C. Camfield, L. Breau, and P. Camfield, "Impact of pediatric epilepsy on the family: a new scale for clinical and research use," *Epilepsia*, vol. 42, no. 1, pp. 104–112, 2001.

[22] V. C. Terra, R. M. Cysneiros, J. S. Schwartzman et al., "Mothers of children with cerebral palsy with or without epilepsy: a quality of life perspective," *Disability and Rehabilitation*, vol. 33, no. 5, pp. 384–388, 2011.

[23] R. Lv, L. Wu, L. Jin et al., "Depression, anxiety and quality of life in parents of children with epilepsy," *Acta Neurologica Scandinavica*, vol. 120, no. 5, pp. 335–341, 2009.

[24] S. Cushner-Weinstein, K. Dassoulas, J. A. Salpekar et al., "Parenting stress and childhood epilepsy: the impact of depression, learning, and seizure-related factors," *Epilepsy and Behavior*, vol. 13, no. 1, pp. 109–114, 2008.

[25] A. M. McNelis, J. Buelow, J. Myers, and E. A. Johnson, "Concerns and needs of children with epilepsy and their parents," *Clinical Nurse Specialist*, vol. 21, no. 4, pp. 195–202, 2007.

[26] K. Snead, J. Ackerson, K. Bailey, M. M. Schmitt, A. Madan-Swain, and R. C. Martin, "Taking charge of epilepsy: the development of a structured psychoeducational group intervention for adolescents with epilepsy and their parents," *Epilepsy and Behavior*, vol. 5, no. 4, pp. 547–556, 2004.

[27] J. Williams, C. Steel, G. B. Sharp et al., "Parental anxiety and quality of life in children with epilepsy," *Epilepsy and Behavior*, vol. 4, no. 5, pp. 483–486, 2003.

[28] P. Hoare, "The quality of life of children with chronic epilepsy and their families," *Seizure*, vol. 2, no. 4, pp. 269–275, 1993.

[29] J. R. Hughes, "Psychosocial well-being of carers of people with epilepsy in Hong Kong," *Epilepsy and Behavior*, vol. 3, no. 2, pp. 147–157, 2002.

[30] F. Tajudeen Nuhu, A. Jika Yusuf, A. Akinbiyi et al., "The burden experienced by family caregivers of patients with epilepsy attending the government psychiatric hospital, Kaduna, Nigeria," *The Pan African Medical Journal*, vol. 5, p. 16, 2010.

[31] P. J. Thompson and D. Upton, "The impact of chronic epilepsy on the family," *Seizure*, vol. 1, no. 1, pp. 43–48, 1992.

[32] J. van Andel, W. Westerhuis, M. Zijlmans, K. Fischer, and F. S. S. Leijten, "Coping style and health-related quality of life in caregivers of epilepsy patients," *Journal of Neurology*, vol. 258, no. 10, pp. 1788–1794, 2011.

[33] J. van Andel, M. Zijlmans, K. Fischer, and F. S. S. Leijten, "Quality of life of caregivers of patients with intractable epilepsy," *Epilepsia*, vol. 50, no. 5, pp. 1294–1296, 2009.

[34] A. C. Westphal-Guitti, N. B. Alonso, R. C. V. P. Migliorini et al., "Quality of life and burden in caregivers of patients with epilepsy," *The Journal of Neuroscience Nursing*, vol. 39, no. 6, pp. 354–360, 2007.

[35] J. U. Ohaeri, A. W. Awadalla, and A. A. Farah, "Quality of life in people with epilepsy and their family caregivers: an Arab experience using the short version of the World Health Organization quality of life instrument," *Saudi Medical Journal*, vol. 30, no. 10, pp. 1328–1335, 2009.

[36] A. T. Beck, N. Epstein, G. Brown, and R. A. Steer, "An inventory for measuring clinical anxiety: psychometric properties," *Journal of Consulting and Clinical Psychology*, vol. 56, no. 6, pp. 893–897, 1988.

[37] A. T. Beck and R. A. Steer, *Manual for the Beck Depression Inventory*, Psychological Corporation, San Antonio, Tex, USA, 1993.

[38] D. W. Loring, K. J. Meador, and G. P. Lee, "Determinants of quality of life in epilepsy," *Epilepsy and Behavior*, vol. 5, no. 6, pp. 976–980, 2004.

[39] M. W. Johns, "A new method for measuring daytime sleepiness: the Epworth sleepiness scale," *Sleep*, vol. 14, no. 6, pp. 540–545, 1991.

[40] A. B. Douglass, R. Bornstein, G. Nino-Murcia et al., "The Sleep Disorders Questionnaire I: creation and multivariate structure of SDQ," *Sleep*, vol. 17, no. 2, pp. 160–167, 1994.

[41] A. S. Giorelli, G. S. D. M. L. Neves, M. Venturi, I. M. Pontes, A. Valois, and M. D. M. Gomes, "Excessive daytime sleepiness in patients with epilepsy: a subjective evaluation," *Epilepsy and Behavior*, vol. 21, no. 4, pp. 449–452, 2011.

[42] C. Piperidou, A. Karlovasitou, N. Triantafyllou et al., "Influence of sleep disturbance on quality of life of patients with epilepsy," *Seizure*, vol. 17, no. 7, pp. 588–594, 2008.

[43] J. A. Cramer, K. Perrine, O. Devinsky, L. Bryant-Comstock, K. Meador, and B. Hermann, "Development and cross-cultural translations of a 31-item quality of life in epilepsy inventory," *Epilepsia*, vol. 39, no. 1, pp. 81–88, 1998.

[44] Z. S. Nasreddine, N. A. Phillips, V. Bédirian et al., "The Montreal Cognitive Assessment, MoCA: a brief screening tool for mild cognitive impairment," *Journal of the American Geriatrics Society*, vol. 53, no. 4, pp. 695–699, 2005.

[45] K. Phabphal and J. Kanjanasatien, "Montreal Cognitive Assessment in cryptogenic epilepsy patients with normal Mini-Mental State Examination scores," *Epileptic Disorders*, vol. 13, no. 4, pp. 375–381, 2011.

[46] S. H. Zarit, K. E. Reever, and J. Bach-Peterson, "Relatives of the impaired elderly: correlates of feelings of burden," *Gerontologist*, vol. 20, no. 6, pp. 649–655, 1980.

[47] J. E. Ware Jr. and B. Gandek, "Overview of the SF-36 Health Survey and the International Quality of Life Assessment (IQOLA) project," *Journal of Clinical Epidemiology*, vol. 51, no. 11, pp. 903–912, 1998.

[48] D. Hirtz, D. J. Thurman, K. Gwinn-Hardy, M. Mohamed, A. R. Chaudhuri, and R. Zalutsky, "How common are the "common" neurologic disorders?" *Neurology*, vol. 68, no. 5, pp. 326–337, 2007.

[49] F. Zimmermann and M. Endermann, "Self-proxy agreement and correlates of health-related quality of life in young adults with epilepsy and mild intellectual disabilities," *Epilepsy and Behavior*, vol. 13, no. 1, pp. 202–211, 2008.

[50] M. Pinquart and S. Sörensen, "Helping caregivers of persons with dementia: which interventions work and how large are their effects?" *International Psychogeriatrics*, vol. 18, no. 4, pp. 577–595, 2006.

[51] M. J. V. Pugh, D. R. Berlowitz, G. Montouris et al., "What constitutes high quality of care for adults with epilepsy?" *Neurology*, vol. 69, no. 21, pp. 2020–2027, 2007.

[52] D. C. Hesdorffer, V. Beck, C. E. Begley et al., "Research implications of the Institute of Medicine Report, epilepsy across the spectrum: promoting health and understanding," *Epilepsia*, vol. 54, no. 2, pp. 207–216, 2013.

27

The Syndrome of Absence Status Epilepsy:
Review of the Literature

Leonilda Bilo,[1] Sabina Pappatà,[2] Roberto De Simone,[1] and Roberta Meo[3]

[1] Epilepsy Center, Department of Neuroscience, School of Medicine, Federico II University of Naples, 80131 Naples, Italy
[2] Institute of Biostructure and Bioimaging, CNR and Department of Biomorphological Sciences, Federico II University, 80131 Naples, Italy
[3] Neurology Outpatients Service, Naples Local Health Unit, 80100 Naples, Italy

Correspondence should be addressed to Leonilda Bilo; leda.bilo@gmail.com

Academic Editor: Louis Lemieux

The authors review the literature for cases fulfilling the criteria for the proposed idiopathic generalized epilepsy syndrome (IGE) of absence status epilepsy described by Genton et al. (2008). Difficulties arising in diagnosing such cases are remarked, and possible overlapping with other proposed IGE syndromes is discussed.

1. Introduction

Absence status epilepticus (AS) is a peculiar epileptic condition which has been defined as a prolonged, generalized absence seizure, lasting at least more than half an hour but usually lasting for hours and even for days [1]; the impairment of consciousness is sometimes associated with automatisms or other subtle myoclonic, tonic, atonic, or autonomic phenomena [2]. AS has been distinguished in "typical," if occurring in the setting of idiopathic generalized epilepsy (IGE) and "atypical" in patients with symptomatic or cryptogenetic generalized epilepsy [3]. During "typical" AS continuous or almost continuous generalized spike wave (SW) or polyspike-wave (PSW) activity at 2–4 Hz is recorded on EEG.

Typical AS may occur sporadically in many IGE syndromes, but it can also occur in a recurrent fashion as the main seizure type. This concept was underlined by Andermann and Robb in 1972 [4], commenting on the findings observed in a series of 38 patients with AS; the authors underlined that this condition could occur as the only seizure pattern or represent the dominant seizure pattern, especially in adult life. Most of the patients with recurring AS observed by these authors were either in the second decade of their life or adults, who had had or still had absence attacks. In adolescents AS was often sporadic, while in adults it had a greater tendency to recur. Generalized tonic clonic seizures

(GTCS) terminating (or, more rarely, preceding) an episode of AS were also reported in this series.

Thirty-six years later, Genton et al. [5] described a series of 11 patients in whom recurrent, unprovoked episodes of typical AS represented the main clinical feature. The patients described in this series presented recurrent AS, with onset in adolescence or adulthood, as the main seizure type. Infrequent GTCS, mostly associated with AS, occurred in the majority of patients, while infrequent typical absences were reported in the minority of cases. While all patients had clinical and laboratory findings consistent with a diagnosis of IGE (normal neuroimaging, interictal EEG showing generalized SW, and PSW 2–4 Hz on a normal background activity), none of them could be included in any of the recognized IGE syndromes with typical absences or GTCS. The authors suggested that this condition may represent a specific and rare epilepsy entity which they proposed to name "absence status epilepsy" (ASE).

Reviewing the literature for eligible cases of ASE is not an easy task. While this may be partly due to the fact that this syndrome is rare, it must also be underlined that reports describing patients with typical AS in adult age do not necessarily give detailed information on recurrence of AS and its predominance among other seizure types. Moreover, especially in earlier reports, it is not always possible to ascertain whether or not a definite recognized IGE syndrome has been diagnosed in patients who presented with recurring AS. Consequently, while in some cases it is possible to evaluate if reported patients fulfill the criteria proposed by Genton et al. [5], in others a definite conclusion can not be reached due to lack of necessary data.

2. Review of the Literature

In reviewing the literature, patients were considered as eligible for a diagnosis of ASE if they satisfied the following criteria: recurrent episodes of unprovoked AS, onset of AS in adolescence or adult age, AS being the main seizure type, and clinical and laboratory findings consistent with a diagnosis of IGE but not suggesting one of the recognized IGE syndromes. We considered that definite cases of ASE are those who fulfilled all the above mentioned criteria and possible cases are those in whom some features were atypical or in whom data were insufficient for a diagnosis of ASE. The main data of reviewed patients are summarized in Table 1.

We performed a literature search using the following keywords, alone or in combination: absence status epilepsy, absence status, nonconvulsive status, recurring/recurrent absence status, recurring/recurrent nonconvulsive status, absence status in adults, and nonconvulsive status in adults. The literature search was performed on PubMed, PubMed Central, and Google Scholar.

On the whole, 106 articles were retrieved. We selected for this review only reports describing recurrent AS with onset in adolescence/adulthood, in which individual patients' data (regarding in particular age at onset of AS, recurrence of AS, characteristics of coexisting seizures, and diagnosis of epilepsy syndrome) were detailed or could be inferred, albeit incompletely in some cases.

Patients eligible for a diagnosis of ASE are more easily found in single case reports, probably because these case presentations include a detailed clinical history in which all the data necessary for a diagnosis are given. This is the case of the patients reported by Nightingale and Welch [6], Zambrelli et al. [7], Bilo et al. [8], and Pro et al. [9], who all fulfill the criteria suggested for diagnosis of ASE.

Nightingale and Welch [6] describe a female patient in whom recurring AS was diagnosed at 66 years. In childhood she had suffered from GTCS, which had recurred after a long remission at 47 years; after this relapse, she had been treated with primidone and phenytoin. No overt epileptic seizures had appeared since then, but at 56 years she had started to present long and recurring episodes of "vagueness," which recurred quite regularly at 4-week intervals and lasted about 48 hours. At the age of 66 a diagnosis of AS was made after recording of ictal EEG showing almost continuous generalized SW activity at 2-3 Hz. Neurological examination was normal; no information on family history is offered. Interictal EEG showed bursts of generalized SW; photosensitivity is not mentioned. The patient refused to increase/modify her previous antiepileptic treatment and continued to present AS episodes.

Zambrelli et al. [7] report a male patient without family history of epilepsy who presented a GTCS at the age of 20.

Successively he presented recurring AS, generally followed by GTCS, which were initially sporadic but became very frequent after the age of 73. No absences are reported. AS lasted from 48 to 72 hours, with ictal patterns characterized by continuous generalized SW at 3 Hz. Interictal EEG showed brief 3-Hz generalized SWD, without photosensitivity. Several AEDs, alone or in association, failed to control the AS episodes; at the time of the report, seizure control had been obtained for 2 years after adding lamotrigine (LTG) to valproate (VPA).

Bilo et al. [8] report a 56-year old male who had been suffering from episodes of clouded consciousness and confusion of long duration (36–48 hours) since adolescence. The episodes were initially rare, but during adulthood their frequency increased progressively up to about 1/month; moreover, he presented 2 GTCS which prompted him to seek medical attention. He had no family history of epilepsy. Interictal EEG showed frequent bursts of generalized SW and PSW, without photosensitivity; ictal EEG showed almost continuous generalized SW or PSW activity at 2-3 Hz. He underwent a [18F]FDG-PET study, which showed relative hypermetabolism in thalami bilaterally, mostly in the anterior nuclei, and relative hypometabolism in bilateral frontal cortex and, to a lesser extent, relative hypermetabolism in the cerebellar vermis and relative hypometabolism in parietal and posterior cingulate cortices and in cerebellar hemispheres. Interictal [18F]FDG-PET was normal. LTG monotherapy was uneffective, and side effects prevented the use of adequate doses of VPA; treatment with LTG and low doses of VPA led to reduction, but not disappearance, of AS episodes [10].

Pro et al. [9] report a female patient who presented recurring episodes of mental confusion and ideomotor slowing since the age of 54, usually lasting 5-6 h, with a frequency of 2/3 per year. Medical observation was sought at 77 years. No other seizures had ever occurred, and no triggering factors for the AS were observed. Interictal EEG showed 3–3.5 Hz generalized SW and PSW and photoparoxysmal response; ictal EEG showed continuous, diffuse 3-4 Hz SW and PSW. LTG treatment controlled the AS episodes. A 16-year-old grandson had had febrile seizures and an episode of loss of consciousness that was not clearly interpreted as epilepsy; his EEG recordings showed epileptiform activity which was focal during sleep and generalized during wakefulness.

Other individual case reports found in the literature describe recurring AS in which, however, some atypical features leave doubts as to their eligibility for a diagnosis of the ASE syndrome as described by Genton et al. [5]. This is the case for the patients described by Terzano et al. [11], Iivanainen et al. [18], and Fernández-Torre and Rebollo [19].

Terzano et al. [11] report a woman with no family history of epilepsy and a normal neurological history until the age of 70. At the age of 70 she presented a GTCS and started treatment with barbiturates and phenytoin. Six years later she began to present recurring confusional episodes which lasted as long as 24 hours, often terminating with GTCS, which led to medical observation. The patient was observed during two distinct episodes; in both she was slowed and confused and presented massive and diffuse myoclonic jerks involving mainly the abdominal muscles and

TABLE 1: Patients with recurrent AS with onset in adolescent/adult age.

Authors	Sex	Age at AS onset (yrs)	Other seizures	Epilepsy family history	Photo sensitivity	AED therapy	Response of AS to AEDs	Notes
Definite cases of ASE								
Nightingale and Welch, 1982 [6]	F	56	GTCS	NS	NS	PRI, PHT	Persistence of seizures	
Zambrelli et al., 2006 [7]	M	>20	GTCS	No	No	LTG, VPA	Seizure free	
Genton et al., 2008 [5]	F	14	GTCS	No	No	VPA	Seizure free	
	F	34	A	No	No	VPA, LTG	Seizure free	
	F	16	GTCS	No	No	VPA, ESM, and CZP	Persistence of seizures	
	M	35	GTCS	No	No	VPA, ESM	Seizure free	
	M	15	GTCS	No	No	VPA	Seizure free	
	M	26	GTCS	No	No	VPA	Seizure free	
	F	26	GTCS	No	No	VPA, PB, and LEV	Persistence of seizures	
	F	65	GTCS	No	No	VPA	Seizure free	
	M	16	A, GTCS	No	No	VPA, LTG	Persistence of seizures	
	M	36	A	No	No	LEV, TPM	Seizure free	
	M	36	GTCS	No	No	LTG, ESM	Seizure free	
Bilo et al., 2010 [8]	M	14	GTCS	No	No	LTG, VPA	Persistence of seizures	
Pro et al., 2011 [9]	F	54	No	Yes	Yes	LTG	Seizure free	
Possible cases of ASE (atypical features)								
Terzano et al., 1978 [11]	F	76	GTCS	No	Yes	?	?	Atypical feature: prominent myoclonic jerks during AS
Possible cases of ASE (insufficient data)								
Lee 1985 [12]	Three patients in this series presented recurring AS, but it is not clear if a defined IGE syndrome and/or other seizures were the main seizure type and/or if AS episodes were situation related.							
Berkovic et al., 1989* [13]	Fourteen patients in this series had recurring AS with onset after the age of 15. An undetermined number of these 14 patients belonged to "the unusual but well-recognized group of IGEs beginning in middle to later life, where AS is a particular prominent seizure type."							
Tomson et al., 1992 [14]	AS was the only seizure type in 5 patients with undetermined IGE. However, it is not clear whether or not AS was recurring in any of these patients.							
Agathonikou et al., 1998 [15] (patients 18, 19, and 20)	M	48	GTCS	NS	NS	VPA, CBZ, and PHT	Seizure free	It is not clear if AS is the main seizure type.
	F	36	A, GTCS	NS	NS	VPA	Seizure free	It is not clear if AS is the main seizure type.
	F	43	A, GTCS	NS	NS	PB, PHT, ESM, and CZP	Seizure free	It is not clear if AS is the main seizure type.
Szucs et al., 2008 [16] (patient 2)	F	45	GTCS	NS	NS	NS	Seizure free	It is not clear if AS is the main seizure type.
Mireles and O'Donovan, 2010 [17] (patients 1, 2, and 3)	NS	49	A	NS	NS	LEV	Seizure free	Possible diagnosis of CAE
	NS	60	GTCS	NS	NS	LEV, LTG, PTH, and VPA	Persistence of seizures	Insufficient clinical data
	NS	47	No	NS	NS	VPA	Seizure free	Insufficient clinical data

TABLE 1: Continued.

Authors	Sex	Age at AS onset (yrs)	Other seizures	Epilepsy family history	Photo sensitivity	AED therapy	Response of AS to AEDs	Notes
Possible cases of ASE (prompt diagnosis may have altered natural history)
Iivanainen et al., 1984 [18] (patient 2)	F	61	A, GTCS	No	No	VPA	Seizure free	This patient had few seizures in her life, among which AS does not stand as the main seizure type. However, its low recurrence may be due to prompt diagnosis and treatment.
Fernández-Torre and Rebollo, 2009 [19]	F	68	GTCS	No	Yes	VPA	Seizure free	Concomitant seizures were rare and disappeared after childhood. AS is not recurrent, but this may be due to prompt diagnosis and treatment.
Cases of AS not fulfilling criteria for ASE
Iivanainen et al., 1984 [18] (patient 1)	F	55	A, GTCS	No	No	VPA, PB		Concomitant seizures were very frequent.
Michelucci et al., 1996 [20] (patients 1 and 4)	F	28	A, GTCS	No	NS	VPA	NS	AS was not the main seizure type.
	M	41	A, GTCS	No	NS	PHT, PB	NS	Diagnosis of JAE.
Agathonikou et al., 1998 [15]	Patients 1–17 had defined IGE syndromes; moreover, patients 9, 10, 16, and 17 had presented only one AS episode.
Baykan et al., 2002 [21]	All 8 patients had recurrent AS but all of them were diagnosed with defined IGE syndromes.
Nguyen Michel et al., 2011 [22] (patient 5)	F	71	A, GTCS	NS	NS	LTG, LEV	?	Diagnosis of CAE.

AS: absence status; ASE: absence status epilepsy.
*This series includes also the patients presented in Andermann and Robb, 1972 [4].
GTCS: generalized tonic clonic seizures; A: absences.
NS: not specified.
AED: antiepileptic drugs; PRI: primidone; PHT: phenytoin; LTG: lamotrigine; VPA: valproate; ESM: ethosuximide; CZP: clonazepam; PB: phenobarbital; LEV: levetiracetam; TPM: topiramate; CBZ: carbamazepine.
IGE: idiopathic generalized epilepsy; JAE: juvenile absence epilepsy; CAE: childhood absence epilepsy.

the antigravitative muscles of the upper limbs. Ictal EEG showed slowed background activity with superimposition of generalized polyspikes and PSW, grouped in continuous and arrhythmical bursts; an increase in the paroxysmal discharges and the myoclonus was produced by intermittent photic stimulation. Interictal EEG showed isolated diffuse PSW and SW. The history of this patient is in agreement with a possible diagnosis of ASE: onset in late adulthood, recurrent AS as the main seizure type, and concomitant GTCS. However, the clinical and EEG features of her status episodes are quite unusual and actually, rather than AS, can be considered as myoclonic absence status epilepticus as defined by the ILAE task force report [23]. However, while AS with prominent myoclonic features is usually seen in IGE patients

who present seizures with myoclonic jerks, this patient only presented GTCS aside from episodes of status. It is possible that in the future the definition of ASE could include also patients with recurring myoclonic absence status, if they share the other features which characterize this condition (recurring absence status as the main seizure type and lack of inclusion in any recognized IGE syndrome). To date, however, the peculiar features of status do not consent to include confidently this patient into the present definition of ASE.

Iivanainen et al. [18] report 2 female patients with recurring AS with onset in adulthood. In both cases, however, AS does not seem as the prominent seizure type. Patient 1 had an undefined IGE with onset of GTCS in childhood, absence seizures appearing at 32, and recurring AS at 55. All seizure types were quite frequent and concomitant seizures persisted at the time of AS onset. Patient 2, conversely, had epilepsy onset at 57 years, with sporadic absences (which successively increased in frequency) and a single GTCS followed from a confusional state, possibly resulting in AS, at the age of 61. No family history for epilepsy is mentioned. A definite AS occurred a couple of weeks later, with hospitalization and recording of continuous generalized SW activity. No photosensitivity was present in ictal and interictal EEGs. She was promptly treated with VPA and became completely seizure free. While the history of this patient closely resembles those of patients in the series of Genton et al. [5] (onset in later life of undetermined IGE, recurring AS, associated sporadic GTCS, and absences), recurrence of AS is too low for these seizures to be considered the main seizure type with regard to absences and GTCS. However, one may argue that the prompt diagnosis and treatment of AS (which occurred after the second episode) may have altered the natural course of the condition in this patient. In fact, in most patients with recurring AS, the diagnosis of status occurs quite late and several episodes occur before an appropriate treatment approach is employed. Similar considerations may be suggested for the case described by Fernández-Torre and Rebollo [19], who report an elderly woman who at the age of 68 presented with an episode of typical AS as late complication of an unrecognised and "nonspecific" picture of IGE. Ictal EEG showed frequent and recurrent generalized paroxysms of 4–6 Hz PSW and SW intermixed with brief periods of normal background activity, while the interictal EEG showed occasional discharges of generalized SW and a photoparoxysmal response. The patient was treated with VPA and remained seizure free during the 2-year follow-up. We have no evidence that this patient could have shown a tendency to AS recurrency and that AS may have resulted in being her main seizure type. However, the possible role of the well documented prompt diagnosis and treatment in influencing the natural history of her epilepsy must be taken into account. Accordingly, the authors remark the similarities between their patient and the one described by Genton et al. [5].

Other individual reports (Szucs et al., 2008; Mireles and O'Donovan, 2010) do not give sufficient data for a definite diagnosis of ASE. Szucs et al. [16] present 3 female patients with AS with onset in adult age. None of them seems to fit into a possible diagnosis of ASE, even if additional information/clarification on their clinical histories would be needed before reaching a definite conclusion. Patient 1 has a diagnosis of juvenile absence epilepsy (JAE), but the onset of her absence seizures is reported at 6 years of age. She suffered from absences and GTCS, whose frequency is not detailed but seems to be quite high. Only one AS was documented at the age of 55. Also patient 3 had a single AS episode occurring at 63 after a convulsive status; she suffered from epilepsy since the age of 15, manifested as frequent GTCS which the authors consider as probable episodes of ASE, without offering any explanation for this diagnosis. Only patient 2, with a diagnosis of undefined IGE with onset around 45 years of age and recurring long confusional states (recognized as

AS at the age of 55 after an ictal recording), could fit into the diagnosis of ASE. However, this patient also presented GTCS probably with high frequency, and the authors do not clarify if AS were the prominent seizure type.

In a report presented as a poster, Mireles and O'Donovan [17] report 3 patients with recurrent AS with onset in adult life and presumed IGE. The limited amount of data typical of a poster presentation does not consent a detailed clinical history; patients' sex is not detailed, but a male preponderance is mentioned in the discussion. Patient 1 had had absences in childhood, responsive to ethosuximide; no additional details are given, so a possible diagnosis of childhood absence epilepsy (CAE) can not be ruled out. At the age of 49 the patient presented recurrent confusional episodes, diagnosed as AS, which failed to respond to several antiepileptic drugs and were finally controlled by levetiracetam. Patient 2 had adult onset (60 years of age) of yearly bouts of AS evolving to GTC status; while convulsive status was controlled, AS was drug resistant. Patients 3 had epilepsy onset at 47, with recurring unusual electrographic generalized status, lasting for days, during which complex neuropsychological testing was performed without difficulty. While apparently in all patients, ictal EEGs consistent with a diagnosis of AS was obtained, the authors underline "lack of correlation between epileptiform patterns on EEG and precise manifestations of altered awareness and seizure frequency rates." Family history and response to intermitted photic stimulation are not reported in any of the patients. To our knowledge these authors have not reported these cases outside the poster presentation. Without additional information on these interesting patients, it is not possible to understand if they might actually represent cases of ASE.

Many authors have reported patient series with recurrent adult onset AS. In most of these reports, no patient is eligible for a diagnosis of ASE because all of them suffer from a definite recognized IGE syndrome and/or have isolated episodes of AS and/or AS is not the main seizure type in their clinical history (Michelucci et al., 1996 [20]; Baykan et al., 2002 [21]; Nguyen Michel et al., 2011 [22]).

In other reports describing patient series, the lack of detailed individual data does not allow to ascertain if ASE could be diagnosed, at least in a minority of patients. Lee [12] describes 11 adult patients with AS without previous history of epileptic seizures, with a follow-up lasting as long as 5 years. Two of these patients are reported to have partial seizures during follow-up, casting some doubts on the previous diagnosis of AS. Moreover, in 7 patients of this series AS was provoked by metabolic imbalance or related to psychotropic treatment, suggesting that they may suffer from "de novo" AS, a condition reported in middle age or in the elderly, without previous history of epilepsy, resulting from the addition of several epileptogenic factors (iatrogenic or metabolic) [24]. Recurrence of status during follow-up is reported in 3 patients, after discontinuation of antiepileptic treatment. However, there is no way of ascertaining if patients with recurring AS had also other generalized (or even focal?) seizures as their main seizure type, if a recognized epilepsy syndrome was diagnosed and if they had had a situation-related provoked status to begin with.

Similarly, no definite conclusion can be drawn from the report by Tomson et al. (1992) [14], describing 32 patients with nonconvulsive status, in some of whom a review of case histories disclosed probable, previously undiagnosed episodes of status. Twenty-one of these patients presented recurrence of AS on follow-up. Eighteen patients had "generalized EEG seizure activity" during the status, but 2 of them were finally diagnosed as suffering from focal epilepsy. Of the remaining 16, 6 had a history of a recognized IGE syndrome, 5 had a diagnosis of undetermined epilepsy due to insufficient information of previous seizures, and 5 had had AS as the only epileptic manifestation. Since it is not possible to ascertain if some of these 5 patients were in the group of previous undiagnosed episodes of status or if they were in the group of patients with recurring status on follow-up, it is not possible to know if these patients had recurring AS and no conclusion can be reached as to the possible diagnosis of ASE.

Other reports describing patient series give more detailed information on individual cases, allowing the proposal of possible diagnosis of ASE in some cases. Berkovic et al. (1989) [13] report the effectiveness of VPA treatment in preventing recurrence of AS in 25 patients (this report includes also the patients with AS discussed, with no individual details, in the paper from Andermann and Robb mentioned above [4]). The series from Berkovic et al. [13] includes 18 patients with IGE, in 16 of whom AS was recurring; in 14 of these 16, the onset of AS was after 15 years of age. In the table no information is given about the specific IGE syndrome presented by individual patients, and it is not specified if AS was the main seizure type in any of these patients. However, in the discussion the authors underline that "the group [with IGE] included patients with typical IGE [···] but other patients were of the unusual but well recognized group of IGEs beginning in middle to later life where AS is a particular prominent seizure type." This definition is more or less identical to the definition of ASE given by Genton et al. [5], and so we must infer that this series most probably includes patients with ASE. It is not possible, however, to gather how many of these patients are presented nor their individual features such as sex, age at onset of AS, family history, and photosensitivity.

In 1998 Agathonikou et al. [15] reported a series of 21 adult IGE patients who had presented one or more episodes of typical AS, with the aim of documenting the relations of AS to the various syndromes of IGEs. The original study population consisted of 136 adult patients with IGE, of whom 21 had presented AS. All these 21 patients had presented typical absences and GTCS besides AS; in most patients AS had recurred, with varying frequency (from 2/life to more than 40/life); precipitating factors for AS were occasionally reported, but only in 3 patients a consistent precipitant was identified. Most patients could be diagnosed with a specific IGE syndrome, with the highest frequency of AS observed in perioral myoclonia with absences (PMA) (57.1% of all PMA adult patients observed in the study population) followed by IGE with phantom absences (IGE-PA) (46,2%). However, half of the patients with PMA presented only one episode of AS in their life, while patients affected by IGE-PA had the highest mean of AS episodes during life. Interestingly,

4 of the 21 patients of this series could not be included in any definite IGE syndrome and were consequently defined as suffering from "unclassified IGE with typical absences." There is no information on family history or photosensitivity in these 4 patients; in all of them AS had recurred, with episodes ranging from 4 in life to more than 30. Three patients (n° 18, 19, and 20) had onset of AS in adult age. All presented other seizure types consisting of absences and GTCS; it is not possible to ascertain if AS was the main seizure type in this group, but this possibility seems likely when AS recurs very frequently. In conclusion, patient number 18 seems a likely candidate for a diagnosis of ASE, with >30 episodes of unprovoked AS with onset at 48 years of age; in patients number 19 (4 episodes of AS) and in patient number 20 (7 episodes of AS) no definite conclusion can be drawn.

3. Conclusions

While the existence of a seizure condition with recurrent, unprovoked AS in adult age has been recognized 40 years ago, only recently this condition has been proposed as a possible definite entity in the IGE group [5]. The proposing authors [5], presenting a homogeneous group of 11 patients with this condition, define its features as recurrent AS with onset in adolescence or adulthood, infrequent GTCS, rarely typical absences, no family history of epilepsy, normal neuroimaging, interictal EEG showing generalized SW and PSW 2–4 Hz on a normal background activity, absence of photoparoxysmal responses, variable response of AS to IV BDZs, and good seizure control with adequate dose of antiabsence drugs, mainly VPA.

Recurrent unprovoked ASs are reported in another proposed adult IGE syndrome, IGE-PA, characterized by phantom absences (PA), infrequent GTCS, and AS in up to 50% of the patients [25]. PAs are absence seizures so mild and short-lasting to be barely perceived by the patient or the observer, with a duration of approximately 2–4 s without other clinical features [26]; they can only be revealed by cognitive tests during video-EEG monitoring. PAs are difficult to diagnose and often escape recognition not only by patients but by physicians as well. Consequently, while we have excluded from our review all reports in which a diagnosis of IGE-PA was proposed, it is not possible to rule out the occurrence of PA in the reports which we have suggested as ASE patients. Genton et al. [5], while underlining that patients in their series present some clinical features overlapping with patients with IGE-PA who also present recurrent AS, find episodes possibly consistent with PA in only one of their patients; they also remark, however, that it is not possible to exclude in their series subtle cognitive deficit during the generalized paroxysmal discharges lasting for more than 3 s. These authors [5] question the recognition of IGE-PA as a specific epilepsy condition: the same doubts, however, may be cast on the recognition of the ASE syndrome, which at present is not considered as a distinct IGE entity. Actually, at present it is probably questionable to consider any of these two conditions as specific IGE syndromes, and it is possible that both may share the same pathophysiologic mechanisms and anatomical substrates of more common phenotypic expressions of IGE. However, it is conceivable that the epileptic conditions characterized essentially by recurring AS as the main seizure type might in the future be considered as a specific IGE entity, with ASE and IGE-PA being viewed as different parts of the same continuum. More reports of patients with recurrent AS, with specific investigations aimed at disclosing PA, are warranted to clarify this point.

Until recently, AS occurring in adult age was often unrecognized and misdiagnosed as complex partial status epilepticus or, especially in the elderly, as a confusional episode related to cerebrovascular disturbances. Emergency EEG is of paramount importance for the diagnosis of AS. Moreover, AS occurring in elderly patients with IGE must also be distinguished from "de novo" AS, a condition first reported by Thomas et al. [24] and occurring in patients without previous history of epilepsy under the influence of several epileptogenic factors. Most commonly, it is caused by withdrawal of psychotropic drugs, usually benzodiazepines; metabolic imbalance or chronic alcoholism may act as cofactors. De novo AS is considered a situation-related epileptic status epilepticus; long term antiepileptic treatment is not required, since there is no recurrence if precipitating factors are avoided. However, as underlined by Fernández-Torre and Rebollo [19], the differential diagnosis between "de novo" AS and AS occurring in patients with IGE may be difficult, since elderly subjects may often overlook a previous history of epilepsy, and the use of psychotropic drugs in these patients is quite common. A detailed clinical history and analysis of interictal EEGs are necessary to avoid misdiagnosis, which may lead to mistreatment and, most often, to recurrence. However, in recent times a better recognition of this entity has led to prompt diagnosis and early appropriate treatment, with a consequent reduction/disappearance of recurrences, as described in some reports [18, 19]. In consideration also of the usual good response to treatment, it is conceivable that in the future one of the cardinal features of this proposed syndrome—recurrence of AS—might gradually disappear.

Conflict of Interests

The authors declare that there is no conflict of interests regarding the publication of this paper.

References

[1] C. P. Panayiotopoulos, "Absence Status Epilepticus," 2011, http://www.medmerits.com/index.php/article/absence_status_epilepticus.

[2] P. Thomas, L. Valton, and P. Genton, "Absence and myoclonic status epilepticus precipitated by antiepileptic drugs in idiopathic generalized epilepsy," *Brain*, vol. 129, no. 5, pp. 1281–1292, 2006.

[3] S. Shorvon and M. Walker, "Status epilepticus in idiopathic generalized epilepsy," *Epilepsia*, vol. 46, no. 9, pp. 73–79, 2005.

[4] F. Andermann and J. P. Robb, "Absence status. A reappraisal following review of thirty-eight patients," *Epilepsia*, vol. 13, no. 1, pp. 177–187, 1972.

[5] P. Genton, E. Ferlazzo, and P. Thomas, "Absence status epilepsy: delineation of a distinct idiopathic generalized epilepsy syndrome," *Epilepsia*, vol. 49, no. 4, pp. 642–649, 2008.

[6] S. Nightingale and J. L. Welch, "Psychometric assessment in absence status," *Archives of Neurology*, vol. 39, no. 8, pp. 516–519, 1982.

[7] E. Zambrelli, M. Terzaghi, E. Sinforiani, and R. Manni, "Non-convulsive status epilepticus and generalised tonic-clonic seizures ersisting in old age in a patient with idiopathic generalised epilepsy: a long-term observation," *Neurological Sciences*, vol. 27, no. 6, pp. 436–438, 2006.

[8] L. Bilo, R. Meo, M. F. D. Leva, C. Vicidomini, M. Salvatore, and S. Pappatà, "Thalamic activation and cortical deactivation during typical absence status monitored using [^{18}F]FDG-PET: a case report," *Seizure*, vol. 19, no. 3, pp. 198–201, 2010.

[9] S. Pro, E. Vicenzini, F. Randi, P. Pulitano, and O. Mecarelli, "Idiopathic late-onset absence status epilepticus: a case report with an electroclinical 14 years follow-up," *Seizure*, vol. 20, no. 8, pp. 655–658, 2011.

[10] L. Bilo, "Absence status epilepsy: una nuova sindrome nell'ambito delle epilessie generalizzate idiopatiche. Descrizione di un caso studiato con [^{18}F]FDG-PET critica," *Epilepsy News*, no. 3, pp. 10–11, 2010.

[11] M. G. Terzano, F. Gemignani, and D. Mancia, "Petit mal status with myoclonus: case report," *Epilepsia*, vol. 19, no. 4, pp. 385–392, 1978.

[12] S. I. Lee, "Nonconvulsive status epilepticus. Ictal confusion in later life," *Archives of Neurology*, vol. 42, no. 8, pp. 778–781, 1985.

[13] S. F. Berkovic, F. Andermann, A. Guberman, D. Hipola, and P. F. Bladin, "Valproate prevents the recurrence of absence status," *Neurology*, vol. 39, no. 10, pp. 1294–1297, 1989.

[14] T. Tomson, U. Lindbom, and B. Y. Nilsson, "Nonconvulsive status epilepticus in adults: thirty-two consecutive patients from a general hospital population," *Epilepsia*, vol. 33, no. 5, pp. 829–835, 1992.

[15] A. Agathonikou, C. P. Panayiotopoulos, S. Giannakodimos, and M. Koutroumanidis, "Typical absence status in adults: diagnostic and syndromic considerations," *Epilepsia*, vol. 39, no. 12, pp. 1265–1276, 1998.

[16] A. Szucs, G. Barcs, R. Jakus et al., "Late-life absence status epilepticus: a female disorder?" *Epileptic Disorders*, vol. 10, no. 2, pp. 156–161, 2008.

[17] P. Mireles and C. O'Donovan, "Consciousness and seizure characteristics in adults with recurrent absence status and generalized epilepsy," *Epilepsy Currents*, vol. 11, no. 2045, Supplement 1, 2010, AES 64th Annual Meeting and 3rd Biennial North American Regional Epilepsy Congress December , 2010, San Antonio, Tex, USA.

[18] M. Iivanainen, L. Bergstrom, A. Nuutila, and M. Viukari, "Psychosis-like absence status of elderly patients: successful treatment with sodium valproate," *Journal of Neurology Neurosurgery and Psychiatry*, vol. 47, no. 9, pp. 965–969, 1984.

[19] J. L. Fernández-Torre and M. Rebollo, "Typical absence status epilepticus as late presentation of idiopathic generalised epilepsy in an elderly patient," *Seizure*, vol. 18, no. 1, pp. 82–83, 2009.

[20] R. Michelucci, G. Rubboli, D. Passarelli et al., "Electroclinical features of idiopathic generalised epilepsy with persisting absences in adult life," *Journal of Neurology Neurosurgery and Psychiatry*, vol. 61, no. 5, pp. 471–477, 1996.

[21] B. Baykan, A. Gökyiğit, C. Gürses, and M. Eraksoy, "Recurrent absence status epilepticus: clinical and EEG characteristics," *Seizure*, vol. 11, no. 5, pp. 310–319, 2002.

[22] V. H. Nguyen Michel, C. Sebban, S. Debray-Meignan et al., "Electroclinical features of idiopathic generalized epilepsies in the elderly: a geriatric hospital-based study," *Seizure*, vol. 20, no. 4, pp. 292–298, 2011.

[23] J. Engel Jr., "Report of the ILAE classification core group," *Epilepsia*, vol. 47, no. 9, pp. 1558–1568, 2006.

[24] P. Thomas, A. Beaumanoir, P. Genton, C. Dolisi, and M. Chatel, "'De novo' absence status of late onset: report of 11 cases," *Neurology*, vol. 42, no. 1, pp. 104–110, 1992.

[25] C. P. Panayiotopoulos, M. Koutroumanidis, S. Giannakodimos, and A. Agathonikou, "Idiopathic generalised epilepsy in adults manifested by phantom absences, generalised tonic-clonic seizures, and frequent absence status," *Journal of Neurology Neurosurgery and Psychiatry*, vol. 63, no. 5, pp. 622–627, 1997.

[26] C. P. Panayiotopoulos, "Syndromes of idiopathic generalized epilepsies not recognized by the international league against epilepsy," *Epilepsia*, vol. 46, no. 9, pp. 57–66, 2005.

28

Adaptive Skills and Somatization in Children with Epilepsy

Nichole Wicker Villarreal,[1] Cynthia A. Riccio,[2] Morris J. Cohen,[3] and Yong Park[3]

[1] *Texas A&M University, College Station, TX 77843-4225, USA*
[2] *Department of Educational Psychology, Texas A&M University, College Station, TX 77843-4225, USA*
[3] *Children's Hospital of Georgia, BT-2601, 1446 Harper Street, Augusta, GA 30912, USA*

Correspondence should be addressed to Cynthia A. Riccio; criccio@tamu.edu

Academic Editor: Joseph I. Sirven

Objective. Children with epilepsy are at risk for less than optimum long-term outcomes. The type and severity of their epilepsy may contribute to educational, psychological, and social outcomes. The objective of this study was to determine the relation between somatization and adaptive skills based on seizure type that could impact on those outcomes. *Methods.* This study examined adaptive functioning and somatization in 87 children with epilepsy using archival data from a tertiary care facility. *Results.* No significant differences in adaptive skills emerged between groups of children diagnosed with complex partial (CP) as compared to CP-secondary generalized (SG) seizures; however, deficits in adaptive behavior were found for both groups. The number of medications, possibly reflecting the severity of the epilepsy, was highly correlated to adaptive function. *Conclusions.* Identification of deficits in adaptive behavior may represent an opportunity for tailored prevention and intervention programming for children with epilepsy. Addressing functional deficits may lead to improved outcomes for these children.

1. Introduction

Among chronic illnesses, epilepsy is the most common neurological condition in childhood [1–3]. Childhood epilepsy is associated with multiple causes including neurological deficit present at birth, cerebrovascular disease, trauma, tumor, or infection. Often the cause is unknown or designated as idiopathic. Not all children experience the same type of seizure and potential effects on educational and psychological outcome may differ by seizure type or etiology. Epilepsy, regardless of seizure type, has been increasingly recognized as a risk factor for potential negative outcomes for children and their families, from childhood into adulthood [3–5]. Specifically, long-term studies have shown that the social and psychological outcomes of adults with childhood onset of epilepsy are poorer than for typical peers with regard to educational level, employment, independent functioning, and socioeconomic status [6–9]. Although it is not uncommon for epilepsy to be associated with lower cognitive functioning, the negative outcomes are not specific to those with impaired cognition. Studies conducted on young adults with normal cognitive ability and a history of childhood epilepsy also found lower than expected levels of educational attainment, greater unemployment, lower socioeconomic status, and lower marriage rates [6, 7, 10, 11].

Studies have highlighted the relationship between seizure variables (e.g., age at onset, time since diagnosis, and medications), psychological well-being, and independent functioning [8, 12–16]. A number of studies have concluded that epilepsy-related factors are not strong predictors of psychopathology in childhood [17, 18]. In contrast, there are indications that demonstration of adaptive behavior may be associated with seizure severity and control [2, 5, 19, 20]. Adaptive behavior encompasses a range of behaviors that are considered essential for everyday functioning, including daily living skills, social competence, functional communication, leadership, and adaptability.

At best, Sillanpää and Cross [5] found that although most individuals with epilepsy were able to function independently, the risk of deficits in independent living was greatest in those with complicated epilepsy. Clary et al. [21] found children and adolescents to evidence significant deficits in both daily living skills and functional communication. When children with normal cognitive ability were considered separately, results still indicated significant deficits across adaptive areas, including socialization, communication, and daily living skills [22]. Other studies found that children with epilepsy evidenced significant adaptive behavior deficits not explained by cognitive deficits [23, 24]. Of the adaptive skills, social and communication skills were found to predict later school performance in children with early-onset epilepsy [25].

In addition to potentially impaired adaptive skills, associated with health and medical concerns, children with epilepsy may exhibit a higher than expected level of somatic complaints, potentially indicative of somatization. From a psychological perspective, somatization is best described as the presentation of a psychological problem (e.g., anxiety or depression) as a physical complaint. Specific behaviors (e.g., complaints of headache or stomach ache and taking medication) in an otherwise healthy individual oftentimes are interpreted in this manner. For children with epilepsy, these behaviors may reflect the medical condition as opposed to (or in addition to) an underlying psychological problem. Somatic complaints have been found to be more common among children with lower cognitive abilities [26]; thus, the cognitive ability differences in a sample could affect results. Notably, Clary et al. [21] did not find elevated mean somatization scores in their sample but reported that 17% of the participants did reach clinically significant levels. Little research has examined the extent to which children and adolescents with epilepsy exhibit somatic complaints or the extent to which somatization is related to adaptive skill development.

Although epilepsy is by far one of the most studied and explored chronic illnesses, research has not examined the relationship between somatization and general adaptive functioning to the same extent that risk for psychopathology has been explored. Existing data suggest that the presence of epilepsy increases the likelihood of somatic complaints and low adaptive skills. The likelihood of these problems developing is increased by poor cognitive functioning and behavioral problems, potentially contributing to social skill deficits [12, 13, 22, 27, 28]. The connection between cognition and behavioral functioning is well established. In contrast, the association between adaptive skills and somatic complaints is not well established. A clearer understanding of levels of adaptive functioning for children with epilepsy and the relationship between adaptive skills and somatic complaints could provide a better framework for working with these children. Moreover, psychosocial and adaptive functioning are not only predictive of long-term outcome, but also have been found to be related to quality of life in children and adolescents with epilepsy [21, 29]. The purpose of this study was to add to the growing literature on the relation of aspects of adaptive functioning, levels of somatization, and epilepsy-related factors. It was hypothesized that there would be differences in level of somatization and adaptive behavior for children with complex partial (CP) seizures as compared to CP-secondary generalized (SG) seizures.

2. Materials and Methods

2.1. Participants. This is a retrospective study using extant data of children and adolescents with epilepsy who were referred to a tertiary care epilepsy center in the south for neuropsychology evaluation between the years of 1997 and 2010. The 87 participants included those individuals with epilepsy who meet the criteria for inclusion. Children were included if (a) they were between the ages of 4 and 17, (b) they had been administered a version of the Behavior Assessment System for Children BASC [30]/BASC-2 [31] Parent Report, and (c) they had a predominant seizure type of complex partial (CP) or complex partial-secondary generalized (SG) epilepsy at least one year prior to the time of the evaluation. The determination of seizure type was made by a pediatric neurologist based upon the seizure characterization and EEG monitoring. CP and SG are the most common types of seizures seen at this facility and it was of interest to see if secondary generalization would further affect functioning. The following exclusionary criteria were used: (a) children with a diagnosis of epilepsy for less than a year, (b) omission of the BASC/BASC-2 parent report, or (c) cognitive ability below 70. Cognitive ability was restricted in order to control for adaptive behavior deficits that could otherwise be associated with intellectual disability. Teacher reports on the BASC/BASC-2 were available on some but not all of the participants. Requiring the teacher form would have significantly reduced the sample size; however, results of the teacher form are reported.

Participants ($N = 87$) were predominantly male (59.77%) and Caucasian (72.41%). The participants had a mean age of 10.65 (SD = 2.89). The participants' cognitive ability ranged from 70 to 115, with a mean IQ of 86.26 (SD = 10.89). Of the participants, 64 (73.56%) had a diagnosis of CP and 23 (26.44%) had a diagnosis of SG. The two groups did not differ in age at the time of assessment or full scale IQ. Seizure variables of interest included age of onset, duration, and number of medications. In particular, number of medications was used as an indicator of severity; number of medications for both groups ranged from 0 to 3. Most frequent antiepileptic medications included one or more of the following: oxcarbazepine (36% of participants), levetiracetam (28%), carbamazepine (22%), lamotrigine (19%), or valproate (16%). No between group differences were found for age at onset, duration, or number of medications. Similarly, chi-square analyses indicated that groups did not differ significantly in sex, race/ethnicity, or reported family income. Table 1 provides the demographic data by seizure type.

2.2. Procedures. This study was a retrospective research project using an existing data base. The primary measures of interest were parent-/guardian- and teacher-rating scales of the child's behaviors, as well as information pertaining to the child's medical history. Approval for the study was obtained from the Medical College of Georgia Institutional Review Board (IRB) and then by the Texas A&M University IRB to use the extant data base. Because the data for this study were archival, collection and coding systems were already established. Demographic information including age,

TABLE 1: Descriptive characteristics by seizure type.

Demographics (n, %)	CP ($n = 64$)	SG ($n = 23$)
Sex		
Male	40 (62.50%)	12 (52.17%)
Female	24 (37.50%)	11 (47.83%)
Ethnicity		
Caucasian	48 (75.00%)	15 (65.22%)
African American	11 (17.19%)	7 (11.48%)
Hispanic/other	5 (7.81%)	1 (4.35%)
Annual income		
>$10,000	7 (10.94%)	2 (8.70%)
$10–20,000	11 (17.19%)	6 (26.09%)
$20–30,000	12 (18.75%)	4 (17.39%)
$30–40,000	7 (10.94%)	1 (4.35%)
$40–50,000	5 (7.81%)	3 (13.04%)
>$50,000	22 (34.38%)	7 (11.48%)
	Mean (SD)	Mean (SD)
Age at testing	10.36 (2.89)	11.42 (2.71)
Full scale IQ	86.42 (11.10)	86.48 (10.70)
Age of onset	5.99 (3.46)	6.14 (3.62)
Duration (years since onset)	4.42 (3.77)	5.33 (3.20)
Number of medications	1.72 (0.85)	1.95 (0.77)

CP: complex partial; SG: complex partial-secondary generalized; FSIQ: full scale intelligence quotient.

race/ethnicity, gender, income, and type of epilepsy, as well as dependent and independent variables used in this study, was provided in the database. Only those cases meeting the inclusion and exclusion criteria were retained. Data were collected from comprehensive neuropsychological reports completed with appropriate parental and child consent at the tertiary care epilepsy center. The dependent variables that were examined in this study were the adaptive skills and level of somatization as reported by parents and teachers, as well as specific epilepsy-related variables.

2.3. Measures. Wechsler Intelligence Scale for Children [32, 33]. The Wechsler scales are commonly used measures of ability for children and adults. Because of the retrospective nature of the study, children had different editions of the Wechsler scales. Each of the participants in this study was given the WISC-III or WISC-IV, as a measure of cognitive ability. For the purposes of this study, the results of the WISC-III and WISC-IV are included for descriptive purposes with consideration of the full scale score only. The correlation of the WISC-IV with the previous version of the WISC-III is high ($r = 0.89$). For this sample, 51 (68.62%) of the participants were administered the WISC-IV.

Behavior Assessment System for Children [30, 31]. The BASC/BASC-2 is used to evaluate the behavior and self-perceptions of children and adults aged 2 through 25 years of age. The BASC/BASC-2 includes forms for preschool, child, and adolescent. The BASC/BASC-2 has been well recognized as an appropriate instrument for the evaluation of behavior

in children and adolescents [34]. There are specific forms of the BASC/BASC-2 based on the age of the individual, as well as the relationship of the rater to the individual (e.g., parent, teacher, and self). The interpretation of the BASC/BASC-2 scales and subscales is based on T-scores. T-scores from 60 through 69 on the clinical scales and 31 through 40 on the adaptive scales are considered at risk. T-scores of 70 and above on clinical scales and 30 and below on adaptive scales are considered clinically significant. The BASC/BASC-2 includes two validity scales such that records likely to be invalid for reasons such as carelessness, inattentiveness, or cognitive limitations could be eliminated. Additionally, the BASC/BASC-2 demonstrates good convergent validity with other measures [34, 35].

For the purposes of this study, the variables of interest included the adaptive skills subscale scores, as well as the somatization subscale from the internalizing composite. The adaptive skills composite includes the following subscales: adaptability, social skills, functional communication, leadership, learning problems (teacher only), study skills (teacher only), and activities of daily living (parent only) depending on the form and version used. The coefficient alpha across forms and version is greater than .80 except for the activities of daily living subscale (.72–.76).

The Somatization subscale assesses the tendency of the child or adolescent to be report physical complaints or seek medical intervention. It is composed of items that cover topics including doctors' visits and physical ailments (e.g., visits school nurse, gets sick, has headaches, is afraid of getting sick, makes frequent visits to the doctor, and so on). The reliability coefficients for the somatization subscale for children aged 6 to 18 range from .79 to .84. Convergent validity for this subscale has been demonstrated as well [30, 31].

For this study, both child and adolescent forms were administered depending upon the child's age. It should be noted that not all forms included all subscales. Further, using retrospective data meant that some participants had the original BASC and others had the BASC-2. Although correlations between the composite scores for the two versions are good (.89–.98), the functional communication subscale was not a component of the BASC. As a result of the differences in forms, the number of participants who had specific scales varies based on age, form (parent/teacher), and version.

3. Results and Discussion

Preliminary analyses were performed to ensure no violation of the assumptions of normality, linearity, and homoscedasticity on the dependent variables. Across BASC/BASC-2 variables and epilepsy variables (onset, duration, and number of medications), no variables violated assumptions. To compare by seizure type, a two-group design was used. It was hypothesized that the two groups, CP and SG, would differ in level of somatic complaints as well as adaptive skills. Correlational analyses were used to examine relations between variables. Alpha was set at .05 so as to reduce the likelihood of type II error, the greater concern in a small clinical sample. All analyses were conducted using SPSS.

		Complex partial (CP)			CP-secondary generalized	
	n	% At risk	% Clinically significant	n	% At risk	% Clinically significant
Parent variables						
Somatization	64	18.76%	26.56%	23	13.04%	30.43%
Adaptability	55	40.00%	1.82%	20	50.00%	5.00%
Social skills	64	32.81%	12.5%	22	27.27%	4.5%
Leadership	61	29.51%	6.56%	22	45.45%	13.64%
ADL	29	41.38%	10.34%	14	28.57%	28.57%
FuncComm	30	40.00%	3.33%	13	7.69%	38.46%
Teacher variables						
Somatization	57	22.81%	33.33%	21	42.86%	9.52%
Learning problems	55	27.27%	10.91%	20	35.00%	30.00%
Adaptability	49	20.41%	4.08%	18	33.33%	5.56%
Social skills	57	17.86%	1.79%	21	23.80%	4.76%
Leadership	52	25.00%	1.92%	20	45.00%	0%
Study skills	53	24.53%	0%	20	45.00%	5.00%
FuncComm	26	15.38%	3.85%	13	38.46%	15.38%

Note. At risk = z-score = ±1; Clinically significant = z-score = ±2; FuncComm: functional communication; ADL: activities of daily living.

3.1. Parent and Teacher Ratings by Seizure Type.

It was hypothesized that the children and adolescents in the SG group would demonstrate more difficulties in adaptive functioning and higher somatization scores than those in the CP group. One-way analysis of variance was used to evaluate the differences between epilepsy groups for the BASC/BASC-2 teacher and parent reports. While no significant between group differences were found for parent reports, the groups differed on the teacher ratings of leadership ($P < .05$, partial eta-squared = .08) and study skills ($P < .05$, partial eta-squared = .09). Specifically, as predicted, the SG group mean scores on these subscales were lower than those of the CP group.

Results were also considered by frequency of at risk and clinically significant scores for each of the variables based on z-scores and standard deviation for the BASC/BASC-2 scores (see Table 2). Notably, for both parent and teacher somatization, more than 40% of each group evidenced an elevated score. As suggested by differences in group means, the frequency of at risk and clinically significant scores is much higher for the SG group (45% and 50%) for leadership and study skills as compared to the CP group (26.92% and 24.53%, resp.). Activities of daily living is only a subscale on the parent-child form, with results only available for a small subsample. It is important to note, however, that of those participants in that age bracket, more than 50% for each group evidenced at risk or clinically significant impairment. Notably, the difficulties in these daily living skills are consistent with prior research [5, 21, 22].

3.2. Relation of Adaptive Skills with Epilepsy Characteristics.

It was hypothesized, for both the parent and teacher reports, that the younger the age at onset of seizures is, the longer

TABLE 3: Correlations for parent/teacher report of adaptive subscales with epilepsy variables (rho) and parent-/teacher-rated somatization (Pearson's r).

	Onset	Duration	Number medications
	r	r	r
Parent variables			
Somatization ($n = 87$)	−.03	−.16	.13
Adaptability ($n = 75$)	.05	−.13	−.28*
Social skills ($n = 87$)	.01	−.16	−.15
Leadership ($n = 83$)	−.01	−.20	−.26*
ADL ($n = 43$)	.23	−.25	−.41**
FuncComm ($n = 43$)	−.01	−.22	−.22
Teacher variables			
Somatization ($n = 78$)	−.04	−.08	.19
Adaptability ($n = 67$)	−.08	−.03	.12
Social skills ($n = 78$)	.03	−.07	−.11
Leadership ($n = 72$)	.02	−.02	−.01
Study skills ($n = 73$)	.01	−.08	−.15
FuncComm ($n = 39$)	.31	−.31	.13

Notes. FuncComm: functional communication; ADL: activities of daily living.
*$P < .05$.
**$P < .01$.

the duration of living with the illness and number of medications taken would be correlated with adaptive skills deficits. Correlation (r) was used to determine the relation between age of onset, duration, and number of medications with each of the adaptive skills subscales for the entire sample, as well as for somatization (see Table 3). No significant correlations

TABLE 4: Relation between somatization and adaptive skills.

	Parent somatization		Teacher somatization	
	r	n	r	n
Parent variables				
Somatization	1.00	87	.30**	78
Adaptability	−.21	75	−.06	68
Social skills	−.04	86	−.27*	77
Leadership	−.07	83	−.30**	74
ADL	−.17	43	−.28	40
FuncComm	−.20	43	−.02	39
Teacher variables				
Somatization	.30**	74	1.00	74
Adaptability	.12	63	−.11	63
Social skills	−.10	74	−.23*	74
Leadership	−.10	68	−.25*	68
Study skills	.01	73	−.31**	69
FuncComm	−.06	39	−.37*	35

Notes. FuncComm: functional communication; ADL: activities of daily living.
*$P < .05$.
**$P < .01$.

were found with age of onset or duration for either parent or teacher ratings. For the parent ratings, there was a significant correlation between number of medications and adaptability ($P > .05$), Leadership, ($P < .05$), and activities of daily living ($P < .01$), with more somatic complaints and lower adaptive skills associated with more medications needed for seizure control (i.e., severity). For teacher ratings, no significant associations were found with epilepsy variables.

3.3. Somatic Complaints and Adaptive Functioning. It was hypothesized that somatization scores would be inversely related to adaptive functioning for both the parent and teacher report, both presumed to reflect severity and impact on functioning. Correlation analysis was conducted to ascertain whether a relationship existed between level of somatic complaints and the adaptive skills subscales as measured by the BASC/BASC-2 parent and teacher reports. The results (see Table 4) indicated that there was relative agreement between parent and teacher ratings of somatization for those children with both respondents information ($n = 78$, $r = .30$, and $P = .007$). The differences between parent and teacher ratings are common [36]. These differences may reflect differences in expectations and contextual demands. Parent-rated somatization was not significantly associated with any of the parent-rated or teacher-rated adaptive skills. In contrast, teacher-rated somatization was significantly related to parent-rated social skills ($P = .02$) and leadership ($P = .01$). Teacher-rated somatization was also significantly correlated with teacher-rated Social Skills ($P < .05$), leadership ($P = .04$), Study Skills ($P = .007$), and functional communication ($P = .02$). In all cases, a higher level of somatic complaints was associated with lower adaptive skills as expected.

4. Conclusions

The long term outcome for children with epilepsy tends to be less than optimum [3, 5, 7, 10, 11, 25]. Not only may they encounter difficulty in academic areas, but also the circumstances of their epilepsy (i.e., age of onset, time since diagnosis, and number of medications) may result in frequent somatic complaints and may limit their participation in social or community activities. Deficits in adaptive behavior [5, 22, 25] can affect school performance and overall adjustment. The findings here on the adaptive skills of children with epilepsy in relation to somatization, as well as epilepsy characteristics (i.e., seizure type, age of onset, duration, and number of medications), provide support to and add to the existing knowledge base.

Parents and teachers identified some differing aspects of adaptive behavior to be of concern; these differences likely reflect the differing contextual demands. Surprisingly, neither age of onset nor time since diagnosis was correlated with the somatization or any of the adaptive skills subscales. In contrast, number of medications was significantly correlated with parent-rated, but not teacher-rated adaptive behavior. For all three significant parent subscales, the ratings were lower as the number of medications (i.e., severity) increased.

When exploring the relation between somatization and adaptive skills, results did not indicate parent ratings of somatization to be related to adaptive skills. In contrast, for teacher ratings, there was an inverse relation such that higher levels of somatic complaints were associated with specific adaptive behaviors (study skills, leadership, and social skills). Because the somatization subscale emphasizes physical aches and pains, medications, and medical treatments, these findings suggest that the higher the degree of symptomology the child is experiencing due to their illness, particularly in the school setting, the less likely they are to actively engage and participate in the classroom.

Somatic complaints may be expected in children and adolescents with epilepsy and other chronic illnesses. As a result, somatization scales may sometimes be elevated for children with epilepsy because of factors related to the seizure disorder rather than because of psychopathology. At the same time, experiencing somatic issues related to epilepsy can have an effect on other areas of development, particularly adaptive skills. Identification of adaptive skills deficits may represent an opportunity for tailored prevention and intervention programming for children with epilepsy to improve their overall outcome. For example, if social competence is the area of concern, implementation of social emotional learning program may be appropriate; if peer relations is the area of concern, a social skills program might be considered. As such, more comprehensive assessment of adaptive skills may be appropriate for children with epilepsy regardless of cognitive ability in order to identify adaptive skills in need of support or intervention [22]. Additional research specific to adaptive skills may better explain the underlying mechanisms related to lower acquisition of these skills for children with epilepsy, as well as the extent to which adaptive skills mediate long-term outcome. A larger, prospective study including a more diverse sample would be useful in identifying moderator and mediator variables for epilepsy-related factors and outcome for children with epilepsy.

Conflict of Interests

The authors declare that there is no conflict of interests regarding the publication of this paper.

References

[1] A. P. Aldenkamp, B. Weber, W. C. G. Overweg-Plandsoen, R. Reijs, and S. van Mil, "Educational underachievement in children with epilepsy: a model to predict the effects of epilepsy on educational achievement," *Journal of Child Neurology*, vol. 20, no. 3, pp. 175–180, 2005.

[2] S. Davies, I. Heyman, and R. Goodman, "A population survey of mental health problems in children with epilepsy," *Developmental Medicine and Child Neurology*, vol. 45, no. 5, pp. 292–295, 2003.

[3] S. A. Russ, K. Larson, and N. Halfon, "A national profile of childhood epilepsy and seizure disorder," *Pediatrics*, vol. 129, no. 2, pp. 256–264, 2012.

[4] C. E. Elger and D. Schmidt, "Modern management of epilepsy: a practical approach," *Epilepsy and Behavior*, vol. 12, no. 4, pp. 501–539, 2008.

[5] M. Sillanpää and J. H. Cross, "The psychosocial impact of epilepsy in childhood," *Epilepsy & Behavior*, vol. 15, pp. S5–S10, 2009.

[6] C. Camfield, P. Camfield, B. Smith, K. Gordon, and J. Dooley, "Biologic factors as predictors of social outcome of epilepsy in intellectually normal children: a population-based study," *Journal of Pediatrics*, vol. 122, no. 6, pp. 869–873, 1993.

[7] M. Jalava, M. Sillanpää, C. Camfield, and P. Camfield, "Social adjustment and competence 35 years after onset of childhood epilepsy: a prospective controlled study," *Epilepsia*, vol. 38, no. 6, pp. 708–715, 1997.

[8] R. Rodenburg, A. M. Meijer, M. Deković, and A. P. Aldenkamp, "Family predictors of psychopathology in children with epilepsy," *Epilepsia*, vol. 47, no. 3, pp. 601–614, 2006.

[9] J. B. Titus, R. Kanive, S. J. Sanders, and L. B. Blackburn, "Behavioral profiles of children with epilepsy: parent and teacher reports of emotional, behavioral, and educational concerns on the BASC-2," *Psychology in the Schools*, vol. 45, no. 9, pp. 893–904, 2008.

[10] J. Kokkonen, E.-R. Kokkonen, A.-L. Saukkonen, and P. Pennanen, "Psychosocial outcome of young adults with epilepsy in childhood," *Journal of Neurology Neurosurgery and Psychiatry*, vol. 62, no. 3, pp. 265–268, 1997.

[11] M. Sillanpää, M. Jalava, O. Kaleva, and S. Shinnar, "Long-term prognosis of seizures with onset in childhood," *The New England Journal of Medicine*, vol. 338, no. 24, pp. 1715–1722, 1998.

[12] J. K. Austin and D. W. Dunn, "Progressive behavioral changes in children with epilepsy," *Progress in Brain Research*, vol. 135, pp. 419–427, 2002.

[13] J. K. Austin, D. W. Dunn, C. S. Johnson, and S. M. Perkins, "Behavioral issues involving children and adolescents with epilepsy and the impact of their families: recent research data," *Epilepsy and Behavior*, vol. 5, supplement 3, pp. S33–S41, 2004.

[14] S. E. Sabbagh, C. Soria, S. Escolano, C. Bulteau, and G. Dellatolas, "Impact of epilepsy characteristics and behavioral problems on school placement in children," *Epilepsy and Behavior*, vol. 9, no. 4, pp. 573–578, 2006.

[15] N. Ellis, D. Upton, and P. Thompson, "Epilepsy and the family: a review of current literature," *Seizure*, vol. 9, no. 1, pp. 22–30, 2000.

[16] C. G. McCusker, P. J. Kennedy, J. Anderson, E. M. Hicks, and D. Hanrahan, "Adjustment in children with intractable epilepsy: importance of seizure duration and family factors," *Developmental Medicine and Child Neurology*, vol. 44, no. 10, pp. 681–687, 2002.

[17] J. K. Austin and R. Caplan, "Behavioral and psychiatric comorbidities in pediatric epilepsy: toward an integrative model," *Epilepsia*, vol. 48, no. 9, pp. 1639–1651, 2007.

[18] A. T. Berg, R. Caplan, and D. C. Hesdorffer, "Psychiatric and neurodevelopmental disorders in childhood-onset epilepsy," *Epilepsy and Behavior*, vol. 20, no. 3, pp. 550–555, 2011.

[19] A. T. Berg, S. N. Smith, D. Frobish et al., "Longitudinal assessment of adaptive behavior in infants and young children with newly diagnosed epilepsy: influences of etiology, syndrome, and seizure control," *Pediatrics*, vol. 114, no. 3, pp. 645–650, 2004.

[20] E. H. Drewel, D. J. Bell, and J. K. Austin, "Peer difficulties in children with epilepsy: association with seizure, neuropsychological, academic, and behavioral variables," *Child Neuropsychology*, vol. 15, no. 4, pp. 305–320, 2009.

[21] L. E. Clary, J. S. Vander Wal, and J. B. Titus, "Examining health-related quality of life, adaptive skills, and psychological functioning in children and adolescents with epilepsy presenting for a neuropsychological evaluation," *Epilepsy and Behavior*, vol. 19, no. 3, pp. 487–493, 2010.

[22] J. M. Buelow, S. M. Perkins, C. S. Johnson et al., "Adaptive functioning in children with epilepsy and learning problems," *Journal of Child Neurology*, vol. 27, pp. 1241–1249, 2012.

[23] J. L. Matson, J. W. Bamburg, E. A. Mayville, and I. Khan, "Seizure disorders in people with intellectual disability: an analysis of differences in social functioning, adaptive functioning and maladaptive behaviours," *Journal of Intellectual Disability Research*, vol. 43, no. 6, pp. 531–539, 1999.

[24] W. van Blarikom, I. Y. Tan, A. P. Aldenkamp, and A. T. G. van Gennep, "Living environment of persons with severe epilepsy and intellectual disability: a prospective study," *Epilepsy and Behavior*, vol. 14, no. 3, pp. 484–490, 2009.

[25] A. T. Berg, R. Caplan, C. B. Baca, and B. G. Vickrey, "Adaptive behavior and later school achievement in children with early onset epilepsy," *Developmental Medicine and Child Neurology*, vol. 55, pp. 661–667, 2013.

[26] J. M. Buelow, J. K. Austin, S. M. Perkins, J. Shen, D. W. Dunn, and P. S. Fastenau, "Behavior and mental health problems in children with epilepsy and low IQ," *Developmental Medicine and Child Neurology*, vol. 45, no. 10, pp. 683–692, 2003.

[27] J. J. Barry, A. Lembke, P. A. Gisbert, and F. Gilliam, "disorders in epilepsy," in *Psychiatric Issues in Epilepsy*, B. Ettinger and A. M. Kanner, Eds., pp. 203–247, Lippincott Williams & Wilkins, Philadelphia, Pa, USA, 2nd edition, 2007.

[28] A. Piazzini and R. Canger, "Depression and anxiety in patients with epilepsy," *Epilepsia*, vol. 42, supplement 2, pp. 29–31, 2001.

[29] C. B. Baca, B. G. Vickrey, R. Caplan, S. D. Vassar, and A. T. Berg, "Psychiatric and medical comorbidity and quality of life outcomes in childhood-onset epilepsy," *Pediatrics*, vol. 128, no. 6, pp. e1532–e1543, 2011.

[30] C. R. Reynolds and R. W. Kamphaus, *Behavioral Assessment System for Children Manual*, American Guidance Service, Circle Pines, Minn, USA, 1997.

[31] C. R. Reynolds and R. W. Kamphaus, *BASC-2: Behavioral Assessment System for Children Manual*, American Guidance Service, Circle Pines, Minn, USA, 2nd edition, 2004.

[32] D. Wechsler, *Wechsler Intelligence for Children*, Technical Manual, Psychological Corporation, San Antonio, Tex, USA, 3rd edition, 1991.

[33] D. Wechsler, *Wechsler Intelligence for Children*, Technical Manual, Psychological Corporation, San Antonio, Tex, USA, 4th edition, 2003.

[34] S. P. Merydith, "Temporal Stability and Convergent Validity of the Behavior Assessment System for Children," *Journal of School Psychology*, vol. 3, pp. 253–265, 2001.

[35] T. M. Achenbach and L. A. Rescorla, *Manual for the ASEBA School-Aged Forms and Profiles*, University of Vermont, Research Center for Children, Youth, & Families, Burlington, Mass, USA, 2001.

[36] T. J. Huberty, J. K. Austin, J. Harezlak, D. W. Dunn, and W. T. Ambrosius, "Informant agreement in behavior ratings for children with epilepsy," *Epilepsy and Behavior*, vol. 1, no. 6, pp. 427–435, 2000.

Permissions

List of Contributors

Joe Yuezhou Yu and Phillip L. Pearl
Department of Neurology, Children's National Medical Center, 111 Michigan Avnue, Washington, DC 20010, USA

Guglielmo Lucchese
Brain and Language Laboratory, Cluster of Excellence "Languages of Emotions", Free University of Berlin, 14195 Berlin, Germany

Jean Pierre Spinosa
Faculty of Biology & Medicine, University of Lausanne, CH-1011 Lausanne, Switzerland

Darja Kanduc
Department of Biosciences, Biotechnologies and Biopharmaceutics, University of Bari, 70125 Bari, Italy

Iván Sánchez Fernández
Division of Epilepsy and Clinical Neurophysiology, Department of Neurology, Harvard Medical School, Boston Children's Hospital, Boston, MA 02115, USA
Department of Child Neurology, Hospital Sant Joan de D´eu, Universidad de Barcelona, 08950 Barcelona, Spain

Kevin E. Chapman
Department of Neurology, Children's Hospital Colorado, University of Colorado, Aurora, CO 80045, USA

Jurriaan M. Peters, Chellamani Harini, Alexander Rotenberg and Tobias Loddenkemper
Division of Epilepsy and Clinical Neurophysiology, Department of Neurology, Harvard Medical School, Boston Children's Hospital, Boston, MA 02115, USA
Department of Child Neurology, Hospital Sant Joan de D´eu, Universidad de Barcelona, 08950 Barcelona, Spain

Taoufik Alsaadi, Haytham Taha and Fatema Al Hammadi
Department of Neurology, Sheikh Khalifa Medical City, Abu Dhabi 51900, UAE

Iordanis Georgiadis
Departments of Neurosurgery, University Hospital of Larisa, Faculty of Medicine, University of Thessaly, Biopolis, Larissa 41110,Greece

Effie Z. Kapsalaki
Departments of Neurosurgery & Diagnostic Radiology, University Hospital of Larisa, Faculty of Medicine, University of Thessaly, Larissa, Greece

Kostas N. Fountas
Departments of Neurosurgery, University Hospital of Larisa, Faculty of Medicine, University of Thessaly, Biopolis, Larissa 41110,Greece

CERETETH, Center for Research and Technology of Thessaly, Larissa 38500, Greece

Lily C. Wong-Kisiel and Katherine Nickels
Division of Child and Adolescent Neurology, Department of Neurology, Mayo Clinic College of Medicine, 200 First St. SW, Rochester, MN55905, USA

Filippo S. Giorgi, Chiara Pizzanelli, Veronica Pelliccia, Elisa Di Coscio, Melania Guida, Elena Iacopini, Alfonso Iudice and Enrica Bonanni
Neurology Unit and Epilepsy Center, Department of Neuroscience, A.O.U.P and Department of Clinical and Experimental Medicine of the University of Pisa, Via Roma 67, 56126 Pisa, Italy

Michelangelo Maestri
Sleep & Epilepsy Center, Neurocenter of the Civic Hospital (EOC) of Lugano, Via Tesserete 46, 6900 Lugano, Switzerland

Leena Kämppi, Jaakko Ritvanen
Clinical Neurosciences, Neurology, University of Helsinki and Helsinki University Hospital, 00029 Helsinki, Finland

Harri Mustonen
Department of Surgery, Helsinki University Central Hospital, 00029 Helsinki, Finland

Seppo Soinila
Division of Clinical Neurosciences/General Neurology, Department of Neurology, Turku University Hospital, University of Turku, 20521 Turku, Finland

Masoomeh Akbarbegloo
Department of Pediatric Nursing, Faculty of Nursing and Midwifery, Urmia University of Medical Sciences, Urmia 51389 47977, Iran
Tabriz University of Medical Sciences, Tabriz 51389 47977, Iran

Leila Valizadeh
Department of Pediatric Nursing, Faculty of Nursing and Midwifery, Tabriz University of Medical Sciences, Tabriz 51389 47977, Iran

Vahid Zamanzadeh
Department of Medical Surgical Nursing, Faculty of Nursing and Midwifery, Tabriz University of Medical Sciences, Tabriz 51389 47977, Iran

Faranak Jabarzadeh
Department of Medical Surgical Nursing, Student Research Committee, Faculty of Nursing and Midwifery, Tabriz University of Medical Sciences, Tabriz 51389 47977, Iran

Amanda G. Jaimes-Bautista
Proyecto de Neurociencias, Facultad de Estudios Superiores Iztacala, Universidad Nacional Autónoma de México, 54090 Ciudad de México, MEX, Mexico
Departamento de Neuropsicología, Instituto Nacional de Neurología y Neurocirugía, 14269 Ciudad de México, DF, Mexico

Mario Rodríguez-Camacho
Proyecto de Neurociencias, Facultad de Estudios Superiores Iztacala, Universidad Nacional Autónoma de México, 54090 Ciudad de México, MEX, Mexico

Iris E. Martínez-Juárez
Clínica de Epilepsia, Instituto Nacional de Neurología y Neurocirugía, 14269 Ciudad de México, DF, Mexico

Yaneth Rodríguez-Agudelo
Departamento de Neuropsicología, Instituto Nacional de Neurología y Neurocirugía, 14269 Ciudad de México, DF, Mexico

Emmanouil Magiorkinis, Aristidis Diamantis and Kalliopi Sidiropoulou
Office for the Study of Hellenic Naval Medicine, Naval Hospital of Athens, Deinokratous 70, 11527 Athens, Greece

Christos Panteliadis
Division of Paediatric Neurology and Developmental Medicine, Aristotle University of Thessaloniki, AHEPA Hospital, Stilp Kiriakidi 1, 54634Thessaloniki, Greece

Suresh Gurbani
Comprehensive Epilepsy Program, Southern California Permanente Medical Group, CA, USA
Department of Neurology, Kaiser Permanente Medical Center, Suite No. 208, 3460 E. La Palma Avenue, Anaheim, CA 92806, USA

Sirichai Chayasirisobhon, Leslie Cahan, SooHo Choi, Bruce Enos, Jane Hwang, Meei Lin and Jeffrey Schweitzer
Comprehensive Epilepsy Program, Southern California Permanente Medical Group, CA, USA

Paul Osemeke Nwani
Clinical Pharmacology andTherapeutics Unit/Neurology Unit, Department of Medicine, Nnamdi Azikiwe University Teaching Hospital, PMB 5025, Nnewi 435101, Anambra State, Nigeria

Maduaburochukwu Cosmas Nwosu
Neurology Unit, Department of Medicine, Nnamdi Azikiwe University Teaching Hospital, PMB 5025, Nnewi 435101, Anambra State, Nigeria

Monica Nonyelum Nwosu
Gastroenterology Unit, Department of Medicine, Nnamdi Azikiwe University Teaching Hospital, PMB 5025, Nnewi 435101, Anambra State, Nigeria

Abdulaziz Alsemari
Department of Neurosciences, King Faisal Specialist Hospital and Research Centre, Riyadh 11211, Saudi Arabia
Neurology Section, Department of Neurosciences, King Faisal Specialist Hospital & Research Centre, MBC.76, P.O. Box 3354, Riyadh 11211, Saudi Arabia

Faisal Al-Otaibi, Salah Baz, Ibrahim Althubaiti, Hisham Aldhalaan, David MacDonald, Tareq Abalkhail, Suad Alyamani, Aziza Chedrawi and Donald Maclean
Department of Neurosciences, King Faisal Specialist Hospital and Research Centre, Riyadh 11211, Saudi Arabia

Miguel E. Fiol
University of Minnesota Medical Center, Fairview, Epilepsy Care Center, Minnesota, MN 55455, USA

Frank Leblanc
University of Calgary, AB, Canada T2N 1N4

Andrew Parrent and John Girvin
London Health Science Center, London, ON, Canada N6G 2V4

Halima Benjelloun
Unit of Cardiology A, Ibn Sina University Hospital, 10000 Rabat, Morocco

Swaroop Hassan Suresh
Cipla Ltd, 117/1, Anjanadri, Pantharapalya, Bangalore 560039, India

Hajar Kiai
Food Sciences Laboratory, Department of Biology, Faculty of Sciences Semlalia, Prince Moulay Abdellah Avenue, 40090 Marrakesh, Morocco

Rokia Ghchime
Physiology Laboratory, Faculty ofMedicine and Pharmacy, Mohammed V-SouissiUniversity, 6203 Rabat, Morocco
Department of Clinical Neurophysiology, Hospital of Specialties, Ibn Sina University Hospital, Rabat Institute, 6220 Rabat, Morocco
Unit of Cardiology A, Ibn Sina University Hospital, 10000 Rabat, Morocco

Halima Belaidi and Fatiha Lahjouji
Physiology Laboratory, Faculty ofMedicine and Pharmacy, Mohammed V-SouissiUniversity, 6203 Rabat, Morocco
Department of Clinical Neurophysiology, Hospital of Specialties, Ibn Sina University Hospital, Rabat Institute, 6220 Rabat, Morocco

Reda Ouazzani
Department of Clinical Neurophysiology, Hospital of Specialties, Ibn Sina University Hospital, Rabat Institute, 6220 Rabat, Morocco

Claudia P.Múnera, Carolina Lomlomdjian, Belen Gori, Verónica Terpiluk and Nancy Medel
Epilepsy Center, Neurology Division, Ramos Mejia Hospital, Gral Urquiza 609, C1221ADC Buenos Aires, Argentina
Center for Clinical and Experimental Neurosciences, Epilepsy , Cognition and Behavior, Institute of Cell Biology and

Patricia Solís and Silvia Kochen
Epilepsy Center, Neurology Division, Ramos Mejia Hospital, Gral Urquiza 609, C1221ADC Buenos Aires, Argentina
Center for Clinical and Experimental Neurosciences, Epilepsy , Cognition and Behavior, Institute of Cell Biology and Neurosciences (IBCN), School of Medicine, UBA-CONICET, 2nd Floor, Paraguay 2155, C1121ABG Buenos Aires, Argentina
National Neuroscience Center, Epilepsy Unit, El Cruce Hospital, Avenue Calchaqu´ı 5401, C1888, Florencio Varela, C1073ABA Buenos Aires, Argentina

Akash Virupakshaiah and Ananya Chakraborty
Department of Pharmacology, Vydehi Institute of Medical Sciences and Research Centre, No. 82 EPIP Area, Whitefield, Bangalore 560037, India

Nithin Kumar
Department of Neurology, Columbia Asia Hospital, Whitefield, Bangalore 560066, India

Agnes Prins, Eddie Chengo and Victor Mung'ala Odera
Centre for Geographic Medicine Research-Coast (CGMRC), Kenya Medical Research Institute (KEMRI), P.O. Box 230, Kilifi 80108, Kenya

Manish Sadarangani
Department of Paediatrics, University ofOxford, Level 2, Children's Hospital, Oxford OX3 9DU,UK
Department of Paediatrics, University of British Columbia & BC Children's Hospital, 4480 Oak Street, Vancouver, BC, Canada V6H3V4

Claire Seaton
Department of Paediatrics, John Radcliffe Hospital, Oxford University Hospitals NHS Trust, Headington, Oxford OX3 9DU, UK

Penny Holding
International Centre for Behavioral Studies, P.O. Box 34307, Mombasa 80118, Kenya

Greg Fegan
Centre for Geographic Medicine Research-Coast (CGMRC), Kenya Medical Research Institute (KEMRI), P.O. Box 230, Kilifi 80108, Kenya
Centre for Clinical Vaccinology and Tropical Medicine, Churchill Hospital, Old Road, Oxford OX3 7LJ, UK

Charles R. Newton
Centre for Geographic Medicine Research-Coast (CGMRC), Kenya Medical Research Institute (KEMRI), P.O. Box 230, Kilifi 80108, Kenya
Neurosciences Unit, Institute of Child Health, University College London, 30 Guilford Street, LondonWC1N 1EH, UK
Department of Psychiatry, University of Oxford, Oxford OX3 7JX, UK

Suvasini Sharma and Puneet Jain
Division of Pediatric Neurology, Department of Pediatrics, Lady Hardinge Medical College and
Associated Kalawati Saran Children's Hospital, New Delhi 110001, India

Marcus Ng
Department of Neurology, Epilepsy Service, Massachusetts General Hospital, 55 Fruit Street, Boston, MA 02114, USA

Milena Pavlova
Department of Neurology, Division of Epilepsy, EEG, and Sleep Neurology, Brigham and Women's-Faulkner Hospital, 1153 Centre Street, Boston, MA 02130, USA

M. Matuszczak
Undergraduate Medicine, University of Manitoba, Winnipeg, MB, Canada R3A 1R9

F. A. Zeiler and C. J. Kazina
Section of Neurosurgery, Department of Sugery, University of Manitoba, Winnipeg, MB, Canada R3A 1R9

Emily A. Greene-Colozzi, Abbey R. Sadowski, Elyza Chadwick, Peter T. Tsai, and Mustafa Sahin
The F.M. Kirby Neurobiology Center, Translational Neuroscience Center, Department of Neurology, Children's Hospital Boston, Harvard Medical School, 300 Longwood Avenue CLSB 14073, Boston, MA 02115, USA

J. Teitelbaum
Section of Neurology, Montreal Neurological Institute, McGill, Montreal, QC, CanadaH3A 2B4

L. M. Gillman
Section of Critical Care Medicine, Department of Medicine, University of Manitoba, Winnipeg, MB, Canada R3A 1R9
Section of General Surgery, Department of Surgery, University of Manitoba, Winnipeg, MB, Canada R3A 1R9

AlirezaMansouri
Division of Neurosurgery, University of Toronto, Toronto, ON, Canada
Toronto Western Hospital, University Health Network, Toronto, ON, CanadaM5T 2S8
Department of Clinical Epidemiology and Biostatistics, McMaster University, Hamilton, ON, Canada L8P 1H1

Abdul rahman Aldakkan
Division of Neurosurgery, University of Toronto, Toronto, ON, Canada
Toronto Western Hospital, University Health Network, Toronto, ON, CanadaM5T 2S8
Division of Neurosurgery, King Saud University, Riyadh, Saudi Arabia

Magda J. Kosicka
Toronto Western Hospital, University Health Network, Toronto, ON, CanadaM5T 2S8

Jean-Eric Tarride
Department of Clinical Epidemiology and Biostatistics, McMaster University, Hamilton, ON, Canada L8P 1H1

Taufik A. Valiante
Division of Neurosurgery, University of Toronto, Toronto, ON, Canada
Toronto Western Hospital, University Health Network, Toronto, ON, CanadaM5T 2S8
Institute of Medical Sciences, University of Toronto, Toronto, ON, Canada
Division of Fundamental Neurobiology, Toronto Western Research Institute, Toronto Western Hospital, Toronto, ON, Canada M5T 2S8
Krembil Neuroscience Center, Toronto, Canada

Edwin E. Eseigbe
Department of Paediatrics, Ahmadu Bello University Teaching Hospital, Zaria 810001, Nigeria

Folorunsho T. Nuhu, Taiwo L. Sheikh and Okechukwu J. Oguizu
Federal Neuropsychiatric Hospital (FNPH), Kaduna, Nigeria

Sam J. Adama
Department of Paediatrics, 44 Nigerian Army Reference Hospital, Kaduna, Nigeria

Patricia Eseigbe
Department of Family Medicine, Ahmadu Bello University Teaching Hospital, Zaria 810001, Nigeria

Ioannis Karakis
Department of Neurology, Emory University School of Medicine, Atlanta, GA, USA

Andrew J. Cole
MGH Epilepsy Service, Massachusetts General Hospital, Harvard Medical School, Boston, MA, USA

Georgia D.Montouris
Department of Neurology, Boston Medical Center, Boston University School of Medicine, Boston, MA, USA

Marta San Luciano
Department of Neurology, University California San Francisco, San Francisco, CA, USA

Charitomeni Piperidou
Department of Neurology, Democritus University of Thrace, Alexandroupolis, Greece

Kimford J.Meador
Department of Neurology, Emory University School of Medicine, Atlanta, GA, USA
Department of Neurology, Stanford School of Medicine, Stanford, CA, USA

Leonilda Bilo and Roberto De Simone
Epilepsy Center, Department of Neuroscience, School of Medicine, Federico II University of Naples, 80131 Naples, Italy

Sabina Pappatà
Institute of Biostructure and Bioimaging, CNR and Department of Biomorphological Sciences, Federico II University, 80131 Naples, Italy

Roberta Meo
Neurology Outpatients Service, Naples Local Health Unit, 80100 Naples, Italy

Nichole Wicker Villarreal
Texas A&M University, College Station, TX 77843-4225, USA

Cynthia A. Riccio
Department of Educational Psychology, Texas A&M University, College Station, TX 77843-4225, USA

Morris J. Cohen and Yong Park
Children's Hospital of Georgia, BT-2601, 1446 Harper Street, Augusta, GA 30912, USA